NURSE'S
POCKET
COMPANION

Springhouse Corporation
Springhouse, Pennsylvania

Staff

Executive Director
Matthew Cahill

Editorial Director
Patricia Dwyer Schull, RN, MSN

Clinical Manager
Judith Schilling McCann, RN, MSN

Art Director
John Hubbard

Senior Editor
H. Nancy Holmes

Clinical Editors
Maryann Foley, RN, BSN *(project manager)*, Paulette Dorney, RN, MSN, CCRN; Mary Jane McDevitt, RN, BS

Editors
Peter H. Johnson, Doris Weinstock

Copy Editors
Cynthia C. Breuninger *(manager)*, Diane Armento, Christine Cunniffe, Brenna Mayer

Designers
Arlene Putterman *(associate art director)*, Matie Patterson *(senior designer)*, Elaine Ezrow, Jacalyn Facciolo, Donald Knauss, Amy Litz, Mary Ludwicki, Susan Hopkins Rodzewich, Jeff Sklarow, Lesley Weissman-Cook

Illustrators
John Carlance, Jean Gardner, Linda Gist, Frank Grobelny, Robert Jackson, Robert Neumann, Judy Newhouse, Robert Phillips, Larry Ward

Typography
Diane Paluba *(manager)*, Joyce Rossi Biletz, Phyllis Marron, Valerie Rosenberger

Manufacturing
Deborah Meiris *(director)*, Pat Dorshaw *(manager)*, T.A. Landis

Production Coordination
Margaret A. Rastiello

Editorial Assistants
Carol Caputo, Beverly Lane, Mary Madden, Jeanne Napier

NPC2-021296

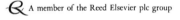 A member of the Reed Elsevier plc group

Library of Congress Cataloging-in-Publication Data
Nurse's pocket companion.
p.   cm.
Includes index.
1. Nursing—Handbooks, manuals, etc.   I. Springhouse Corporation.
[DNLM: 1. Nursing Care—handbooks. 2. Nursing—handbooks. WY 39 N97362 1997]
RT51.N846 1997
610.73—dc20
DNLM/DLC   96-06927
ISBN 0-87434-655-X   CIP

Contents

Foreword

In medicine, as in other areas of human action, it seems the dominant idea is to get one's tools to work faster and do more things than before. Greater ease of use allows complex tasks to be performed more efficiently and quickly. Publishers of the *Nurse's Pocket Companion,* Second Edition, see things much the same way. If there's any way to give speedy access to vital health care information between the covers of a book, they're up to the job. This new edition is only slightly larger than its predecessor, yet it includes a lot of new information: There's a new chapter on dealing with dangerous complications of disorders and treatments and another on home care nursing—our next frontier.

The rest of the book has been thoroughly reviewed and updated. All of the first edition's useful features have been retained, including hundreds of easy-to-read charts, diagrams, and illustrations and quick-reference thumb tabs to guide you to the appropriate subjects. Usability is enhanced by two new graphic symbols in the text: An *Age Alert* symbol draws attention to aspects of procedures and care that are particularly relevant to pediatric or elderly patients, and a *Teaching Tip* symbol highlights information that's valuable for patient education as well as for discharge planning.

Chapter 1 gives directions for the most effective performance of physical assessment, with a review of all organ systems and tips for patients with differing disease etiologies. Chapter 2 explores the 25 most common complaints and concludes with a section on spotting the most frequently overlooked problems. Chapter 3 explains how to interpret any ECG, and Chapter 4 gives reference values for common laboratory tests, significance of abnormal results, and procedure-related nursing care. Chapter 5 helps you formulate nursing diagnoses based on the presenting medical diagnoses and using human response patterns.

Chapter 6 reviews preoperative and postoperative patient care, including patient-teaching needs and discharge planning. This chapter also includes a succinct review of anesthetic agents, their effects on the patient, and pertinent nursing interventions. Chapter 7 reviews bedside procedures in intensive care areas as well as in general care units.

Chapter 8 covers prevention and control of contagious diseases. It reviews universal precautions, lists reportable diseases, and provides a handy chart of specific barrier precautions for dozens of clinical situations. Chapter 9 tells you how to troubleshoot equipment problems.

Chapters 10, 11, and 12 review methods of safely administering medications by all appropriate routes, calculating dosages correctly, and avoiding common hazards of medication administration. These chapters also include nursing interventions for drug reactions, overdoses, and interactions.

Chapter 13, new to this edition, provides the latest information on how to detect and treat life-threatening conditions, such as air embolism, atelectasis, cardiac tamponade, hyperglycemic crisis, and thyroid storm. Each entry gives a description of the complication, causes, signs and symptoms to watch for, and appropriate nursing interventions. Chapter 14 provides examples of commonly used documentation forms, with hints on how to use them effectively. The chapter includes a thorough discussion of patient-discharge planning and instructions, documenting patients' refusal of treatment, and utilizing incident reports correctly. Chapter 15, also new to this edition, is a compact review of the home care field that covers ethical and legal aspects of home care, how to ensure safe home care visits (for the nurse as well as the patient), working with home health aides, understanding documentation and reimbursement, and case management and quality improvement issues. Finally, Chapter 16 provides a handy guide to current medical abbreviations and acronyms.

Nurses found the first edition of the *Nurse's Pocket Companion* to be an indispensable personal reference, one that was easily carried wherever their nursing career took them. This edition will continue to serve most nurses' needs for a compact, single-volume reference. Current information that's easily read and understood remains this book's hallmark.

GINNY WACKER GUIDO, RN, MSN, JD
Professor and Chair, Department of Nursing
Eastern New Mexico University
Portales

CHAPTER 1

Assessment:
Reviewing the techniques

Assessing the eyes, ears, nose, and throat

Reviewing assessment techniques

▶

Performing a 10-minute assessment

You won't always want or need to assess a patient in 10 minutes. But rapid assessment is crucial when you must intervene quickly—such as when a hospitalized patient complains of a change in his condition or when you or a family member notices a change in his physical, mental, or emotional status.

You may also perform a rapid assessment to confirm a diagnostic finding. For example, if arterial blood gas analysis indicates a low oxygen content, you'll quickly assess the patient for other signs of oxygen deprivation, such as an increased respiratory rate and cyanosis.

General guidelines

Try to assess your patient not only quickly but also systematically. To save time, cover some of the assessment components simultaneously. For example, make your general observations while checking the patient's vital signs or asking history questions.

Be flexible. You won't necessarily use the same sequence each time. Let the patient's chief complaint and your initial observations guide your assessment. Sometimes, you may not be able to obtain a quick history and instead will have to rely on your observations and the information on the patient's chart.

Keep the patient calm and cooperative. If you don't know him, first introduce yourself by name and title. Remain calm, and reassure him that you can help. If your demeanor can reduce his anxiety, he's more likely to give you accurate information.

Avoid drawing quick conclusions. In particular, don't assume that the patient's current complaint is related to his admitting diagnosis.

When every minute counts, follow these steps.

Assess airway, breathing, and circulation

This, your first priority, may consist of just a momentary observation. But when a patient appears to be unconscious or has difficulty breathing, you'll assess more thoroughly to detect the problem and intervene immediately.

Make general observations

Note the patient's mental status, general appearance, and level of consciousness for clues to the nature and severity of his condition.

Assess vital signs

Take the patient's body temperature, pulse, respirations, and blood pressure. They provide a quick overview of physiologic condition, and provide valuable information on the heart, lungs, and blood vessels. The seriousness of the patient's chief complaint as well as your general observations of his condition will determine how extensively you measure vital signs.

AGE ALERT A patient's age, activity level, and physical and emotional condition may affect his vital signs. Compare with the patient's baseline, if available.

Conduct the health history

Use pointed questions to explore the patient's perception of his chief complaint. Find out what's bothering him the most. Ask him to quantify the problem. Does he, for instance, feel worse today than he did yesterday? Such questions will help you focus your assessment. To save time, or if the patient can't respond, obtain information from other sources, such as family members, medical history, admission forms, and the patient's chart.

Perform the physical examination

Begin by concentrating on areas related to the patient's chief complaint – the abdomen, for example, if the patient complains of abdominal pain. Compare the results with baseline data, if available.

Sometimes, you may have to perform a complete head-to-toe or body systems assessment – for instance, if a patient is unresponsive (yet has no breathing or circulatory problems) or is confused and thus unreliable. But in most cases, your physical assessment will be guided by the chief complaint as well as by your general observations and vital signs findings.

Guidelines for an effective interview

When you have time for a full assessment, you'll begin by interviewing the patient. Developing an effective interviewing technique will help you collect pertinent health history information efficiently. Use these guidelines to enhance your interviewing skills.

Be prepared

• Before the interview, review all available information. Read current clinical records and, if applicable, previous records. This will focus the interview, prevent tiring the patient, and save you time.
• Review with the patient what you've learned to be sure the information is correct. Keep in mind that the patient's current complaint may be unrelated to his history.

Create a pleasant interviewing atmosphere

• Select a quiet, well-lighted, and relaxed setting. Keep in mind that extraneous noise and activity can interfere with concentration, as can excessive or insufficient light. A relaxed atmosphere eases the patient's anxiety, promotes comfort, and conveys your willingness to listen.
• Ensure privacy. Some patients won't share personal information if they suspect that others can overhear. You may, however, let friends or family members remain if the patient requests it or if he needs their help.
• Be sure the patient feels as comfortable as possible. If the patient is tired, short of breath, or frightened, you should provide care and reschedule the history taking.
• Take your time. If you appear rushed, you may distract the patient. Give him your undivided attention. If you have little time, you should focus on specific areas of interest and return later instead of hurrying through the entire interview.

Establish a good rapport

• Sit and chat with the patient for a few minutes before the interview. Standing may suggest that you're in a hurry and lead the patient to rush, omitting important information.
• Be sure to explain the interview's purpose. Emphasize how the patient benefits when the health care team has the information needed to diagnose and treat a disorder.
• Show your concern for the patient's story. Maintain eye contact, and occasionally repeat what he tells you. If you seem preoccupied

or disinterested, he may choose not to confide in you.

• Encourage the patient to help you develop a realistic plan of care that will serve his perceived needs.

Set the tone and focus

• Encourage the patient to talk about his chief complaint. This helps you focus on his most troublesome signs and symptoms and provides an opportunity to assess the patient's emotional state and level of understanding.

• Keep the interview informal but professional. Allow the patient time to answer questions fully and to add his own perceptions.

• Speak clearly and simply. Avoid using medical terms.

 Be sure the patient understands you, especially if he's elderly. If you think he doesn't, ask him to restate what you've discussed.

• Pay close attention to the patient's words and actions, interpreting not only what he says but also what he doesn't say.

 If the patient is a child, direct as many questions as possible to him. Rely on the parents for information if the child is very young.

Choose your words carefully

• Ask open-ended questions to encourage the patient to provide complete and pertinent information. Avoid yes-or-no–type questions.

• Listen carefully to the patient's answers. Use his words in your subsequent questions to encourage him to elaborate on his signs, symptoms, and other problems.

Take notes

• Avoid documenting everything during the interview, but make sure to jot down important information, such as dates, times, and key words or phrases. Use these to help you

recall the complete history for the medical record.

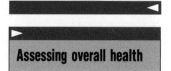

Assessing overall health

For a quick look at your patient's overall health, ask these questions.

• Has your weight changed? Do your clothes, rings, or shoes fit?

• Do you have nonspecific symptoms, such as weakness, fatigue, night sweats, or fever?

• Can you keep up with normal daily activities?

• Have you had any unusual symptoms or problems recently?

• How many colds or other minor illnesses have you had in the last year?

• What prescription and over-the-counter drugs do you take?

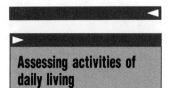

Assessing activities of daily living

For a comprehensive look at your patient's health and health history, ask these questions.

Diet and elimination

• How would you describe your appetite?

• What do you normally eat in a 24-hour period?

• What foods do you like and dislike? Is your diet restricted at all?

• How much fluid do you drink during an average day?

• Are you allergic to any foods?

• Do you prepare your meals, or does someone prepare them for you?

• Do you go to the grocery store, or does someone else shop for you?

• Do you snack and, if so, on what?
• Do you eat a variety of foods?
• Do you have enough money to purchase the groceries you need?
• When do you usually go to the bathroom? Has this pattern recently changed?
• Do you take any foods, fluids, or drugs to maintain your normal elimination patterns?

Exercise and sleep

• Do you have any special exercise program? What is it? How long have you been following it? How do you feel after exercising?
• How many hours do you sleep each day? When? Do you feel rested afterward?
• Do you fall asleep easily?
• Do you take any drugs or do anything special to help you fall asleep?
• What do you do when you can't sleep?
• Do you wake up during the night?
• Do you have sleepy spells during the day? When?
• Do you take naps routinely?
• Do you have any recurrent and disturbing dreams?
• Have you ever been diagnosed with a sleep disorder, such as narcolepsy or sleep apnea?

Recreation

• What do you do when you're not working?
• What kind of nonpaid work do you do for enjoyment?
• How much leisure time do you have?
• Are you satisfied with what you can do in your leisure time?
• Do you and your family share leisure time?
• How do your weekends differ from your weekdays?

Tobacco, alcohol, and drugs

• Do you use tobacco? If so, what kind? How much do you use each day? Each week? For how long have you used it? Have you ever tried to stop?
• Do you drink any alcoholic beverages? If so, what kind (beer, wine, whiskey)?
• How much alcohol do you drink each day? Each week? What time of day do you usually drink?
• Do you usually drink alone or with others?
• Do you drink more when you're under stress?
• Has drinking ever hampered your job performance?
• Do you or your family worry about your drinking?
• Do you feel dependent on alcohol?
• Do you feel dependent on coffee, tea, or soft drinks? How much of these beverages do you drink in an average day?
• Do you use any drugs not prescribed by a doctor (marijuana, sleeping pills, tranquilizers)?

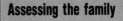

Assessing the family

When assessing how and to what extent the patient's family fulfills its functions, remember to assess both the family into which the patient was born (family of origin) and, if different, the current family.

Because the following questions target a nuclear family — that is, mother, father, and children — you may need to modify them somewhat for single-parent families, families that include grandparents, patients who live alone, or unrelated individuals who live as a family. Remember, you're assessing the *patient's perception* of family function.

Affective function

To assess how family members regard each other, ask these questions.
• How do the members of your family treat each other?
• How do they feel about each other?
• How do they regard each other's needs and wants?
• How are feelings expressed in your family?
• Can family members safely express both positive and negative feelings?
• What happens in the family when members disagree?
• How do family members deal with conflict?

Socialization and social placement

To assess the flexibility of family responsibilities, which aids discharge planning, ask these questions.
• How satisfied are you and your partner with your roles as a couple?
• How did you decide to have (or not to have) children?
• Do you and your partner agree about how to bring up the children? If not, how do you work out differences?
• Who is responsible for taking care of the children? Is this mutually satisfactory?
• How well do you feel your children are growing up?
• Are family roles negotiable within the limits of age and ability?
• Do you share cultural values and beliefs with the children?

Health care function

To identify the family caregiver and thus facilitate discharge planning, ask these questions.
• Who takes care of family members when they're sick? Who makes doctor appointments?
• Are your children learning personal hygiene, healthful eating habits, and the importance of sleep and rest?
• How does your family adjust when a member is ill and unable to fulfill expected roles?

Family and social structures

To assess the value the patient places on family and other social structures, ask these questions.
• How important is your family to you?
• Do you have any friends that you consider family?
• Does anyone other than your immediate family (for example, grandparents) live with you?
• Are you involved in community affairs? Do you enjoy the activities?

Economic function

To explore money issues and their relation to power roles within the family, ask these questions.
• Does your family income meet the family's basic needs?
• Do you consider family needs in relation to individual needs when allocating money?
• Who makes decisions about family money allocation?

Performing palpation techniques

Palpation uses pressure to assess structure size, placement, pulsation, and tenderness. Ballottement, a variation, involves bouncing tissues against the hand to assess rebound of floating structures.

Light palpation

To perform light palpation, press gently on the skin, indenting it ½" to ¾" (1 to 2 cm). Use the lightest touch possible; too much pressure blunts your sensitivity. Close your eyes to concentrate on feeling.

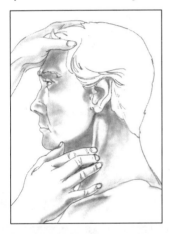

Deep palpation

To perform deep palpation, indent the skin about 1½" (4 cm). Place your other hand on top of the palpating hand to control and guide your movements. To perform a variation of deep palpation that allows pinpointing an inflamed area, press firmly with one hand, then lift your hand away quickly. If the patient complains of increased pain as you release the pressure, you have identified rebound tenderness.

Use both hands (bimanual palpation) to trap a deep, underlying, hard-to-palpate organ (such as the kidney or spleen) or to fix or stabilize an organ (such as the uterus) while palpating with the other hand.

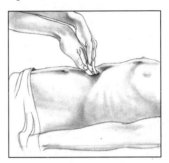

Light ballottement

To perform light ballottement, apply light, rapid pressure from quadrant to quadrant of the patient's abdomen. Keep your hand on the skin surface to detect tissue rebound.

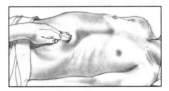

Deep ballottement

To perform deep ballottement, apply abrupt, deep pressure; then release, but maintain contact.

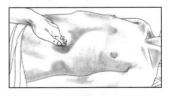

▶

Performing percussion techniques

Percussion has two basic purposes: to produce percussion sounds and to elicit tenderness. It involves three types: indirect, direct, and blunt percussion.

Indirect percussion

The most commonly used method, indirect percussion produces clear, crisp sounds when performed correctly. To perform indirect percussion, use the second finger of your nondominant hand as the pleximeter (the mediating device used to receive the taps) and the middle finger of your dominant hand as the plexor (the device used to tap the pleximeter). Place the pleximeter finger firmly against a body surface, such as the upper back. With your wrist flexed loosely, use the tip of your plexor finger to deliver a crisp blow just beneath the distal joint of the pleximeter. Be sure to hold the plexor perpendicular to the pleximeter. Tap lightly and quickly, removing the plexor as soon as you have delivered each blow.

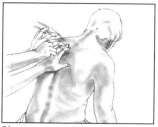

Direct percussion

To perform direct percussion, tap your hand or fingertip directly against the body surface as shown at the top of the next page. This method helps assess an adult's sinuses for tenderness.

▶

Identifying percussion sounds

Percussion produces sounds that vary according to the tissue being percussed. This chart shows important percussion sounds along with their characteristics and typical locations.

SOUND	INTENSITY	PITCH	DURATION
Resonance	Moderate to loud	Low	Long
Tympany	Loud	High	Moderate
Dullness	Soft to moderate	High	Moderate
Hyperresonance	Very loud	Very low	Long
Flatness	Soft	High	Short

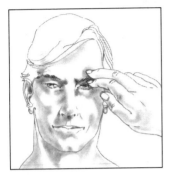

sound—over such organs as the kidneys, gallbladder, or liver. (Another blunt percussion method, used in the neurologic examination, involves tapping a rubber-tipped reflex hammer against a tendon to create a reflexive muscle contraction.)

Blunt percussion

To perform blunt percussion, strike the ulnar surface of your fist against the body surface. Alternatively, you may use both hands by placing the palm of one hand over the area to be percussed and then making a fist with the other hand and using it to strike the back of the first hand. Both techniques aim to elicit tenderness—not to create a

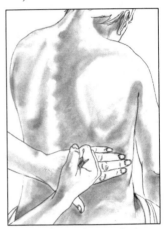

QUALITY	SOURCE
Hollow	Normal lung
Drumlike	Gastric air bubble; intestinal air
Thudlike	Liver; full bladder; pregnant uterus
Booming	Hyperinflated lung (as in emphysema)
Flat	Muscle

Performing auscultation

Auscultation of body sounds — particularly those produced by the heart, lungs, blood vessels, stomach, and intestines — detects both high-pitched and low-pitched sounds. Although you can perform auscultation directly over a body area, using only your ears, you'll typically perform it indirectly, using a stethoscope.

Assessing high-pitched sounds

To properly assess high-pitched sounds, such as breath sounds and S_1 and S_2, use the diaphragm of the stethoscope. Make sure you place the diaphragm's entire surface firmly on the patient's skin. If the area is excessively hairy, improve diaphragm contact and reduce extraneous noise by applying water or water-soluble jelly to the skin before auscultating.

Assessing low-pitched sounds

To assess low-pitched sounds, such as heart murmurs and S_3 and S_4, lightly place the bell of the stethoscope on the appropriate area. Don't exert pressure. If you do, the patient's chest will act as a diaphragm and you'll miss low-pitched sounds. If the patient is extremely thin or emaciated, use a stethoscope with a pediatric chestpiece.

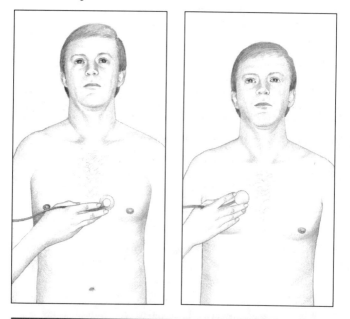

Assessing the cardiovascular system

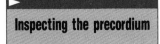

Initial cardiovascular questions

• Ask your patient about cardiac problems, such as palpitations, tachycardia or other irregular rhythms, chest pain, dyspnea on exertion, paroxysmal nocturnal dyspnea, and cough.
• Explore vascular problems. Does the patient experience cyanosis, edema, ascites, intermittent claudication, cold extremities, or phlebitis?
• Ask about postural hypotension, hypertension, rheumatic fever, varicose veins, and peripheral vascular diseases.
• Ask when, if ever, the patient had his last electrocardiogram.

Inspecting the precordium

• First, place the patient in a supine position, with his head flat or elevated for his respiratory comfort. If you're examining an obese patient or one with large breasts, have the patient sit upright. This will bring the heart closer to the anterior chest wall and make any pulsations more visible. If time allows, you can use tangential lighting to cast shadows across the chest. This makes it easier to see any abnormalities.
• Standing to the patient's right (unless you're left handed), remove the clothing covering his chest wall. Quickly identify the following anatomic sites, named for their underlying structures: the sternoclavicular, pulmonary, aortic, right ventricular, epigastric, and left ventricular areas.
• Make a visual sweep of the chest wall, watching for movement, pulsations, and exaggerated lifts or heaves (strong outward thrusts over the chest during systole).

Measuring blood pressure

When you assess your patient's blood pressure, you're measuring the fluctuating force that blood exerts against arterial walls as the heart contracts and relaxes. To measure accurately, follow these steps.

Preparing the patient
Before beginning, make sure the patient is relaxed and has not eaten or exercised in the past 30 minutes. The patient can sit, stand, or lie down during blood pressure measurement.

Applying the cuff and stethoscope
• To obtain a reading in an arm (the most common measurement site), wrap the sphygmomanometer cuff snugly around the upper arm above the antecubital area (the inner aspect of the elbow), with the cuff bladder centered over the brachial artery.

 When taking an infant's or child's blood pressure, be sure to use the appropriate size cuff. Because blood pressure may be inaudible in children under age 2, consider using an electronic stethoscope to get a more accurate measurement.

ASSESSMENT

• Most cuffs have arrows that should be placed over the brachial artery. Be sure to use the proper-sized cuff for the patient.

• Keep the mercury manometer at eye level; if your sphygmomanometer has an aneroid gauge, place it level with the patient's arm. Keep the patient's arm level with the heart by placing it on a table or a chair arm or by supporting it with your hand. Rest a recumbent patient's arm at his side. Don't use the patient's muscle strength to hold up the arm; tension from muscle contraction can elevate systolic pressure and distort your findings.

• Next, palpate the brachial pulse just below and slightly medial to the antecubital area. Place the earpieces of the stethoscope in your ears, and position the stethoscope head over the brachial artery, just distal to the cuff or slightly beneath it.

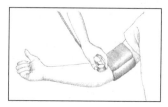

Generally, you will use the easy-to-handle, flat diaphragm to auscultate the pulse; however, you may need to use the bell if the patient has a diminished or hard-to-locate pulse because the bell detects the low-pitched sound of arterial blood flow more effectively.

Obtaining the blood pressure reading

• Watching the manometer, pump the bulb until the mercury column or aneroid gauge reaches about 20 mm Hg above the point at which the pulse disappeared. Then, slowly open the air valve and watch the mercury drop or the gauge needle descend. Release the pressure at a rate of about 3 mm Hg per second, and listen for pulse sounds (Korotkoff's sounds). These sounds, which determine the blood pressure measurement, are classified as follows:

Phase I
Onset of clear, faint tapping, with intensity that increases to a thud or louder tap

Phase II
Tapping that changes to a soft, swishing sound

Phase III
Return of clear, crisp tapping sound

Phase IV (first diastolic sound)
Sound becomes muffled and takes on a blowing quality

Phase V (second diastolic sound)
Sound disappears.

• As soon as you hear blood begin to pulse through the brachial artery, note the reading on the aneroid dial or mercury column. Reflecting phase I (the first Korotkoff's sound), this sound coincides with the patient's systolic pressure. Continue deflating the cuff, noting the point at which pulsations diminish or become muffled – phase IV (the fourth Korotkoff's sound) – and then disappear – phase V (the fifth Korotkoff's sound). For children and highly active adults, many authorities consider phase IV the most accurate reflection of blood pressure.

The American Heart Association and the World Health Organization recommend documenting phases I, IV, and V. To avoid confusion and to make your measurements more useful, follow this format for recording blood pressure: systolic/muffling/disappearance (for example, 120/80/76).

Positioning the patient for cardiac auscultation

During auscultation, you'll typically stand to the right of the patient, who is in a supine position. The patient may lie flat or at a comfortable elevation.

If heart sounds seem faint or undetectable, try repositioning the patient. Alternate positioning may enhance the sounds or make them seem louder by bringing the heart closer to the surface of the chest. Common alternate positions include a seated, forward-leaning position and the left-lateral decubitus position.

Forward-leaning position

This position is best for hearing high-pitched sounds related to semilunar valve problems, such as aortic and pulmonic valve murmurs. To auscultate these sounds, help the patient to the forward-leaning position, and place the diaphragm of the stethoscope over the aortic and pulmonic areas in the right and left second intercostal space.

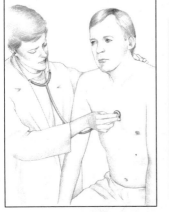

Left-lateral decubitus position

This position is best for hearing low-pitched sounds related to atrio-ventricular valve problems, such as mitral valve murmurs and extra heart sounds. To auscultate these sounds, help the patient to the left-lateral decubitus position, and place the bell of the stethoscope over the apical area. If these positions do not enhance heart sounds, try auscultating with the patient standing or squatting.

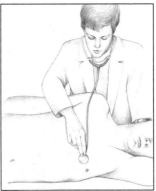

ASSESSMENT

Auscultating heart sounds

Using a stethoscope with 10″ to 12″ (25- to 30-cm) tubing, follow these steps to auscultate heart sounds.
• Locate the four different auscultation sites, as illustrated below.

In the aortic area, blood moves from the left ventricle during systole, crossing the aortic valve and flowing through the aortic arch. In the pulmonic area, blood ejected from the right ventricle during systole crosses the pulmonic valve and flows through the main pulmonary artery. In the tricuspid area, sounds reflect blood movement from the right atrium across the tricuspid valve, filling the right ventricle during diastole. In the mitral, or apical, area, sounds represent blood flow across the mitral valve and the left ventricular filling during diastole.

ing diastole. In the mitral, or apical, area, sounds represent blood flow across the mitral valve and the left ventricular filling during diastole.
• Begin auscultation in the aortic area, placing the stethoscope in the second intercostal space along the right sternal border.
• Then move to the pulmonic area, located in the second intercostal space at the left sternal border.
• Next, assess in the tricuspid area, which lies in the fifth intercostal space along the left sternal border.
• Finally, listen in the mitral area, located in the fifth intercostal space near the midclavicular line.

Note: If the patient's heart is enlarged, the mitral area may be closer to the anterior axillary line.

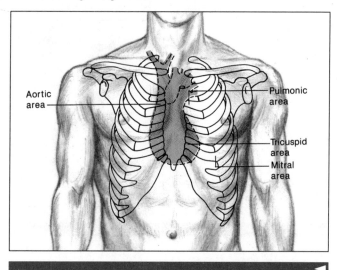

Aortic area

Pulmonic area

Tricuspid area

Mitral area

Palpating arterial pulses

To palpate arterial pulses, you'll apply pressure with your index and middle fingers positioned as shown below.

Carotid pulse
Lightly place your fingers just medial to the trachea and below the jaw angle.

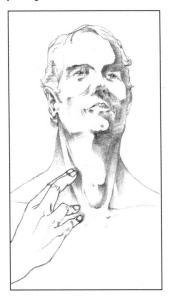

Brachial pulse
Position your fingers medial to the biceps tendon.

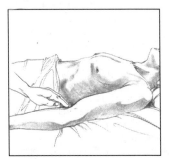

Radial pulse
Apply gentle pressure to the medial and ventral side of the wrist just below the thumb.

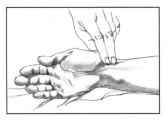

Femoral pulse
Press relatively hard at a point inferior to the inguinal ligament. For an obese patient, palpate in the crease of the groin halfway between the pubic bone and the hip bone.

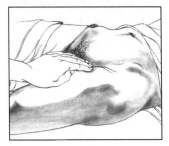

Popliteal pulse
Press firmly against the popliteal fossa at the back of the knee.

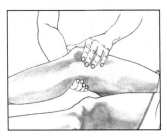

ASSESSMENT

Posterior tibial pulse

Apply pressure behind and slightly below the malleolus of the ankle.

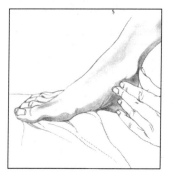

Dorsalis pedis pulse

Place your fingers on the medial dorsum of the foot while the patient points the toes down. In this site, the pulse is difficult to palpate and may seem to be absent in some healthy patients.

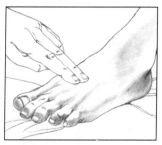

Assessing the respiratory system

Initial respiratory questions

• Inquire about dyspnea or shortness of breath. Does your patient have breathing problems after physical exertion? Also ask him about pain, wheezing, paroxysmal nocturnal dyspnea, and orthopnea (number of pillows used).
• Ask whether the patient experiences cough, sputum production, hemoptysis, or night sweats.
• Find out if he has emphysema, pleurisy, bronchitis, tuberculosis, pneumonia, asthma, or frequent respiratory infections.

Inspecting the chest

Position the patient to allow access to his posterior and anterior chest. If his condition permits, have him sit on the edge of a bed or examining table or on a chair, leaning forward with his arms folded across his chest. If this isn't possible, place him in semi-Fowler's position for the anterior chest examination. Then ask him to lean forward slightly and use the side rails or mattress for support while you quickly examine his posterior chest. If he can't lean forward, place him in a lateral position or ask another staff member to help him sit up.

Systematically compare one side of the chest to the other.
• First, inspect the patient's chest for obvious problems, such as draining, open wounds, bruises, abrasions, scars, and cuts. Also look for less obvious problems, such as rib deformities, fractures, lesions, or masses.
• Examine the shape of the patient's

chest wall. Observe the anteroposterior and transverse diameters.

• Note the patient's respiratory pattern, watching for characteristics such as pursed-lip breathing.

• Observe chest movement during respirations. The chest should move upward and outward symmetrically on inspiration. Factors that may affect movement include pain, poor positioning, and abdominal distention. Watch for paradoxical movement (possibly resulting from fractured ribs or flail chest) and asymmetrical expansion (atelectasis or underlying pulmonary disease).

• Check for accessory muscle use and retraction of intercostal spaces during inspiration (possibly indicating respiratory distress). You may note sudden, violent intercostal retraction (airway obstruction or tension pneumothorax); retraction of abdominal muscles during expiration (chronic obstructive pulmonary disease and other obstructive disorders); inspiratory intercostal bulging (cardiac enlargement or aneurysm); or localized expiratory bulging (rib fracture or flail chest).

Palpating the thorax

Palpation of the anterior and posterior thorax can detect structural and skin abnormalities, areas of pain, and chest asymmetry. To perform this technique, use the fingertips and palmar surfaces of one or both hands, palpating systematically and in a circular motion. Alternate palpation from one side of the thorax to the other.

Anterior thorax

Begin palpation in the supraclavicular area (#1 in the diagram below). Then follow the sequence: infraclavicular, sternal, xiphoid, rib, and axillary areas.

Posterior thorax

Begin palpation in the supraclavicular area, move to the area between the scapulae (interscapular), then below the scapulae (infrascapular), and finally down to the lateral walls of the thorax.

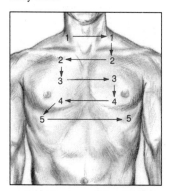

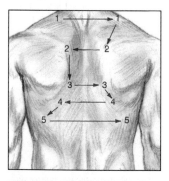

Palpating for tactile fremitus

Because sound travels more easily through solid structures than through air, assessing for tactile fremitus—which involves palpating for voice vibrations—provides valuable information about the contents of the lungs. Follow this procedure.
• Place your open palm flat against the patient's chest without touching the chest with your fingers.

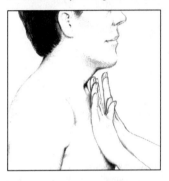

• Ask the patient to repeat a resonant phrase like "ninety-nine" as you systematically move your hands over his chest from the central airways to the lung periphery and back. Always proceed in a systematic manner from the top of the suprascapular area to the interscapular, infrascapular, and hypochondriac areas (found at the level of the 5th and 10th intercostal spaces to the right and left of midline).
• Repeat this procedure on the posterior thorax. You should feel vibrations of equal intensity on either side of the chest. The fremitus normally occurs in the upper chest, close to the bronchi, and feels strongest at the second intercostal space on either side of the sternum. Little or no fremitus should occur in the lower chest. The intensity of the vibrations varies according to the thickness and structure of the patient's chest wall as well as the patient's voice intensity and pitch.

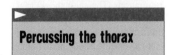

Percussing the thorax

Thorax percussion helps determine the boundaries of the lungs and how much gas, liquid, or solid exists in the lungs. Percussion can effectively assess structures as deep as 1¾" to 3" (4.5 to 8 cm).

To percuss a patient's thorax, always use indirect percussion, which involves striking one finger with another. Proceed systematically, percussing the anterior, lateral, and posterior chest over the intercostal spaces.

Avoid percussing over bones, such as over the manubrium, sternum, xiphoid, clavicles, ribs, vertebrae, or scapulae. Because of their denseness, bones produce a dull sound on percussion and, therefore, yield no useful information.

As you percuss, always follow the same sequence, comparing sound variations from one side to the other. This helps ensure consistency and prevents you from overlooking any important findings.

Anterior thorax
Place your hands over the lung apices in the supraclavicular area. Then proceed downward, moving from side to side at 1½" to 2" (3- to 5-cm) intervals as shown at the top of the next page. Anterior chest percussion should produce resonance from below the clavicle to the fifth intercostal space on the right (where dullness occurs close to the liver) and to the third intercostal space on the left (where dullness occurs near the heart).

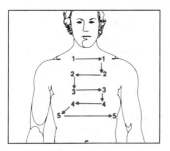

Posterior thorax
Progress in a zigzag fashion from the suprascapular to the interscapular to the infrascapular areas, avoiding the vertebral column and the scapulae, as shown below. Posterior percussion should sound resonant to the level of T10.

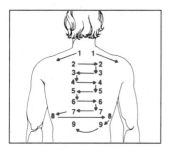

Lateral thorax
Starting at the axilla, move down the side of the rib cage, percussing between the ribs as shown below. Lateral chest percussion should produce resonance to the sixth or eighth intercostal space.

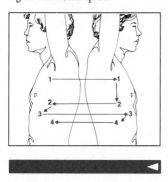

Auscultating breath sounds

An important step in physical assessment, auscultating breath sounds helps you detect abnormal fluid or mucus accumulation as well as obstructed air passages.

To detect breath sounds, auscultate the anterior, lateral, and posterior thorax, following the same sequence as that used for thorax percussion. Begin at the upper lobes, and move from side to side and down, comparing findings.

AGE ALERT If the patient is a child, begin just below the right clavicle, moving to the midsternum, left clavicle, left nipple, and finally the right nipple. Assess one full breath (inspiration and expiration) at each point.

Auscultate the lungs for normal, abnormal, and absent breath sounds. Classify breath sounds by location, intensity, pitch, and duration during inspiratory and expiratory phases.

Assessing the neurologic system

Initial neurologic questions

• Investigate the character of any headaches (frequency, intensity, location, and duration).
• Determine whether your patient has vertigo or syncope.
• Ask about a history of seizures or use of anticonvulsant medication.
• Explore any cognitive disturbances, including recent or remote

memory loss, hallucinations, disorientation, speech and language dysfunction, or inability to concentrate.

• Ask if the patient has a history of sensory disturbances, including tingling, numbness, and sensory loss.
• Explore any motor problems, including problems with gait, balance, coordination, tremor, spasm, or paralysis.
• Find out if his activities of daily living have been impeded by cognitive, sensory, or motor symptoms.

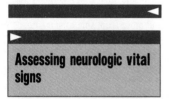

Assessing neurologic vital signs

A supplement to routine measurement of temperature, pulse, and respirations, neurologic vital signs are used to evaluate the patient's level of consciousness (LOC), pupillary activity, and level of orientation to place, time, date, situation, and person.

LOC reflects brain stem function and usually provides the first sign of central nervous system deterioration. Changes in pupillary activity may signal increased intracranial pressure (ICP). Level of orientation evaluates higher cerebral functions. Evaluating muscle strength and tone, reflexes, and posture also may help identify nervous system damage. Finally, respiratory rate and pattern can help locate brain lesions and determine their size.

Equipment

• Penlight • thermometer • stethoscope • sphygmomanometer • pupil size chart.

Implementation

• Explain the procedure to the patient, even if he's unresponsive.

• Assess LOC.
• Ask the patient his full name. If he responds appropriately, assess his orientation to place, time, date, situation, and person. Assess the quality of his replies.
• Assess the patient's ability to understand and follow one-step commands that require a motor response. For example, ask him to open and close his eyes. Note whether he can maintain his LOC.
• If the patient doesn't respond to commands, squeeze the nail beds on his fingers and toes with moderate pressure and note his response. Check motor responses bilaterally to rule out monoplegia and hemiplegia.

Examine pupils and eye movement

• Ask the patient to open his eyes. If he's unresponsive, lift his upper eyelids. Inspect pupils for size and shape, and compare for equality. To evaluate more precisely, use a chart showing the various pupil sizes.
• Test the patient's direct light response. First, darken the room. Hold each eyelid open in turn, keeping the other eye covered. Swing the penlight from the patient's ear toward the midline of the face. Shine the light directly into the eye. Normally, the pupil constricts immediately when exposed to light and then dilates immediately when the light is removed. Wait 20 seconds before testing the other pupil to allow it to recover from reflex stimulation.
• Test consensual light response. Hold both eyelids open, but shine the light into one eye only. Watch for constriction in the other pupil, which indicates proper nerve function.
• Brighten the room and have the conscious patient open his eyes. Observe eyelids for ptosis or drooping. Then check extraocular

movements. Hold up one finger and ask the patient to follow it with his eyes as you move your finger up, down, laterally, and obliquely. See if the patient's eyes track together to follow your finger (conjugate gaze). Watch for involuntary jerking or oscillating eye movements (nystagmus).

• Check accommodation. Hold up one finger midline to the patient's face and several feet away. Have the patient focus on your finger as you move it toward his nose. His eyes should converge, and his pupils should constrict equally.

• Test the corneal reflex by rapidly moving the palm of your hand toward the patient's open eyes. This forces air against the corneas and normally causes a blink reflex.

• If the patient is unconscious, test the oculocephalic (doll's eye) reflex. Hold the patient's eyelids open. Quickly but gently turn the patient's head to one side and then the other. If the patient's eyes move in the opposite direction from the side to which you turn the head, the reflex is intact.

Note: Never test this reflex if you know or suspect that the patient has a cervical spine injury.

Evaluate motor function

• If the patient is conscious, test his grip strength in both hands at the same time. Extend your hands, ask the patient to squeeze your fingers as hard as he can, and compare the strength of each hand. Grip strength is usually slightly stronger in the dominant hand.

• Test arm strength by having the patient close his eyes and hold his arms straight out in front of him with palms up. See if either arm drifts downward or pronates, which indicates weakness. Test leg strength by having the patient raise his legs, one at a time, against gen-

tle downward pressure from your hand.

• If the patient is unconscious, exert pressure on each fingernail bed. If the patient withdraws, compare the strength of each limb.

Note: If decorticate or decerebrate posturing develops in response to painful stimuli, notify the doctor immediately.

• Flex and extend the extremities on both sides to evaluate muscle tone.

• Test the plantar reflex in all patients. Stroke the lateral aspect of the sole of the patient's foot with your thumbnail. Normally, this elicits flexion of all toes. Watch for a positive Babinski's sign – dorsiflexion of the great toe with fanning of the other toes – which indicates an upper motor neuron lesion.

• Test for Brudzinski's and Kernig's signs in patients suspected of having meningitis.

Complete the neurologic examination

• Take the patient's temperature, pulse rate, respiration rate, and blood pressure. Especially note pulse pressure – the difference between systolic and diastolic pressure – because widening pulse pressure can indicate increasing ICP.

Special considerations

Note: If the previously stable patient suddenly develops a change in neurologic or routine vital signs, assess his condition further and notify the doctor immediately.

▶

Performing the Mini–Mental State examination

This examination offers a quick way to quantify cognitive function and screen for cognitive loss. It tests the patient's orientation, registration, attention, calculation, recall, and language and motor skills. To give the examination, seat the patient in a quiet, well-lighted room. Ask him to answer each question as accurately as he can.

Don't time the test, but do score it right away. In the section on attention and calculation, include either items 14 to 18 or item 19, not both. The patient can receive a maximum total score of 30 points. Usually a score below 24 indicates cognitive impairment, although this may not be an accurate cutoff for highly or poorly educated patients. A score below 20 usually appears in patients with delirium, dementia, schizophrenia, or affective disorder and not in normal elderly people or in patients with neurosis or personality disorder.

Orientation

Ask the patient for the date. Then ask for any missing information (year, month, day of the week). Ask if he knows what season it is. Ask him to name the hospital and the floor he's currently on. Finally, ask for the town or city, the county, and the state. Give a point for each right answer (maximum score: 10).

1. Date _____
2. Year _____
3. Month _____
4. Day _____
5. Season _____
6. Hospital _____
7. Floor _____
8. Town or city _____
9. County _____
10. State _____

Registration

Tell the patient that you'd like to test his memory. Then say "ball," "flag," and "tree" clearly and slowly, taking about 1 second to say each word. After you've said all three words, ask him to repeat them. The first repetition determines the score (0 to 3), but keep saying the words (up to six trials) until he can repeat all three. If he doesn't eventually say all three, recall can't be meaningfully tested.

11. Ball _____
12. Flag _____
13. Tree _____
Number of trials _____

Attention and calculation

You may perform this section of the test in one of two ways. Begin by asking the patient to count backward from 100 in increments of 7. Stop after he's said five numbers (93, 86, 79, 72, 65). Score one point for each correct number.

14. 93 _____
15. 86 _____
16. 79 _____
17. 72 _____
18. 65 _____

Performing the Mini–Mental State examination *(continued)*

Attention and calculation *(continued)*

If the patient can't or won't perform this task, ask him to spell "world" backward (D, L, R, O, W). Assign one point for each correctly placed letter. For example, DLROW = 5, DLORW = 3. Record how the patient spelled "world" backward: _____

19. Number of correctly placed letters _____

Recall

Ask the patient to recall the three words you previously asked him to remember (in the registration section). Give a point for each correct answer.

20. Ball _____
21. Flag _____
22. Tree _____

Language and motor skills

This section of the assessment has six parts.

Naming

Show the patient a wristwatch and ask, "What is this?" Repeat the question when holding a pencil. Give one point for each object named correctly.

23. Watch _____
24. Pencil _____

Repetition

Ask the patient to repeat "no ifs, ands, or buts." Allow only one try, and give one point for correct repetition.

25. Repetition _____

Three-stage command

Hand the patient a piece of blank paper and say, "Take the paper in your right hand, fold it in half, and put it on the floor." Score one point for each action performed correctly.

26. Takes in right hand ___
27. Folds in half _____
28. Places on floor _____

Reading

On a blank piece of paper, print "close your eyes" in letters large enough for the patient to see clearly. Ask him to read it and do what it says. Score one point only if he actually closes his eyes.

29. Closes eyes _____

(continued)

Performing the Mini–Mental State examination *(continued)*

Writing
Give the patient a blank piece of paper, and ask him to make up a sentence and write it. Evaluate whether the sentence contains a subject and a verb and whether it makes sense. Correct grammar and punctuation aren't necessary.

30. Writes sentence _____

Copying
On a clean piece of paper, draw intersecting pentagons with each side about 1″ (2.5 cm) long. Ask the patient to copy your drawing exactly as it appears. All 10 angles must be present and 2 must intersect for the patient to receive a point. Ignore tremor and rotation.
Example:

31. Draws pentagons _____

Total score _____

Assessing cerebellar function

To evaluate cerebellar function, you'll test the patient's whole-body coordination and extremity coordination.

Heel-to-toe walking
To assess balance, ask the patient to walk heel to toe. Although he may be slightly unsteady, he should be able to walk and maintain his balance.

Romberg test
To perform this test, ask the patient to stand with his feet together, his eyes open, and his arms at his side. Hold your outstretched arms on either side of him so you can support him if he sways to one side or the other. Observe his balance; then ask him to close his eyes. Note whether he loses his balance or sways. If he falls to one side, the Romberg test is positive. Patients with cerebellar dysfunction have difficulty maintaining their balance with their eyes closed because they cannot use the visual cues that orient them to the upright position.

Point-to-point movements

To evaluate the patient's extremity coordination, test point-to-point movements. Have the patient sit about 2′ (0.6 m) away from you. Hold your index finger up, and ask him to touch the tip of his index finger to the tip of yours and then to touch his nose. Now, move your finger and ask him to repeat the manuever. Gradually, have him increase his speed as you repeat the test. Then test his other hand. Expect the patient to be more accurate with his dominant hand. A patient with cerebellar dysfunction will overshoot his target, and his movements will be jerky.

Rapid skilled movements

To further evaluate the patient's extremity coordination, test rapid skilled movements. Ask the patient to touch the thumb of his right hand to his right index finger and then to each of his remaining fingers. Then instruct him to increase his speed. Observe his movements for smoothness and accuracy. Repeat the test on his left hand.

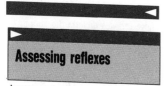

Assessing reflexes

Assessment of deep tendon and superficial reflexes provides information about the intactness of the sensory receptor organ. It also evaluates how well the afferent nerve relays the sensory message to the spinal cord, the spinal cord or brain stem segment mediates the reflex, the lower motor neurons transmit messages to the muscles, and the muscles respond to the motor message.

To evaluate your patient's reflexes, you'll need to test deep tendon and superficial reflexes as well as observe for primitive reflexes.

Deep tendon reflexes

Before you test a deep tendon reflex, be sure the limb is relaxed and the joint is in midposition; for instance, the knee or elbow should be flexed at a 45-degree angle. Then distract the patient by asking him to focus on an object across the room. If he focuses on his performance, the cerebral cortex may dampen his response. You can also distract the patient by using Jendrassik's maneuver. Simply instruct him to clench his teeth or to squeeze his thigh. Be sure to document which technique you used to distract the patient.

Always move from head to toe in testing deep tendon reflexes, and compare contralateral reflexes. To elicit the reflex, tap the tendon lightly but firmly with the reflex hammer. Then grade the briskness of the response: 0 (no response), 2+ (normal), 4+ (hyperactive).

Biceps reflex

Position the patient's arm so his elbow is flexed at a 45-degree angle and his arm is relaxed. Place your thumb or index finger over the biceps tendon and your remaining fingers loosely over the triceps muscle. Strike your thumb or index finger with the pointed tip of the reflex hammer, and watch and feel for contraction of the biceps muscle and flexion of the forearm.

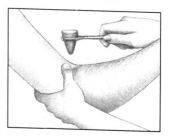

Triceps reflex

Have the patient abduct his arm and place his forearm across his chest. Strike the triceps tendon about 2″ (5 cm) above the olecranon process on the extensor surface of the upper arm. Watch for contraction of the triceps muscle and extension of the forearm.

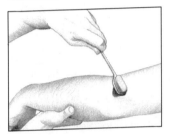

Brachioradialis reflex

Instruct the patient to rest the ulnar surface of his hand on his knee and to partially flex his elbow. With the tip of the hammer, strike the radius about 2″ (5 cm) proximal to the radial styloid. Watch for supination of the hand and flexion of the forearm at the elbow.

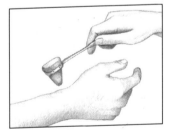

Patellar reflex

Have the patient sit on the side of the bed with his legs dangling freely. If he can't sit up, flex his knee at a 45-degree angle and place your nondominant hand behind it for support. Strike the patellar tendon just below the patella, and look for contraction of the

quadriceps muscle in the anterior thigh and for extension of the leg.

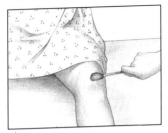

Achilles reflex

Slightly flex the foot and support the plantar surface. Using the pointed end of the reflex hammer, strike the Achilles tendon. Watch for plantar flexion of the foot at the ankle.

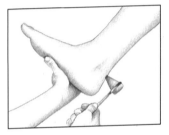

Superficial reflexes

These reflexes include the abdominal, cremasteric, and plantar reflexes. To elicit these reflexes, you'll stimulate the patient's skin or mucous membranes. To document your findings, use a plus sign (+) to indicate that a reflex is present and a minus sign (−) to indicate that it's absent.

Abdominal reflex

Place the patient in the supine position, with his arms at his sides and his knees slightly flexed. Using the tip of the reflex hammer, a key, or an applicator stick, briskly stroke both sides of the abdomen above and below the umbilicus, moving from the periphery toward the midline. After each stroke, watch for abdominal muscle contraction and movement of the umbilicus toward the stimulus. If you're evaluating an obese patient, retract the umbilicus to the side opposite the stimulus and note whether it pulls toward the stimulus. Aging and diseases of the upper and lower motor neurons cause an absent abdominal reflex.

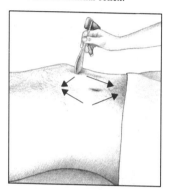

Cremasteric reflex

With a male patient, use an applicator stick to lightly stimulate the inner thigh. Watch for contraction of the cremaster muscle in the scrotum and prompt elevation of the testicle on the side of the stimulus. This reflex may be absent in upper or lower motor neuron disease.

Plantar reflex

Using an applicator stick, a tongue blade, or a key, slowly stroke the lateral side of the patient's sole from the heel to the great toe. The normal response is plantar flexion of the toes. In an elderly patient, this normal response may be diminished because of arthritic deformities of the toe or foot.

In patients with disorders of the pyramidal tract (such as cerebrovascular accident), the Babinski's re-

flex, an abnormal response, is elicited. The patient responds to the stimulus by dorsiflexion of his great toe. You may also see a more pronounced response in which the other toes extend and abduct. In some cases, you may even see dorsiflexion of the ankle, knee, and hip.

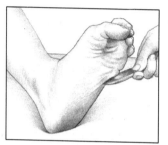

Primitive reflexes

Although normal in infants, primitive reflexes are pathologic in adults.

Grasp reflex

Apply gentle pressure to the patient's palm with your fingers. If he grasps your fingers between his thumb and index finger, suspect cortical (premotor cortex) damage.

Snout reflex

Tap lightly on the patient's upper lip. Lip pursing indicates frontal lobe damage.

Sucking reflex

If the patient begins sucking while you're feeding him or suctioning his mouth, you've elicited a reflex that indicates cortical damage characteristic of advanced dementia.

Glabellar reflex

Repeatedly tap the bridge of the patient's nose. A persistent blinking response indicates diffuse cortical dysfunction.

Assessing the cranial nerves

Cranial nerve assessment provides valuable information about the condition of the central nervous system, particularly the brain stem. Because disorders can affect any of the cranial nerves, knowing how to test each nerve is important. The techniques vary according to the nerve being tested.

CRANIAL NERVE AND ASSESSMENT TECHNIQUE	NORMAL FINDINGS
Olfactory (CN I) After checking the patency of the patient's nostrils, have him close both eyes. Then occlude one nostril, and hold a familiar, pungent substance, such as coffee, tobacco, soap, or peppermint, under the patient's nose and ask its identity. Repeat this technique with the other nostril.	The patient should be able to detect and identify the smell correctly. If he reports detecting the smell but cannot name it, offer a choice, such as, "Do you smell lemon, coffee, or peppermint?"
Optic (CN II) and oculomotor (CN III) To assess the optic nerve, check visual acuity, visual fields, and the retinal structures. To assess the oculomotor nerve, check pupil size, pupil shape, and pupillary response to light.	The pupils should be equal, round, and reactive to light. When assessing pupil size, be especially alert for any trends. For example, watch for a gradual increase in the size of one pupil or the appearance of unequal pupils in a patient whose pupils were previously equal.
Oculomotor (CN III), trochlear (CN IV), and abducens (CN VI) To test the coordinated function of these three nerves, assess them simultaneously by evaluating the patient's extraocular eye movement.	The eyes should move smoothly and in a coordinated manner through all six directions of eye movement. Observe each eye for rapid oscillation (nystagmus), movement not in unison with that of the other eye, or inability to move in certain directions (ophthalmoplegia). Also note any complaint of double vision (diplopia).

Assessing the cranial nerves *(continued)*

CRANIAL NERVE AND ASSESSMENT TECHNIQUE	NORMAL FINDINGS

Trigeminal (CN V)

To assess the sensory portion of the trigeminal nerve, gently touch the right, then the left, side of the patient's forehead with a cotton ball while his eyes are closed. Instruct him to state the moment the cotton touches the area. Compare the patient's response on both sides. Repeat the technique on the right and left cheek and on the right and left jaw. Next, repeat the entire procedure using a sharp object. The cap of a disposable ballpoint pen can be used to test light touch (dull end) and sharp stimuli (sharp end). (If an abnormality appears, also test for temperature sensation by touching the patient's skin with test tubes filled with hot and cold water and asking him to differentiate between them.)

The patient with a normal trigeminal nerve should report feeling both light touch and sharp stimuli in all three areas (forehead, cheek, and jaw) on both sides of his face.

To assess the motor portion of the trigeminal nerve, ask the patient to clench his jaws. Palpate the temporal and masseter muscles bilaterally, checking for symmetry. Try to open the patient's clenched jaws. Next, watch for symmetry as the patient opens and closes his mouth.

The jaws should clench symmetrically and remain closed against resistance.

Then assess the corneal reflex.

The lids of both eyes should close when a wisp of cotton is lightly stroked across a cornea.

Facial (CN VII)

To test the motor portion of the facial nerve, ask the patient to wrinkle his forehead, raise and lower his eyebrows, smile to show teeth, and puff out his cheeks. Also, with the patient's eyes tightly closed, attempt to open the eyelids. With each of these movements, observe closely for symmetry.

Normal facial movements are symmetrical.

(continued)

Assessing the cranial nerves *(continued)*

CRANIAL NERVE AND ASSESSMENT TECHNIQUE	NORMAL FINDINGS
Facial (CN VII) *(continued)* To test the sensory portion of the facial nerve, which supplies taste sensation to the anterior two-thirds of the tongue, first prepare four marked, closed containers: one containing salt; another, sugar; a third, vinegar (or lemon); and a fourth, quinine (or bitters). Then, with the patient's eyes closed, place salt on the anterior two-thirds of his tongue using a cotton swab or dropper. Ask him to identify the taste as sweet, salty, sour, or bitter. Rinse the patient's mouth with water. Repeat this procedure, alternating flavors and sides of the tongue until all four flavors have been tested on both sides. Taste sensations to the posterior third of the tongue are supplied by the glossopharyngeal nerve (CN IX) and are usually tested at the same time.	Normal taste sensations are symmetrical.
Acoustic (CN VIII) To assess the acoustic portion of this nerve, test the patient's hearing acuity.	The patient should be able to hear a whispered voice or a watch tick.
To assess the vestibular portion of this nerve, observe for nystagmus and disturbed balance and note reports of dizziness or the room spinning.	The patient should display normal eye movement and balance and have no dizziness or vertigo.
Glossopharyngeal (CN IX) and vagus (CN X) To assess these nerves, which have overlapping functions, first listen to the patient's voice for indications of a hoarse or nasal quality. Then watch the patient's soft palate when he says "ah." Next, test the gag reflex after warning the patient. To evoke this reflex, touch the posterior wall of the pharynx with a cotton swab or tongue depressor.	The patient's voice should sound strong and clear. The soft palate and the uvula should rise when he says "ah," and the uvula should remain midline. The palatine arches should remain symmetrical during movement and at rest. The gag reflex should be intact. If

Assessing the cranial nerves *(continued)*

CRANIAL NERVE AND ASSESSMENT TECHNIQUE	NORMAL FINDINGS
Glossopharyngeal (CN IX) and vagus (CN X) *(continued)*	the gag reflex appears decreased or the pharynx moves asymmetrically, evaluate each side of the posterior wall of the pharynx to confirm integrity of both cranial nerves.
Spinal accessory (CN XI) To assess, press down on the patient's shoulders while he attempts to shrug against this resistance. Note shoulder strength and symmetry while inspecting and palpating his trapezius muscle. Then apply resistance to the patient's turned head while he attempts to return it to a midline position. Note neck strength while inspecting and palpating the sternocleidomastoid muscle. Repeat for the opposite side.	Normally, both shoulders should be able to overcome the resistance equally well. The neck should overcome resistance in both directions.
Hypoglossal (CN XII) To assess, observe the patient's protruded tongue for deviation from midline, atrophy, or fasciculations (very fine muscle flickerings indicative of lower motor neuron disease). Next, ask the patient to move the tongue rapidly from side to side with the mouth open, then to curl the tongue up toward the nose, and then to curl the tongue down toward the chin. Then use a tongue depressor or folded gauze pad to apply resistance to the patient's protruded tongue and ask him to try to push the depressor to one side. Repeat on the other side and note tongue strength. Listen to the patient's speech for the sounds d, l, n, and t, which require use of the tongue. If general speech suggests a problem, have the patient repeat a phrase or series of words containing these sounds.	Normally, the tongue should be midline and the patient should be able to move it right to left equally, as well as up and down. Pressure exerted by the tongue on the tongue depressor should be equal on either side. Speech should be clear.

Assessing the pupils

Pupillary changes can signal different conditions. Use these illustrations and lists of causes to help you detect problems.

Bilaterally equal and reactive

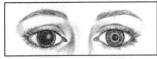

• Normal

Unilateral, dilated (4 mm), fixed, and nonreactive

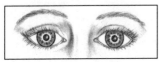

• Uncal herniation with oculomotor nerve damage
• Brain stem compression from an expanding lesion or an aneurysm
• Increased intracranial pressure
• Tentorial herniation
• Head trauma with subsequent subdural or epidural hematoma
• May be normal in some people

Bilateral, dilated (4 mm), fixed, and nonreactive

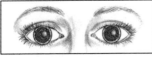

• Severe midbrain damage
• Cardiopulmonary arrest (hypoxia)
• Anticholinergic poisoning

Bilateral, midsized (2 mm), fixed, and nonreactive

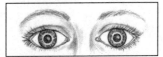

• Midbrain involvement caused by edema, hemorrhage, infarctions, lacerations, contusions

Unilateral, small (1.5 mm), and nonreactive

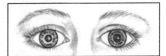

• Disruption of sympathetic nerve supply to the head caused by spinal cord lesion above T1

Bilateral, pinpoint (less than 1 mm), and usually nonreactive

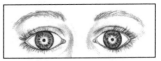

• Lesion of pons, usually after hemorrhage, leading to blocked sympathetic impulses
• Opiates, such as morphine (pupils may be reactive)

Using the Glasgow Coma Scale

The Glasgow Coma Scale provides an objective way to evaluate a patient's level of consciousness and to detect changes from the baseline. To use this scale, evaluate and score your patient's best eye-opening response, verbal response, and motor response. A total score of 15 indicates that he is alert; oriented to person, place, and time; and can follow simple commands. A comatose patient will score 7 points or less. A score of 3 indicates deep coma and a poor prognosis.

Eye-opening response
• Open spontaneously (Score: 4)
• Open to verbal command (Score: 3)
• Open to pain (Score: 2)
• No response (Score: 1)

Verbal response
• Oriented and converses (Score: 5)
• Disoriented and converses (Score: 4)
• Uses inappropriate words (Score: 3)
• Makes incomprehensible sounds (Score: 2)
• No response (Score: 1)

Motor response
• Obeys verbal command (Score: 6)
• Localizes painful stimulus (Score: 5)
• Flexion, withdrawal (Score: 4)
• Flexion, abnormal—decorticate rigidity (Score: 3)
• Extension—decerebrate rigidity (Score: 2)
• No response (Score: 1)

Assessing the gastrointestinal system

Initial GI questions

• Explore signs and symptoms, such as appetite and weight changes, dysphagia, nausea, vomiting, heartburn, stomach or abdominal pain, frequent belching or flatulence, hematemesis, and jaundice. Has your patient had ulcers?
• Determine whether your patient uses laxatives frequently. Ask about hemorrhoids, rectal bleeding, character of stools (color, odor, and consistency), and changes in bowel habits. Does he have a history of diarrhea or constipation?
• Ask if he's had hernias, gallbladder disease, or liver disease such as hepatitis.
• Find out if he's experienced abdominal swelling or ascites.
• If the patient is over age 50, inquire about the date and results of his last Hemoccult test.

Inspecting the abdomen

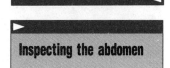

Place the patient in the supine position with his arms at his sides and his head on a pillow to help relax the abdominal muscles.

Mentally divide the abdomen into quadrants or regions. Systematically inspect all areas, if time and the patient's condition permit, concluding with the symptomatic area.

Then examine the patient's entire abdomen, observing overall contour, color, and skin integrity. Look for any rashes, scars, or incisions from past surgeries. Observe the umbilicus for protrusions or discoloration.

Note any visible abdominal asymmetry, masses, pulsations, or peristalsis. You can detect masses — especially hepatic and splenic — more easily by inspecting the areas while the patient takes a deep breath and holds it. This forces the diaphragm downward, increasing intra-abdominal pressure and reducing the size of the abdominal cavity.

Finally, examine the rectal area for redness, irritation, or hemorrhoids.

Note: If your patient is pregnant, vary the assessment position depending on the stage of pregnancy. For example, in the final weeks, the supine position can impair respiratory excursion and blood flow. To enhance comfort, have the patient lie on her side or assume semi-Fowler's position. Also during the assessment, remember the normal variations: increased pigmentation of the abdominal midline, purplish striae, and upward displacement of the abdominal organs and the umbilicus.

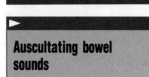

Auscultating bowel sounds

Auscultate the abdomen to detect sounds that provide information on bowel motility and the condition of abdominal vessels and organs.

To auscultate bowel sounds, which result from air and fluid movement through the bowel, press the diaphragm of the stethoscope against the abdomen and listen carefully. Auscultate the quadrants systematically.

Normally, air and fluid moving through the bowel by peristalsis create soft, bubbling sounds with no regular pattern, often with soft clicks and gurgles interspersed. A hungry patient normally may have a familiar "stomach growl," a condition of hyperperistalsis called borborygmi. Rapid, high-pitched, loud, and gurgling bowel sounds are hyperactive, which may occur normally in a hungry patient. Sounds occurring at a rate of one every minute or longer are hypoactive and normally occur after bowel surgery or when the colon is filled with feces.

Be sure to describe bowel sounds accurately — for example, as quiet or loud gurgles, occasional gurgles, fine tinkles, or loud tinkles.

In a routine complete assessment, auscultate for a full 5 minutes before determining that bowel sounds are absent. However, if you're pressed for time, perform a rapid assessment. If you can't hear bowel sounds within 2 minutes, suspect a serious problem. Even if subsequent palpation stimulates peristalsis, still report a long silence in that quadrant.

Before reporting absent bowel sounds, make sure the patient has an empty bladder; a full bladder may obsure the sounds. Gently pressing on the abdominal surface may initiate peristalsis and audible bowel sounds, as will having the patient eat or drink something.

Next, lightly apply the bell of the stethoscope to each quadrant to auscultate for vascular sounds, such as bruits and venous hums, and for friction rubs. Normally, you should not hear vascular sounds.

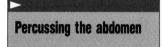

Percussing the abdomen

Abdominal percussion helps determine the size and location of abdominal organs and helps you identify areas of tenderness, gaseous distention, ascites, or solid masses.

To perform this technique, percuss in all four quadrants, moving clockwise to the percussion sites in each quadrant, as shown below. Keep approximate organ locations in mind as you progress. However, if the patient complains of pain in a particular quadrant, adjust the percussion sequence to percuss that quadrant last. When tapping, move your right finger away quickly so you do not inhibit vibrations.

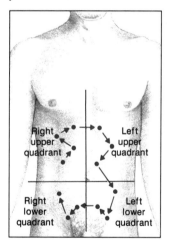

When assessing a tender abdomen, have the patient cough; then lightly percuss where the cough produced the pain, helping to localize the involved area. As you percuss, note areas of dullness, tympany, and flatness as well as any patient complaints of tenderness.

Percussion sounds vary depending on the density of underlying structures; usually, you will detect dull notes over solids and tympanic notes over air. The predominant abdominal percussion sound is tympany, created by percussion over an air-filled stomach or intestine. Dull sounds normally occur over the liver and spleen, a lower intestine filled with feces, and a bladder filled with urine. Distinguishing abdominal percussion notes may be difficult in obese patients.

Note: Keep in mind that abdominal percussion or palpation is contraindicated in patients with abdominal organ transplants or suspected abdominal aortic aneurysm. Perform it cautiously in patients with suspected appendicitis.

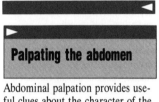

Palpating the abdomen

Abdominal palpation provides useful clues about the character of the abdominal wall; the size, condition, and consistency of abdominal organs; the presence and nature of any abdominal masses; and the presence, degree, and location of abdominal pain. For a rapid assessment, palpate primarily to detect areas of pain and tenderness, guarding, rebound tenderness, and costovertebral-angle tenderness.

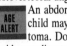 An abdominal mass in a child may be a nephroblastoma. Don't palpate it, to avoid spreading tumor cells.

Light palpation
Use light palpation to detect tenderness, areas of muscle spasm or rigidity, and superficial masses. To palpate for superficial masses in the abdominal wall, have the patient raise his head and shoulders to tighten the abdominal muscles. The tension obscures a deep mass, but a wall mass remains palpable.

This technique also may help you determine whether pain originates from the abdominal muscles or from deeper structures.

If you detect tenderness, assess for involuntary guarding, or abdominal rigidity. As the patient exhales, palpate the abdominal rectus muscles. Normally, they should soften and relax on exhalation; note abnormal muscle tension or inflexibility. Involuntary guarding points to peritoneal irritation. In generalized peritonitis, rigidity is severe and diffuse, commonly described as a "boardlike" abdomen.

A tense or ticklish patient may exhibit voluntary guarding. Help him relax with deep breathing, inhaling through his nose and exhaling through his mouth.

If a patient complains of abdominal pain, check for rebound tenderness. Because this maneuver can be painful, perform it near the end of your abdominal assessment. Press your fingertips into the site where the patient reports pain or tenderness. As you quickly release the pressure, the abdominal tissue will rebound. If the patient reports pain as the tissue springs back, you've elicited rebound tenderness.

Deep palpation

If time permits, perform deep abdominal palpation to detect deep tenderness or masses and to evaluate organ size. If you feel a mass, note its size, shape, consistency, and location. If the patient complains of pain or tenderness, note if the location is generalized or localized. Also note any guarding the patient exhibits during deep palpation. You may feel a tensing of a small or large area of abdominal musculature directly below your fingers.

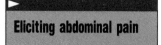

Eliciting abdominal pain

Rebound tenderness and the iliopsoas and obturator signs can indicate conditions such as appendicitis or peritonitis. During assessment, you can elicit these signs of abdominal pain.

Rebound tenderness

Place the patient in the supine position with the knees flexed to relax the abdominal muscles. Place your hands gently on the right lower quadrant at McBurney's point, located about midway between the umbilicus and the anterior superior iliac spine. Slowly and deeply dip your fingers into the area.

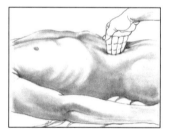

Now release the pressure in a quick, smooth motion. Pain on release — rebound tenderness — is a positive sign. The pain may radiate to the umbilicus. *Caution:* Do not repeat this maneuver, to minimize the risk of rupturing an inflamed appendix.

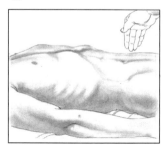

Iliopsoas sign

Place the patient in the supine position with the legs straight. Instruct the patient to raise the right leg upward as you exert slight downward pressure with your hand.

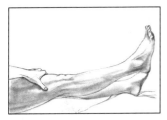

Repeat the maneuver with the left leg. Increased abdominal pain, with testing on either leg, is a positive result, indicating irritation of the psoas muscle.

Obturator sign

Place the patient in the supine position with the right leg flexed 90 degrees at the hip and knee. Hold the patient's leg just above the knee and at the ankle; then rotate the leg laterally and medially. Pain in the hypogastric region is a positive sign, indicating irritation of the obturator muscle.

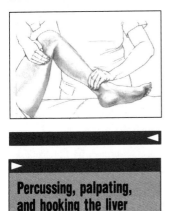

Percussing, palpating, and hooking the liver

You can estimate the size and position of the liver through percussion and palpation (or, in some cases, hooking). The following illustrations show you the correct hand positions for these three techniques.

Liver percussion

Begin by percussing the abdomen along the right midclavicular line, starting below the level of the umbilicus. Move upward until the percussion notes change from tympany to dullness, usually at or slightly below the costal margin. Mark the point of change with a felt-tip pen.

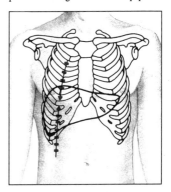

Percuss along the right midclavicular line, starting above the nipple. Move downward until percussion notes change from normal lung resonance to dullness, usually at the fifth to seventh intercostal space. Again, mark the point of change with a felt-tip pen. Estimate liver size by measuring the distance between the two marks.

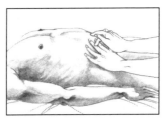

Liver palpation

Place one hand on the patient's back at the approximate height of the liver. Place your other hand below your mark of liver fullness on the right lateral abdomen. Point your fingers toward the right costal margin, and press gently in and up as the patient inhales deeply. This maneuver may bring the liver edge down to a palpable position.

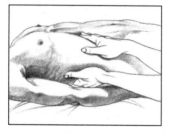

Liver hooking

If liver palpation is unsuccessful, try hooking the liver. To do so, stand on the patient's right side, below the area of liver dullness, as shown. As the patient inhales deeply, press your fingers inward and upward, attempting to feel the liver with the fingertips of both hands.

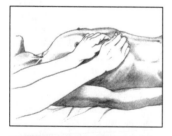

Palpating for indirect inguinal hernia

To assess for an indirect inguinal hernia, examine the patient while he stands. Then examine the patient in the supine position with his knee flexed on the side you're ex-

amining. Place your gloved index finger on the neck of the patient's scrotum and gently push upward into the inguinal canal, as shown. When you've inserted your finger as far as possible, ask the patient to bear down and cough. A hernia will feel like a mass of tissue that withdraws when met by the finger.

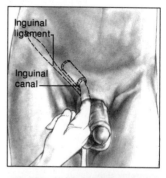

Inguinal ligament

Inguinal canal

Assessing the urinary system

Initial urinary questions

• Ask about urine color, oliguria, and nocturia. Does your patient experience incontinence, dysuria, frequency, urgency, or difficulty with urinary stream (such as reduced flow or dribbling)?
• Find out about pyuria, urine retention, and passage of calculi.
• Ask about a history of bladder, kidney, or urinary tract infections.

AGE ALERT If your patient is a child, ask his parents if they've had any problems with toilet training or bed-wetting.

Evaluating urine color

For important clues to your patient's current health status, be sure to ask about any urine color changes. Such changes can result from fluid intake, medications, and dietary factors as well as from various disorders.

APPEARANCE	INDICATION
Amber or straw color	Normal
Cloudy	Infection, inflammation, glomerular nephritis, vegetarian diet
Colorless or pale straw color (dilute urine)	Excess fluid intake, anxiety, chronic renal disease, diabetes insipidus, diuretic therapy
Dark brown or black	Acute glomerulonephritis, drugs (such as nitrofurantoin and chlorpromazine)
Dark yellow or amber (concentrated urine)	Low fluid intake, acute febrile disease, vomiting or diarrhea causing large fluid loss
Green-brown	Bile duct obstruction
Orange-red to orange-brown	Urobilinuria, drugs (such as phenazopyridine), obstructive jaundice (tea-colored urine)
Red or red-brown	Porphyria, hemorrhage, drugs (such as doxorubicin)

Inspecting the urethral meatus

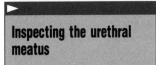

Put on gloves before examining the urethral meatus.

To inspect a male patient's urethral meatus, have him lie in the supine position and drape him, exposing only his penis. Then compress the tip of the glans to open the urethral meatus, which should be located in the center of the glans. Check for swelling, discharge, signs of urethral infection, and ulcerations, which can signal a sexually transmitted disease (STD).

To inspect a female patient's urethral meatus, help her into the dorsal lithotomy position and drape her, exposing only the area to be assessed. Then spread the labia and look for the urethral meatus. It should be a pink, irregular, slitlike opening located at the midline just above the vagina. Check for swelling, discharge, signs of urethral infection, a cystocele, and ulcerations, a sign of an STD.

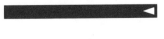

Percussing the urinary organs

Percuss the kidneys to elicit pain or tenderness, and percuss the bladder to elicit percussion sounds. Before you start, be sure to tell the patient what you're going to do. Otherwise, he may be startled, and you could mistake his reaction for a feeling of acute tenderness.

Kidney percussion

With the patient sitting upright, percuss each costovertebral angle (the angle over each kidney whose borders are formed by the lateral and downward curve of the lowest rib and the spinal column). To perform direct percussion, place your left palm over the costovertebral angle and gently strike it with your right fist as shown below. Use just enough force to cause a painless but perceptible thud. To perform indirect percussion, gently strike your fist over each costovertebral angle. The normal patient will feel a thudding sensation or pressure during percussion. Be sure to percuss both sides of the body to assess both kidneys. Pain or tenderness suggests a kidney infection.

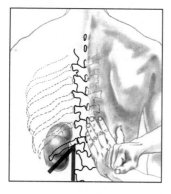

Bladder percussion

Before percussing the bladder, have the patient urinate. Then ask the patient to lie in the supine position. Next, using direct percussion, percuss the area over the bladder, beginning 2″ (5 cm) above the symphysis pubis as shown below. To detect differences in sound, percuss toward the base of the bladder. Percussion normally produces a tympanic sound. (Over a urine-filled bladder, it produces a dull sound.)

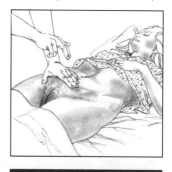

Palpating the urinary organs

Bimanual palpation of the kidneys and bladder may detect tenderness, lumps, and masses. In the normal adult, the kidneys usually cannot be palpated because of their location deep within the abdomen. However, they may be palpable in a thin patient or in one with reduced abdominal muscle mass. (Because the right kidney is slightly lower than the left, it may be easier to palpate.) Keep in mind that both kidneys descend with deep inhalation.

If palpable, the bladder normally feels firm and relatively smooth. However, keep in mind that an adult's bladder may not be palpable.

Kidney palpation

Help the patient lie in the supine position, and expose the abdomen from the xiphoid process to the symphysis pubis. Standing at the patient's right side, place your left hand under the back, midway between the lower costal margin and the iliac crest, as shown below.

Next, place your right hand on the patient's abdomen, directly above your left hand. Angle this hand slightly toward the costal margin. To palpate the right lower edge of the right kidney, press your right fingertips about 1½" (4 cm) above the right iliac crest at the midinguinal line; press your left fingertips upward into the right costovertebral angle, as shown below.

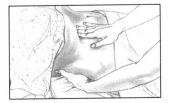

Instruct the patient to inhale deeply so that the lower portion of the right kidney can move down between your hands. If it does, note the shape and size of the kidney. Normally, it feels smooth, solid, and firm, yet elastic. Ask the patient if palpation causes tenderness.

Note: Avoid using excessive pressure to palpate the kidney because this may cause intense pain.

To assess the left kidney, move to the patient's left side and position your hands as described above, but with this change: place your right hand 2" (5 cm) above the left iliac crest. Then apply pressure with both hands as the patient inhales. If the left kidney can be palpated, compare it to the right kidney; it should be the same size.

Bladder palpation

Before palpating the bladder, make sure the patient has voided. Then locate the edge of the bladder by pressing deeply in the midline about 1" to 2" (2.5 to 5 cm) above the symphysis pubis, as shown below.

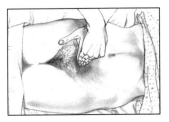

As the bladder is palpated, note its size and location and check for lumps, masses, and tenderness. The bladder normally feels firm and relatively smooth. (Keep in mind that an adult's bladder may not be palpable.) During deep palpation, the patient may report the urge to urinate — a normal response.

Assessing the male reproductive system

Initial questions for the male patient

• Ask your patient about penile discharge or lesions and testicular pain or lumps.
• Determine whether your patient performs testicular self-examinations. Has he had a vasectomy?
• Ask about sexually transmitted diseases and other infections. Assess his knowledge of how to prevent sexually transmitted disease, including acquired immunodeficiency syndrome.

• Find out if the patient has a history of prostate problems.
• Ask if he's satisfied with his sexual function. Does he have any concerns about impotence or sterility? Also inquire about his contraceptive practices.

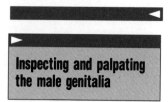

Inspecting and palpating the male genitalia

First, ask the patient to disrobe from the waist down and to cover himself with a drape. Then put on gloves and examine his penis, scrotum and testicles, inguinal and femoral areas, and prostate gland.

Penis

Observe the penis. Its size will depend on the patient's age and overall development. The penile skin should be slightly wrinkled and pink to light brown in a white patient and light brown to dark brown in a black patient. Check the penile shaft and glans for lesions, nodules, inflammation, and swelling. Also check the glans for smegma, a cheesy secretion. Then gently compress the glans and inspect the urethral meatus for discharge, inflammation, and lesions, specifically genital warts. If you note any discharge, obtain a culture specimen.

Using your thumb and forefinger, palpate the entire penile shaft. It should be somewhat firm, and the skin should be smooth and movable. Note any swelling, nodules, or indurations.

Scrotum and testicles

Have the patient hold his penis away from his scrotum so that you can observe the scrotum's general size and appearance. The skin will

be darker than the rest of the body. Spread the surface of the scrotum, and examine the skin for swelling, nodules, redness, ulceration, and distended veins. You'll probably notice some sebaceous cysts—firm, white to yellow, nontender cutaneous lesions. Also, check for pitting edema, a sign of cardiovascular disease. Spread the pubic hair and check the skin for lesions and parasites.

Gently palpate both testicles between your thumb and first two fingers. Assess their size, shape, and response to pressure (typically, a deep visceral pain). The testicles should be equal in size. They should feel firm, smooth, and rubbery and should move freely in the scrotal sac. If you note any hard, irregular areas or lumps, transilluminate the testicle by darkening the room and pressing the head of a flashlight against the scrotum, behind the lump. The testicle will appear as an opaque shadow, as will any lumps, masses, warts, or blood-filled areas. Transilluminate the other testicle to compare your findings.

Next, palpate the epididymis, usually located in the posterolateral area of the testicle. It should be smooth, discrete, nontender, and free of swelling or induration.

Finally, palpate each spermatic cord, located above each testicle. Begin palpating at the base of the epididymis and continue to the inguinal canal. The vas deferens is a smooth, movable cord inside the spermatic cord. If you feel any swelling, irregularity, or nodules, transilluminate the problem area, as described above. If serous fluid is present, you'll see a red glow; if tissue and blood are present, you won't see this glow.

Prostate gland

Usually, a doctor performs prostate palpation as part of a rectal assessment. However, if the patient has not scheduled a separate rectal assessment, you may palpate the prostate during the reproductive system assessment. Because palpation of the prostate usually is uncomfortable and may embarrass the patient, begin by explaining the procedure and reassuring the patient that the procedure should not be painful.

Have the patient urinate to empty the bladder and reduce discomfort during the examination. Then ask him to stand at the end of the examination table, with his elbows flexed and his upper body resting on the table. If he can't assume this position because he's unable to stand, have him lie on his left side with his right knee and hip flexed or with both knees drawn up toward his chest.

Inspect the skin of the perineal, anal, and posterior scrotal surfaces. The skin should appear smooth and unbroken, with no protruding masses.

Apply water-soluble lubricant to your gloved index finger. Then introduce the finger, pad down, into the patient's rectum. Instruct the patient to relax to ease passage of the finger through the anal sphincter.

Using the pad of your index finger, palpate the prostate on the anterior rectal wall, located just past the anorectal ring. The prostate should feel smooth and rubbery. Normal size varies but usually is about that of a walnut. The prostate should not protrude into the rectal lumen. The proximal portions of the seminal vesicles sometimes may be palpated, as corrugated structures, above the superolateral to midpoint section of the gland.

Assessing the female reproductive system

Initial questions for the female patient

• Ask your patient about her age at menarche and the character of menstrual periods (frequency, regularity, and duration). What was the date of her last period? Does she have a history of menorrhagia, metrorrhagia, or amenorrhea? If she's postmenopausal, find out the date of menopause.
• Ask if she has irregular or painful vaginal bleeding, dyspareunia, or frequent vaginal infections.
• Ask about the character of any pregnancies (number, durations, deliveries, and abortions, either spontaneous or induced). Has she had any problems with infertility?
• Find out what birth control method she uses.
• Determine the dates of her last gynecologic examination and Papanicolaou (Pap) test.
• Ask about sexually transmitted diseases and other infections. Assess her knowledge of how to prevent sexually transmitted disease, including acquired immunodeficiency syndrome.
• Explore the patient's satisfaction with her sexual function.

Inspecting the female genitalia

Before starting the examination, ask the patient to urinate. Next, help her into the dorsal lithotomy position and drape her. After putting on gloves, examine the patient's external and internal genitalia and her breasts, as appropriate.

Inspecting the external genitalia

Observe the skin and hair distribution of the mons pubis. Spread the hair with your fingers to check for lesions and parasites.

Next, inspect the skin of the labia majora, spreading the hair to examine for lesions, parasites, and genital warts. The skin should be slightly darker than the rest of the body, and the labia majora should be round and full. Examine the labia minora, which should be dark pink and moist. In nulliparous women, the labia majora and minora are close together; in women who have experienced vaginal deliveries, they may gape open.

Closely observe each vulvar structure for syphilitic chancres and cancerous lesions. Examine the area of Bartholin's and Skene's glands and ducts for swelling, erythema, duct enlargement, or discharge. Next, inspect the urethral opening. It should be slitlike and the same color as the mucous membranes. Look for erythema, polyps, and discharge.

Inspecting the internal genitalia

First, select a speculum that's appropriate for the patient. In most cases, you'll use a Graves speculum. However, if the patient is a virgin or nulliparous or if she has a contracted introitus due to menopause, you should use a Pederson speculum.

Hold the speculum's blades under warm running water. This warms the blades and helps to lubricate them, making insertion easier and more comfortable for the patient. Don't use any commercial lubricants—they're bacteriostatic and will distort cells on Pap tests. Sit or stand at the foot of the examination table. Tell the patient that she'll feel some pressure; then insert the speculum.

While inserting and withdrawing the speculum, note the color, texture, and mucosal integrity of the vagina and any vaginal secretions. A white, odorless, thin discharge is normal.

With the speculum in place, examine the cervix for color, position, size, shape, mucosal integrity, and discharge. The cervix should be smooth, round, rosy pink, and free of ulcerations and nodules. A clear, watery discharge is normal during ovulation; a slightly bloody discharge is normal just before menstruation. Obtain a culture specimen of any other discharge. After inspecting the cervix, obtain a specimen for a Pap test.

When you've completed your examination, unlock the speculum blades and close them slowly while you begin withdrawing the instrument. Close the blades completely before they reach the introitus. Then withdraw the speculum from the vagina.

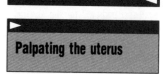

Palpating the uterus

To palpate the uterus bimanually, insert the index and middle fingers of one gloved hand into the patient's vagina, and place your other hand on the abdomen between the umbilicus and symphysis pubis. Press the abdomen in and down while you elevate the cervix and uterus with your two fingers, as shown at the top of the next page. Try to grasp the uterus between your hands.

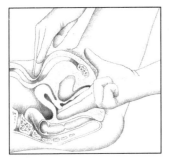

With the patient seated, palpate the axillae. Palpate the right axilla with the middle three fingers of one hand while supporting the patient's arm with your other hand. You can usually palpate one or more soft, small, nontender, central nodes. If the nodes feel large or hard or are tender, or if the patient has a suspicious-looking lesion, try to palpate the other groups of lymph nodes.

Then slide your fingers farther into the anterior fornix and palpate the body of the uterus between your hands. Note its size, shape, surface characteristics, consistency, and mobility. Note any tenderness of the uterine body and fundus. Also note fundal position.

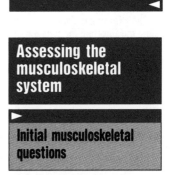

Assessing the musculoskeletal system

Initial musculoskeletal questions

Palpating the breasts and axillae

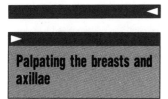

With the patient supine, place a pillow under the shoulder on the side you're examining. Ask him or her to raise that arm above the head. Using your finger pads, palpate the breast in concentric circles from the center to the periphery.

Note the consistency of breast tissue. Check for nodules or unusual tenderness. In females, nodularity may increase before menstruation; tenderness may result from premenstrual fullness, cysts, or cancer. Any lump or mass that feels different from the rest of the breast may represent a pathologic change.

Palpate the areola and nipple, and compress the nipple between your thumb and index finger to detect discharge. If you see any, note the color, consistency, and quantity.

• Ask if your patient experiences muscle pain, joint pain, swelling, tenderness, or difficulty with balance or gait. Does he have joint stiffness? If so, find out when it occurs and its duration.
• Inquire whether your patient has noticed noise with joint movement.
• Find out if he has arthritis or gout.
• Ask about a history of fractures, injuries, back problems, and deformities. Also ask about weakness and paralysis.
• Explore any limitations on walking, running, or participation in sports. Do muscle or joint problems interfere with activities of daily living?

 If the patient is a child, ask the parents if developmental milestones, such as sitting up, crawling, and walking, have been achieved.

Assessing range of motion

Assessment of joint range of motion (ROM) tests the joint function. To assess joint ROM, ask the patient to move specific joints through the normal ROM. If he can't do so, move the joints through passive ROM.

The following pages show each joint and illustrate the tests for ROM, including the expected degree of motion for each joint.

Shoulders

To assess forward flexion and backward extension, have the patient bring his straightened arm forward and up, then behind him.

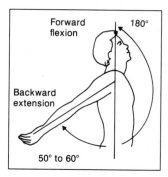

Elbows

Assess flexion by having the patient bend his arm and attempt to touch his shoulder. Assess extension by having him straighten his arm.

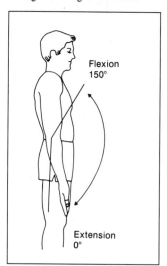

Assess abduction and adduction by asking the patient to bring his straightened arm to the side and up, then in front of him.

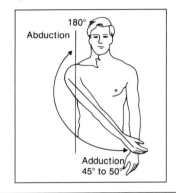

To assess external and internal rotation, have the patient abduct his arm with his elbow bent. Then ask him first to place his hand behind his head, then behind the small of his back.

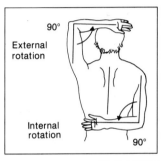

To assess pronation and supination, hold the patient's elbow in a flexed position and ask him to rotate his arm until his palm faces the floor, then rotate his hand back until his palm faces upward.

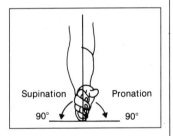

Wrists

To assess flexion, ask the patient to bend his wrist downward; assess extension by having him straighten his wrist. To assess hyperextension, ask him to bend his wrist upward.

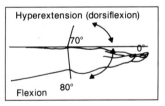

Assess radial and ulnar deviation by asking the patient to move his hand first toward the radial side, then toward the ulnar side.

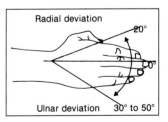

Fingers

To assess abduction and adduction, have the patient first spread his fingers and then bring them together. There should be 20 degrees between the fingers in abduction; in adduction, the fingers should touch.

To assess extension and flexion, ask the patient first to straighten his fingers and then to make a fist with his thumb remaining straight.

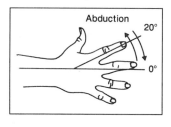

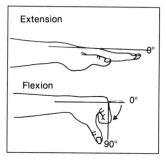

Hips

Assess flexion by asking the patient to bend his knee to his chest while keeping his back straight. If he's undergone total hip replacement, don't perform this movement without the surgeon's permission; motion can dislocate the prosthesis.

Assess extension by having the patient straighten his knee. To assess hyperextension, ask him to extend his leg backward with his knee straight. This motion can be performed with the patient prone or standing.

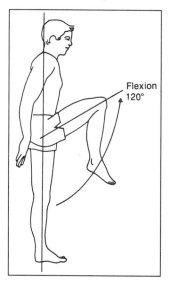

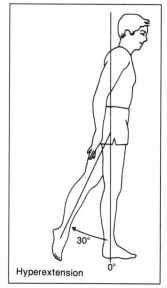

Thumbs

Assess extension by having the patient straighten his thumb. To assess flexion, have him bend his thumb at the top joint, then at the bottom.

Assess adduction by having the patient extend his hand, bringing his thumb first to the index finger and then to the little finger.

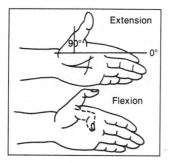

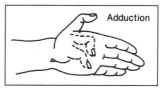

To assess abduction, have the patient move his straightened leg away from the midline.

To assess adduction, instruct the patient to move his leg toward the midline.

To assess internal and external rotation, ask the patient to bend his knee and turn his leg inward. Then have him turn his leg outward.

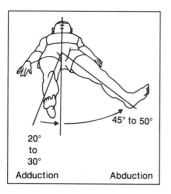

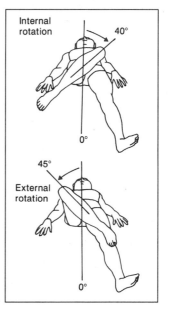

Knees

Ask the patient to straighten his leg at the knee to demonstrate extension; ask him to bend his knee and bring his foot up to touch his buttock to demonstrate flexion.

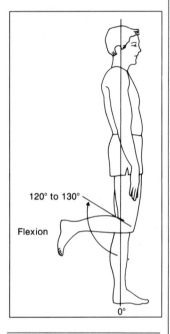

Toes

Assess extension and flexion by asking the patient to straighten and then curl his toes. Then check hyperextension by asking him to straighten his toes and point them upward.

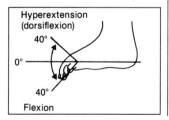

Ankles and feet

Have the patient demonstrate plantar flexion by bending his foot downward, and hyperextension by bending his foot upward.

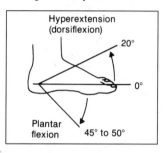

To assess eversion and inversion, ask the patient to point his toes. Have him turn his foot inward, then outward.

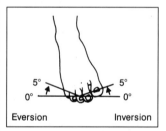

To assess forefoot adduction and abduction, stabilize the patient's heel while he turns his foot first inward, then outward.

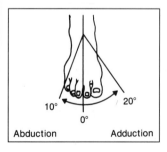

▶

Testing muscle strength

Assess your patient's motor function by testing his strength in the affected limb. Have him attempt normal range-of-motion (ROM) movements against your resistance. (Before you begin muscle strength tests, find out whether the patient is right- or left-handed because the dominant arm is usually stronger.) Note the strength that the patient exerts against your resistance. If the muscle group is weak, you should lessen your resistance or provide no resistance to permit an accurate assessment. If necessary, position the patient so his limb doesn't have to resist gravity, and repeat the test.

Rate muscle strength on a scale from 0 to 5 (to minimize subjective interpretations of test findings), as follows:

0 = No visible or palpable contraction felt; paralysis
1 = Slight palpable contraction felt
2 = Passive ROM maneuvers when gravity is removed
3 = Active ROM against gravity
4 = Active ROM against gravity and light resistance
5 = Active ROM against full resistance; normal strength

Deltoid

With your patient's arm fully extended, place one hand over his deltoid muscle and the other on his wrist. Have him abduct his arm to a horizontal position against your resistance; as he does, palpate for deltoid contraction.

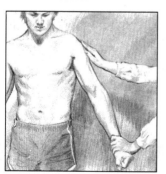

Biceps

With your hand on the patient's fist, have him flex his forearm against your resistance; observe for biceps contraction.

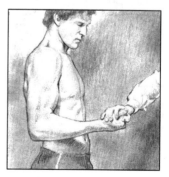

ASSESSMENT

Triceps

Have the patient abduct and hold his arm midway between flexion and extension. Hold and support his arm at the wrist, and ask him to extend it against your resistance. Observe for triceps contraction.

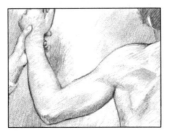

Dorsal interosseous

Have him extend and spread his fingers and resist your attempt to squeeze them together.

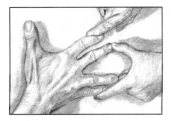

Forearm and hand (grip)

Have the patient grasp your middle and index fingers and squeeze them as hard as he can.

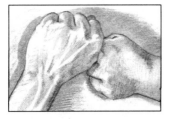

Psoas

While you support his leg, have the patient raise his knee and flex his hip against your resistance. Observe for psoas contraction.

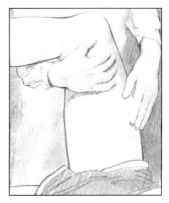

Quadriceps

Have the patient bend his knee slightly while you support his lower leg. Then ask him to extend his knee against your resistance; as he's doing so, palpate for quadriceps contraction.

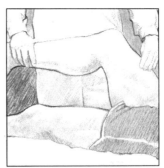

Gastrocnemius

With the patient on his side, support his foot and ask him to plantar-flex his ankle against your resistance. Palpate for gastrocnemius contraction.

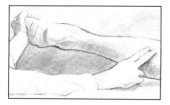

Anterior tibial

With the patient sitting on the side of the exam table with his legs dangling, place your hand on his foot and ask him to dorsiflex his ankle against your resistance.

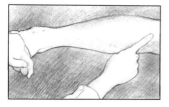

Extensor hallucis longus

With your finger on his great toe, have him dorsiflex the toe against your resistance. Palpate for extensor hallucis contraction.

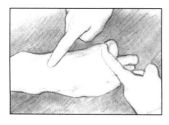

Assessing the skin

▶ Initial skin questions

• Determine if your patient has any known skin disease, such as psoriasis.
• Ask him to describe any changes in skin pigmentation, temperature, moisture, or hair distribution.
• Explore skin symptoms, such as itching, rashes, or scaling. Is his skin excessively dry or oily?
• Find out if the skin reacts to hot or cold weather. If so, how?
• Ask if your patient has noticed easy bruising or bleeding, changes in warts or moles, or lumps. Ask about the presence and location of scars, sores, and ulcers.

▶ Inspecting and palpating the skin

Before beginning your examination, make sure the lighting is adequate for inspection; then put on a pair of gloves. To examine the patient's skin, you'll use both inspection and palpation—sometimes simultaneously. During your examination, focus on such skin tissue characteristics as color, texture, turgor, moisture, and temperature. Also evaluate any skin lesions.

Color

Begin by systematically inspecting the skin's overall appearance. Remember, skin color reflects the patient's nutritional, hematologic, cardiovascular, and pulmonary status.

Observe general coloring and pigmentation, keeping in mind racial differences as well as normal variations from one part of the body to another. Examine all exposed areas of the skin, including the face, ears, back of the neck, axillae, and backs of the hands and arms.

Note the location of any bruising, discoloration, or erythema. Look for pallor, a dusky appearance, jaundice, and cyanosis. Ask the patient if he has noticed any changes in skin color anywhere on his body.

Texture

Inspect and palpate the texture of the skin, noting thickness and mobility. Does the skin feel rough, smooth, thick, fragile, or thin? Changes can indicate local irritation or trauma, or they can be a result of problems in other body systems. For example, rough, dry skin is common in hypothyroidism; soft, smooth skin is common in hyperthyroidism. To determine if the skin over a joint is supple or taut, have the patient bend the joint as you palpate.

Turgor

Assessing the turgor, or elasticity, of the patient's skin helps you evaluate hydration. To assess turgor, gently squeeze the skin on the forearm. If it quickly returns to its original shape, the patient has normal turgor. If it resumes its original shape slowly or maintains a tented shape, the skin has poor turgor.

 Decreased turgor occurs with dehydration as well as with aging. Increased turgor is associated with progressive systemic sclerosis.

To accurately assess skin turgor in an elderly patient, try squeezing the skin of the sternum or forehead instead of using the forearm. In an elderly patient, the skin of the forearms tends to be flaccid, so using this site to assess skin turgor wouldn't give you an accurate evaluation of the patient's hydration.

Moisture

Observe the skin for excessive dryness or moisture. If the patient's skin is too dry, you may see reddened or flaking areas. Elderly patients frequently have dry, itchy skin. Moisture that appears shiny may result from oiliness.

If the patient is overhydrated, the skin may be edematous and spongy. Localized edema can occur in response to trauma or skin abnormalities, such as ulcers. When you palpate local edema, be sure to document any associated discoloration or lesions.

Temperature

To assess skin temperature, touch the surface using the backs of your fingers. Inflamed skin will feel warm because of increased blood flow. Cool skin results from vasoconstriction. With hypovolemic shock, for instance, the skin feels cool and clammy.

Make sure you distinguish between generalized and localized warmth or coolness. Generalized warmth, or hyperthermia, is associated with fever stemming from a systemic infection or hyperthyroidism. Localized warmth occurs with a burn or localized infection. Generalized coolness occurs with hypothyroidism; localized coolness, with arteriosclerosis.

Skin lesions

During your inspection, you may note vascular changes in the form of red, pigmented lesions. Among the most common are hemangiomas, telangiectases, petechiae, purpura, and ecchymoses. Keep in mind that these lesions may or may not indicate disease. You'll see telangiectases, for instance, in pregnant patients as well as in those with hepatic cirrhosis.

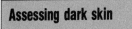

Evaluating skin color variations

COLOR	DISTRIBUTION	POSSIBLE CAUSE
Absent	Small, circumscribed areas	Vitiligo
	Generalized	Albinism
Blue	Around lips (circumoral pallor) or generalized	Cyanosis. (*Note:* In blacks, bluish gingivae are normal.)
Deep red	Generalized	Polycythemia vera (increased red blood cell count)
Pink	Local or generalized	Erythema (superficial capillary dilation and congestion)
Tan to brown	Facial patches	Chloasma of pregnancy; butterfly rash of lupus erythematosus
Tan to brown-bronze	Generalized (not related to sun exposure)	Addison's disease
Yellow	Sclera or generalized	Jaundice from liver dysfunction. (*Note:* In blacks, yellowish brown pigmentation of the sclera is normal.)
Yellow-orange	Palms, soles, and face; not sclera	Carotenemia (carotene in the blood)

Assessing dark skin

Be prepared for certain color variations when assessing dark-skinned patients. For example, some dark-skinned patients have a pigmented line, called Futcher's line, extending diagonally from the shoulder to the elbow. This is normal. Also normal are deeply pigmented ridges in the palms.

To detect color variations in dark-skinned and black patients, examine the sclerae, conjunctivae, buccal mucosa, tongue, lips, nail beds, palms, and soles. A yellowish brown color in dark-skinned patients or an ash-gray color in black patients indicates pallor, which results from a lack of the underlying pink and red tones normally present in dark skin.

Among dark-skinned blacks, yellowish pigmentation isn't necessarily an indication of jaundice. To detect jaundice in these patients, examine the hard palate and the sclerae.

Look for petechiae by examining areas with lighter pigmentation, such as the abdomen, gluteal areas, and the volar aspect of the forearm. To distinguish petechiae and ecchymoses from erythema in dark-skinned patients, apply pressure to the area. Erythematous areas will blanch, but petechiae or ecchymoses won't. Because erythema is commonly associated with an increased skin temperature, you can also palpate the skin for warmth.

When you assess edema in dark skin, remember that the affected area may have decreased color because fluid expands the distance between the pigmented layers and the external epithelium. When you palpate the affected area, it may feel tight.

Cyanosis can be difficult to identify in both white and black patients. Because the lips and nail beds are often affected by factors such as cold, be sure you also assess the conjunctivae, palms, soles, buccal mucosa, and tongue.

To detect rashes in black or dark-skinned patients, you'll need to palpate the area for skin texture changes.

Assessing the eyes, ears, nose, and throat

▶

Initial EENT questions

Eyes
• Ask your patient about visual problems, such as myopia, hyperopia, blurred vision, or double vision. Does he wear corrective lenses?
• Find out when his last eye examination was.
• Ask if he's noticed any visual disturbances, such as rainbows around lights, blind spots, or flashing lights.
• Ask if he experiences excessive tearing, dry eyes, itching, burning, pain, inflammation, swelling, color blindness, or photophobia.
• Elicit any history of eye infections, eye trauma, glaucoma, cataracts, detached retina, or other eye disorders.
• If he's over age 50 or has a family history of glaucoma, inquire about the date and results of his last check for glaucoma.

Ears
• Find out if your patient has hearing problems, such as deafness, poor hearing, tinnitus, or vertigo. Is he abnormally sensitive to noise? Has he noticed any recent changes in his hearing?
• Inquire about ear discharge, pain, or tenderness behind the ears.
• Ask about frequent or recent ear infections or ear surgery.
• Determine the date and result of his last hearing test.
• Ask if he uses a hearing aid.

• Determine his ear care habits, including use of cotton-tipped swabs for ear wax removal.

Nose
• Explore any nasal problems, including sinusitis, discharge, colds, coryza (more than four times a year), rhinitis, trauma, or frequent sneezing.
• Determine whether your patient has an obstruction, breathing problems, or an inability to smell. Has he had nosebleeds?
• Ask if he ever had surgery on his nose or sinuses. If so, explore when, why, and what type.

Mouth and throat
• Investigate whether your patient has sores in the mouth or on the tongue. Does he have a history of oral herpes infection?
• Find out if he has toothaches, bleeding gums, loss of taste, voice changes, dry mouth, or frequent sore throats.
• If the patient has frequent sore throats, ask when they occur. Are they associated with fever or difficulty swallowing? How have the sore throats been treated medically?
• Ask if the patient ever had a problem swallowing. If so, does he have trouble swallowing solids or liquids? Is the problem constant or intermittent? What precipitates the swallowing difficulty? What makes it go away?
• Determine whether he has dental caries or tooth loss? Ask if he wears dentures or bridges.
• Ask about the date and result of his last dental examination.
• Explore his use of proper dental hygiene, including fluoride toothpaste.

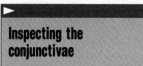

Inspecting the conjunctivae

Bulbar conjunctiva
While wearing gloves, gently evert the patient's lower eyelid with the thumb or index finger, as shown below. Ask the patient to look up, down, left, and right as you examine the bulbar conjunctiva. It should be clear and shiny.

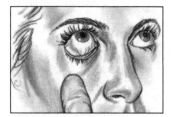

Palpebral conjunctiva
Check the palpebral conjunctiva only if you suspect a foreign body or if the patient complains of eyelid pain. To perform this examination, ask the patient to look down while you gently pull the medial eyelashes forward and upward with your thumb and index finger.

While holding the eyelashes, press on the tarsal border with a cotton-tipped applicator to evert the eyelid, as shown below. Hold the lashes against the brow and examine the conjunctiva, which should be pink with no swelling.

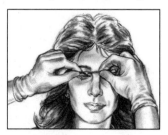

To return the eyelid to its normal position, release the eyelashes and ask the patient to look upward. If this doesn't invert the eyelid, grasp the eyelashes and gently pull them forward.

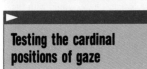

Testing the cardinal positions of gaze

This test of coordinated eye movements evaluates the oculomotor, trigeminal, and abducens nerves as well as the extraocular muscles. To perform the test, sit directly in front of the patient and ask him to remain still. Hold a small object, such as a pencil, directly in front of his nose at a distance of about 18″ (46 cm). Ask him to follow the object with his eyes without moving his head.

Then, move the object to each of the six cardinal positions, returning it to midpoint after each movement. The patient's eyes should remain parallel as they move. Note any abnormal findings, such as nystagmus or the failure of one eye to follow the object.

Test each of the six cardinal positions of gaze: the left superior, the left lateral, the left inferior, the right inferior, the right lateral, and the right superior. The illustrations at right show tests of the three left positions.

Left superior

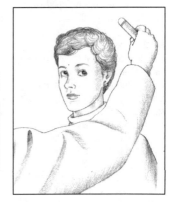

Left lateral

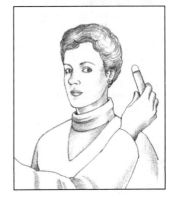

Left inferior

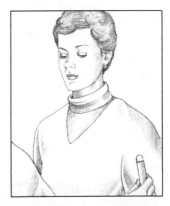

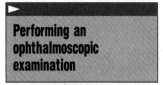

Performing an ophthalmoscopic examination

To use an ophthalmoscope to help identify inner eye abnormalities, follow these steps.
• Place the patient in a darkened or semi-darkened room, with neither you nor the patient wearing glasses unless you are very myopic or astigmatic. However, either of you may wear contact lenses.
• Sit or stand in front of the patient with your head about 18″ (46 cm) in front of and about 15 degrees to the right of the patient's line of vision in the right eye. Hold the ophthalmoscope in your right hand with the viewing aperture as close to your right eye as possible. Place your left thumb on the patient's right eyebrow to prevent hitting the patient with the ophthalmoscope as you move in close. Keep your right index finger on the lens selector to adjust the lens as necessary, as shown below. To examine the left eye, perform these steps on the patient's left side.

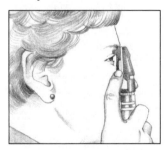

• Instruct the patient to look straight ahead at a fixed point on the wall. Next, approaching from an oblique angle about 15″ (38 cm) out and with the diopter set at 0, focus a small circle of light on the pupil, as shown at top right.

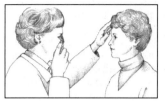

Look for the orange-red glow of the red reflex, which should be sharp and distinct through the pupil. The red reflex indicates that the lens is free from opacity and clouding.
• Move closer to the patient, changing the lens selector with your forefinger to keep the retinal structures in focus, as shown below.

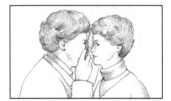

• Change the lens selector to a positive diopter to view the vitreous humor, observing for any opacity.
• Next, view the retina using a strong negative lens setting. Look for a retinal blood vessel, and follow that vessel toward the patient's nose, rotating the lens selector to keep the vessel in focus. Carefully examine all the retinal structures, including the retinal vessels, the optic disk, the retinal background, the macula, and the fovea centralis retinae.
• Examine the vessels for their color, the size ratio of arterioles to veins, the arteriole light reflex, and the arteriovenous (AV) crossing. The crossing points should be smooth, without nicks or narrowings, and the vessels should be free of exudate, bleeding, and narrowing. Retinal vessels normally have an AV ratio of 2:3 or 4:5.

• Evaluate the color of the retinal structures. The retina should be light yellow to orange and the background free from hemorrhages, aneurysms, and exudates. The optic disk, located on the nasal side of the retina, should be orange-red with distinct margins. The physiologic cup is normally yellow-white and readily visible.

• Examine the macula last, and as briefly as possible, because it is very light sensitive. The macula, which is darker than the rest of the retinal background, is free of vessels and located temporally to the optic disk. The fovea centralis retinae is a slight depression in the center of the macula.

 AGE ALERT For an infant or a toddler, grasp the auricle and pull it down and back.

Hold the otoscope as shown below, with the handle parallel to the patient's head. Avoid hitting the ear canal with the speculum.

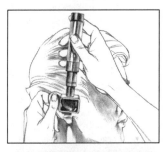

Using the otoscope

Perform an otoscopic examination to assess the external auditory canal, tympanic membrane, and malleus. Before inserting the speculum into the patient's ear, check the canal opening for foreign particles or discharge. Palpate the tragus and pull up the auricle. If this area is tender, don't insert the speculum; the patient may have external otitis, and inserting the speculum could be painful.

If the ear canal is clear, straighten the canal by grasping the auricle and pulling it up and back, as shown below. Then insert the speculum.

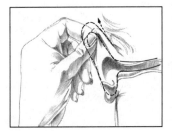

Performing Weber's test

If you've detected a hearing deficit, you can evaluate bone conduction using Weber's test. To do so, use a tuning fork that's within the frequency of normal human speech (512 cycles/second). Strike it against your hand, so it vibrates lightly, then place it on the patient's forehead at the midline, as shown below. (Alternatively, you can place the tuning fork on top of the patient's head.)

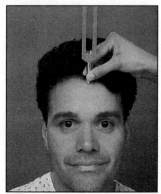

If the patient hears tone equally well in both ears, record this normal finding as a negative Weber's test. If he hears the tone better in one ear, record the result as right or left lateralization. With this abnormality, the tone actually sounds louder in the ear with more hearing loss because the bone conducts the tone to this ear. Because the unaffected ear picks up other sounds, it doesn't hear the tone as clearly.

Inspecting the nostrils

For direct inspection of the nostrils, you'll need a nasal speculum and a small flashlight or penlight.

Have the patient sit in front of you and tilt his head back. Then insert the tip of the closed speculum into one of his nostrils until you reach the point where the blade widens. Slowly open the speculum as wide as you can without causing discomfort. Now shine the flashlight in the nostril to illuminate the area. The illustration below shows proper placement of the nasal speculum. The inset shows the structures that should be visible during an examination of the left nostril.

Note the color and patency of the nostril and the presence of any exudate. The mucosa should be moist, pink to red, and free of lesions and polyps. Normally, you won't see any drainage, edema, or inflammation of the nasal mucosa, although some tissue enlargement is normal in a pregnant patient.

You should see the choana (posterior air passage), cilia, and the middle and inferior turbinates. Below each turbinate will be a groove, or meatus, where the paranasal sinuses drain.

When you've completed your inspection of one nostril, close the speculum and remove it. Then inspect the other nostril.

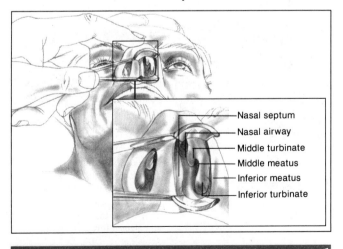

Nasal septum
Nasal airway
Middle turbinate
Middle meatus
Inferior meatus
Inferior turbinate

▶ Inspecting and palpating the frontal and maxillary sinuses

During an inspection, you'll be able to examine the frontal and maxillary sinuses, but not the ethmoidal and sphenoidal sinuses. However, if the frontal and maxillary sinuses are infected, you can assume that the ethmoidal and sphenoidal are as well.

Begin by inspecting for swelling around the eyes, especially over the sinus area. Then palpate the frontal and maxillary sinuses for tenderness and warmth.

To palpate the frontal sinuses, place your thumbs above the patient's eyes, just under the bony ridges of the upper orbits. Place your fingertips on his forehead and apply gently pressure.

To palpate the maxillary sinuses, place your thumbs as shown below. Then apply gentle pressure by pressing your thumbs (or index and middle fingers) on each side of the nose just below the zygomatic bone (cheekbone).

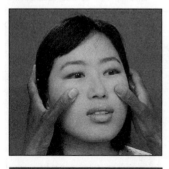

▶ Inspecting and palpating the thyroid gland

To locate the thyroid gland, observe the lower third of the patient's anterior neck. With the patient's neck extended slightly, look for masses or asymmetry in the gland. Ask him to sip water, with his neck still slightly extended. Watch the thyroid rise and fall with the trachea. You should see slight, symmetrical movement. A fixed thyroid lobe may indicate a mass.

Next, palpate the thyroid gland while standing in front of the patient. Locate the cricoid cartilage first; then move one hand to each side to palpate the thyroid lobes. The lobes can be difficult to feel because of their location and overlying tissues.

To evaluate the size and texture of the thyroid gland, ask the patient to tilt his head to the right. Then gently displace the thyroid toward the right. Have the patient swallow as you palpate the thyroid's lateral lobes, as shown below. Displace the thyroid toward the left to examine the left side.

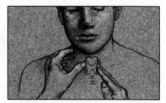

An enlarged thyroid may feel well-defined and finely lobulated. Thyroid nodules feel like a knot, protuberance, or swelling; a firm, fixed nodule may be a tumor. Do not confuse thick neck muscles with an enlarged thyroid or goiter.

CHAPTER 2

Assessment findings:
Distinguishing health from disease

Compendium of normal findings

Exploring the 25 most common chief complaints

Detecting commonly overlooked problems

Compendium of normal findings

To distinguish between health and disease, you must be able to recognize normal assessment findings in each part of the body. When you perform a physical examination, use this head-to-toe roster of normal findings as a reference. It's designed to help you quickly zero in on physical abnormalities and evaluate your patient's overall condition.

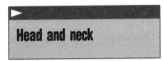

Head and neck

Inspection
• a symmetrical, lesion-free skull
• symmetrical facial structures with no cyanosis or vascular lesions
• unrestricted range of motion in the neck
• an ability to shrug the shoulders, a sign of an adequately functioning cranial nerve XI (accessory nerve)
• no bulging of the thyroid
• symmetrical, unswollen lymph nodes.

Palpation
• no lumps or tenderness on the head
• symmetrical strength in the facial muscles, a sign of adequately functioning cranial nerves V and VII (trigeminal and facial nerves)
• symmetrical sensation when you stroke a wisp of cotton on each cheek
• mobile, soft lymph nodes less than ½″ (1 cm) with no tenderness
• symmetrical pulses in the carotid arteries
• a palpable, symmetrical, lesion-free thyroid and absence of thyroid tenderness

• midline location of the trachea and absence of tracheal tenderness
• no crepitus, tenderness, or lesions in the cervical spine
• symmetrical muscle strength in the neck.

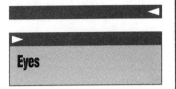

Eyes

Inspection
• no edema, scaling, or lesions on eyelids
• eyelids completely covering the corneas when closed
• eyelid color the same as surrounding skin color
• palpebral fissures of equal height
• margin of upper lid falling between superior pupil margin and superior limbus
• symmetrical, lesion-free upper eyelids that don't lag or droop when the patient opens his eyes
• evenly distributed eyelashes that curve outward
• globe of eye neither protruding from nor sunken into orbit
• eyebrows with equal size, color, and distribution
• absence of nystagmus
• clear conjunctiva with visible small blood vessels and no signs of drainage
• white sclera visible through conjunctiva
• symmetrical irises of the same color
• a transparent anterior chamber that contains no visible material when you shine a penlight into the side of the eye
• transparent, smooth, and bright cornea with no visible irregularities or lesions
• closing of the lids of both eyes when you stroke each cornea with a wisp of cotton, a test of cranial

nerve V (trigeminal nerve)
• round, equal-sized pupils that react normally to light and accommodation
• constriction of both pupils when you shine a light on one
• lacrimal structures free of exudate, swelling, and excessive tearing
• proper eye alignment
• parallel eye movement in each of the six cardinal fields of gaze.

Palpation
• absence of eyelid swelling or tenderness
• globes that feel equally firm without feeling overly hard or spongy
• lacrimal sacs that don't regurgitate fluid.

Ears

Inspection
• bilaterally symmetrical, proportionately sized auricles that have a vertical measurement between 1½″ and 4″ (4 to 10 cm)
• tip of ear crossing eye-occiput line (an imaginary line extending from the lateral aspect of the eye to the occipital protuberance)
• long axis of ear perpendicular to (or no more than 10 degrees from perpendicular to) the eye-occiput line
• color match between ears and facial skin
• no signs of inflammation, lesions, or nodules
• no cracking, thickening, scaling, or lesions behind the ear when you bend the auricle forward
• no visible discharge from auditory canal
• a patent external meatus
• skin color on the mastoid process

that matches the skin color of the surrounding areas
• no redness or swelling.

Palpation
• no masses or tenderness on the auricle
• no tenderness on the auricle or tragus during manipulation
• either small, nonpalpable lymph nodes on the auricle or discrete, mobile lymph nodes with no signs of tenderness
• well-defined, bony edges on the mastoid process with no signs of tenderness.

Nose and mouth

Inspection
• a symmetrical, lesion-free nose with no deviation of the septum or discharge
• little or no nasal flaring
• nonedematous frontal and maxillary sinuses
• an ability to identify familiar odors
• pinkish red nasal mucosa with no visible lesions and no purulent drainage
• no evidence of foreign bodies or dried blood in the nose
• pink lips with no dryness, cracking, lesions, or cyanosis
• symmetrical facial structures
• an ability to purse the lips and puff out the cheeks, a sign of an adequately functioning cranial nerve VII (facial nerve)
• an ability to easily open and close the mouth
• light pink, moist oral mucosa with no ulcers or lesions
• visible salivary ducts with no inflammation

- a white hard palate
- a pink soft palate
- pink gums with no tartar, inflammation, or hemorrhage
- all teeth intact with no signs of occlusion, caries, or breakage
- a pink tongue with no swelling, coating, ulcers, or lesions
- a tongue that moves easily and without tremor, a sign of a properly functioning cranial nerve XII (hypoglossal nerve)
- no swelling or inflammation on anterior and posterior arches
- no lesions or inflammation on posterior pharynx
- lesion-free tonsils that are the right size for the patient's age
- a uvula that moves when the patient says "ah" and a gag reflex when a tongue blade touches the posterior pharynx. These are signs of properly functioning cranial nerves IX and X.

Palpation

- no structural deviation, tenderness, or swelling in the external nose
- no tenderness or edema on the frontal and maxillary sinuses
- lips free from pain and induration
- no lesions, unusual color, tenderness, or swelling on the posterior and lateral surfaces of the tongue
- no tenderness, nodules, or swelling on the floor of the mouth.

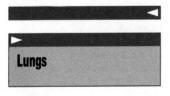

Lungs

Inspection

- side-to-side symmetrical chest configuration
- anteroposterior diameter less than the transverse diameter, with a 1:2 to 5:7 ratio in an adult

- normal chest shape, with no deformities, such as a barrel chest, kyphosis, retraction, sternal protrusion, or depressed sternum
- costal angle less than 90 degrees, with the ribs joining the spine at a 45-degree angle
- quiet, unlabored respirations with no use of accessory neck, shoulder, or abdominal muscles. You should also see no intercostal, substernal, or supraclavicular retractions.
- symmetrically expanding chest wall during respiration
- normal adult respiratory rate of 16 to 20 breaths/minute. Expect some variation depending on the age of your patient.
- regular respiratory rhythm, with expiration taking about twice as long as inspiration. Men and children breathe diaphragmatically, whereas women breathe thoracically.
- skin color that matches the rest of the body's complexion.

Palpation

- warm, dry skin
- no tender spots or bulges in the chest.

Percussion

- resonant percussion sounds over the lungs.

Auscultation

- loud, high-pitched bronchial breath sounds over the trachea
- intense, medium-pitched bronchovesicular breath sounds over the mainstem bronchi, between the scapulae, and below the clavicles
- soft, breezy, low-pitched vesicular breath sounds over most of the peripheral lung fields.

Heart

Inspection
• no visible pulsations, except at the point of maximal impulse (PMI)
• no lifts (heaves) or retractions in the four valve areas of the chest wall.

Palpation
• no detectable vibrations or thrills
• no lifts
• no pulsations, except at the PMI and epigastric area. At the PMI, a localized (<½″ [1.25-cm] diameter area) tapping pulse may be felt at the start of systole. In the epigastric area, pulsation from the abdominal aorta may be palpable.

Auscultation
• an S_1 sound—the "lub" sound heard best with the diaphragm of the stethoscope over the mitral area when the patient is in a left lateral position. It sounds longer, lower, and louder there than S_2 sounds. S_1 splitting may be audible in the tricuspid area.
• an S_2 sound—the "dub" sound heard best with the diaphragm of the stethoscope in the aortic area while the patient sits and leans over. It sounds shorter, sharper, higher, and louder there than S_1 sounds. Normal S_2 splitting may be audible in the pulmonic area on inspiration.
• an S_3 sound in children and slender, young adults with no cardiovascular disease is normal. It usually disappears when adults reach 25 to 35 years of age. In an older adult it may signify ventricular failure. S_3 may be heard best with the bell of the stethoscope over the mitral area with the patient supine and exhaling. It sounds short, dull, soft, and low.
• murmurs may be functional in children and young adults, but are abnormal in older adults. Innocent murmurs are soft, short, and vary with respirations and patient position. They occur in early systole and are heard best in pulmonic or mitral areas with the patient supine.

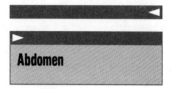

Abdomen

Inspection
• skin free from vascular lesions, jaundice, surgical scars, and rashes
• faint venous patterns (except in thin patients)
• flat, round, or scaphoid abdominal contour
• symmetrical abdomen
• umbilicus positioned midway between the xiphoid process and the symphysis pubis, with a flat or concave hemisphere
• no variations in the color of the patient's skin
• no apparent bulges
• abdominal movement apparent with respiration
• pink or silver-white striae from pregnancy or weight loss.

Auscultation
• high-pitched, gurgling bowel sounds, heard every 5 to 15 seconds through the diaphragm of the stethoscope
• vascular sounds heard through the bell of the stethoscope
• venous hum over the inferior vena cava
• no bruits, murmurs, friction rubs, or other venous hums.

Percussion
• tympany predominantly over hollow organs including the stomach, intestines, bladder, abdominal aorta, and gallbladder

• dullness over solid masses including the liver, spleen, pancreas, kidneys, uterus, and a full bladder.

Palpation
• no tenderness or masses
• abdominal musculature free from tenderness and rigidity
• no guarding, rebound tenderness, distention, or ascites
• unpalpable liver except in children. (If palpable, liver edge is regular, sharp, and nontender and is felt no more than ¾" [2 cm] below the right costal margin.)
• unpalpable spleen
• unpalpable kidneys except in thin patients or those with a flaccid abdominal wall. (Right kidney is felt more commonly than left.)

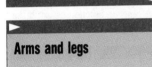

Arms and legs

Inspection
• no gross deformities
• symmetrical body parts
• good body alignment
• no involuntary movements
• a smooth gait
• active range of motion in all muscles and joints
• no pain with active range of motion
• no visible swelling or inflammation of joints or muscles
• equal bilateral limb length and symmetrical muscle mass.

Palpation
• a normal shape with no swelling or tenderness
• equal bilateral muscle tone, texture, and strength
• no involuntary contractions or twitching
• equally strong bilateral pulses.

Exploring the 25 most common chief complaints

A patient's chief complaint is the starting point for almost every initial assessment. To evaluate the complaint thoroughly, you'll need to ask the right health history questions, conduct a physical examination based on the history data you collect, and analyze possible causes of the problem.

This alphabetized list examines the 25 complaints most frequently encountered in nursing practice. For each one, you'll find a concise description, detailed questions to ask during the history, areas to focus on during the physical examination, and common causes to consider.

Cough, nonproductive

A nonproductive cough is a noisy, forceful expulsion of air from the lungs that doesn't yield sputum or blood. One of the most common symptoms of a respiratory disorder, a nonproductive cough can be ineffective and cause damage, such as airway collapse, rupture of the alveoli, or blebs.

A nonproductive cough that later becomes productive is a classic sign of a progressive respiratory disease. An acute nonproductive cough has a sudden onset and may be self-limiting. A nonproductive cough that persists beyond 1 month is considered chronic; often, such a cough results from cigarette smoking.

Health history
• When did the cough begin? Does any body position or specific activ-

ity relieve or exacerbate it? Does it get better or worse at certain times of the day? How does the cough sound? Does it occur often? Is it paroxysmal?
• Is the cough accompanied by pain?
• Have you noticed any recent changes in your appetite, energy level, exercise tolerance, or weight? Have you had surgery recently? Do you have any allergies? Do you smoke? Have you been exposed recently to fumes or chemicals?
• What medications are you taking?

Physical examination

Note whether the patient appears agitated, anxious, confused, diaphoretic, flushed, lethargic, nervous, pale, or restless. Is his skin cold or warm, clammy or dry?

Observe the rate and depth of his respirations, noting any abnormal patterns. Then examine his chest configuration and chest wall motion.

Check the patient's nose and mouth for congestion, drainage, inflammation, and signs of infection. Then inspect his neck for vein distention and tracheal deviation.

As you palpate the patient's neck, note any enlarged lymph nodes or masses. Next, percuss his chest while listening for dullness, flatness, and tympany. Finally, auscultate his lungs for crackles, decreased or absent breath sounds, pleural friction rubs, rhonchi, and wheezes.

Causes
Asthma

Typically, an asthma attack occurs at night, starting with a nonproductive cough and mild wheezing. Then, it progresses to audible wheezing, chest tightness, a cough that produces thick mucus, and severe dyspnea. Other signs include accessory muscle use, cyanosis, diaphoresis, flaring nostrils, flushing,

intercostal and supraclavicular retractions on inspiration, prolonged expirations, tachycardia, and tachypnea.

Interstitial lung disease

With this disorder, the patient has a nonproductive cough and progressive dyspnea. He may also be cyanotic and fatigued, and have fine crackles, finger clubbing, chest pain, and a recent weight loss.

Other causes

A nonproductive cough may stem from an airway occlusion, atelectasis, common cold, hypersensitivity pneumonitis, pericardial effusion, pleural effusion, pulmonary embolism, *Hantavirus* infection, and sinusitis. Also, incentive spirometry, intermittent positive-pressure breathing, and suctioning can bring on a nonproductive cough.

Cough, productive

With productive coughing, the airway passages are cleared of accumulated secretions that normal mucociliary action doesn't remove. The sudden, forceful, noisy expulsion contains sputum, blood, or both.

Usually caused by a cardiopulmonary disorder, productive coughing typically stems from an acute or chronic infection that causes inflammation, edema, and increased mucus production in the airways. Such coughing can also result from inhaling antigenic or irritating substances; in fact, its most common cause is cigarette smoking.

Health history

• When did the cough begin? How much sputum do you cough up daily? Is sputum production associated with time of day, meals, activities, or environment? Has it increased since coughing began? What are the color, odor, and consistency of the sputum? How does the cough sound and feel? Have you ever had a productive cough before?

• Have you noticed any recent changes in your appetite or weight?

• Do you have a history of recent surgery or allergies? Do you smoke or drink alcohol? If so, how much? Do you work around chemicals or respiratory irritants?

• What medications are you taking?

Physical examination

As you examine the patient's mouth and nose for congestion, drainage, and inflammation, note his breath odor. Then inspect his neck for vein distention. As he breathes, observe the chest for accessory muscle use, intercostal and supraclavicular retractions, and uneven expansion.

Palpate his neck for enlarged lymph nodes, masses, and tenderness. Next, percuss his chest, listening for dullness, flatness, and tympany. Finally, auscultate for abnormal breath sounds, crackles, pleural friction rubs, rhonchi, and wheezes.

Causes
Bacterial pneumonia

With this disorder, an initially dry cough becomes productive. Rust-colored sputum appears in pneumococcal pneumonia; brick red or currant-jelly sputum, in *Klebsiella* pneumonia; salmon-colored sputum, in staphylococcal pneumonia; and mucopurulent sputum, in streptococcal pneumonia.

Lung abscess

The cardinal sign of a ruptured lung abscess is coughing that produces copious amounts of purulent, foul-smelling and, possibly, blood-

tinged sputum. A ruptured abscess can also cause anorexia, diaphoresis, dyspnea, fatigue, fever with chills, halitosis, headache, inspiratory crackles, pleuritic chest pain, tubular or amphoric breath sounds, and weight loss.

Other causes

A productive cough can result from acute bronchiolitis, aspiration and chemical pneumonitis, bronchiectasis, common cold, cystic fibrosis, lung cancer, pertussis, pulmonary embolism, pulmonary edema, and tracheobronchitis. Also, expectorants, incentive spirometry, and intermittent positive-pressure breathing can cause a productive cough.

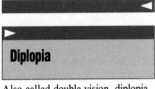

Diplopia

Also called double vision, diplopia occurs when the extraocular muscles fail to work together, causing images to fall on noncorresponding parts of the retina. Diplopia can result from orbital lesions, eye surgery, or impaired function of the cranial nerves that supply the extraocular muscles.

Classified as binocular or monocular, diplopia is usually intermittent at first or affects near or far vision exclusively. Binocular diplopia usually results from ocular deviation or displacement, or retinal surgery. Monocular diplopia may result from an early cataract, retinal edema or scarring, or poorly fitting contact lenses. Diplopia may also occur with hysteria or malingering.

Health history

• When did you first notice your double vision? Are the images side by side (horizontal), one above the other (vertical), or both? Is the dip-

lopia intermittent or constant? Are both eyes affected or just one? Is near or far vision affected? Does the diplopia occur only when you gaze in certain directions? Has the problem worsened, remained the same, or subsided? Does it worsen as the day progresses? Can you correct the problem by tilting your head? If so, ask the patient to show you, and note the direction of the tilt.
• Do you have eye pain?
• Have you had recent eye surgery? Do you wear contact lenses?
• Have you had any previous vision problems? Has anyone in your family?
• What medications are you taking?

Physical examination
Observe the patient for conjunctival infection, exophthalmos, lid edema, ocular deviation, and ptosis. Have him occlude one eye at a time; if he sees double with only one eye, he has monocular diplopia. Test his visual acuity and extraocular muscle function.

Causes
Botulism
Hallmark signs and symptoms of botulism are diplopia, dysarthria, dysphagia, and ptosis. Early findings include diarrhea, dry mouth, sore throat, and vomiting. Later, descending weakness or paralysis of extremity and trunk muscles causes dyspnea and hyporeflexia.

Intracranial aneurysm
A life-threatening disorder, intracranial aneurysm initially produces diplopia and eye deviation, perhaps accompanied by a dilated pupil on the affected side and ptosis. Other findings include a decreased level of consciousness; dizziness; neck and spinal pain and rigidity; a severe, unilateral, frontal headache, which becomes violent after rupture

of the aneurysm; tinnitus; unilateral muscle weakness or paralysis; and vomiting.

Other causes
Alcohol intoxication, brain tumors, diabetes mellitus, encephalitis, eye surgery, head injury, migraine, multiple sclerosis, and orbital tumors may also cause diplopia.

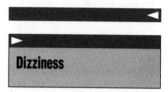

Dizziness

A common symptom, dizziness is a sensation of imbalance or faintness sometimes associated with blurred or double vision, confusion, and weakness. Dizziness may be mild or severe, have an abrupt or gradual onset, and be aggravated by standing up quickly and alleviated by lying down. Episodes are usually brief.

Dizziness typically results from inadequate blood flow and oxygen supply to the cerebrum and spinal cord. It may occur with anxiety, respiratory and cardiovascular disorders, and postconcussion syndrome. Dizziness is also a key symptom of certain serious disorders, such as hypertension and vertebrobasilar artery insufficiency.

Health history
• When did the dizziness start? How severe is it? How often does it occur, and how long does each episode last? Does the dizziness abate spontaneously? Is it triggered by standing up suddenly or bending over?
• Do you have blurred vision, chest pain, a chronic cough, diaphoresis, a headache, or shortness of breath?
• Have you ever had hypertension or another cardiovascular disorder? What about diabetes mellitus, ane-

mia, respiratory or anxiety disorders, or head injury?
• What medications are you taking?

Physical examination

Assess the patient's level of consciousness, respirations, and body temperature. As you observe his breathing, look for accessory muscle use or barrel chest. Look also for finger clubbing, cyanosis, dry mucous membranes, and poor skin turgor. Then, evaluate the patient's motor and sensory functions and reflexes.

Palpate the extremities for peripheral edema and capillary refill. Then, auscultate the patient's heart rate and rhythm and his breath sounds. Take his blood pressure while he's lying down, sitting, and standing. If the diastolic pressure exceeds 100 mm Hg, notify the doctor immediately and have the patient lie down.

Causes

Cardiac arrhythmias

Dizziness lasts for several minutes or longer and may precede fainting. Other signs and symptoms include blurred vision; confusion; hypotension; palpitations; paresthesia; weakness; and an irregular, rapid, or thready pulse.

Hypertension

Dizziness may precede fainting but may be relieved by rest. Other findings include blurred vision; elevated blood pressure; headache; and retinal changes, such as hemorrhage, exudate discharge, and papilledema.

Transient ischemic attack

Dizziness of varying severity occurs during a transient ischemic attack. Lasting from a few seconds to 24 hours, an attack may be triggered by turning the head to the side and typically signals an impending cerebrovascular accident. During an at-

tack, blindness or visual field deficits, diplopia, hearing loss, numbness, paresis, ptosis, and tinnitus may also occur.

Other causes

Dizziness may result from anemia, generalized anxiety disorder, orthostatic hypotension, panic disorder, and postconcussion syndrome. Also, dizziness may be an adverse reaction to certain drugs, including antianxiety agents, central nervous system depressants, narcotic analgesics, decongestants, antihistamines, antihypertensives, and vasodilators.

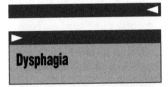

Dysphagia

Difficulty swallowing, or dysphagia, is the most common—and sometimes the only—symptom of esophageal disorders. This symptom may also result from oropharyngeal, respiratory, and neurologic disorders, and from exposure to toxins. Patients with dysphagia have an increased risk of aspiration and choking, and of malnutrition and dehydration.

Health history

• When did your trouble swallowing start? Is swallowing painful? If so, is the pain constant or intermittent? Can you point to the spot where you have the most trouble swallowing? Does eating alleviate or aggravate the problem? Do you have more trouble swallowing solids or liquids? Does the problem disappear after you try to swallow a few times? Is swallowing easier if you change position?
• Have you or anyone in your family ever had an esophageal, oropharyngeal, respiratory, or neurologic disorder? Have you recently had a

tracheotomy or been exposed to a toxin?

Physical examination
Evaluate the patient's swallowing and his cough and gag reflexes. As you listen to his speech, note any signs of muscle, tongue, or facial weakness; aphasia; or dysarthria. Is his voice nasal or hoarse? Check his mouth for dry mucous membranes and thick secretions.

Causes
Airway obstruction
A life-threatening condition, upper airway obstruction is marked by respiratory distress. Dysphagia occurs along with gagging and dysphonia.

Esophageal carcinoma
Typically, painless dysphagia accompanies rapid weight loss. As the carcinoma advances, dysphagia becomes painful and constant. The patient complains of a cough with hemoptysis, hoarseness, sore throat, and steady chest pain.

Esophagitis
A patient with corrosive esophagitis will have dysphagia accompanied by excessive salivation, fever, hematemesis, intense pain in the mouth and anterior chest, and tachypnea. Monilial esophagitis will produce dysphagia and sore throat. In reflux esophagitis, dysphagia is a late symptom that usually accompanies stricture.

Hiatal hernia
The patient with a hiatal hernia may complain of belching, dysphagia, dyspepsia, flatulence, heartburn, regurgitation, and retrosternal or substernal chest pain aggravated by lying down or bending over.

Other causes
Dysphagia results from botulism, esophageal diverticula, external

esophageal compression, hypocalcemia, laryngeal nerve damage, and Parkinson's disease. Radiation therapy and a tracheotomy may also cause dysphagia.

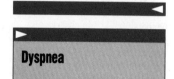

Dyspnea

Patients typically describe dyspnea as shortness of breath, but this symptom also refers to difficult or uncomfortable breathing. Its severity varies greatly and is often unrelated to the seriousness of the underlying cause. Dyspnea may arise suddenly or slowly and may subside rapidly or persist for years.

Health history
• When did the dyspnea first occur? Did it begin suddenly or gradually? Is it constant or intermittent? Does it occur during activity or while you're resting? Does anything seem to trigger, exacerbate, or relieve it? Have you ever had dyspnea before?
• Do you have a productive or nonproductive cough or chest pain?
• Have you recently had an upper respiratory tract infection or experienced trauma? Do you smoke? If so, how much and for how long? Have you been exposed to any allergens? Do you have any known allergies?
• What medications are you taking?

Physical examination
Observe the patient's respirations, noting their rate and depth, and any breathing difficulties or abnormal respiratory patterns. Check too for flaring nostrils, grunting respirations, inspiratory stridor, intercostal retractions during inspiration, and pursed-lip expirations.

Also examine the patient for barrel chest, diaphoresis, neck vein distention, finger clubbing, and peripheral edema. Note the color, consistency, and odor of any sputum.

Palpate his chest for asymmetrical expansion, decreased diaphragmatic excursion, tactile fremitus, and subcutaneous crepitation. Also check the rate, rhythm, and intensity of his peripheral pulses.

As you percuss the lung fields, note dull, hyperresonant, or tympanic percussion sounds. Auscultate the lungs for bronchophony, crackles, decreased or absent unilateral breath sounds, egophony, pleural friction rubs, rhonchi, whispered pectoriloquy, and wheezing. Then auscultate the heart for abnormal sounds or rhythms, such as ventricular or atrial gallop, and for pericardial friction rubs and tachycardia. Be sure to monitor the patient's blood pressure and pulse pressure.

Causes
Adult respiratory distress syndrome
In adult respiratory distress syndrome (ARDS), acute dyspnea is followed by accessory muscle use, crackles, grunting respirations, progressive respiratory distress, rhonchi, and wheezes. In the late stages, anxiety, cyanosis, decreased mental acuity, and tachycardia occur. Severe ARDS can produce signs of shock, such as cool, clammy skin and hypotension. The typical patient has no history of underlying cardiac or pulmonary disease but has sustained a recent pulmonary or systemic insult.

Airway obstruction (partial)
Inspiratory stridor and acute dyspnea occur as the patient tries to overcome the obstruction. Related findings include accessory muscle use, anxiety, asymmetrical chest expansion, cyanosis, decreased or absent breath sounds, diaphoresis, hypotension, and tachypnea. The patient may have aspirated vomitus or a foreign body, or been exposed to an allergen.

Asthma
Acute dyspneic attacks occur along with accessory muscle use, apprehension, dry cough, flushing or cyanosis, intercostal retractions, tachypnea, and tachycardia. On palpation, you'll detect decreased tactile fremitus. Hyperresonance occurs on chest percussion. On auscultation, you'll note wheezing and rhonchi or, during a severe episode, decreased breath sounds.

Congestive heart failure
Dyspnea usually develops gradually or occurs as chronic paroxysmal nocturnal dyspnea. In ventricular failure, dyspnea occurs with basilar crackles, dependent peripheral edema, distended neck veins, fatigue, orthopnea, tachycardia, ventricular or atrial gallop, and weight gain. The patient may have a history of cardiovascular disease or may be taking drugs that can precipitate congestive heart failure (CHF), such as amiodarone (Cordarone), certain beta blockers, or corticosteroids.

Myocardial infarction
Sudden dyspnea occurs with crushing substernal chest pain that may radiate to the back, neck, jaw, and arms. The patient's history may include heart disease, hypertension, hypercholesterolemia, or use of drugs that can precipitate a myocardial infarction (MI), such as cocaine, dextrothyroxine sodium (Choloxin), estramustine phosphate sodium (Emcyt), or aldesleukin (Proleukin).

Pneumonia
Dyspnea occurs suddenly, usually accompanied by fever, pleuritic chest pain that worsens with deep

inspiration, and shaking chills. The patient also has a dry or productive cough, depending on the stage and type of pneumonia. Sputum may be discolored and foul-smelling. Crackles, decreased breath sounds, dullness on percussion, and rhonchi may also be present. The history may include exposure to a contagious organism, hazardous fumes, or air pollution.

Pulmonary edema
In this disorder, severe dyspnea is often preceded by signs of CHF, such as crackles in both lung fields, cyanosis, tachycardia, tachypnea, and marked anxiety. The patient may have a dry cough or one that produces copious amounts of pink, frothy sputum. The history may reveal cardiovascular disease, cyanosis, fatigue, and pallor.

Pulmonary embolism
Severe dyspnea occurs with intense angina-like or pleuritic pain aggravated by deep breathing and thoracic movement. Other findings include crackles, cyanosis, diffuse wheezing, dull percussion sounds, low-grade fever, nonproductive cough, pleural friction rubs, restlessness, tachypnea, and tachycardia. The patient's history may include acute MI, CHF, hip or leg fractures, oral contraceptive use, pregnancy, thrombophlebitis, or varicose veins.

Other causes
Dyspnea may also result from anemia, anxiety, cardiac arrhythmias, cor pulmonale, inhalation injury, lung cancer, pleural effusion, and sepsis.

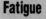

Fatigue

A common symptom, fatigue is a feeling of excessive tiredness, lack of energy, or exhaustion, accompanied by a strong desire to rest or sleep. Fatigue differs from weakness, which involves the muscles, but may accompany it.

A normal response to physical overexertion, emotional stress, and sleep deprivation, fatigue can also result from psychological and physiologic disorders, especially viral infections and endocrine, cardiovascular, or neurologic disorders.

Health history
• When did the fatigue begin? Is it constant or intermittent? If it's intermittent, when does it occur? Does the fatigue worsen with activity and improve with rest, or vice versa? (The former usually signals a physiologic disorder; the latter, a psychological disorder.)
• Have you experienced any recent stressful changes at home or at work?
• Have you changed your eating habits? Have you recently lost or gained weight?
• Have you or anyone in your family been diagnosed with any cardiovascular, endocrine, or neurologic disorders? What about viral infections or psychological disorders?
• What medications are you taking?

Physical examination
Observe the patient's general appearance for signs of depression or organic illness. Is he unkempt? Expressionless? Tired or unhealthy looking? Is he slumped over? Assess his mental status, noting especially any agitation, attention deficits, mental clouding, or psychomotor impairment.

Causes

Anemia

Fatigue after mild activity is often anemia's first symptom. Other signs and symptoms typically include dyspnea, pallor, and tachycardia.

Cancer

Unexplained fatigue is often the earliest indication of cancer. Related signs and symptoms reflect the type, location, and stage of the tumor, and usually include abnormal bleeding, anorexia, nausea, pain, a palpable mass, vomiting, and weight loss.

Chronic infection

In a patient with a chronic infection, fatigue is usually the most prominent symptom—and sometimes the only one.

Congestive heart failure

Persistent fatigue and lethargy are characteristic symptoms of congestive heart failure. Left ventricular failure produces exertional and paroxysmal nocturnal dyspnea, orthopnea, and tachycardia. Right ventricular failure causes neck vein distention and, sometimes, a slight but persistent nonproductive cough.

Depression

Chronic depression is almost always accompanied by persistent fatigue that's unrelated to exertion. The patient may also complain of anorexia, constipation, headache, and sexual dysfunction.

Diabetes mellitus

The most common symptom in this disorder, fatigue may begin insidiously or abruptly. Related findings include polydipsia, polyphagia, polyuria, and weight loss.

Myasthenia gravis

The cardinal symptoms of this disorder are easy fatigability and muscle weakness that worsen with exertion and abate with rest. These symptoms are related to the specific muscle groups affected.

Other causes

Fatigue can be caused by anxiety, myocardial infarction, rheumatoid arthritis, systemic lupus erythematosus, and malnutrition. Certain drugs—notably antihypertensives and sedatives—and most types of surgery also cause fatigue.

Fever

An abnormal elevation of body temperature above 98.6° F (37° C), fever (or pyrexia) is a common sign arising from disorders that affect virtually every body system. As a result, fever alone has little diagnostic value. However, persistently high fever is a medical emergency.

Fever can be classified as low (oral reading of 99° to 100.4° F [37.2° to 38° C]), moderate (100.5° to 104° F [38° to 40° C]), or high (above 104° F [40° C]). Fever above 108° F (42.2° C) causes unconsciousness and, if prolonged, brain damage.

Health history

• When did the fever begin? How high did it reach? Is the fever constant, or does it disappear and then reappear later?
• Do you also have chills, fatigue, or pain?
• Have you had any immunodeficiency disorders, infections, recent trauma or surgery, or diagnostic tests? Have you traveled recently?
• What medications are you taking? Have you recently had anesthesia?

Causes
Infectious and inflammatory disorders
Fever may be low, as in Crohn's disease and ulcerative colitis, or extremely high, as in bacterial pneumonia. It may be remittent, as in infectious mononucleosis; sustained, as in meningitis; or relapsing, as in malaria. Fever may arise abruptly, as in Rocky Mountain spotted fever, or insidiously, as in mycoplasmal pneumonia. Typically, it accompanies a self-limiting disorder, such as the common cold.

Medications
Fever and rash commonly result from hypersensitivity to quinidine, methyldopa (Aldomet), procainamide hydrochloride (Pronestyl), phenytoin (Dilantin), anti-infectives, barbiturates, iodides, and some antitoxins. Fever can also result from the use of chemotherapeutic agents and medications that decrease sweating, such as anticholinergics. Plus, toxic doses of salicylates, amphetamines, and tricyclic antidepressants can cause fever.

Other causes
Fever may also result from an injection of contrast media used in diagnostic tests, from surgery, and from blood transfusion reactions.

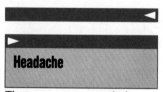

Headache

The most common neurologic symptom, a headache may be mild to severe, localized or generalized, constant or intermittent. About 90% of all headaches are benign and can be described as vascular, muscle-contraction, or a combination of both.

Occasionally, this symptom indicates a severe neurologic disorder. A generalized, pathologic headache may result from disorders associated with intracranial inflammation, increased intracranial pressure (ICP), meningeal irritation, or a vascular disturbance. A headache may also result from eye and sinus disorders and from the effects of drugs, tests, and treatments.

Health history
• When did the headache first occur? Is the pain mild, moderate, or severe? Is it localized or generalized? If it's localized, where does it occur? Is it constant or intermittent? If it's intermittent, what's the duration? How would you describe the pain; for example, is it stabbing, dull, throbbing, or viselike? Does anything seem to trigger it, exacerbate it, or relieve it?
• Have you also experienced confusion, dizziness, drowsiness, eye pain, fever, muscle twitching, nausea, photophobia, seizures, speaking or walking difficulties, neck stiffness, visual disturbances, vomiting, or weakness?
• Have you been under unusual stress at home or at work? For family members: Have you noticed any changes in the patient's behavior or personality?
• Do you have a history of blood dyscrasia, cardiovascular disease, glaucoma, hemorrhagic disorders, hypertension, poor vision, seizures, or smoking? Have you had any recent traumatic injuries; dental work; or sinus, ear, or systemic infections?
• What medications are you taking?

Physical examination
Observe the rate and depth of the patient's respirations, noting any breathing difficulty or abnormal patterns. Then inspect his head for bruising, swelling, and sinus bleeding. Check also for Battle's sign,

neck stiffness, otorrhea, and rhinorrhea.

Assess the patient's level of consciousness (LOC). Is he drowsy, lethargic, or comatose? Examine his eyes, noting pupil size, equality, and response to light. With the patient both at rest and active, note any tremors.

Gently palpate the skull and sinuses for tenderness. Unless head trauma has occurred, slowly move the neck to check for nuchal rigidity or pain. Then assess the patient's motor strength. Palpate his peripheral pulses, noting their rate, rhythm, and intensity.

Check for a positive Babinski's reflex. As you percuss for other reflexes, note any hyperreflexia. Then auscultate over the temporal artery, listening for bruits. Be sure to monitor the patient's blood pressure and pulse pressure.

Causes

Brain abscess

A headache stemming from a brain abscess typically intensifies over a few days, localizes to a particular spot, and is aggravated by straining. The headache may be accompanied by a decreased LOC (drowsiness to deep stupor), focal or generalized seizures, nausea, and vomiting. Depending on the abscess site, the patient may also have aphasia, ataxia, impaired visual acuity, hemiparesis, personality changes, or tremors. Signs of an infection may or may not appear. The patient's history may include systemic, chronic middle ear, mastoid, or sinus infection; osteomyelitis of the skull or a compound fracture; or a penetrating head wound.

Brain tumor

Initially, the headache develops near the tumor site and becomes generalized as the tumor grows. Pain is usually intermittent, deep-seated, dull, and most intense in the morning. It's aggravated by coughing, stooping, Valsalva's maneuver, and changes in head position.

Cerebral aneurysm (ruptured)

This headache is sudden and excruciating. It may be unilateral and usually peaks within minutes of the rupture. The headache may be accompanied by nausea, vomiting, and signs of meningeal irritation. The patient may lose consciousness. His history may include hypertension or other cardiovascular disorders, a stressful life-style, or smoking.

Encephalitis

The patient has a severe, generalized headache accompanied by a deteriorating LOC over a 48-hour period. Fever, focal neurologic deficits, irritability, nausea, nuchal rigidity, photophobia, seizures, and vomiting may also develop. His history may reveal exposure to the viruses that commonly cause encephalitis, such as mumps or herpes simplex.

Epidural hemorrhage (acute)

A progressively severe headache immediately follows a brief loss of consciousness. Then the patient's LOC rapidly and steadily declines. Accompanying signs and symptoms include increasing ICP, ipsilateral pupil dilation, nausea, and vomiting. The patient's history usually reveals head trauma within the past 24 hours.

Glaucoma (acute angle-closure)

An ophthalmic emergency, glaucoma may cause an excruciating headache. Other signs and symptoms include blurred vision, cloudy cornea, halo vision, moderately dilated and fixed pupil, photophobia, nausea, and vomiting.

Hypertension

Patients with hypertension may have a slightly throbbing occipital headache on awakening. Then, during the day, the severity may decrease. But if the patient's diastolic blood pressure exceeds 120 mm Hg, the headache remains constant.

Meningitis

The patient experiences a severe, constant, generalized headache that starts suddenly and worsens with movement. He may also have chills, fever, hyperreflexia, nuchal rigidity, and positive Kernig's and Brudzinski's signs. His history may include recent systemic or sinus infection, dental work, or exposure to bacteria or viruses that commonly cause meningitis, such as *Haemophilus influenzae*, *Streptococcus pneumoniae*, enteroviruses, and mumps.

Migraine

A severe, throbbing headache, migraine may follow a 5- to-15-minute prodrome of dizziness; tingling of the face, lips, or hands; unsteady gait; and visual disturbances. Other signs and symptoms include anorexia, nausea, photophobia, and vomiting.

Sinusitis (acute)

Patients with sinusitis have a dull, periorbital headache that's typically aggravated by bending over or touching the face. They may also have fever, malaise, nasal discharge, nasal turbinate edema, sinus tenderness, and sore throat. Sinusitis is relieved by sinus drainage.

Subarachnoid hemorrhage

The hallmarks of this disorder are a sudden, violent headache along with dizziness, hypertension, ipsilateral pupil dilation, nausea, nuchal rigidity, seizures, vomiting, and an altered LOC that may rapidly progress to coma. The patient's history may include congenital vascular defects, arteriovenous malformation, cardiovascular disease, smoking, or excessive stress.

Subdural hematoma

A severe, localized headache usually follows head trauma that causes an immediate loss of consciousness, a latent period of drowsiness, confusion or personality changes, and agitation. Later, signs of increased ICP may develop. If the head trauma occurred within 3 days of the onset of signs and symptoms, the hematoma is acute; within 3 weeks, subacute; after more than 3 weeks, chronic. About 50% of patients with this disorder have no history of head trauma.

Other causes

Cervical traction, lumbar puncture, myelography, use of vasodilators, and withdrawal from vasopressors or sympathomimetic drugs can also cause headache. So can indomethacin (Indocin); digoxin (Lanoxin); nitroglycerin (Nitrostat), isosarbide dinitrate (Isordil), and other vasodilators.

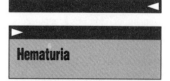

Hematuria

A cardinal sign of renal and urinary tract disorders, hematuria is the presence of blood in the urine. Hematuria may be evident or confirmed by a urine test for occult blood.

The bleeding may be continuous or intermittent, is often accompanied by pain, and may be aggravated by prolonged standing or walking. Dark or brownish blood indicates renal or upper urinary tract bleeding; bright red blood, lower urinary tract bleeding.

Health history
• When did you first notice blood in your urine? Does it occur every time you urinate? Are you passing any clots? Have you ever had this problem before?
• Do you have any pain? If so, does the pain occur only when you urinate, or is it continuous?
• Do you have bleeding hemorrhoids? Have you had any recent trauma or performed any strenuous exercise? Do you have a history of renal, urinary, prostatic, or coagulation disorders? For women patients: are you menstruating?
• What medications are you taking?

Physical examination
Check the urinary meatus for any bleeding or abnormalities. Then, palpate the abdomen and flanks, noting any pain or tenderness. Finally, percuss the abdomen and flanks, especially the costovertebral angle, to elicit any tenderness.

Causes
Bladder cancer
A primary cause of gross hematuria in men, bladder cancer may produce pain in the bladder, rectum, pelvis, flank, back, or legs. You may also note signs of urinary tract infection.

Calculi
Both bladder and renal calculi produce hematuria, which may be accompanied by signs and symptoms of urinary tract infection. Bladder calculi usually produce gross hematuria, pain referred to the penile or vulvar area and, in some patients, bladder distention. Renal calculi may produce either microscopic or gross hematuria.

Glomerulonephritis
Usually, acute glomerulonephritis begins with gross hematuria. It may also produce anuria or oliguria,

flank and abdominal pain, and increased blood pressure. Chronic glomerulonephritis typically causes microscopic hematuria accompanied by generalized edema, increased blood pressure, and proteinuria.

Nephritis
Acute nephritis causes fever, a maculopapular rash, and microscopic hematuria. In chronic interstitial nephritis, the patient may have dilute, almost colorless urine along with polyuria.

Pyelonephritis (acute)
A typical sign of pyelonephritis is microscopic or macroscopic hematuria that progresses to grossly bloody hematuria. After the infection resolves, microscopic hematuria may persist for a few months. Other findings include flank pain, high fever, and signs and symptoms of a urinary tract infection.

Renal infarction
Patients with renal infarction usually have gross hematuria. Other signs and symptoms include anorexia; costovertebral angle tenderness; and constant, severe flank and upper abdominal pain.

Other causes
Hematuria may result from benign prostatic hyperplasia, bladder trauma, obstructive nephropathy, polycystic kidney disease, renal trauma, and urethral trauma. Also, diagnostic tests – such as cystoscopy and renal biopsy – and drugs – such as anticoagulants; chemotherapeutic agents such as aldesleukin (Proleukin), BCG intravesical (TheraCys), ifosfamide (Ifex), leuprolide (Lupron); etretinate (Tegison); and thiabendazole (Mintezol) – may cause hematuria.

Hemoptysis

The expectoration of blood or bloody sputum from the lungs or tracheobronchial tree is known as hemoptysis. Usually resulting from a tracheobronchial tree abnormality, hemoptysis is associated with inflammatory conditions or lesions that cause erosion and necrosis of bronchial tissues and blood vessels.

Sometimes, hemoptysis is confused with bleeding from the mouth, throat, nasopharynx, or GI tract. Severe hemoptysis requires emergency endotracheal intubation and suctioning.

Health history

• When did you begin expectorating blood? How much blood or sputum are you expectorating? How often?
• Did you recently have a flulike syndrome? Have you had any recent invasive pulmonary procedures or chest trauma?
• Do you smoke? Did you ever smoke? If so, how much? Have you ever been diagnosed with a cardiac, respiratory, or bleeding disorders?
• What medications are you taking? Are you taking anticoagulants?

Physical examination

After assessing the patient's level of consciousness, examine his nose, mouth, and pharynx for sources of bleeding. Observe the rate and depth of his respirations, noting any breathing difficulty or abnormal breathing patterns. Also, as he breathes, look for abnormal chest movement, accessory muscle use, and retractions. Inspect the skin for central and peripheral cyanosis, diaphoresis, lesions, and pallor.

Palpate the rate, rhythm, and intensity of the peripheral pulses. Then feel the chest, noting abnormal pulsations, diaphragmatic tenderness, and fremitus. Check for respiratory excursion. If the patient has a history of trauma, carefully check the position of the trachea and note any edema.

As you percuss over the lung fields, note any dullness, flatness, hyperresonance, or tympany. Then auscultate the lungs for crackles, rhonchi, and wheezes, and the heart for bruits, gallops, murmurs, and pleural friction rubs. Be sure to monitor the patient's blood pressure and pulse pressure.

Causes

Bronchitis (chronic)

With this disorder, the patient usually has a productive cough that lasts at least 3 months and leads to expectoration of blood-streaked sputum. Other respiratory signs include dyspnea, prolonged expiration, scattered rhonchi, and wheezing.

Lung abscess

A patient with a lung abscess expectorates copious amounts of bloody, purulent, foul-smelling sputum. He also has anorexia, chills, diaphoresis, fever, headache, and pleuritic or dull chest pain. Lung auscultation may reveal tubular breath sounds or crackles. Percussion reveals dullness on the affected side. The patient may have a history of a recent pulmonary infection or evidence of poor oral hygiene with dental or gingival disease.

Lung cancer

Ulceration of the bronchus commonly causes recurring hemoptysis (an early sign), which can vary from blood-streaked sputum to blood. Related findings include anorexia, chest pain, dyspnea, fever, a productive cough, weight loss, and wheezing.

Pulmonary edema

A patient with pulmonary edema may expectorate copious amounts of frothy, blood-tinged, pink sputum. He may also complain of dyspnea and orthopnea. On examination, you may detect diffuse crackles in both lung fields and a ventricular gallop.

Tracheal trauma

With tracheal trauma, the bleeding appears to come from the back of the throat. Accompanying signs and symptoms include airway occlusion, dysphagia, hoarseness, neck pain, and respiratory distress.

Other causes

Hemoptysis may also result from bronchiectasis, coagulation disorders, cystic fibrosis, lung or airway injuries from diagnostic procedures, and primary pulmonary hypertension.

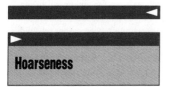

Hoarseness

A rough or harsh-sounding voice, hoarseness can be acute or chronic. It may result from infections or inflammatory lesions or exudates in the larynx, from laryngeal edema, from compression or disruption of the vocal cords or recurrent laryngeal nerve damage, or from irritating polyps on the vocal cords. Hoarseness can also occur with aging because the laryngeal muscles and mucosa atrophy, leading to diminished control of the vocal cords. Hoarseness may be exacerbated by excessive alcohol intake, smoking, inhalation of noxious fumes, excessive talking, and shouting.

Health history

• When did the hoarseness start? Is it constant or intermittent? Does anything relieve or exacerbate it? Have you been overusing your voice?
• Have you also had a cough, a dry mouth, difficulty swallowing dry food, shortness of breath, or a sore throat?
• Have you ever had cancer or other disorders? Do you regularly drink alcohol or smoke? If so, how much?

Physical examination

Inspect the patient's mouth and throat for redness or exudate, possibly indicating an upper respiratory tract infection. Ask him to stick out his tongue: If he can't, the hypoglossal nerve (cranial nerve XII) may be impaired.

As the patient breathes, observe for asymmetrical chest expansion, intercostal retractions, nasal flaring, stridor, and other signs of respiratory distress.

Palpate the patient's neck for masses and the cervical lymph nodes and thyroid gland for enlargement. Then palpate the trachea to assess for deviation.

As you percuss the chest wall, note any dullness. Then, auscultate the lungs for crackles, rhonchi, tubular sounds, or wheezes. To detect bradycardia, auscultate the heart.

Causes
Inhalation injury

Exposure to a fire or an explosion can cause an inhalation injury, which produces coughing, hoarseness, orofacial burns, singed nasal hair, and soot-stained sputum. Subsequent signs and symptoms include crackles, rhonchi, wheezes, and respiratory distress.

Laryngitis

Persistent hoarseness may be the only sign of chronic laryngitis. In acute laryngitis, hoarseness or a complete loss of voice develops suddenly. Related findings include cough, fever, pain (especially during swallowing or speaking), profuse diaphoresis, rhinorrhea, and sore throat.

Vocal cord polyps

With this disorder, a raspy hoarseness will be the chief complaint. The patient may also have a chronic cough and a crackling voice.

Other causes

Hoarseness may result from hypothyroidism, pulmonary tuberculosis, rheumatoid arthritis, and laryngeal cancer (most common in men ages 50 to 70). Prolonged intubation, surgical severing of the recurrent laryngeal nerve, and a tracheostomy may also produce hoarseness.

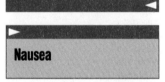

Nausea

A profound feeling of revulsion to food, or a signal of impending vomiting, nausea is usually accompanied by anorexia, diaphoresis, hypersalivation, pallor, tachycardia, tachypnea, and vomiting. A common symptom of GI disorders, nausea may also result from electrolyte imbalances; infections; metabolic, endocrine, and cardiac disorders; early months of pregnancy; drug therapy; surgery; and radiation therapy. Also, severe pain, anxiety, alcohol intoxication, overeating, and ingestion of something distasteful can trigger nausea.

Health history

• When did the nausea begin? Is it intermittent or constant? How severe is it?
• Do you have any other symptoms, such as abdominal pain, loss of appetite, changes in bowel habits, excessive belching or gas, weight loss, or vomiting?
• For female patients: Are you pregnant or could you be? Have you ever had GI, endocrine, or metabolic disorders? Have you had any recent infections? Have you ever had cancer or radiation therapy or chemotherapy?
• What medications are you taking? Do you drink alcohol and, if so, how much?

Physical examination

Examine the patient's skin for bruises, jaundice, poor turgor, and spider angiomas. Then inspect his abdomen for distention.

Because palpation and percussion can affect the frequency and intensity of bowel sounds, you should auscultate the abdomen first. Listen for bowel sounds in each quadrant. Then, using the bell of the stethoscope, listen for abdominal bruits.

As you palpate the abdomen, note any rigidity, tenderness, or rebound tenderness. Next, palpate the size of the liver. Then, percuss the abdomen and liver for any abnormalities.

Causes

Appendicitis

The patient with appendicitis will feel nauseated and may vomit. He'll also have vague epigastric or periumbilical discomfort that localizes in the right lower quadrant.

Cholecystitis (acute)

In this disorder, nausea commonly follows severe right upper quadrant pain that may radiate to the back or shoulders. Associated findings include abdominal tenderness, vomiting and, possibly, abdominal rigidity and distention, diaphoresis, and fever with chills.

Gastritis

Patients with gastritis often have nausea, especially after ingestion of alcohol, aspirin, spicy foods, or caffeine. Belching, epigastric pain, fever, malaise, and vomiting of mucus or blood may also occur.

Other causes

Nausea may result from cirrhosis, electrolyte imbalances, labyrinthitis, metabolic acidosis, myocardial infarction, renal and urologic disorders, and ulcerative colitis. Use of anesthetics, antibiotics, antineoplastics, ferrous sulfate, oral potassium, and quinidine, and overdoses of digitalis glycosides and theophylline may also trigger nausea, as may radiation therapy and surgery—especially abdominal surgery.

Pain, abdominal

Usually, abdominal pain results from GI disorders, but it can also stem from reproductive, genitourinary, musculoskeletal, or vascular disorders, from drug use, or from the effects of toxins. Abdominal pain may originate in the abdominopelvic viscera, the parietal peritoneum, or the capsules of the liver, kidneys, or spleen. The pain may be acute or chronic, diffuse or localized.

Health history

• When did the pain begin? What does it feel like? How long does it last? Where exactly is it? Does it radiate to other areas, such as the chest or back? Does it get better or worse when you change position, move, exert yourself, cough, eat, or have a bowel movement?
• Does fever occur during episodes of pain? Do you have appetite changes, constipation, diarrhea, nausea, pain with urination, pink or cloudy urine, vomiting, or urinary frequency or urgency?
• Do you have a history of adrenal disease, heart disease, recent infection, or recent blunt trauma to the abdomen, flank, or chest? Have you had any condition that could predispose you to emboli or that could narrow an arterial lumen? Have you recently undergone a urinary tract procedure or surgery? Have you traveled to a foreign country recently?
• For women of childbearing age: what was the date of your last menses? Has your menstrual pattern changed? Could you be pregnant?
• Have you ever used I.V. drugs? Do you drink alchohol? If so, how much and how often? What prescription drugs do you take?

Physical examination

After assessing the patient's level of consciousness, observe his skin for diaphoresis, jaundice, and turgor. Then check for coolness, discoloration, and edema of the arms and legs. Inspect the abdomen and chest for signs of trauma: A bluish discoloration around the umbilicus (Cullen's sign) and around the flank area (Turner's sign) can indicate blunt trauma. Obtain and record a baseline measurement of abdominal girth at the umbilicus.

After inspecting for neck vein distention, observe the rate and depth of respirations, noting any abnormal patterns. Observe the color and odor of the patient's urine.

Because palpation and percussion can affect the frequency and intensity of bowel sounds, you should auscultate the abdomen first. Listen for bowel sounds in each quadrant, noting whether the sounds are high-pitched and tinkling, hyperactive, or absent.

Then, listen to the patient's heart and breath sounds for abnormalities. Be sure to monitor his blood pressure and pulse pressure.

As you systematically palpate the abdominal, pelvic, flank, and epigastric areas, note any enlarged organs, masses, rigidity, tenderness, rebound tenderness, or tenderness with guarding. Check the patient's peripheral pulses for rate, rhythm, and intensity.

Percuss each abdominal quadrant, noting tenderness, increased pain, and percussion sounds. Dull percussion sounds indicate free fluid; hollow sounds, air.

Causes
Abdominal aortic aneurysm (dissecting)
Constant, dull upper abdominal pain radiating to the lower back typically accompanies rapid aneurysm enlargement and may herald a rupture. Palpation may reveal an epigastric mass that pulsates before rupture. On auscultation, you may detect a systolic bruit over the aneurysm. You may also note abdominal rigidity, increasing abdominal girth, and signs of hypovolemic shock.

Abdominal trauma
The patient may have generalized or localized abdominal pain along with abdominal ecchymosis, abdominal tenderness, or vomiting. If he is hemorrhaging into the peritoneal cavity, you may note abdominal rigidity, dullness on percussion, and increasing abdominal girth. You may hear hollow bowel sounds if an abdominal organ has been perforated, or bowel sounds may be absent. Bowel sounds heard in the chest cavity usually signal a diaphragmatic tear.

Appendicitis
The patient with appendicitis may have sudden pain in the epigastric or umbilical region that increases over a few hours or days, along with flulike symptoms. Anorexia, constipation or diarrhea, nausea, and vomiting precede the pain, which may be dull or severe. Pain localizes at McBurney's point in the right lower quadrant. Abdominal rigidity and rebound tenderness may also occur.

Ectopic pregnancy
Lower abdominal pain may be sharp, dull, or cramping, and either constant or intermittent. The pain may be accompanied by breast tenderness, nausea, vaginal bleeding, vomiting, and urinary frequency. The patient typically has a 1- to 2-month history of amenorrhea. Rupture of the fallopian tube produces sharp lower abdominal pain, which may radiate to the shoulders and neck and become extreme on cervical or adnexal palpation.

Hepatitis
Liver enlargement from any type of hepatitis causes discomfort or dull pain and tenderness in the right upper quadrant.

Intestinal obstruction
With an intestinal obstruction, short episodes of intense, colicky, cramping pain alternate with pain-free periods.

Pancreatitis
The characteristic symptom of pancreatitis is fulminating, continuous upper abdominal pain that may radiate to both flanks and to the back.

Renal calculi
Depending on the location of the calculi, the patient may feel severe abdominal or back pain. However, the classic symptom of renal calculi is colicky pain that travels from the costovertebral angle to the flank, the suprapubic region, and the external genitalia.

Other causes
Abdominal pain may result from adrenal crisis, cholecystitis, congestive heart failure, diabetic ketoacidosis, diverticulitis, hepatic abscess, mesenteric artery ischemia, myocardial infarction, an ovarian cyst, a perforated ulcer, peritonitis, pneumonia, pneumothorax, pyelonephritis, renal infarction, and splenic infarction. Also, salicylates and nonsteroidal anti-inflammatory drugs can produce abdominal pain.

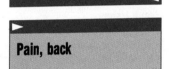

Pain, back

Back pain may be acute, chronic, constant, or intermittent. It also may remain localized in the back or radiate along the spine or down one or both legs. A patient's pain may be exacerbated by activity (most commonly, stooping or lifting) and alleviated by rest. Or it may be unaffected by either.

Intrinsic back pain results from muscle spasm, nerve root irritation, fracture, or a combination of these causes. It usually occurs in the lower back or lumbosacral area. Back pain may also be referred from the abdomen, possibly signaling a life-threatening disorder.

Health history
• When did the pain first occur? What does it feel like? Is it mild, moderate, or severe? Is it constant or intermittent? Where exactly is it? Is it associated with activity? What relieves or exacerbates it? For women of childbearing age: Does the pain occur before or during your menses?
• Have you had recent episodes of abdominal tenderness or rigidity, fever, nausea, or vomiting? Do you feel any unusual sensations in your legs? Have you had urinary frequency or urgency or painful urination?
• Do you have a history of trauma, back surgery, or urinary tract surgery, procedures, obstructions, or infections?
• What medications are you taking?

Physical examination
Observe the rate and depth of respirations, noting any breathing difficulty or abnormal breathing patterns. Check the skin for diaphoresis, discoloration, edema, mottling, and pallor. Then inspect the back, legs, and abdomen for signs of trauma. After checking for abdominal distention, take a baseline abdominal girth measurement.

Because palpation and percussion can affect the frequency and intensity of bowel sounds, you should auscultate the abdomen first. Listen for bowel sounds in each quadrant. Then listen over the abdominal aorta for bruits and over the lungs for crackles. Be sure to monitor the patient's blood pressure and pulse pressure.

Palpate the abdominal, epigastric, and pelvic areas for abdominal rigidity, enlarged organs, masses, and tenderness. If you feel any pulsations, don't palpate deeply. Check the peripheral pulses for rate, rhythm, and intensity. Then gently palpate the painful area, noting contractions, excessive muscle tone, or spasm.

Finally, percuss each abdominal quadrant, noting any abnormal sounds, increased pain, or tenderness.

Causes
Abdominal aortic aneurysm (dissecting)
Low back pain and dull upper abdominal pain often accompany a rapidly enlarging aneurysm and may indicate the early stages of

rupture. On palpation, you may detect tenderness over the aneurysm area and a pulsating epigastric mass. Other signs include absent femoral and pedal pulses, mottling of the skin below the waist, and signs of hypovolemic shock.

Pancreatitis
Fulminating, continuous abdominal pain that may radiate to the back and both flanks characterizes pancreatitis. You may also note abdominal tenderness, rigidity, and distention; fever; hypoactive bowel sounds; pallor; tachycardia; and vomiting. The history may include alcohol abuse, use of thiazide diuretics, gallbladder disease, or trauma.

Pyelonephritis (acute)
The patient with acute pyelonephritis has progressive back pain or tenderness in the flank area, accompanied by costovertebral angle pain and abdominal pain in one or two quadrants. Associated signs and symptoms include dysuria, high fever, hematuria, nocturia, shaking chills, vomiting, and urinary frequency and urgency. The history may reveal a recent urinary tract procedure, urinary tract infection or obstruction, compromised renal function, or neurogenic bladder.

Other causes
Back pain may also result from appendicitis, cholecystitis, a lumbosacral sprain, osteoporosis, a perforated ulcer, renal calculi, tumors, and vertebral osteomyelitis.

Pain, chest

Patients describe chest pain in many ways. They may report a dull ache, a sensation of heaviness or fullness, a feeling of indigestion, or a sharp, shooting pain. The pain may be constant or intermittent, may radiate to other body parts, and may arise suddenly or gradually. Patients may say that stress, anxiety, exertion, deep breathing, or certain foods seem to trigger the pain.

Chest pain may indicate several acute and life-threatening cardiopulmonary and GI conditions. But it can also result from musculoskeletal and hematologic disorders, anxiety, and certain drugs.

Health history
• When did the chest pain begin? Did it develop suddenly or gradually? Is the pain localized or diffuse? Does it radiate to the neck, jaw, arms, or back? Is the pain sharp and stabbing or dull and aching? Is it constant or intermittent? Does breathing, changing positions, or eating certain foods exacerbate or relieve the pain?
• Do you have any other symptoms, such as coughing, shortness of breath, headache, nausea, palpitations, vomiting, or weakness?
• Have you ever had cardiac or respiratory disease, cardiac surgery, chest trauma, or intestinal disease? Do you have a family history of cardiac disease?
• Do you drink alcohol or use any illicit drugs? What medications are you taking?

Physical examination
Assess the patient's skin temperature, color, and general appearance, noting coolness, cyanosis, diaphoresis, mottling below the waist, pallor, peripheral edema, and prolonged capillary refill time. Look too for facial edema, jugular vein distention, and tracheal deviation. And note any signs of altered level of consciousness, anxiety, dizziness, or restlessness.

Then observe the rate and depth of the patient's respirations, noting any abnormal patterns or breathing difficulty. If the patient has a productive cough, examine the sputum.

Palpate the patient's neck, chest, and abdomen. Note any asymmetrical chest expansion, masses, subcutaneous crepitation, tender areas, tracheal deviation, or tactile fremitus. Also, palpate his peripheral pulses, and record their rate, rhythm, and intensity.

As you percuss over an affected lung, note any dullness. Then auscultate the lungs to identify crackles, diminished or absent breath sounds, pleural friction rubs, rhonchi, or wheezes. Auscultate the heart for clicks, gallops, murmurs, and pericardial friction rub. To check for abdominal bruits, apply the bell of the stethoscope over the abdominal aorta. Be sure to monitor the patient's blood pressure closely.

Causes
Angina
Anginal pain usually begins gradually, builds to a peak, and then slowly subsides. The pain can last from 2 to 10 minutes. It occurs in the retrosternal region and radiates to the neck, jaw, and arms. Associated signs and symptoms include diaphoresis, dyspnea, nausea, vomiting, palpitations, and tachycardia. On auscultation, you may detect an atrial gallop (or S_4 heart sound), or a murmur. Attacks may occur at rest or be provoked by exertion, emotional stress, or a heavy meal.

Aortic aneurysm (dissecting)
A patient with a dissecting aortic aneurysm complains of sudden, excruciating, tearing pain in the chest and neck, radiating to the upper back, lower back, and abdomen. Other signs and symptoms include abdominal tenderness; heart murmurs; jugular vein distention; systolic bruits; tachycardia; weak or absent femoral or pedal pulses; and pale, cool, diaphoretic, mottled skin below the waist.

Cholecystitis
With this disorder, the patient has sudden epigastric or right upper quadrant pain, which may be steady or intermittent, radiate to the back, and be sharp or intense. Other signs and symptoms include chills, diaphoresis, nausea, and vomiting. Palpation of the right upper quadrant may reveal distention, rigidity, tenderness, and a mass.

Myocardial infarction
Usually, the patient has severe, crushing substernal pain that radiates to the left arm, jaw, or neck. The pain may be accompanied by anxiety, clammy skin, diaphoresis, dyspnea, a feeling of impending doom, nausea, vomiting, pallor, and restlessness. The patient may have an atrial gallop (or S_4 heart sound), crackles, hypotension or hypertension, murmurs, and a pericardial friction rub. A history of heart disease, hypertension, hypercholesterolemia, or cocaine abuse is common.

Peptic ulcer
A sharp, burning pain arising in the epigastric region, usually hours after eating, characterizes peptic ulcer. Other signs and symptoms include epigastric tenderness, nausea, and vomiting. Food or antacids usually relieve the pain.

Pneumothorax
A collapsed lung produces a sudden, sharp, severe chest pain that's often unilateral and increases with chest movement. You may detect decreased breath sounds, hyperresonant or tympanic percussion sounds, and subcutaneous crepita-

tion. Other signs and symptoms include accessory muscle use, anxiety, asymmetrical chest expansion, nonproductive cough, tachycardia, and tachypnea. The history may include chronic obstructive pulmonary disease, lung cancer, diagnostic or therapeutic procedures involving the thorax, or thoracic trauma.

Pulmonary embolism
Typically, the patient experiences sudden dyspnea with an intense angina-like or pleuritic ischemic pain aggravated by deep breathing and thoracic movement. Other findings include anxiety, cough with blood-tinged sputum, crackles, dull percussion sounds, restlessness, and tachycardia. If the embolism is large, the cardiovascular, pulmonary, and neurologic systems may be compromised. The patient's history may reveal thrombophlebitis, a hip or leg fracture, acute myocardial infarction, congestive heart failure, pregnancy, or the use of oral contraceptives.

Other causes
Chest pain may also result from abrupt withdrawal of beta blockers, acute bronchitis, anxiety, esophageal spasm, lung abscess, muscle strain, pancreatitis, pneumonia, a rib fracture, or tuberculosis.

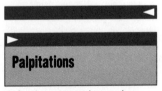

Palpitations

Defined as a person's conscious awareness of his own heartbeat, palpitations are usually felt over the precordium or in the throat or neck. The patient may describe his heart as pounding, jumping, turning, fluttering, flopping, or missing or skipping beats. Palpitations may be regular or irregular, fast or slow, and paroxysmal or sustained. Besides cardiac causes, palpitations may stem from anxiety, drug reactions, hypertension, thyroid hormone deficiency, and several other problems.

Health history
• When did the palpitations start? Where do you feel them? How would you describe them? What were you doing when they started? How long did they last? Have you ever had palpitations before?
• Do you have chest pain, dizziness, or weakness along with the palpitations?
• Are you under unusual stress at home or at work? Have you recently undergone multiple blood transfusions or an infusion of phosphate?
• Have you ever had thyroid disease, calcium or vitamin D deficiency, malabsorption syndrome, bone cancer, renal disease, hypoglycemia, or cardiovascular or pulmonary disorders that may produce arrhythmias or hypertension?
• What medications are you taking? Are you taking an over-the-counter drug that contains caffeine or a sympathomimetic, such as a cough, cold, or allergy preparation? Do you smoke or drink alcohol? If so, how much?

Physical examination
Assess the patient's level of consciousness, noting any anxiety, confusion, or irrational behavior. Check his skin for pallor and diaphoresis. Then observe the eyes for exophthalmos.

Note the rate and depth of his respirations, checking for abnormal patterns and breathing difficulty. Also, inspect the fingertips for capillary nail bed pulsations.

To check for thyroid gland enlargement, gently palpate the patient's neck. Then palpate his muscles for weakness and twitching. Evaluate his peripheral pulses, noting the rate, rhythm, and intensity. And assess his reflexes for hyperreflexia.

Auscultate the heart for gallops and murmurs, and the lungs for abnormal breath sounds. Be sure to monitor blood pressure and pulse pressure.

Causes

Acute anxiety attack

Palpitations may be accompanied by diaphoresis, facial flushing, and trembling. The patient usually hyperventilates, which may lead to dizziness, syncope, and weakness.

Cardiac arrhythmias

Paroxysmal or sustained palpitations may occur with dizziness, fatigue, and weakness. Other signs and symptoms include chest pain; confusion; decreased blood pressure; diaphoresis; pallor; and an irregular, rapid, or slow pulse rate. The patient may be using drugs that can cause cardiac arrhythmias — for instance, antihypertensives, sympathomimetics, ganglionic blockers, anticholinergics, or methylxanthines.

Thyrotoxicosis

In this disorder, sustained palpitations may accompany diaphoresis, diarrhea, dyspnea, heat intolerance, nervousness, tachycardia, tremors, and weight loss despite increased appetite. Exophthalmos and an enlarged thyroid gland may also develop.

Other causes

Palpitations may also arise from anemia, aortic insufficiency, hypocalcemia, hypertension, hypoglycemia, mitral valve stenosis or prolapse, and pheochromocytoma.

Paresthesia

Paresthesia is an abnormal sensation, commonly described as a numbness, prickling, or tingling, that's felt along peripheral nerve pathways. It may develop suddenly or gradually and be transient or permanent. A common symptom of many neurologic disorders, paresthesia may also occur in certain systemic disorders and with the use of certain drugs.

Health history

• When did the paresthesia begin? What does it feel like? Where does it occur? Is it transient or constant?
• Have you had recent trauma, surgery, or an invasive procedure that may have injured peripheral nerves? Have you been exposed to industrial solvents or heavy metals? Have you had long-term radiation therapy? Do you have any neurologic, cardiovascular, metabolic, renal, or chronic inflammatory disorders, such as arthritis or lupus erythematosus?
• What medications are you taking?

Physical examination

Focus on the patient's neurologic status, assessing his level of consciousness and cranial nerve function. Also note his skin color and temperature.

Test muscle strength and deep tendon reflexes in the extremities affected by paresthesia. Systematically evaluate light touch, pain, temperature, vibration, and position sensation. Then palpate his pulses.

Causes

Arterial occlusion (acute)

A patient with a saddle embolus may complain of sudden paresthesia and coldness in one or both legs. Aching pain at rest, intermittent claudication, and paresis are also characteristic. The leg becomes mottled, and a line of temperature and color demarcation develops at the level of the occlusion. Pulses are absent below the occlusion and capillary refill time is diminished.

Brain tumor
Tumors that affect the parietal lobe may cause progressive contralateral paresthesia accompanied by agnosia, agraphia, apraxia, homonymous hemianopia, and loss of proprioception.

Herniated disk
Herniation of a lumbar or cervical disk may cause acute or gradual paresthesia along the distribution pathways of the affected spinal nerves. Other neuromuscular effects include muscle spasms, severe pain, and weakness.

Herpes zoster
Paresthesia, an early symptom of herpes zoster, occurs in the dermatome supplied by the affected spinal nerve. Within several days, this dermatome is marked by a pruritic, erythematous, vesicular rash accompanied by sharp, shooting pain.

Spinal cord injury
Paresthesia may occur in a partial spinal cord transection after spinal shock resolves. The paresthesia may be unilateral or bilateral and occur at or below the level of the lesion.

Other disorders
Paresthesia may result from arthritis, a cerebrovascular accident, migraine headache, multiple sclerosis, peripheral neuropathies, vitamin B_{12} deficiency, hypocalcemia, and heavy metal or solvent poisoning. Also, long-term radiation therapy, parenteral gold therapy, and certain drugs — such as chemotherapeutic agents, guanadrel (Hylorel), interferons, and isoniazid (Laniazid) — may cause paresthesia.

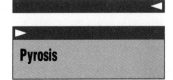

Pyrosis

A substernal burning sensation that rises in the chest and may radiate to the neck or throat, pyrosis results from the reflux of gastric contents into the esophagus. Usually, it is accompanied by regurgitation. Because increased intra-abdominal pressure contributes to reflux, pyrosis commonly occurs with pregnancy, ascites, or obesity, but it may also be caused by GI disorders, connective tissue disease, and certain drugs.

In most cases, pyrosis develops after meals or when a person lies down, bends over, lifts heavy objects, or exercises vigorously. It usually worsens with swallowing and improves when the person sits upright or takes antacids. Some patients confuse pyrosis with a myocardial infarction (MI), but a patient who is having an MI typically has other symptoms besides a burning sensation.

When a patient complains of pyrosis, you'll obtain a health history, but you won't perform a physical examination.

Health history
• When did the pyrosis start? Do certain foods or beverages seem to trigger it? Does stress or fatigue seem to aggravate it? Do movement, certain body positions, or very hot or cold liquids worsen or relieve it? Where exactly is the burning sensation? Does it radiate to other areas? Does it cause you to regurgitate sour- or bitter-tasting

fluids? Have you ever had pyrosis before?

• Do you have a history of GI problems or connective tissue disease? For women of child-bearing age: are you pregnant?

• What medications are you taking?

Causes
Esophageal cancer
Pyrosis may be a sign of esophageal cancer. The first symptom is usually painless dysphagia that progressively worsens. Eventually, partial obstruction and rapid weight loss occur. The patient may complain of a feeling of substernal fullness, hoarseness, nausea, sore throat, steady pain in the posterior and anterior chest, and vomiting.

Gastroesophageal reflux
Severe, chronic pyrosis is the most common symptom of this disorder. The pyrosis usually occurs within 1 hour after eating and may be triggered by certain foods or beverages. It worsens when the person lies down or bends over and abates when he sits, stands, or ingests antacids. Other findings include a dull retrosternal pain that may radiate, dysphagia, flatulent dyspepsia, and postural regurgitation.

Peptic ulcer
Pyrosis and indigestion usually signal the onset of a peptic ulcer attack. Most patients experience a gnawing, burning pain in the left epigastrium, although some report sharp pain. The pain typically occurs when the stomach is empty and is often relieved by taking antacids. The pain may also occur after the patient ingests coffee, aspirin, or alcohol.

Scleroderma
A connective tissue disease, scleroderma may cause esophageal dysfunction resulting in pyrosis, bloating after meals, odynophagia, the sensation of food sticking behind the sternum, and weight loss. Other GI effects include abdominal distention, constipation or diarrhea, and malodorous, floating stools.

Other disorders
Pyrosis may also be caused by esophageal diverticula, obesity, and several drugs, including aspirin, nonsteroidal anti-inflammatory drugs, anticholinergic agents, inhalational corticosteroids or inhalational beta-adrenergic agents, and drugs having anticholinergic effects.

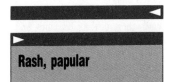

Rash, papular

Consisting of small, raised, circumscribed and, possibly, discolored lesions, a papular rash can erupt anywhere on the body and in various configurations. A characteristic sign of many cutaneous disorders, a papular rash may also result from allergies or from infectious, neoplastic, or systemic disorders.

Health history
• When and where did the rash erupt? What did it look like? Has it spread or changed in any way? If so, when and how did it spread?

• Does the rash itch or burn? Is it painful or tender?

• Have you had a fever, GI distress, or a headache? Do you have any allergies? Have you had any previous skin disorders, infections, sexually transmitted diseases, or tumors? What childhood diseases have you had?

• Have you recently been bitten by an insect or a rodent or exposed to anyone with an infectious disease?

• What medications are you taking? Have you applied any topical agents to the rash and, if so, when was the last application?

Physical examination
Observe the color, configuration, and location of the rash.

Causes
Acne vulgaris
The rupture of enlarged comedones produces inflamed and, possibly, painful and pruritic papules, pustules, nodules, or cysts. They may appear on the face, shoulders, chest, and back.

Insect bites
Venom from insect bites – especially those of ticks, lice, flies, and mosquitoes – may cause an allergic reaction that produces a papular, macular, or petechial rash. Associated findings include fever, headache, lymphadenopathy, myalgia, nausea, and vomiting.

Kaposi's sarcoma
A neoplastic disorder most commonly found in patients with acquired immunodeficiency syndrome, Kaposi's sarcoma produces purple or blue papules or macules on the extremities, ears, and nose. Firm pressure causes these lesions to decrease in size, but they return to their original size within 10 to 15 seconds. The lesions may become scaly, ulcerate, and bleed.

Psoriasis
In this disorder, small, erythematous, pruritic papules appear on the scalp, chest, elbows, knees, back, buttocks, and genitalia. The papules may be painful. They enlarge and coalesce, forming elevated, red, plaques covered by silver scales, except in moist areas, such as the genitalia. The scales may flake off easily or thicken, covering the plaque. Other common findings include pitted fingernails and arthralgia.

Other causes
Infectious mononucleosis or sarcoidosis may produce a papular rash. Such a rash may also be caused by nonsteroidal anti-inflammatory drugs, succimer (Chemet), and interferons.

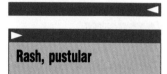

Rash, pustular

Crops of pustules (small, elevated, circumscribed lesions), vesicles (small blisters), and bullae (large blisters) filled with purulent exudate make up a pustular rash. The lesions vary in size and shape and may be generalized or localized (limited to the hair follicles or sweat glands).

Pustules may result from skin disorders, systemic disorders, ingestion of certain drugs, and exposure to skin irritants. Although many pustular lesions are sterile, a pustular rash usually indicates infection.

Health history
• When and where did the rash erupt? Did another type of skin lesion precede the pustules?
• What does the rash look like? Has it spread or changed in any way? If so, how and where did it spread?
• Have you ever had a skin disorder? Do you have any allergies? What about family members?
• What medications are you taking? Have you applied any topical medication to the rash and, if so, when did you last apply it?

Physical examination
Examine the entire skin surface, noting if it's dry, oily, moist, or greasy. Record the exact location, distribution, color, shape, and size of the lesions.

Causes

Folliculitis

A bacterial infection of the hair follicles, folliculitis produces individual pustules, each pierced by a hair. The patient may also suffer from pruritus. Hot-tub folliculitis is characterized by pustules on the area covered by a bathing suit.

Scabies

Threadlike channels or burrows under the skin characterize scabies, a disorder that can also produce pustules, vesicles, and excoriations. The lesions are 1 to 10 cm long, with a swollen nodule or red papule containing the itch mite. In men, crusted lesions often develop on the glans and shaft of the penis and on the scrotum. In women, lesions may form on the nipples. Other common sites include the wrists, elbows, axillae, and waist.

Other causes

A pustular rash may result from blastomycosis, furunculosis, and pustular psoriasis. Also, certain drugs – such as bromides, iodides, corticotropin (ACTH), corticosteroids, lithium (Eskalith), phenytoin (Dilantin), phenobarbital (Luminal), isoniazid (Laniazid), and oral contraceptives – can cause a pustular rash.

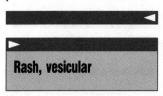

Rash, vesicular

The lesions in a vesicular rash are scattered or linear vesicles that are sharply circumscribed and usually less than 0.5 cm in diameter. They may be filled with clear, cloudy, or bloody fluid. Lesions larger than 0.5 cm in diameter are called bullae. A vesicular rash may be mild or severe, transient or permanent.

Health history

• When and where did the rash erupt? Did other skin lesions precede the vesicles?
• What does the rash look like? Has it spread or changed in any way? If so, how and where did it spread?
• Do you have a history of allergies or skin disorders? Does anyone else in your family?
• Have you recently had an infection or been bitten by an insect?

Physical examination

Examine the patient's skin and note the location, general distribution, color, shape, and size of the lesions. Check for crusts, macules, papules, scales, scars, and wheals. Note whether the outer layer of epidermis separates easily from the basal layer.

Palpate the vesicles or bullae to determine whether they're flaccid or tense.

Causes

Burns

Thermal burns that affect the epidermis and part of the dermis often cause vesicles and bullae, along with erythema, moistness, pain, and swelling.

Herpes zoster

First, fever and malaise occur. Then, the vesicular rash appears along a dermatome. This rash is accompanied by pruritus, deep pain, and paresthesia or hyperesthesia, usually of the trunk and sometimes of the arms and legs. The vesicles erupt, dry up, and form scabs in about 10 days. Occasionally, herpes zoster involves the cranial nerves; such involvement produces dizziness, eye pain, facial palsy, hearing loss, impaired vision, and loss of taste.

Other causes

Other causes of vesicular rashes include dermatitis, herpes simplex, insect bites, pemphigus, scabies, tinea pedis, and toxic epidermal necrolysis.

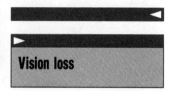

Vision loss

Vision loss can occur suddenly or gradually, be temporary or permanent, and may range from a slight impairment to total blindness. It may result from eye, neurologic, and systemic disorders, as well as from trauma and reactions to certain drugs.

Health history

• When did the loss first occur? Did it occur suddenly or gradually? Does it affect one or both eyes? Does it affect all or part of the visual field?
• Are you experiencing blurred vision, halo vision, nausea, pain, photosensitivity, or vomiting with the vision loss?
• Have you had a recent facial or eye injury?
• Have you ever had cardiovascular or endocrine disorders, infections, or allergies? Does anyone in your family have a history of vision loss or other eye problems?
• What medications are you taking?

Physical examination

Observe the patient's eyes for conjunctival or scleral redness, drainage, edema, foreign bodies, and signs of trauma. With a flashlight, examine the cornea and iris. Observe the size, shape, and color of the pupils. Then test direct and consensual light reflexes and visual accommodation, extraocular muscle function, and visual acuity. Gently palpate each eye, noting any hardness. Then auscultate over the neck and temple for carotid bruits.

Causes

Glaucoma

Acute angle-closure glaucoma may cause rapid blindness. Findings include halo vision, nonreactive pupillary response, photophobia, rapid onset of unilateral inflammation and pain, and reduced visual acuity. By contrast, chronic open-angle glaucoma progresses slowly. Usually bilateral, it causes aching eyes, halo vision, peripheral vision loss, and reduced visual acuity.

Eye trauma

Sudden unilateral or bilateral vision loss may occur after an eye injury. The loss may be total or partial, permanent or temporary. The eyelids may be reddened, edematous, and lacerated.

Other causes

Vision loss may also be caused by congenital rubella or syphilis, herpes zoster, Marfan's syndrome, a pituitary tumor, retrolental fibroplasia, and drugs such as digitalis glycosides, indomethacin (Indocin), ethambutol hydrochloride (Myambutol), quinine sulfate (Quinamm), and methanol.

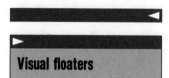

Visual floaters

Particles of blood or cellular debris that move about in the vitreous humor appear as spots or dots when they enter the visual field. Chronic floaters commonly occur in elderly or myopic patients. But the sudden onset of visual floaters often signals retinal detachment, an ocular emergency.

Health history
• When did the floaters first appear? What do they look like? Did they appear suddenly or gradually? If they appeared suddenly, did you also see flashing lights and have a curtainlike loss of vision?
• Are you nearsighted, and do you wear corrective lenses?
• Do you have a history of eye trauma or other eye disorders, allergies, granulomatous disease, diabetes mellitus, or hypertension?
• What medications are you taking?

Physical examination
Inspect the eyes for signs of injury, such as bruising or edema. Then assess the patient's visual acuity, using the Snellen alphabet or "E" chart.

Causes
Retinal detachment
Floaters and light flashes appear suddenly in the portion of the visual field where the retina has detached. As retinal detachment progresses (a painless process), gradual vision loss occurs, with the patient seeing a "curtain" falling in front of his eyes. Ophthalmoscopic examination reveals a gray, opaque, detached retina with an indefinite margin. Retinal vessels appear almost black.

Vitreous hemorrhage
Rupture of retinal vessels produces a shower of red or black dots or a red haze across the visual field. Vision blurs suddenly in the affected eye, and visual acuity may be greatly reduced.

Other causes
Visual floaters may also result from posterior uveitis.

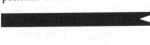

Weight loss

Weight loss can reflect decreased food intake, increased metabolic requirements, or a combination of the two. Its causes include endocrine, neoplastic, GI, and psychological disorders; nutritional deficiencies; infections; and neurologic lesions that cause paralysis and dysphagia. Weight loss may also accompany conditions that prevent sufficient food intake, such as painful oral lesions, ill-fitting dentures, and the loss of teeth. Weight loss may stem from poverty, adherence to fad diets, excessive exercise, or drug use.

Health history
• When did you first notice you were losing weight? How much weight have you lost? Was the loss intentional? If not, can you think of any reason for it?
• What do you usually eat in a day? Have your eating habits changed recently? Why?
• Have your stools changed recently? For instance, have you noticed bulky, floating stools or have you had diarrhea? What about abdominal pain, excessive thirst, excessive urination, heat intolerance, nausea, or vomiting?
• Have you felt anxious or depressed? If so, why?
• What medications are you taking? Do you take diet pills or laxatives to lose weight?

Physical examination
Record the patient's height and weight. As you take his vital signs, note his general appearance. Does he appear well-nourished? Do his clothes fit? Is muscle wasting evident?

Next, examine his skin for turgor

and abnormal pigmentation, especially around the joints. Does he have jaundice or pallor? Examine his mouth, including the condition of his teeth or dentures. Also check his eyes for exophthalmos and his neck for swelling.

Finally, palpate the patient's abdomen for liver enlargement, masses, and tenderness.

Causes

Anorexia nervosa

A psychogenic disorder, anorexia nervosa is most common in young women and is characterized by a severe, self-imposed weight loss. This may be accompanied by amenorrhea, blotchy or sallow skin, cold intolerance, constipation, frequent infections, loss of fatty tissue, loss of scalp hair, and skeletal muscle atrophy.

Cancer

Weight loss is frequently a sign of cancer. Associated signs and symptoms reflect the type, location, and stage of the tumor, and typically include abnormal bleeding, anorexia, fatigue, nausea, pain, a palpable mass, and vomiting.

Crohn's disease

Weight loss occurs with abdominal pain, anorexia, and chronic cramping. Other findings include abdominal distention, tenderness, and guarding; diarrhea; hyperactive bowel sounds; pain; and tachycardia.

Depression

In severe depression, weight loss may occur along with anorexia, apathy, fatigue, feelings of worthlessness, and insomnia or hypersomnia. Other signs and symptoms include incoherence, indecisiveness, and suicidal thoughts or behavior.

Leukemia

Acute leukemia causes a progressive weight loss accompanied by bleeding tendencies, high fever, and severe prostration. Chronic leukemia causes a progressive weight loss with anemia, anorexia, bleeding tendencies, an enlarged spleen, fatigue, fever, pallor, and skin eruptions.

Other causes

Weight loss may result from adrenal insufficiency, diabetes mellitus, gastroenteritis, cryptosporidiosis, lymphoma, ulcerative colitis, and thyrotoxicosis. Drugs such as amphetamines, chemotherapeutic agents, laxatives, and thyroid preparations can also cause weight loss.

◄

Detecting commonly overlooked problems

Not every disorder can be detected by systematically assessing a patient's chief complaint. Sometimes, a patient's signs and symptoms are so subtle or insidious that an underlying clinical problem can be easily missed.

What makes certain disorders hard to detect? The reasons vary, but in many cases, not even the patient knows something is wrong. For example, a woman with early-stage ovarian cancer may be asymptomatic, whereas a hypothyroid patient may dismiss overt symptoms as an inevitable result of old age.

The key to detecting hidden illness is to heighten your awareness of the risk factors for disorders and the early signs and symptoms. Review the disorders described below, which head the list of commonly overlooked problems. Then, when you encounter patients with risk factors for any of these conditions, use your assessment skills to check for abnormal findings. Typically, you'll also need to examine test results to form an accurate diagnostic impression.

▶

Adult respiratory distress syndrome

Difficult to recognize, adult respiratory distress syndrome (ARDS) can quickly lead to acute respiratory failure. Prompt and accurate assessment is essential, because the syndrome can prove fatal within 48 hours of its onset if not promptly detected and treated.

A form of pulmonary edema, ARDS may follow direct or indirect lung injury. Increased permeability of the alveolocapillary membranes allows fluid to accumulate in the lung interstitium, alveolar spaces, and small airways, causing the lung to stiffen. This impairs ventilation, reducing oxygenation of pulmonary capillary blood.

Although this four-stage syndrome can progress to intractable and fatal hypoxemia, patients who recover may have little or no permanent lung damage. The sooner the patient is assessed and correctly diagnosed, the better his chances for complete recovery.

In some patients, the syndrome may coexist with disseminated intravascular coagulation. Whether ARDS stems from disseminated intravascular coagulation or develops independently remains unclear.

Assessment
As you conduct your assessment, be alert for the patient's particular stage of ARDS. Each has typical signs.

Stage I
The patient may complain of dyspnea, especially on exertion. Respiratory and pulse rates are normal to high. Auscultation may reveal diminished breath sounds.

Stage II
Respiratory distress becomes more apparent. The patient may use accessory muscles to breathe and appear pallid, anxious, and restless. He may have a dry cough with thick, frothy sputum and bloody, sticky secretions. Palpation may disclose cool, clammy skin. Tachycardia and tachypnea may accompany elevated blood pressure. Auscultation may detect basilar crackles.

Be aware that stage II signs and symptoms are often incorrectly attributed to other causes, such as multiple trauma.

Stage III
You'll observe the patient struggling to breathe. A check of vital signs reveals tachypnea (more than 30 breaths/minute), tachycardia with arrhythmias (usually premature ventricular contractions), and a labile blood pressure. Inspection may reveal a productive cough and pale, cyanotic skin. Auscultation may disclose crackles and rhonchi. The patient will need intubation and ventilation.

Stage IV
The patient has acute respiratory failure with severe hypoxia. His mental status is deteriorating, and he may become comatose. His skin appears pale and cyanotic. Spontaneous respirations are not evident. Bradycardia with arrhythmias accompanies hypotension. Metabolic and respiratory acidosis develop. When ARDS reaches this stage, the patient is at high risk for fibrosis. Pulmonary damage becomes life-threatening.

ASSESSMENT FINDINGS

Diagnostic tests

• Arterial blood gas (ABG) analysis (with the patient breathing room air) initially shows a reduced partial pressure of oxygen (PaO_2) (less than 60 mm Hg) and a decreased partial pressure of carbon dioxide ($PaCO_2$) (less than 35 mm Hg). Hypoxemia despite increased supplemental oxygen is the hallmark of ARDS. The resulting blood pH usually reflects respiratory alkalosis. As ARDS worsens, ABG values show respiratory acidosis (increasing $PaCO_2$ [more than 45 mm Hg]) and metabolic acidosis (decreasing HCO^-_3 levels [less than 22 mEq/liter]) and declining PaO_2 despite oxygen therapy.

• Pulmonary artery catheterization helps identify the cause of pulmonary edema by measuring pulmonary artery wedge pressure (PAWP). This procedure also allows collection of samples of pulmonary artery, mixed venous blood that show decreased oxygen saturation, reflecting tissue hypoxia. Normal PAWP values in ARDS are 12 mm Hg or less.

• Serial chest X-rays in early stages show bilateral infiltrates. In later stages, findings demonstrate lung fields with a ground-glass appearance and, eventually (with irreversible hypoxemia), "whiteouts" of both lung fields.

Differential diagnosis must rule out cardiogenic pulmonary edema, pulmonary vasculitis, and diffuse pulmonary hemorrhage. Etiologic tests may involve sputum analyses (including Gram stain and culture and sensitivity); blood cultures (to identify infectious organisms); toxicology tests (to screen for drug ingestion); and various serum amylase tests (to rule out pancreatitis).

Bulimia nervosa

Although 5% to 15% of adult women have some symptoms of bulimia nervosa, many are never diagnosed or treated. Why? Because unlike anorexia nervosa, which causes patients to become emaciated, bulimic patients often manage to keep their weight within the normal range. Also, because bulimic patients tend to practice their habits in private, this eating disorder often remains hidden.

The essential features of bulimia nervosa include eating binges followed by feelings of guilt, humiliation, and self-deprecation. These feelings precipitate self-induced vomiting, the use of laxatives or diuretics, or strict dieting or fasting to overcome the effects of the binges. Unless the patient devotes an excessive amount of time to binging and purging, bulimia nervosa seldom is incapacitating.

Bulimia nervosa usually begins in adolescence or early adulthood and can occur simultaneously with anorexia nervosa. It affects nine females for every one male.

Assessment
Health history

Ask questions to elicit information about eating disorders, especially if your patient is an adolescent or young adult woman. Use nonthreatening questions, such as "Many young women have concerns about their weight or about food. Do you have any concerns about weight or food?" Also, pay particular attention to overt psychological clues. These include:

• peculiar eating habits or rituals
• frequent weighing
• distorted body image
• difficulties with impulse control

- chronic depression
- exaggerated sense of guilt
- low tolerance for frustration
- recurrent anxiety
- feelings of alienation
- self-consciousness
- difficulty expressing feelings, such as anger
- impaired social or occupational adjustment.

In bulimic patients, episodic binge eating may occur up to several times a day. The patient commonly reports a binge-eating episode during which she continues eating until abdominal pain, sleep, or the presence of another person interrupts her. The preferred food usually is sweet, soft, and high in calories and carbohydrates.

Signs and symptoms

Be alert for the following complaints or signs:
- abdominal and epigastric pain, resulting from acute gastric dilation
- amenorrhea
- painless swelling of the salivary glands, hoarseness, throat irritation or lacerations, and dental erosion — all signs of repetitive vomiting
- calluses of the knuckles or abrasions and scars on the dorsum of the hand, resulting from tooth injury during self-induced vomiting.

Diagnostic criteria

Diagnosis is made when the patient meets the *Diagnostic and Statistical Manual IV* criteria for this disorder: recurrent episodes of binge eating (rapid consumption of a large amount of food in a discrete period of time) and recurrent episodes of inappropriate compensatory behavior to prevent weight gain (self-induced vomiting; misuse of laxatives, enemas, or other medications; fasting). Both of these behaviors must occur at least twice a week for 3 months.

The following tests help to detect complications or determine the course of therapy:
- The Beck Depression Inventory may identify coexisting depression.
- Laboratory tests can help determine the presence and severity of complications.
- A baseline electrocardiogram should be done if tricyclic antidepressants will be prescribed.

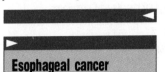

Esophageal cancer

Most common in men over age 60, esophageal cancer usually is advanced when diagnosed. Surgery and other treatments are palliative, not curative. As a result, the prognosis for this cancer is poor: 5-year survival rates are less than 5%, and most patients die within 6 months of diagnosis. Recognition of early signs and symptoms during GI assessment could help to improve the prognosis.

Esophageal tumors are usually rapidly growing and infiltrating. In most cases, the tumor partially constricts the lumen of the esophagus. Regional metastasis occurs early by way of submucosal lymphatics, often fatally invading adjacent intrathoracic organs. If the patient survives primary extension, the liver and lungs are the usual sites of distant metastases. Most esophageal cancers (98%) arise in squamous cell epithelium, although a few are adenocarcinomas and fewer still, melanomas and sarcomas.

Assessment
Early signs and symptoms

Early in the disease, the patient may report a feeling of fullness, pressure, indigestion, or substernal burning. He may also tell you he uses antacids to relieve GI upset. Because these symptoms are often mistaken for heartburn, the disease often goes undiagnosed in its early stages, when it can be most successfully treated. To promote early detection, refer patients with chronic or recurring heartburn for complete diagnostic workups.

Later signs and symptoms

The patient may complain of dysphagia and weight loss. The degree of dysphagia varies, depending on the extent of disease. At first, the dysphagia is mild, occurring only after the patient eats solid foods, especially meat. Later, he has difficulty swallowing coarse foods and, in some cases, liquids.

As the disease progresses, your assessment also may detect these signs and symptoms:
• hoarseness, resulting from laryngeal nerve involvement
• chronic cough, possibly from aspiration
• anorexia, vomiting, and regurgitation of food—all signs that the tumor's size has exceeded the limits of the esophagus
• pain on swallowing or pain that radiates to the back
• extreme weight loss, cachexia, and dehydration—signs of late-stage disease.

Diagnostic tests

• X-rays of the esophagus, with barium swallow and motility studies, delineate structural and filling defects and reduced peristalsis.
• Chest X-rays or esophagography may reveal pneumonitis.
• Esophagoscopy, punch or brush biopsies, and exfoliative cytologic tests confirm esophageal tumors.
• Bronchoscopy (usally performed after esophagoscopy) may reveal tumor growth in the tracheobronchial tree.
• Endoscopic ultrasonography of the esophagus combines endoscopy and ultrasound technology to measure the depth of penetration of the tumor.
• Computed tomography scan may help diagnose and monitor esophageal lesions.
• Magnetic resonance imaging scan permits evaluation of the esophagus and adjacent structures.
• Liver function studies and other laboratory tests may reveal abnormalities. If so, a liver scan and mediastinal tomography scan can help reveal the extent of the disease.

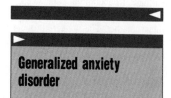

Generalized anxiety disorder

A rational response to a real threat, occasional anxiety is a normal part of life. However, overwhelming anxiety can result in generalized anxiety disorder—uncontrollable, unreasonable worry that persists for at least 6 months and narrows perceptions or interferes with normal functioning.

Recent evidence shows that the prevalence of generalized anxiety disorder is greater than previously thought and may even exceed that of depression. However, because many patients aren't aware that anxiety is a treatable disorder like depression, they may not seek appropriate therapy or understand the nature of their symptoms. Astute nursing assessment can help patients to recognize and obtain treatment.

Assessment

Psychological or physiologic symptoms of anxiety vary with the severity of the symptom. Use these criteria to help you recognize and quantify anxiety in your patient.

Mild anxiety

The patient reports slight discomfort. He is alert, asks questions, seeks help, and can solve problems. Mild anxiety mainly causes psychological symptoms, with unusual self-awareness and alertness to the environment.

Moderate anxiety

The moderately anxious patient is irritable, may speak rapidly, and appears restless and shaky. The patient needs help to focus on the presenting problem. Moderate anxiety leads to selective inattention, yet with the ability to concentrate on a single task.

Severe anxiety

The patient with severe anxiety can't cope with his situation; for example, he may say, "I can't think" or "I don't know what to do." He may not hear or pay attention to directions or information. Severe anxiety causes an inability to concentrate on more than scattered details of a task.

Panic

In this state, the patient's behavior projects great emotional pain and disorganization. He may be unresponsive or run about wildly. He's unable to focus his attention to solve problems. Panic with acute anxiety causes a complete loss of concentration, often with unintelligible speech.

Physical examination may reveal symptoms of motor tension, including trembling, muscle aches and spasms, headaches, and an inability to relax. Autonomic signs and symptoms include shortness of breath, tachycardia, sweating, and abdominal complaints.

In addition, the patient may startle easily and complain of feeling apprehensive, fearful, or angry and of having difficulty concentrating, eating, and sleeping. The medical, psychiatric, and psychosocial histories fail to identify a specific physical or environmental cause of the anxiety.

Diagnostic criteria

When the patient's symptoms match criteria documented in the *Diagnostic and Statistical Manual IV,* the diagnosis of generalized anxiety disorder is confirmed. The criteria include the following:
• The patient has unrealistic or excessive anxiety and worry about a number of events or activities for 6 months (or longer), during which he has been bothered most days by these concerns. In children and adolescents, this may take the form of anxiety and worry about academic, athletic, and social performance.
• The patient finds it difficult to control the worry.
• The focus of the anxiety and worry is not confined to features of an Axis I disorder.
• The anxiety, worry, or physical symptoms cause clinically significant distress or impairment in social, occupational, or other important areas of functioning.
• The disturbance is not due to the direct physiologic effects of a substance or a general medical condition and does not occur exclusively during a mood disorder, a psychotic disorder, or a pervasive developmental disorder.
• The anxiety and worry are associated with at least three of the following six symptoms:
– restlessness or feeling keyed up or on the edge
– easy fatigability
– difficulty concentrating or mind going blank
– irritability
– muscle tension
– sleep disturbances (difficulty falling or staying asleep, or restless, unsatisfying sleep).

Laboratory tests must exclude organic causes of the patient's signs and symptoms, such as hyperthyroidism, pheochromocytoma, coronary artery disease, supraventricular tachycardia, and Ménière's disease.

Because anxiety is the central symptom of other mental disorders, psychiatric evaluation must rule out phobias, obsessive-compulsive disorders, depression, and acute schizophrenia.

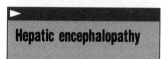

Hepatic encephalopathy

A neurologic syndrome, hepatic encephalopathy develops as a complication of aggressive fulminant hepatitis or chronic hepatic disease. Most common in patients with cirrhosis, this syndrome may be acute and self-limiting or chronic and progressive.

Prognosis is best if the syndrome is detected and treated promptly. However, because early symptoms are so subtle, they're typically overlooked. In advanced stages, the prognosis is extremely poor despite vigorous treatment. When you encounter patients at risk for hepatic encephalopathy, such as those with cirrhosis, routinely assess them for signs and symptoms of this syndrome. Be especially alert to slight changes in behavior or mental status that may signal early-stage symptoms.

Assessment

Clinical features vary, depending on the severity of neurologic involvement. The disorder usually progresses through four stages, but the patient's symptoms can fluctuate from one stage to another. Be on the lookout for characteristic signs

and symptoms of these major stages.

Prodromal stage

Although symptoms may not be obvious in this stage, suspect hepatic encephalopathy in high-risk patients who exhibit the following signs and symptoms:
• trouble concentrating or thinking clearly
• fatigue or drowsiness
• slurred or slowed speech
• slight tremor
• slight personality changes, such as agitation, belligerence, disorientation, or forgetfulness.

Impending stage

The patient undergoes continuing mental changes. Watch for confusion and disorientation as to time, place, and person. Inspection continues to reveal tremors that have progressed to asterixis. The hallmark of hepatic encephalopathy, asterixis refers to quick, irregular extensions and flexions of the wrists and fingers, when the wrists are held out straight and the hands flexed upward. On inspection, you may observe lethargy and aberrant behavior. Some patients demonstrate apraxia. When asked, the patient is unable to reproduce a simple design, such as a star.

Stuporous stage

The patient shows marked confusion. On inspection, he appears drowsy and stuporous. Yet he can still be aroused and is often noisy and abusive when aroused. Hyperventilation, muscle twitching, and asterixis are also evident.

Comatose stage

The patient cannot be aroused and is obtunded with no asterixis. Seizures, though uncommon, may occur. Palpation may reveal hyperactive reflexes and demonstrate a positive Babinski's sign. The patient often has fetor hepaticus (musty odor of the breath and urine). Fetor hepaticus may occur in other stages also.

Diagnostic tests
• Serum ammonia levels in venous and arterial samples are elevated and, together with characteristic clinical features, strongly suggest hepatic encephalopathy.
• Electroencephalography shows slowing waves as the disease progresses.

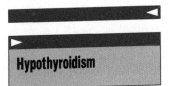

Hypothyroidism

When a patient complains of feeling tired, run-down, and out of sorts, don't overlook the possibility of hypothyroidism. Vague and varied, the symptoms of hypothyroidism are easy to miss, and up to half of cases go undiagnosed.

In hypothyroidism, metabolic processes slow down because of a deficiency of the thyroid hormones triiodothyronine (T_3) or thyroxine (T_4). Hypothyroidism is classified as primary or secondary. Primary hypothyroidism stems from a disorder of the thyroid gland itself. Secondary hypothyroidism stems from a failure to stimulate normal thyroid function or by a failure of target tissues to respond to normal blood levels of thyroid hormones. Either type may progress to myxedema, which is considered a medical emergency.

Hypothyroidism is most prevalent in women; in North America, its incidence is rising significantly in persons ages 40 to 50.

Assessment
Health history
The patient may simply complain that she feels "old" or "run-down." Many patients dismiss symptoms such as fatigue, forgetfulness, and joint stiffness as inevitable signs of aging. Other common complaints include energy loss, sensitivity to cold, unexplained weight gain, constipation, anorexia, decreased libido, menorrhagia, paresthesia, and muscle cramping.

Inspection
You'll observe characteristic alterations in the patient's overall appearance and behavior. These changes include decreased mental stability (slight mental slowing to severe obtundation) and a thick, dry tongue, causing hoarseness and slow, slurred speech.

You'll probably note dry, flaky, inelastic skin; puffy face, hands, and feet; periorbital edema; and drooping upper eyelids. Hair may be dry and sparse with patchy hair loss and loss of the outer third of the eyebrow. Nails may be thick and brittle with visible transverse and longitudinal grooves. You may also find ataxia, intention tremor, and nystagmus.

Palpation
You may detect rough, doughy skin that feels cool; a weak pulse and bradycardia; muscle weakness; sacral or peripheral edema; and delayed reflex relaxation time (especially in the Achilles tendon). The thyroid tissue itself may not be easily palpable unless a goiter is present.

Auscultation
You may note absent or decreased bowel sounds, hypotension, a gallop or distant heart sounds, and adventitious breath sounds.

Percussion and palpation may detect abdominal distention or ascites.

Diagnostic tests

Hypothyroidism is confirmed when radioimmunoassay with radioactive iodine (^{131}I) shows low serum levels of thyroid hormones and when a thorough history and physical examination show characteristic signs and symptoms. A differential diagnosis may reveal these results:

• Serum TSH levels determine the primary or secondary nature of the disorder. An increased serum TSH level with hypothyroidism results from thyroid insufficiency; a decreased TSH level results from hypothalamic or pituitary insufficiency.

• Serum antithyroid antibodies are elevated in autoimmune thyroiditis.

• Radioisotope scans of thyroid tissue reveal ectopic thyroid tissue.

• Skull X-ray, computed tomography scan, and magnetic resonance imaging help locate pituitary or hypothalamic lesions that may be the underlying cause of hypothyroidism.

AGE ALERT In untreated infants, ECG changes, such as bradycardia and flat or inverted T waves, are seen. Hip, knee, and thigh X-rays reveal absence of the femoral or tibial epiphyseal line and delayed skeletal development that is markedly inappropriate for the child's chronologic age.

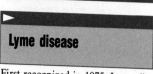

Lyme disease

First recognized in 1975, Lyme disease results from the bite of a tick that's infected with a microorganism called *Borrelia burgdorferi*. Assessment of this disorder is difficult. Because Lyme disease occurs in stages and affects multiple body systems, it may be misdiagnosed as another disorder, such as arthritis. Symptoms of Lyme disease vary from person to person and may be vague. What's more, the infected person may not even remember being bitten by a tick.

Typically, the infection begins in summer or early fall with the classic skin lesion called erythema chronicum migrans. Weeks or months later, cardiac, neurologic, or joint abnormalities develop, possibly followed by arthritis. The incidence has risen in most states over the past 8 years. Although Lyme disease used to be limited to the northeastern United States, outbreaks are spreading west, so it's more important than ever to learn to detect the insidious symptoms.

Assessment
Health history

A thorough exploration of the patient's history is the starting point for detecting Lyme disease. Ask the patient these or similar questions.

• Has he recently been in tick-infested woods or outdoor areas? Does he live, work, play, or take vacations in wooded areas where Lyme disease is endemic?

• Can he recall being bitten by a tick?

• Does he remember noticing a skin rash (erythema chronicum migrans) around the time his symptoms started?

• When did his symptoms first start? (Typically, patients report the onset of symptoms in warmer months, when the ticks are active.)

Early signs and symptoms

Initial symptoms tend to be flulike, including fatigue, malaise, and migratory myalgias and arthralgias. Nearly 10% of patients report cardiac symptoms, such as palpitations and mild dyspnea, especially in the early stage. Severe headache and stiff neck, suggestive of meningeal irritation, also may occur.

More than half of patients get a telltale skin rash called erythema chronicum migrans. The rash begins as a red macule or papule at the tick-bite site and may grow as large as 2″ (5 cm) in diameter. The patient may describe the lesion as hot and pruritic. Characteristic lesions (not seen in all patients) have bright red outer rims and white centers. They usually appear on the axilla, thigh, and groin. Within a few days, other lesions may erupt, as may a migratory, ringlike rash and conjunctivitis. In 3 to 4 weeks, the lesions fade to small red blotches, which persist for several more weeks.

Especially in children, body temperature may rise to 104° F (40° C) in the early stage and be accompanied by chills.

Later signs and symptoms
Bell's palsy may be seen in the second stage and may occur alone. Also during the later stage, inspection may disclose signs and symptoms of intermittent arthritis: joint swelling, redness, and limited movement. Typically, the disease affects one or only a few joints, especially large ones, such as the knee. In the later stage, the patient also may report neurologic symptoms, such as memory loss.

Related signs and symptoms
You may detect tachycardia or an irregular heartbeat. During the first or second stage, you may palpate regional lymphadenopathy as well. The patient may complain of tenderness at the lesion site or the posterior cervical area. Generalized lymphadenopathy is less common.

If the patient has neurologic involvement, Kernig's and Brudzinski's signs usually aren't positive,

and neck stiffness usually occurs only with extreme flexion.

Diagnostic tests
Blood tests, including antibody titers to identify the causative spirochete, *B. burgdorferi*, are the most practical diagnostic tools. Or an enzyme-linked immunosorbent assay (ELISA) may be ordered because of its greater sensitivity and specificity. However, serologic test results don't always confirm the diagnosis — especially in Lyme disease's early stages before the body produces antibodies — or seropositivity for *B. burgdorferi*. Also, the validity of test results depends on laboratory techniques and interpretation.

Other findings
Mild anemia in addition to elevated erythrocyte sedimentation rate, white blood cell count, serum immunoglobulin M levels, and aspartate aminotransferase (formerly called SGOT) levels support the diagnosis.

A lumbar puncture may be ordered if Lyme disease involves the central nervous system. Analysis of cerebrospinal fluid may detect antibodies to *B. burgdorferi*.

Nephrotic syndrome

This syndrome is characterized by marked proteinuria, hypoalbuminemia, hyperlipidemia, and edema. Because the patient with nephrotic syndrome may complain only of lethargy and depression, an underlying kidney disorder may be overlooked.

Nephrotic syndrome results from a glomerular defect that affects the vessels' permeability and indicates renal damage. The prognosis is highly variable, depending on the underlying cause of the glomerular defect. Because some forms of nephrotic syndrome may eventually progress to end-stage renal failure, early assessment is important so that treatment can be implemented before irreversible kidney damage occurs.

Assessment

When you inspect the patient, check closely for edema, a common problem. You may notice periorbital edema, which occurs primarily in the morning and is more common in children; mild-to-severe dependent edema of the ankles or sacrum; or pitting edema. When edema is severe, brawny edema may develop. The tissues swell so that fluid can't be displaced, making pitting impossible. Subcutaneous tissue becomes fibrotic and rock-hard to the touch.

To assess for pitting edema, press your index finger for 5 to 10 seconds over a bony surface, such as the subcutaneous part of the tibia, fibula, sacrum, or sternum. Then remove your finger and note how long the depression remains. Document your observation on a scale from +1 (barely detectable depression) to +4 (persistent pit, 1″ or 2.5 cm), as shown at right.

+1 pitting edema

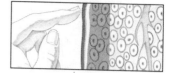

+4 pitting edema

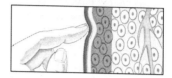

Brawny edema

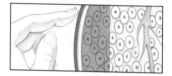

In your assessment you also may note orthostatic hypotension, ascites, swollen external genitalia, signs of pleural effusion, anorexia, and pallor.

Diagnostic tests

The patient's diagnostic workup typically reveals these findings.
• Consistent, heavy proteinuria (levels over 3.5 mg/dl for 24 hours). Examination of urine also reveals an increased number of hyaline, granular, and waxy, fatty casts as well as oval fat bodies.
• Increased serum levels of cholesterol, phospholipids (especially low-density and very-low-density lipoproteins), and triglycerides, and decreased albumin levels.
• Histologic identification of the glomerular lesion, following renal biopsy.

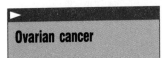

Ovarian cancer

Delay in diagnosing ovarian cancer – the fourth most common cause of cancer deaths among American women – is common. Early detection is difficult, because early-stage disease may not produce symptoms. Or, the disease may cause vague complaints that are easily mistaken for other ailments. What's more, ovarian cancer has no reliable screening test, unlike cervical or breast cancer, which can be detected early by a Papanicolaou test or mammography, respectively.

Because of these obstacles, a careful nursing assessment is especially important. A complete health history can identify women at high risk for this disease, who then can be monitored with both standard and investigational diagnostic techniques. A thorough diagnostic workup also may detect early-stage cancer in patients with vague, but suspicious symptoms.

The prognosis varies with the histologic type and staging of the disease, but it's often poor because of few warning signs and rapid progression. Although about 40% of women with ovarian cancer survive for 5 years, no major improvement in the overall survival rate has been made in the past 30 years.

Incidence is higher in women of upper socioeconomic status between the ages of 20 and 54. However, the disease may occur during childhood or even pregnancy.

Assessment
Health history
Ask the patient if she has one or more first-degree relatives (mother, sister, or daughter) who have had a confirmed diagnosis of the disease. Women with close relatives who have had ovarian cancer are at much greater risk for the disease than those without a familial history. Also explore the patient's health history. A woman with a history of breast, colon, or endometrial cancer also has an increased risk of developing ovarian cancer. Other risk factors include a high-fat diet, smoking, alcohol, perianal use of talcum powder, nulliparity, infertility, and anovulation.

Women who are at high risk for the disease, especially those with a familial history, may be referred for investigational screening tests.

Signs and symptoms
Because ovarian cancer is seldom diagnosed early, the tumor usually has metastasized before a diagnosis is made. Signs and symptoms vary with the tumor's size and the extent of metastasis.

In early-stage disease, the patient may complain of vague abdominal discomfort, indigestion, and other mild GI disturbances. In later stages, the history may disclose urinary frequency, constipation, pelvic discomfort, distention, and weight loss. The patient may complain of pain, possibly associated with tumor rupture, torsion, or infection. In a young patient, the pain may mimic that of appendicitis.

In late-stage disease, you'll typically observe a patient who is alert but gaunt. Inspection often discloses a grossly distended abdomen accompanied by ascites – typically the sign that prompts the patient to seek treatment.

You may feel masses as you palpate the abdominal organs and peritoneum. On palpation, an ovarian tumor may vary from a rocky hardness to a rubbery or cyst-like quality. Postmenopausal women who have palpable, premenopausal-size ovaries require further evaluation for an ovarian tumor.

Diagnostic tests
Screening tests

Although no suitable test has been devised to routinely screen asymptomatic, healthy women, some experts recommend that women at high risk for ovarian cancer be regularly screened with investigational techniques. These diagnostic screening tools include the biochemical marker, CA 125, and transvaginal color Doppler ultrasonography.

• The CA 125 antigen test, used primarily to evaluate the efficacy of treatment in patients with advanced disease, also may have a role in early detection. Some experts recommend that women with a strong family history of ovarian cancer receive this screening test every 6 months. However, elevation of CA 125 levels is not a certain indication of ovarian cancer; levels also may rise in early pregnancy, as well as endometriosis and other disorders. Morever, the test fails to detect early-stage cancer in some patients.

• Transvaginal Doppler ultrasonography produces more detailed pictures of the ovaries than standard abdominal ultrasonography. In this procedure, the ultrasound probe is placed inside the vagina.

Other tests

Tests ordered to help assess the patient's condition may include a complete blood count, blood chemistries, electrocardiography, and the following tests.

• Exploratory laparotomy, including lymph node evaluation and tumor resection, is required for accurate diagnosis and staging.

• Abdominal ultrasonography, computed tomography scan, or X-rays delineate tumor size.

• Excretory urography provides information on renal function and possible urinary tract obstruction.

• Chest X-rays can help identify distant metastasis and pleural effusions.

• Barium enema (especially in patients with GI symptoms) may reveal obstruction and tumor size.

• Lymphangiography can show lymph node involvement.

• Mammography can rule out primary breast cancer.

• Liver function studies or a liver scan can help identify metastasis with ascites.

• Aspiration of ascitic fluid can reveal atypical cells.

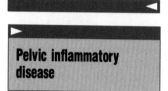

Pelvic inflammatory disease

An umbrella term, pelvic inflammatory disease (PID) refers to any acute, subacute, recurrent, or chronic infection of the oviducts and ovaries, with adjacent tissue involvement. PID includes inflammation of the uterus (endometritis), fallopian tubes (salpingitis), and ovaries (oophoritis), which can extend to the connective tissue lying between the broad ligaments (parametritis).

Although some patients may have acute symptoms of the disease, others are asymptomatic or have mild, insidious symptoms. In these patients, PID may go undiagnosed until a serious complication arises, such as infertility, recurrent pelvic pain, or ectopic pregancy.

Because one in four women diagnosed with PID suffers complications, which can be life-threatening, accurate and early detection is important. Early diagnosis and treatment help prevent damage to the reproductive system as does well-planned nursing care.

Neisseria gonorrhoeae and *Chlamydia trachomatis* are the usual causes of PID, although aerobic and anaerobic bacteria from the lower genitourinary tract also may be involved. In particular, *C. trachomatis* often goes undiagnosed, because it may be completely asymptomatic.

Assessment
Health history
Because PID does not always produce symptoms, carefully assess the patient's history for risk factors. Some experts recommend routine diagnostic screening of high-risk patients. Risk factors include:
• age younger than 30
• failure to use barrier contraceptives
• multiple sex partners or a new sex partner within the previous 2 months
• sex partner with gonorrhea or *C. trachomatis* infection.

Signs and symptoms
The patient with PID may have a high fever and severe abdominal, adnexal, or cervical motion pain. The patient may complain of profuse, purulent vaginal discharge, sometimes accompanied by low-grade fever and malaise (particularly if gonorrhea is the cause). She may also describe lower abdominal pain and vaginal bleeding. Vaginal examination may reveal pain during movement of the cervix or palpation of the adnexa.

Diagnostic tests
These tests help to confirm the diagnosis and determine the course of treatment.
• Gram stain of secretions from the endocervix or cul-de-sac determines the causative agent.
• Culture and sensitivity testing aids selection of the appropriate antibiotic. Urethral and rectal secretions may also be cultured.
• Ultrasonography, computed tomography scan, and magnetic resonance imaging may help to identify

and locate an adnexal or uterine mass.
• Culdocentesis obtains peritoneal fluid or pus for culture and sensitivity testing.

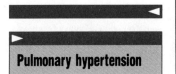

Pulmonary hypertension

Pulmonary hypertension occurs when pulmonary artery pressure (PAP) rises above normal and is not attributable to the effects of aging or altitude. It is indicated by a resting systolic PAP of 25 mm Hg or higher. The primary form is so difficult to detect that it's sometimes diagnosed only at autopsy.

Primary or idiopathic pulmonary hypertension is characterized by increased PAP and increased pulmonary vascular resistance, both of which occur without an obvious cause. This form is most common in women between ages 20 and 40 and is usually fatal within 3 to 4 years; mortality is highest in pregnant women.

Secondary pulmonary hypertension results from existing cardiac or pulmonary disease or both. The prognosis in secondary pulmonary hypertension depends on the severity of the underlying disorder.

Assessment
Assessing the patient with primary pulmonary hypertension is difficult, because he may have no signs or symptoms until lung damage becomes severe. Because pulmonary hypertension may ultimately lead to cardiac failure, focus your assessment on detecting signs and symptoms of left or right ventricular failure.

Usually, a patient with pulmonary hypertension complains of increasing dyspnea on exertion, weakness, syncope, and fatigue. He may also have difficulty breathing, feel short of breath, and report that breathing causes pain. Such signs may result from left ventricular failure.

Inspection
You may observe signs of right ventricular failure, including ascites and neck vein distention. The patient may appear restless and agitated and have a decreased level of consciousness. He may even be confused and have memory loss. You may observe decreased diaphragmatic excursion and respiration, and the point of maximal impulse may be displaced beyond the midclavicular line.

Palpation
You may also note signs of right ventricular failure, such as peripheral edema. The patient typically has an easily palpable right ventricular lift and a reduced carotid pulse. He may also have a palpable and tender liver and tachycardia.

Auscultation
Findings are specific to the underlying disorder but may include a systolic ejection murmur, a widely split S2 sound, and S3 and S4 sounds. You may also hear decreased breath sounds and loud tubular sounds. The patient may have decreased blood pressure.

Diagnostic tests
• Arterial blood gas (ABG) studies reveal hypoxemia (decreased partial pressure of oxygen PaO_2).
• Electrocardiography in right ventricular hypertrophy shows right axis deviation and tall or peaked P waves in inferior leads.
• Cardiac catheterization discloses increased PAP, with a systolic pressure above 30 mm Hg. It may also show an increased pulmonary artery wedge pressure (PAWP) if the

underlying cause is left atrial myxoma, mitral stenosis, or left ventricular failure; otherwise, PAWP is normal.
• Pulmonary angiography detects filling defects in pulmonary vasculature, such as those that develop with pulmonary emboli.
• Pulmonary function tests may show decreased flow rates and increased residual volume in underlying obstructive disease; in underlying restrictive disease, they may show reduced total lung capacity.
• Radionuclide imaging allows assessment of right and left ventricular functioning.
• Open lung biopsy may determine the type of disorder.
• Echocardiography allows the assessment of ventricular wall motion and possible valvular dysfunction. It can also demonstrate right ventricular enlargement, abnormal septal configuration consistent with right ventricular pressure overload, and a reduction in left ventricular cavity size.
• Perfusion lung scan may produce normal or abnormal results, with multiple patchy and diffuse filling defects that don't suggest pulmonary thromboembolism.

Right ventricular infarction

When you care for a patient with a myocardial infarction (MI), do you routinely assess for damage to the right ventricle? A right ventricular infarction (RVI) develops from blockage in the right coronary artery, which supplies the right ventricle and the lower left ventricle. So, an RVI usually involves the heart's inferior wall. Here are insights into a cardiac problem that's often overlooked.

Assessment
Besides having the classic signs of acute inferior wall MI, the patient may show other signs that offer clues to an RVI.

Jugular vein distention
An RVI weakens the right ventricle, preventing it from pumping efficiently. As blood pools in the ventricle, right ventricular filling pressures rise. These increased pressures affect the right atrium and the superior vena cava and eventually distend the jugular veins.

Kussmaul's sign
Inspiration will accentuate jugular vein distention.

Clear lungs
Because the right ventricle's pumping action is impaired, blood backs up in the heart's right side and the peripheral venous system. Less blood reaches the lungs, so pulmonary congestion doesn't develop.

Hypotension
Ultimately, the left ventricle receives less blood, too. Inadequate left ventricular filling causes cardiac output to drop; hypotension develops.

Heart block
For most people, the right coronary artery supplies blood to the atrioventricular node. A flow interruption disrupts normal electrical conduction, causing varying degrees of heart block.

Ventricular gallop
Also called S_3, ventricular gallop develops when blood rushes into the dilated ventricle during diastole. The ventricle distends rapidly, causing the abnormal vibrations you hear as ventricular gallop.

Diagnostic tests
Because right precordial electrocardiogram (ECG) tracings provide the most specific information about right ventricular conduction, they may confirm an RVI. Place the six right precordial (VR) leads as shown below.

ASSESSMENT FINDINGS

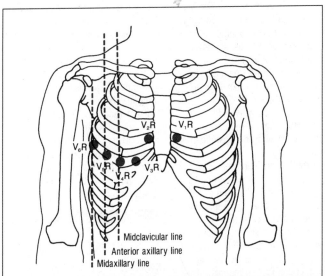

Midclavicular line
Anterior axillary line
Midaxillary line

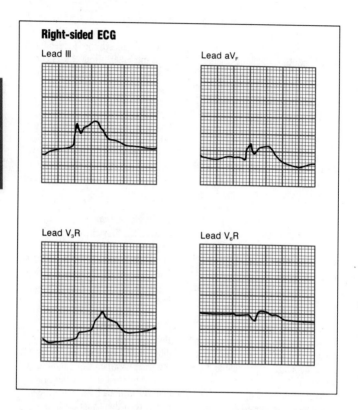

Right-sided ECG

Lead III

Lead aV_F

Lead V₃R

Lead V₆R

When ECG changes already signal an acute inferior or posterior MI, monitor ST segments. Ongoing elevations of these segments in the right precordial leads, as shown above, confirm an RVI.

Typically, an RVI patient's diagnostic workup also shows the following changes:
• elevated cardiac enzymes
• increased right atrial pressure and right ventricular end-diastolic pressure
• normal or below-normal PAP
• subnormal cardiac output
• right ventricular dilation and abnormal ventricular and septal wall motion on echocardiography.

Radionuclide scanning may be used to locate the infarction site. In this test, the radioactive isotope technetium Tc 99m pyrophosphate migrates to necrotic tissue after being injected intravenously. The infarcted area appears as a "hot spot" on the scan. This test is most useful when performed 16 hours to 6 days after the onset of signs and symptoms.

Multiple-gated acquisition scanning may be used to evaluate ventricular function. Using the radioactive isotope technetium Tc 99m pertechnetate, this test focuses on ventricular wall motion and ventricular size. The scan can be used to calculate the ventricular ejection fraction.

CHAPTER 3

ECGs:
Interpreting them with ease and accuracy

Normal ECG

How to read any ECG: An 8-step guide

An electrocardiogram (ECG) waveform has three basic elements: a P wave, a QRS complex, and a T wave. These are joined by five other useful diagnostic elements: the PR interval, the U wave, the ST segment, the J point, and the QT interval. The diagram below shows how they're related.

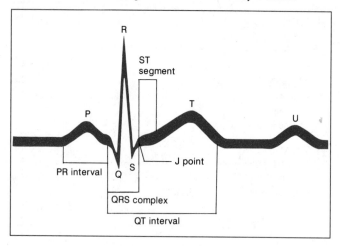

The following 8-step guide will enable you to read any ECG.

Step 1: Evaluate the P wave

Observe the P wave's size, shape, and location in the waveform. If the P wave consistently precedes the QRS complex, the electrical impulse is being initiated by the sinoatrial node, as it should be.

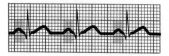

Step 2: Evaluate the atrial rhythm

The P wave should occur at regular intervals, with only small variations associated with respiration. Using a pair of calipers, you can easily measure the interval between P waves (the P-P interval). Compare the P-P intervals in several ECG cycles. Make sure the calipers are set at the same point – at the beginning of the wave or on its peak. Instead of lifting the calipers, rotate one of its legs to the next P wave, to ensure accurate measurements.

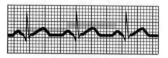

Step 3: Determine the atrial rate

To determine the atrial rate quickly, count the number of P waves in two 3-second segments. Multiply this number by 10.

For a more accurate determination, count the number of small squares between two P waves using either the apex of the wave or the initial upstroke of the wave. Each small square equals 0.04 second; 1,500 squares equal 1 minute (0.04 × 1,500 = 60 seconds). So, divide 1,500 by the number of squares you counted between the P waves. This gives you the atrial rate — the number of contractions per minute.

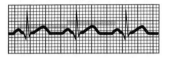

Step 4: Calculate duration of the PR interval

Count the number of small squares between the beginning of the P wave and the beginning of the QRS complex. Multiply the number of squares by 0.04 second. The normal interval is between 0.12 and 0.20 second, or between 3 and 5 small squares wide. A wider interval indicates delayed conduction of the impulse to the ventricles.

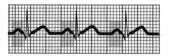

Step 5: Evaluate the ventricular rhythm

Use the calipers to measure the R-R intervals. Remember to place the calipers on the same point of the QRS complex. If the R-R intervals remain consistent, the ventricular rhythm is regular.

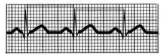

Step 6: Determine the ventricular rate

To determine the ventricular rate, use the same formula as in Step 3. In this case, however, count the number of small squares between two R waves to do the calculation. Also check that the QRS complex is shaped appropriately for the lead you're monitoring.

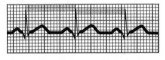

Step 7: Calculate the duration of the QRS complex

Count the number of squares between the beginning and the end of the QRS complex and multiply by 0.04 second. A normal QRS complex is less than 0.12 second, or less than 3 small squares wide. Some references specify 0.06 to 0.10 second as the normal duration for the QRS complex.

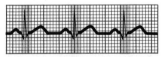

Step 8: Calculate the duration of the QT interval

Count the number of squares from the beginning of the QRS complex to the end of the T wave. Multiply this number by 0.04 second. The normal range is 0.36 to 0.44 second, or 9 to 11 small squares wide.

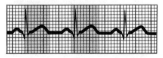

Normal sinus rhythm

When the heart functions normally, the sinoatrial (SA) node acts as the primary pacemaker, initiating the electrical impulses that set the rhythm for cardiac contractions. The SA node assumes this role because its automatic firing rate exceeds that of the heart's other pacemakers, allowing cells to depolarize spontaneously. Two factors account for increased automaticity: First, during the resting phase of the depolarization-repolarization cycle, SA node cells have the least negative charge. Second, depolarization actually begins during the resting phase.

Based on an electrical disturbance's location, arrhythmias can be classified as sinus, atrial, junctional, or ventricular arrhythmias or atrioventricular (AV) blocks. Functional disturbances in the SA node produce sinus arrhythmias. Enhanced automaticity of atrial tissue or reentry may produce atrial arrhythmias, the most common arrhythmias.

Junctional arrhythmias originate in the area around the AV node and the bundle of His. These arrhythmias usually result from a suppressed higher pacemaker or blocked impulses at the AV node.

Ventricular arrhythmias originate in ventricular tissue below the bifurcation of the bundle of His. These rhythms may result from reentry or enhanced automaticity, or after depolarization.

An AV block results from an abnormal interruption or delay of atrial impulse conduction to the ventricles. It may be partial or total and may occur in the AV node, the bundle of His, or the Purkinje system.

Lead II

Regular rhythm ——————————————   P wave — ┌ QRS complex

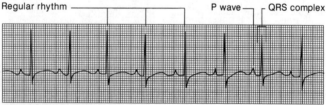

Characteristics and interpretation

Atrial rhythm: regular
Ventricular rhythm: regular
Atrial rate: 60 to 100 beats/minute. On this strip, it's 80 beats/minute.
Ventricular rate: 60 to 100 beats/minute. Rate shown: 80 beats/minute.
P wave: normally shaped. All P waves have similar size and shape; P wave precedes each QRS complex.
PR interval: within normal limits (0.12 to 0.20 second) and constant.

Duration shown: 0.20 second.
QRS complex: within normal limits (0.06 to 0.10 second). All QRS complexes have the same configuration. Duration shown: 0.12 second.
T wave: normally shaped (upright and rounded). Each QRS complex is followed by a T wave.
QT interval: within normal limits (0.36 to 0.44 second) and constant. Duration shown: 0.44 second.

Arrhythmias

Sinus arrhythmia

In sinus arrhythmia, the heart rate stays within normal limits but the rhythm is irregular and corresponds to the respiratory cycle and variations of vagal tone. During inspiration, an increased volume of blood returns to the heart, reducing vagal tone and increasing sinus rate. During expiration, venous return decreases, vagal tone increases, and sinus rate slows.

Conditions unrelated to respiration may also produce sinus arrhythmia. These conditions include an inferior wall myocardial infarction, digitalis toxicity, and increased intracranial pressure.

Sinus arrhythmia is easily recognized in elderly, pediatric, and sedated patients. The patient's pulse rate increases with inspiration and decreases with expiration. Usually, the patient will be asymptomatic.

Intervention
Treatment usually isn't necessary, unless the patient is symptomatic or the sinus arrhythmia stems from an underlying cause. When the patient is symptomatic, atropine may be administered if the heart rate falls below 40 beats/minute.

Lead II
Cyclic, irregular rhythm

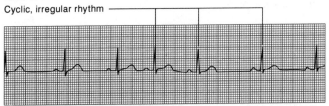

Characteristics and interpretation

Atrial rhythm: irregular, corresponding to the respiratory cycle
Ventricular rhythm: irregular, corresponding to the respiratory cycle
Atrial rate: within normal limits; varies with respiration. On this strip, it's 60 beats/minute.
Ventricular rate: within normal limits; varies with respiration. On this strip, it's 60 beats/minute.
P wave: normal size and configuration. One P wave precedes each QRS complex.

PR interval: within normal limits. On this strip, it's 0.16 second and constant.
QRS complex: normal duration and configuration. On this strip, the duration is 0.06 second.
T wave: normal size and configuration
QT interval: within normal limits. On this strip, it's 0.36 second.
Other: phasic slowing and quickening of the rhythm.

ECGs

Sinus bradycardia

Characterized by a sinus rate of less than 60 beats/minute, sinus bradycardia usually occurs as the normal response to a reduced demand for blood flow. It's common among athletes, whose well-conditioned hearts can maintain stroke volume with reduced effort. It may also be caused by drugs, such as digitalis glycosides, calcium channel blockers, and beta blockers.

Sinus bradycardia may occur after an inferior wall myocardial infarction involving the right coronary artery, which provides the blood supply to the sinoatrial node. The rhythm may develop during sleep and in patients with elevated intracranial pressure. It may also result from vagal stimulation caused by vomiting or defecating. Pathologic sinus bradycardia may occur with sick sinus syndrome.

The patient with sinus bradycardia will be asymptomatic if he's able to compensate for the drop in heart rate by increasing stroke volume. If not, he may have signs and symptoms of decreased cardiac output, such as hypotension, syncope, confusion, and blurred vision.

Intervention

If the patient is asymptomatic, treatment isn't necessary. If he has signs and symptoms, treatment aims to identify and correct the underlying cause. The heart rate may be increased with such drugs as atropine or dopamine (Intropin). A temporary or permanent pacemaker may be inserted if the bradycardia persists.

Lead II

Regular rhythm with rate less than 60 beats/minute

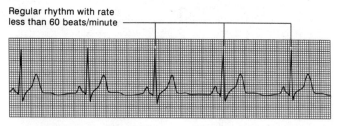

Characteristics and interpretation

Atrial rhythm: regular
Ventricular rhythm: regular
Atrial rate: less than 60 beats/minute. Rate shown: 50 beats/minute.
Ventricular rate: less than 60 beats/minute. Rate shown: 50 beats/minute.
P wave: normal size and configuration. One P wave precedes each QRS complex.
PR interval: within normal limits and constant. Duration shown: 0.14 second.
QRS complex: normal duration and configuration. Duration shown: 0.08 second.
T wave: normal size and configuration
QT interval: within normal limits. Interval shown: 0.40 second.

Sinus tachycardia

A normal response to cellular demands for increased oxygen delivery and blood flow commonly produces sinus tachycardia. Conditions causing such a demand include congestive heart failure (CHF), shock, anemia, exercise, fever, hypoxia, pain, and stress. Drugs that stimulate the beta$_1$-receptors in the heart will also cause sinus tachycardia. These include isoproterenol (Isuprel), aminophylline (Aminophyllin), and inotropic agents, such as dobutamine. Alcohol, caffeine, and nicotine may also produce sinus tachycardia.

An elevated heart rate increases myocardial oxygen demands. If the patient can't meet these demands (for example, because of coronary artery disease), ischemia and further myocardial damage may occur. If tachycardia exceeds 140 beats/minute for longer than 30 minutes, ECG may show ST-segment and T-wave changes, indicating ischemia.

Intervention
Treatment focuses on finding the primary cause. If it's high catecholamine levels, a beta blocker may slow the heart rate. After myocardial infarction, persistent sinus tachycardia may precede CHF or cardiogenic shock.

Lead II

Regular rhythm with rate greater than 100 beats/minute

Characteristics and interpretation
Atrial rhythm: regular
Ventricular rhythm: regular
Atrial rate: 100 to 160 beats/minute. Rate shown: 110 beats/minute.
Ventricular rate: 100 to 160 beats/minute. Rate shown: 110 beats/minute.

P wave: normal size and configuration. One P wave precedes each QRS complex. As the sinus rate reaches about 150 beats/minute, the P wave merges with the preceding T wave and may be difficult to identify. Examine the descending slope of the preceding T wave closely for notches, indicating the presence of the P wave. P wave shown: normal.

PR interval: within normal limits and constant. Duration shown: 0.16 second.

QRS complex: normal duration and configuration. Duration shown: 0.10 second.

T wave: normal size and configuration

QT interval: within normal limits and constant. Duration shown: 0.36 second.

Other: gradual onset and cessation.

▶

Sinus arrest

Failure of the sinoatrial node to generate an impulse interrupts the sinus rhythm, producing "sinus pause" when one or two beats are dropped, or "sinus arrest" when three or more beats are dropped. Such failure may result from an acute inferior wall myocardial infarction, increased vagal tone, or use of certain drugs (digitalis glycosides, calcium channel blockers, or beta blockers). The arrhythmia may also be linked to sick sinus syndrome.

The patient will have an irregular pulse rate associated with the sinus rhythm pauses. If the pauses are infrequent, the patient will be asymptomatic. If they occur frequently and last for several seconds, the patient may have signs of decreased cardiac output.

Intervention

For a symptomatic patient, treatment focuses on maintaining cardiac output and discovering the cause of the sinus arrest. If indicated, atropine may be given or a temporary or permanent pacemaker may be inserted.

Lead II

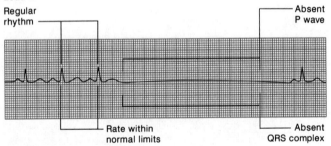

Regular rhythm — / Absent P wave

Rate within normal limits / Absent QRS complex

Characteristics and interpretation

Atrial rhythm: regular, except for the missing complex

Ventricular rhythm: regular, except for the missing complex

Atrial rate: within normal limits, but varies because of the pauses. On this strip, it's 94 beats/minute.

Ventricular rate: within normal limits, but varies because of pauses. On this strip, it's 94 beats/minute.

P wave: normal size and configuration. One P wave precedes each QRS complex but is absent during a pause.

PR interval: within normal limits and constant when P wave is present; unmeasurable when P wave is absent. On this strip, the duration is 0.20 second on all complexes surrounding the arrest.

QRS complex: normal duration and configuration. QRS complex absent during a pause. On this strip, the duration is 0.08 second.

T wave: normal size and configuration; absent during a pause.

QT interval: within normal limits; unmeasurable during pause. On this strip, it's 0.40 second and constant.

◀

Type I second-degree sinoatrial block

In a sinoatrial (SA) block, the SA pacemaker generates an impulse but some impulses are delayed or blocked from reaching the atria. Based on the length of the delay or block, SA blocks are divided into three categories: first-, second-, and third-degree. Second-degree block is further divided into Type I (Mobitz I or Wenckebach) and Type II (Mobitz II).

First-degree SA block consists of a delay between SA node firing and atrial depolarization. Because an ECG doesn't show sinus activity, you can't detect a first-degree SA block. But you can detect the other three types.

In Type I second-degree SA block, conduction time between the SA node and atrial tissue progressively lengthens until an entire cycle of P-QRS-T is dropped. Such an arrhythmia may be associated with increased vagal tone, myocardial infarction, acute myocarditis, hypokalemia or hyperkalemia, or use of certain sympatholytics, beta blockers, calcium channel blockers, Class 1A and 1C antiarrhythmic drugs, and cholinergics.

The patient will have an irregular pulse rate associated with the dropped beats. If the dropped beats become frequent, he may experience signs of decreased cardiac output.

Intervention
For a symptomatic patient, treatment focuses on maintaining cardiac output and identifying the arrhythmia's cause. Atropine may be given.

Lead I

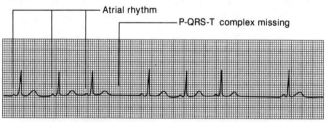

Atrial rhythm — P-QRS-T complex missing

Characteristics and interpretation
Atrial rhythm: irregular; P-P interval progressively shorter until pause
Ventricular rhythm: irregular; R-R interval progressively shorter until pause
Atrial rate: usually normal
Ventricular rate: usually normal
P wave: periodically absent
PR interval: can't be measured on missing complex; otherwise usually normal

QRS complex: periodically missing QRS complex; otherwise usually normal
T wave: periodically absent T wave; otherwise usually normal
QT interval: periodically absent; otherwise usually normal
Other: pause is less than twice the shortest P-P interval.

ECGs

Type II second-degree sinoatrial block

In Type II second-degree sinoatrial (SA) block, conduction time between the SA node and atrial tissue is normal until an impulse is blocked. Such an arrhythmia may be associated with increased vagal tone, myocardial infarction, acute myocarditis, hypokalemia or hyperkalemia; or the use of certain drugs (sympatholytics, beta blockers, calcium channel blockers, Class 1A and 1C antiarrhythmic agents, and cholinergics).

The patient will have an irregular pulse rate associated with the dropped beats. If the dropped beats become frequent, the patient may experience signs and symptoms of decreased cardiac output, including hypotension, confusion, syncope, and blurred vision.

Intervention

An asymptomatic patient needs no treatment. For a symptomatic patient, treatment focuses on maintaining cardiac output and identifying the cause of the arrhythmia. If indicated, atropine may be administered.

Lead II

P-QRS-T complex missing

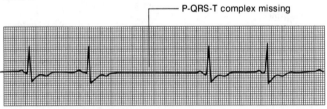

Characteristics and interpretation

Atrial rhythm: regular except for the pause

Ventricular rhythm: regular, except for the pause

Atrial rate: usually within normal limits

Ventricular rate: usually within normal limits

P wave: periodically absent

PR interval: can't be measured on missing complex; otherwise usually within normal limits

QRS complex: periodically missing QRS complex; otherwise usually within normal limits

T wave: periodically absent T wave; otherwise usually within normal limits

QT interval: periodically absent; otherwise usually within normal limits

Other: pause is a multiple of the normal P-P interval.

Third-degree sinoatrial block

Third-degree sinoatrial (SA) block looks similar to sinus arrest. But a block results from failure to conduct impulses, whereas sinus arrest results from failure to generate impulses from the SA node. Such an arrhythmia may be associated with increased vagal tone, myocardial infarction, or certain drugs, such as sympatholytics, beta blockers, calcium channel blockers, Class 1A and 1C antiarrhythmic agents, and cholinergics.

The patient will have an irregular pulse rate associated with the dropped beats. If the dropped beats become frequent, the patient may experience signs and symptoms of decreased cardiac output, including hypotension, confusion, syncope, and blurred vision.

Intervention
An asymptomatic patient needs no treatment. For a symptomatic patient, treatment focuses on maintaining cardiac output and identifying the cause of the arrhythmia. If indicated, atropine may be administered or a pacemaker inserted.

Lead II

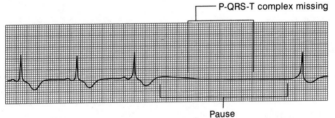

P-QRS-T complex missing

Pause

Characteristics and interpretation

Atrial rhythm: regular until pause; may be regular or irregular if an escape rhythm occurs

Ventricular rhythm: regular until pause; may be regular or irregular if an escape rhythm occurs

Atrial rate: usually within normal limits until pause; may be abnormal if an escape rhythm occurs

Ventricular rate: usually within normal limits until pause; may be abnormal if an escape rhythm occurs

P wave: periodically absent

PR interval: usually within normal limits until pause; may be unmeasurable if an escape rhythm occurs

QRS complex: usually within normal limits until pause; may be abnormal if an escape rhythm occurs

T wave: usually within normal limits until pause; present if an escape rhythm occurs

QT interval: periodically absent; usually within normal limits until pause; present if an escape rhythm occurs

Other: pause isn't a multiple of the P-P interval; pause may end with an escape rhythm or a normal sinus rhythm.

ECGs

ECGs

▶
Premature atrial contractions

Premature atrial contractions (PACs) usually result from an irritable focus in the atria that supersedes the sinoatrial node as the pacemaker for one or two beats. Although PACs commonly occur in normal hearts, they're also associated with coronary and valvular heart disease. In an inferior wall myocardial infarction (MI), PACs may indicate a concomitant right atrial infarct. In an anterior wall MI, PACs are an early sign of left ventricular failure. They also may warn of a more severe atrial arrhythmia, such as atrial flutter or fibrillation.

Possible causes include digitalis toxicity, hyperthyroidism, elevated catecholamine levels, acute respiratory failure, and chronic obstructive pulmonary disease.

Intervention
Symptomatic patients may be treated with digoxin (Lanoxin), procainamide (Pronestyl), propranolol (Inderal), and verapamil (Calan, Isoptin).

Lead II

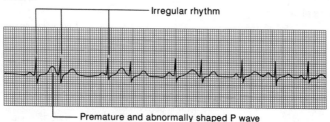

Irregular rhythm

Premature and abnormally shaped P wave

Characteristics and interpretation

Atrial rhythm: irregular. Incomplete compensatory pause follows PAC. Underlying rhythm may be regular.

Ventricular rhythm: irregular. Incomplete compensatory pause follows PAC. Underlying rhythm may be regular.

Atrial rate: varies with underlying rhythm. On this strip, it's 90 beats/minute.

Ventricular rate: varies with underlying rhythm. On this strip, it's 90 beats/minute.

P wave: premature and abnormally shaped; possibly lost in previous T wave. Varying configurations indicate multiform PACs.

PR interval: usually normal but may be shortened or slightly prolonged, depending on origin of ectopic focus. On this strip, the PR interval is 0.16 second and constant.

QRS complex: usually normal duration and configuration. On this strip, it's 0.08 second and constant.

T wave: usually normal configuration; may be distorted if P wave is hidden in previous T wave

QT interval: usually normal. On this strip, it's 0.36 second and constant.

Other: may occur in bigeminy or in couplets.

◀

Atrial tachycardia

In this arrhythmia, the atrial rhythm is ectopic and the atrial rate is rapid, shortening diastole. This results in a loss of atrial kick, reduced cardiac output, reduced coronary perfusion, and ischemic myocardial changes.

Although atrial tachycardia occurs in healthy patients, it's usually associated with high catecholamine levels, digitalis toxicity, myocardial infarction, cardiomyopathy, hyperthyroidism, hypertension, and valvular heart disease. Three types of atrial tachycardia exist: atrial tachycardia with block, multifocal atrial tachycardia, and paroxysmal atrial tachycardia.

Intervention

If the patient is symptomatic, prepare for immediate cardioversion. If the patient is stable, the doctor may perform carotid sinus massage (if no bruits are present) or order drug therapy, such as adenosine (Adenocard), verapamil (Calan), digoxin (Lanoxin), beta blockers, or diltiazem (Cardizem). If these measures fail, cardioversion may be necessary.

ECGs

Lead II

Regular rhythm ——————

Rate between 160 and 250 beats/minute

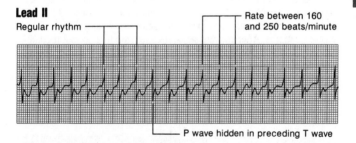

P wave hidden in preceding T wave

Characteristics and interpretation

Atrial rhythm: regular
Ventricular rhythm: regular
Atrial rate: three or more successive ectopic atrial beats at a rate of 160 to 250 beats/minute. On this strip, it's 210 beats/minute.
Ventricular rate: varies with atrioventricular conduction ratio. On this strip, it's 210 beats/minute.
P wave: 1:1 ratio with QRS complex, though often indiscernible due to rapid rate. May be hidden in previous ST segment or T wave.
PR interval: may be unmeasurable if P wave can't be distinguished from preceding T wave. If P wave is present, PR interval often exceeds

0.20 second due to rapid rate and intrinsic refractoriness of AV node. On this strip, the PR interval isn't discernible.
QRS complex: usually normal unless aberrant intraventricular conduction is present. On this strip, the duration is 0.10 second.
T wave: may be normal or inverted if ischemia is present. On this strip, the T waves are inverted.
QT interval: usually normal but may be shorter due to rapid rate. On this strip, it's 0.20 second.
Other: ST-segment and T-wave changes appear if tachyarrhythmia persists longer than 30 minutes.

Atrial flutter

Characterized by an atrial rate of 300 or more beats/minute, atrial flutter results from multiple reentry circuits within the atrial tissue. Causes include conditions that enlarge atrial tissue and elevate atrial pressures. Atrial flutter is associated with myocardial infarction, increased catecholamine levels, hyperthyroidism, and digitalis toxicity. A ventricular rate of 300 beats/minute suggests the presence of an anomalous pathway.

If the patient's pulse rate is normal, he usually has no symptoms. If his pulse rate is high, he'll probably have signs and symptoms of decreased cardiac output, such as hypotension and syncope.

Intervention

The doctor may perform vagal stimulation to slow the ventricular response and demonstrate the presence of flutter waves. This is contraindicated if carotid bruit is present. If the patient is symptomatic, prepare for immediate cardioversion.

Drugs that may be ordered to slow atrioventricular conduction include calcium channel blockers (diltiazem, verapamil) and beta blockers (esmolol, metoprolol). Digoxin may be ordered, but some experts question its use for urgent treatment. After the rate slows, if conversion to a normal rhythm has not occurred, procainamide (Pronestyl) or quinidine (Quinidex) may be ordered.

Lead II

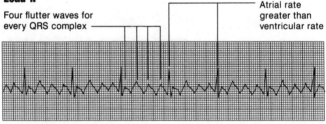

Four flutter waves for every QRS complex

Atrial rate greater than ventricular rate

Characteristics and interpretation

Atrial rhythm: regular

Ventricular rhythm: may be regular or irregular, depending on the conduction ratio. On this strip, it's regular.

Atrial rate: 300 to 350 beats/minute. On this strip, it's 300 beats/minute.

Ventricular rate: variable. On this strip, it's 70 beats/minute.

P wave: atrial activity seen as flutter waves, often with a saw-toothed appearance

PR interval: not measurable

QRS complex: usually normal, but can be distorted by the underlying flutter waves. On this strip, the duration is 0.10 second and normal.

T wave: not identifiable

QT interval: can't be measured.

Atrial fibrillation

Defined as chaotic, asynchronous electrical activity in the atrial tissue, atrial fibrillation results from impulses in many reentry pathways. These impulses cause the atria to quiver instead of contract regularly. With this arrhythmia, blood may pool in the left atrial appendage and form thrombi that can be ejected into the systemic circulation. An associated rapid ventricular rate can decrease cardiac output.

Possible causes include valvular disorders, hypertension, coronary artery disease, myocardial infarction, and the use of certain drugs, such as aminophylline (Aminophyllin) and digitalis glycosides.

Intervention

If the patient is symptomatic, synchronized cardioversion should be used immediately. Vagal stimulation may be used to slow the ventricular response, but it won't convert the arrhythmia. Drugs that may be ordered to slow atrioventricular conduction include calcium channel blockers (diltiazem) and beta blockers (metoprolol). Digoxin may be ordered if the patient is stable. After the rate slows, if conversion to a normal sinus rhythm has not occurred, procainamide (Pronestyl) or quinidine (Quinidex) may be ordered. If atrial fibrillation is of several days' duration, anticoagulant therapy is recommended before pharmacologic or electrical conversion.

Lead MCL₁

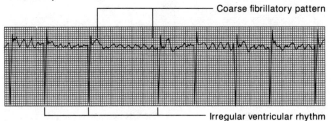

Coarse fibrillatory pattern

Irregular ventricular rhythm

Characteristics and interpretation

Atrial rhythm: grossly irregular
Ventricular rhythm: grossly irregular
Atrial rate: greater than 400 beats/minute
Ventricular rate: 60 to 150 beats/minute, depending on treatment. On this strip, it's 80 beats/minute.
P wave: absent; erratic baseline f waves (fibrillatory waves) appear in their place. When the f waves are pronounced, the arrhythmia is called coarse atrial fibrillation.

When the f waves aren't pronounced, the arrhythmia is known as fine atrial fibrillation. On this strip, the f waves are pronounced.
PR interval: indiscernible
QRS complex: duration usually within normal limits, with aberrant intraventricular conduction. On this strip, the duration is 0.08 second.
T wave: indiscernible
QT interval: unmeasurable.

ECGs

Junctional rhythm

This arrhythmia occurs in the atrioventricular junctional tissue, producing retrograde depolarization of the atrial tissue and antegrade depolarization of the ventricular tissue. It results from conditions that depress sinoatrial node function, such as an inferior wall myocardial infarction (MI), digitalis toxicity, and vagal stimulation. The arrhythmia may also stem from increased automaticity of the junctional tissue, which can be brought about by digitalis toxicity or ischemia associated with an inferior wall MI.

A junctional rhythm with a ventricular rate of 60 to 100 beats/minute is known as an accelerated junctional rhythm. If the ventricular rate exceeds 100 beats/minute, the arrhythmia is called junctional tachycardia.

Intervention
Treatment aims to identify and manage the arrhythmia's primary cause. If the patient is symptomatic, treatment may include atropine to increase the sinus or junctional rate. Or the doctor may insert a pacemaker to maintain an effective heart rate.

Lead II

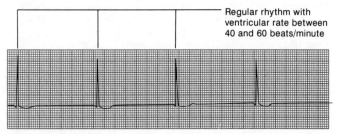

Regular rhythm with ventricular rate between 40 and 60 beats/minute

Characteristics and interpretation

Atrial rhythm: regular
Ventricular rhythm: regular
Atrial rate: if discernible, 40 to 60 beats/minute. On this strip, the rate isn't discernible.
Ventricular rate: 40 to 60 beats/minute. On this strip, the rate is 40 beats/minute.
P wave: usually inverted; may precede, follow, or fall within the QRS complex; may be absent. On this strip, the P wave is absent.
PR interval: if the P wave precedes the QRS complex, the PR interval will be less than 0.12 second and constant; otherwise it can't be measured. On this strip, it can't be measured.
QRS complex: duration normal; configuration usually normal. On this strip, the duration is 0.08 second.
T wave: usually normal configuration
QT interval: usually normal. On this strip, duration is 0.32 second.

Premature junctional contractions

In premature junctional contractions (PJCs), a junctional beat occurs before the next normal sinus beat. Ectopic beats, PJCs commonly result from increased automaticity in the bundle of His or the surrounding junctional tissue, which interrupts the underlying rhythm. The patient may complain of palpitations if PJCs are frequent.

PJCs most commonly result from digitalis toxicity. Their other causes include ischemia associated with an inferior wall myocardial infarction, excessive caffeine ingestion, and excessive levels of amphetamines.

Intervention
In most cases, treatment is directed at the underlying cause.

Lead II

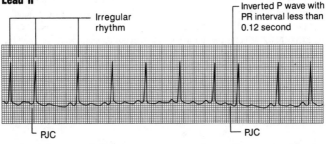

Irregular rhythm

Inverted P wave with PR interval less than 0.12 second

PJC

PJC

Characteristics and interpretation

Atrial rhythm: irregular with PJC, but underlying rhythm may be regular

Ventricular rhythm: irregular with PJC, but underlying rhythm may be regular

Atrial rate: follows the underlying rhythm. On this strip, the rate is 100 beats/minute.

Ventricular rate: follows the underlying rhythm. On this strip, the rate is 100 beats/minute.

P wave: usually inverted; may precede, follow, or fall within the QRS complex; may be absent. On this strip, it precedes the QRS complex.

PR interval: if P wave precedes the QRS complex, PR interval will be less than 0.12 second on the PJC; otherwise, it can't be measured. On this strip, it's 0.14 second and constant on the underlying rhythm, and 0.06 second on the PJC.

QRS complex: normal duration and configuration. On this strip, the duration is 0.06 second.

T wave: usually normal configuration

QT interval: usually within normal limits. On this strip, it's 0.30 second.

ECGs

Premature ventricular contractions

Among the most common arrhythmias, premature ventricular contractions (PVCs) occur in both healthy and diseased hearts. These ectopic beats may occur singly or in clusters of two or more. They also occur in bigeminy.

PVCs may result from the use of digitalis glycosides and sympathomimetic drugs or from electrolyte imbalances, such as hypokalemia and hypocalcemia. They may also result from exercise or ingestion of caffeine, tobacco, or alcohol. What's more, the arrhythmia may result from hypoxia, myocardial infarction, and myocardial irritation by pacemaker electrodes.

When you detect PVCs, you must determine whether they appear in a pattern that indicates danger. *Paired PVCs,* for instance, can produce ventricular tachycardia because the second PVC usually meets refractory tissue. A *salvo,* three or more PVCs in a row, is considered a run of ventricular tachycardia. *Multiform PVCs* look different from one another and arise from different ventricular sites; alternately, they may arise from the same site but be abnormally conducted. In *R-on-T phenomenon,* the PVC occurs so early that it falls on the T wave of the preceding beat. Because the cells haven't fully depolarized, ventricular tachycardia or fibrillation can result.

When palpating the peripheral pulse in a patient with PVCs, you may feel a longer than normal pause immediately after the PVC, depending on how early in the cardiac cycle the beat occurs. The earlier the beat, the shorter the diastolic filling time, and the lower the stroke volume. Some patients complain of palpitations with frequent PVCs.

Intervention

If the PVCs are thought to result from a serious cardiac problem, the doctor will order a drug, such as lidocaine (Xylocaine), to suppress ventricular irritability or other antiarrhythmics, such as procainamide (Pronestyl) and quinidine (Quinidex, Quinamm). When a patient's PVCs are thought to result from a noncardiac problem, treatment aims at correcting the underlying cause — correcting an acid-base or electrolyte disturbance, discontinuing an antiarrhythmic, treating hypothermia, or correcting high catecholamine levels.

Lead MCL₁

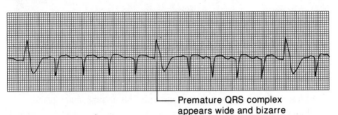

└─── Premature QRS complex
appears wide and bizarre

ECGs

Characteristics and interpretations

Atrial rhythm: irregular during PVC; underlying rhythm may be regular

Ventricular rhythm: irregular during PVC; underlying rhythm may be regular

Atrial rate: follows underlying rhythm. On this strip, it's 120 beats/minute.

Ventricular rate: follows underlying rhythm. On this strip, it's 120 beats/minute.

P wave: atrial activity is independent of the PVC; if retrograde atrial depolarization exists, a retrograde P wave will distort the ST segment of the PVC. On this strip, no P wave appears before the PVC, but one occurs with each QRS complex.

PR interval: determined by underlying rhythm; not associated with the PVC. On this strip, the underlying PR interval is 0.12 second and constant.

QRS complex: occurs earlier than expected; duration exceeds 0.12 second and complex has a bizarre configuration. May be normal in the underlying rhythm. On this strip, it's 0.08 second in the normal beats; it's bizarre and 0.12 second in the PVC.

T wave: occurs in the direction opposite that of the QRS complex; normal in the underlying complexes

QT interval: not usually measured in the PVC, but may be within normal limits in the underlying rhythm. On this strip, the QT interval is 0.28 second in the underlying rhythm.

► LIFE-THREATENING ARRHYTHMIA

Ventricular tachycardia

This arrhythmia develops when three or more premature ventricular contractions occur in a row and the rate exceeds 100 beats/minute. It may result from enhanced automaticity or reentry within the Purkinje system. The rapid ventricular rate reduces ventricular filling time, and because atrial kick is lost, cardiac output drops. This puts the patient at risk for ventricular fibrillation.

Ventricular tachycardia usually results from acute myocardial infarction, coronary artery disease, valvular heart disease, heart failure, or cardiomyopathy. The arrhythmia can also stem from an electrolyte imbalance or from toxic levels of a drug, such as a digitalis glycoside, procainamide (Pronestyl), or quinidine (Quinidex, Quinamm). You may detect two variations of this arrhythmia: R-on-T phenomenon and torsades de pointes.

Intervention

This rhythm often degenerates into ventricular fibrillation and cardiovascular collapse, requiring immediate cardiopulmonary resuscitation and defibrillation. If the patient is symptomatic, prepare for immediate cardioversion, followed by antiarrhythmic therapy. Lidocaine (Xylocaine) is usually administered immediately. If it proves ineffective, procainamide (Pronestyl) or bretylium (Bretylol) is used instead.

Lead MCL₁

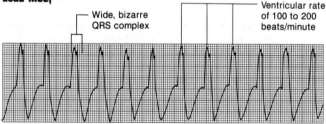

Wide, bizarre QRS complex

Ventricular rate of 100 to 200 beats/minute

Characteristics and interpretation

Atrial rhythm: independent P waves may be discernible with slower ventricular rates. On this strip, the P waves aren't visible.

Ventricular rhythm: usually regular, but may be slightly irregular. On this strip, it's regular.

Atrial rate: can't be determined

Ventricular rate: usually 100 to 200 beats/minute. On this strip, it's 120 beats/minute.

P wave: usually absent; may be obscured by the QRS complex; retrograde P waves may be present.

PR interval: not measurable

QRS complex: duration greater than 0.12 second; bizarre appearance, usually with increased amplitude. On this strip, the duration is 0.16 second.

T wave: opposite the terminal forces of the QRS complex

QT interval: not measurable.

► LIFE-THREATENING ARRHYTHMIA

Ventricular fibrillation

Defined as chaotic, asynchronous electrical activity within the ventricular tissue, ventricular fibrillation results in death if the rhythm isn't stopped immediately. Conditions leading to ventricular fibrillation include myocardial ischemia, hypokalemia, cocaine toxicity, hypoxia, hypothermia, severe acidosis, and severe alkalosis.

Patients with myocardial infarctions have the greatest risk of ventricular fibrillation during the first 2 hours after the onset of chest pain. Those who experience ventricular fibrillation will have a reduced risk of recurrence as healing progresses and scar tissue forms.

In ventricular fibrillation, a lack of cardiac output results in a loss of consciousness, pulselessness, and respiratory arrest. Initially, you may see coarse fibrillatory waves on the electrocardiogram strip. As the acidosis develops, the waves become fine and progress to asystole, unless defibrillation restores cardiac rhythm.

Intervention

Perform cardiopulmonary resuscitation until the patient can receive defibrillation. Administer epinephrine if initial defibrillation is unsuccessful. Other drugs that may be used include lidocaine (Xylocaine), bretylium (Bretylate), and procainamide (Pronestyl). Magnesium sulfate may be used for torsades de pointes or refractory ventricular fibrillation.

Lead MCL,

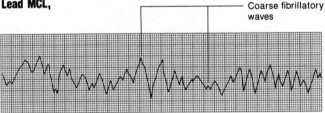

Coarse fibrillatory waves

Characteristics and interpretation

Atrial rhythm: can't be determined
Ventricular rhythm: irregular
Atrial rate: can't be determined
Ventricular rate: can't be determined
P wave: indiscernible

PR interval: can't be measured
QRS complex: replaced with fibrillatory waves; the duration can't be determined.
T wave: can't be determined
QT interval: can't be measured.

► LIFE-THREATENING ARRHYTHMIA

Idioventricular rhythm

This arrhythmia acts as a safety mechanism when all potential pacemakers above the ventricles fail to discharge or when a block prevents supraventricular impulses from reaching the ventricles.

The slow ventricular rate and loss of atrial kick associated with this arrhythmia will markedly reduce the patient's cardiac output. In turn, this will cause hypotension, confusion, vertigo, and syncope.

Intervention

Treatment aims to identify and manage the primary problem that triggered this safety mechanism.

Atropine or dopamine (Intropin) may be given to increase the patient's atrial rate. A pacemaker may also be inserted to increase the heart rate and thereby improve cardiac output.

Lead II

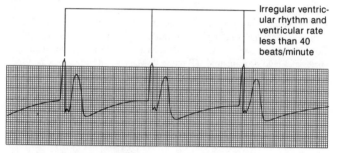

Irregular ventricular rhythm and ventricular rate less than 40 beats/minute

Characteristics and interpretation

Atrial rhythm: unable to be determined

Ventricular rhythm: usually regular, except with isolated escape beats. On this strip, the rhythm is irregular.

Atrial rate: unable to be determined

Ventricular rate: less than 40 beats/minute. On this strip, it's 30 beats/minute.

P wave: absent

PR interval: usually not measurable

QRS complex: duration greater than 0.12 second; complex is wide and has a bizarre configuration. On this strip, the complex is 0.20 second and bizarre.

T wave: directed opposite terminal forces of QRS complex

QT interval: usually greater than 0.44 second. On this strip, it's 0.46 second.

▶ LIFE-THREATENING ARRHYTHMIA

Accelerated idioventricular rhythm

When the pacemaker cells above the ventricles fail to generate an impulse or when a block prevents supraventricular impulses from reaching the ventricles, idioventricular rhythms result. When the rate of an idioventricular rhythm ranges from 40 to 100 beats/minute, it's considered accelerated idioventricular rhythm, denoting a rate greater than the inherent pacemaker.

In this rhythm, the cells of the His-Purkinje system operate as pacemaker cells. The characteristic waveform results from an area of enhanced automaticity within the ventricles, which may be associated with myocardial infarction, digitalis toxicity, or metabolic imbalances. In addition, the arrhythmia commonly occurs during myocardial reperfusion following thrombolytic therapy.

The patient may or may not be symptomatic, depending on his heart rate and ability to compensate for the loss of the atrial kick. If symptomatic, he may experience signs and symptoms of decreased cardiac output, including hypotension, confusion, syncope, and blurred vision.

Intervention

An asymptomatic patient needs no treatment. For a symptomatic patient, treatment focuses on maintaining cardiac output and identifying the cause of the arrhythmia. The patient may require an atrial pacemaker to enhance cardiac output. Remember, this rhythm protects the heart from ventricular standstill and never should be treated with lidocaine (Xylocaine) or other antiarrhythmic agents.

Lead V₁

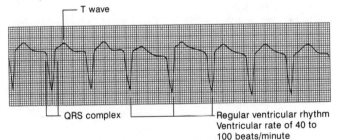

Characteristics and interpretation

Atrial rhythm: can't be determined
Ventricular rhythm: usually regular
Atrial rate: can't be determined
Ventricular rate: 40 to 100 beats/minute
P wave: absent
PR interval: can't be measured

QRS complex: duration greater than 0.12 second; wide and bizarre configuration
T wave: deflection usually opposite that of QRS complex
QT interval: may be within normal limits or may be prolonged.

ECGs

First-degree atrioventricular block

Defined as delayed conduction velocity through the atrioventricular (AV) node or His-Purkinje system, first-degree AV block is associated with an inferior wall myocardial infarction and the effects of digitalis glycosides or amiodarone (Cordarone). The arrhythmia is also associated with chronic degeneration of the conduction system.

Usually, patients with first-degree AV block are asymptomatic.

Intervention
Management of first-degree AV block includes identifying and treating the underlying cause as well as monitoring the patient for signs of progressive AV block.

Lead II

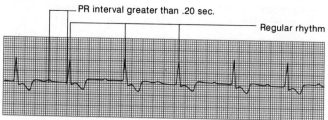

PR interval greater than .20 sec.

Regular rhythm

Characteristics and interpretation
Atrial rhythm: regular
Ventricular rhythm: regular
Atrial rate: usually within normal limits. On this strip, it's 60 beats/minute.
Ventricular rate: usually within normal limits. On this strip, it's 60 beats/minute.
P wave: normal size and configuration. One P wave precedes each QRS complex.
PR interval: greater than 0.20 sec-

ond and constant. On this strip, the duration is 0.32 second.
QRS complex: usually normal duration and configuration. On this strip, the duration is 0.08 second and the configuration is normal.
T wave: normal size and configuration
QT interval: usually within normal limits. On this strip, it's 0.32 second.

Type I second-degree atrioventricular block

In Type I (Wenckebach or Mobitz I) second-degree atrioventricular (AV) block, diseased AV node tissues conduct impulses to the ventricles increasingly later, until one of the atrial impulses fails to be conducted or is blocked. Type I block most commonly occurs at the level of the AV node and is caused by an inferior wall myocardial infarction, vagal stimulation, or digitalis toxicity.

The arrhythmia usually doesn't cause symptoms. However, a patient may have signs and symptoms of decreased cardiac output, such as hypotension, confusion, and syncope. These effects occur especially if the patient's ventricular rate is slow.

Intervention

If the patient is asymptomatic, no intervention is required other than monitoring the electrocardiogram frequently to see if a more serious form of AV block develops.

If the patient is symptomatic, the doctor may order atropine to increase the rate and to stop the decremental conduction through the AV node. Occasionally, the doctor may insert a temporary pacemaker to maintain an effective cardiac output.

Lead II

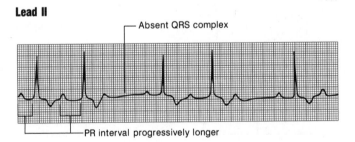

Absent QRS complex

PR interval progressively longer

Characteristics and interpretation

Atrial rhythm: regular
Ventricular rhythm: irregular
Atrial rate: determined by the underlying rhythm. Rate shown: 80 beats/minute.
Ventricular rate: slower than the atrial rate. Rate shown: 50 beats/minute.
P wave: normal size and configuration
PR interval: progressively prolonged with each beat until a P wave appears

without a QRS complex
QRS complex: normal duration and configuration; periodically absent. Duration shown: 0.08 second.
T wave: normal size and configuration
QT interval: usually within normal limits. Interval shown: 0.46 second and constant.
Other: usually distinguished by a pattern of group beating, referred to as the footprints of Wenckebach.

ECGs

► LIFE-THREATENING ARRHYTHMIA

Type II second-degree atrioventricular block

Produced by a conduction disturbance in the His-Purkinje system, a Type II (Mobitz II) second-degree atrioventricular (AV) block causes an intermittent absence of conduction. In Type II block, two or more atrial impulses are conducted to the ventricles with constant PR intervals, when suddenly, without warning, the atrial impulse is blocked. This type of block occurs in an anterior wall myocardial infarction, severe coronary artery disease, and chronic degeneration of the conduction system.

Intervention

If the patient is hypotensive, treatment aims at increasing his heart rate to improve cardiac output. Because the conduction block occurs in the His-Purkinje system, drugs that act directly on the myocardium usually prove more effective than those that increase the atrial rate. As a result, dopamine (Intropin) instead of atropine may be ordered to increase the ventricular rate.

If the patient has an anterior wall MI, the doctor will immediately insert a temporary pacemaker to prevent ventricular asystole. For long-term management, the patient will usually need a permanent pacemaker.

Lead II

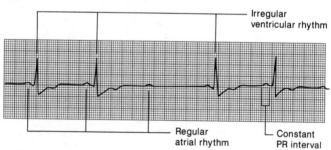

Irregular ventricular rhythm

Regular atrial rhythm

Constant PR interval

Characteristics and interpretation

Atrial rhythm: regular
Ventricular rhythm: regular or irregular
Atrial rate: usually within normal limits. Rate shown: 60 beats/minute.
Ventricular rate: may be within normal limits but less than the atrial rate. Rate shown: 40 beats/minute.
P wave: normal size and configuration. Not all P waves will be followed by a QRS complex.

PR interval: constant and frequently within normal limits for all conducted beats
QRS complex: usually greater than 0.16 second due to the presence of a preexisting bundle-branch heart block. Complex shown: 0.12 second.
T wave: usually normal size and configuration
QT interval: usually within normal limits. Interval shown: 0.44 second.

> ► LIFE-THREATENING ARRHYTHMIA

Third-degree atrioventricular block

Also called complete heart block, third-degree atrioventricular (AV) block occurs when all supraventricular impulses are prevented from reaching the ventricles. If this type of block originates at the AV node, a junctional escape rhythm occurs; if it originates below the AV node, an idioventricular escape rhythm occurs.

Third-degree AV block involving the AV node may result from an inferior wall myocardial infarction (MI) or digitalis toxicity. Third-degree AV block below the AV node may result from an anterior wall MI or chronic degeneration of the conduction system.

Intervention

If cardiac output isn't adequate or the patient's condition is deteriorating, the doctor will order therapy to improve the ventricular rhythm. Initially, atropine or dopamine (Intropin) may be ordered to increase the ventricular rate and improve cardiac output until a pacemaker is available. Dopamine should be titrated carefully because it places the patient at risk for ventricular tachycardia.

Lead MCL₁

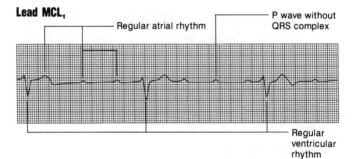

Regular atrial rhythm

P wave without QRS complex

Regular ventricular rhythm

Characteristics and interpretation

Atrial rhythm: usually regular
Ventricular rhythm: usually regular
Atrial rate: usually within normal limits. Rate shown: 90 beats/minute.
Ventricular rate: slow. Rate shown: 30 beats/minute.
P wave: normal size and configuration
PR interval: can't be measured because the atria and ventricles beat independently of each other
QRS complex: determined by the site of the escape rhythm. With a junctional escape rhythm, the duration and configuration are normal; with an idioventricular escape rhythm, the duration is greater than 0.12 second and the complex is distorted. Complex shown: duration 0.16 second, configuration abnormal, and complex distorted.
T wave: normal size and configuration
QT interval: may or may not be within normal limits. Interval shown: 0.56 second.

> ► LIFE-THREATENING ARRHYTHMIA

Ventricular asystole

With ventricular asystole (or standstill), electrical activity in the ventricles stops. What you see on an electrocardiogram (ECG) strip is an almost-flat line. Some activity may be evident in the atria, but the atrial impulse isn't conducted to the ventricles. P waves may continue for a time, but the QRS complexes have disappeared.

Asystole is life-threatening, caused by cardiac or noncardiac conditions that cause inadequate blood flow. Without ventricular electrical activity, ventricular contraction doesn't occur. Consequently, there's no cardiac output or perfusion.

The same ECG pattern may appear if the patient's electrodes fall off or the monitor isn't turned on, but you should evaluate the patient before checking anything else.

Intervention

A patient with asystole needs immediate treatment including cardiopulmonary resuscitation (CPR) and other life-support measures. If he has a temporary demand pacemaker, turn it on.

Treatment includes the following steps: If the rhythm is unclear but ventricular fibrillation may be present, defibrillate the patient. If asystole appears, confirm its presence in two leads. Continue CPR and establish I.V. access. Intubate when possible. Consider immediate transcutaneous pacing. Give the patient epinephrine 1:10,000, 1 mg I.V. push, every 3 to 5 minutes. Give atropine 1 mg I.V. push (repeat in 3 to 5 minutes) up to 0.04 mg/kg. If the patient fails to respond, consider terminating efforts.

Keep in mind that sodium bicarbonate isn't recommended for a routine cardiac arrest.

Lead II

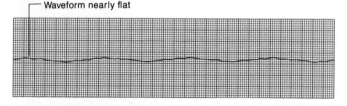

Waveform nearly flat

Characteristics and interpretation

Atrial rhythm: usually indiscernible
Ventricular rhythm: none
Atrial rate: usually indiscernible
Ventricular rate: none
P wave: may or may not be present
PR interval: not measurable

QRS complex: absent
T wave: absent
QT interval: not measurable
Other: waveform is an almost-flat line.

CHAPTER 4

Common laboratory tests:
Giving care and interpreting results

LAB TESTS

Specimen identification

Guide to color-top collection tubes

The color of the specimen collection tube you use indicates the type of test to be performed, as shown below.

COLOR AND DRAW VOLUME	ADDITIVE	TEST PURPOSE
Red (2 to 20 ml)	None	Serum studies
Lavender (2 to 10 ml)	EDTA	Whole blood studies
Green (2 to 15 ml)	Heparin (sodium, lithium, or ammonium)	Plasma studies
Blue (2.7 or 4.5 ml)	Sodium citrate and citric acid	Coagulation studies on plasma
Black (2.7 or 4.5 ml)	Sodium oxalate	Coagulation studies on plasma
Gray (3 to 10 ml)	Glycolytic inhibitor, such as sodium fluoride, powdered oxalate salt, or glycolytic microbial inhibitor	Glucose determinations on serum or plasma
Marble-top	Silicone gel	Serum separation

LAB TESTS

Laboratory tests

Activated partial thromboplastin time

The activated partial thromboplastin time (APTT) test evaluates all the clotting factors of the intrinsic pathway, except platelets. Relying on an activator, such as kaolin, to shorten clotting time, this test measures the time needed to form a fibrin clot after calcium and phospholipid emulsion are added to a plasma sample.

Purpose
• To screen for clotting factor deficiencies in the intrinsic pathway
• To monitor heparin therapy.

Procedure-related nursing care
Explain the purpose of the test to the patient, and tell him the test requires a blood sample. Inform a patient who's receiving heparin therapy that the test may be repeated at regular intervals to assess his response to treatment.

Perform a venipuncture, collecting a blood sample in a 7-ml blue-top tube.

Reference values

A fibrin clot should form 25 to 36 seconds after a reagent is added.

Abnormal results

A prolonged APTT may indicate a deficiency of certain plasma clotting factors or the presence of heparin, fibrin split products, fibrinolysin, or circulating anticoagulants that act as antibodies to specific clotting factors.

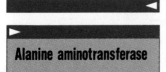

Alanine aminotransferase

Alanine aminotransferase (ALT) is one of two specialized enzymes called aminotransferases that catalyze a reversible amino group transfer in the Krebs cycle and that can accumulate in the bloodstream when liver cells are injured. ALT serves as an indicator of hepatic disease. It appears primarily in the cytoplasm of liver cells with smaller amounts in the kidneys, heart, and skeletal muscles. This test is also referred to as alanine transaminase or serum glutamic-pyruvic transaminase (SGPT).

Purpose

• To help detect and evaluate treatment of hepatic disease — especially hepatitis, and cirrhosis without jaundice
• To help distinguish between myocardial and hepatic tissue damage (when used with the aspartate aminotransferase test)
• To assess hepatotoxicity of certain drugs.

Procedure-related nursing care

Explain the purpose of the test to the patient, and tell him you'll need to take a blood sample.

Perform a venipuncture, collect-ing the sample in a 7-ml red-top tube. If necessary, you can store the serum sample for up to 3 days at room temperature.

Reference values

Serum ALT levels range from 10 to 35 units/liter.

Abnormal results

Extremely high levels of ALT (up to 50 times normal) suggest viral or severe drug-induced hepatitis, or another hepatic disease with extensive necrosis.

Moderate to high elevations may indicate infectious mononucleosis, chronic hepatitis, intrahepatic cholestasis or cholecystitis, early or improving acute viral hepatitis, or severe hepatic congestion caused by heart failure.

Slight to moderate elevations may appear in any condition that produces acute hepatocellular injury, such as active cirrhosis and drug-induced or alcoholic hepatitis. Marginal elevations occasionally occur in acute myocardial infarction, reflecting secondary hepatic congestion or release of some ALT from myocardial tissue.

Aldosterone, serum

This test measures serum levels of aldosterone, the principal mineralocorticoid secreted by the zona glomerulosa of the adrenal cortex. Aldosterone regulates ion transport across cell membranes in the renal tubules, helping to maintain blood pressure and volume and to regulate fluid and electrolyte balance.

Aldosterone secretion is controlled primarily by the renin-angiotensin system, serum potassium level, and corticotropin. Hyponatremia, hypovolemia, and other disorders that provoke renin release stimulate aldosterone secretion. Similarly, high potassium levels trigger aldosterone secretion through a potent feedback system.

Purpose
• To help diagnose primary and secondary aldosteronism, hypoaldosteronism, and salt-losing syndrome.

Procedure-related nursing care
Explain the purpose of the test to the patient, and tell him the test requires two blood samples. Instruct him to maintain a low-carbohydrate, normal-sodium (3 g/day or 135 μ/mol) diet for at least 2 weeks (preferably 30 days) before the test.

If the patient is premenopausal, specify the phase of her menstrual cycle on the laboratory slip. (Aldosterone levels may fluctuate during the menstrual cycle.) If aldosterone levels will be measured using radioimmunoassay, make sure the patient hasn't undergone a radioactive scan during the week preceding the test.

Perform a venipuncture in the morning while the patient is still supine after a night's rest. Collect the sample in a 7-ml red-top tube. Note the time and the patient's position during venipuncture on the laboratory slip.

Draw another sample 4 hours later after the patient has been up and about and while he stands. Use another 7-ml red-top collection tube, noting the time and the patient's position on the laboratory slip. Tell the patient he can resume his normal diet.

Reference values
Normally, serum aldosterone levels (in a standing, nonpregnant patient) range from 1 to 16 ng/dl. The range for an adult who has been standing for at least 2 hours is 4 to 31 ng/dl. Values in females are variable.

Abnormal results
Excessive aldosterone secretion points to primary or secondary aldosteronism. Primary aldosteronism (Conn's syndrome) may result from adrenocortical adenoma, bilateral adrenal hyperplasia or, less commonly, cancer. Secondary aldosteronism can result from conditions that increase renin-angiotensin activity, such as sodium depletion, potassium excess, renovascular hypertension, congestive heart failure, cirrhosis, nephrotic syndrome, and idiopathic edema. Other causes include corticotropin treatment and pregnancy (third trimester).

Depressed aldosterone levels may indicate primary hypoaldosteronism, salt-losing syndrome, toxemia of pregnancy, Addison's disease, renin deficiency, or hypokalemia.

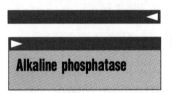

Alkaline phosphatase

This test measures serum levels of alkaline phosphatase (ALP), which are particularly sensitive to mild biliary obstruction.

An enzyme that's most active at a pH of about 9.0, alkaline phosphatase influences bone calcification and lipid and metabolite transport. Total serum levels reflect the combined activity of several alkaline phosphatase isoenzymes found in the liver, bones, kidneys, intestinal lining, and placenta.

Purpose
• To detect focal hepatic lesions causing biliary obstruction, such as tumors or abscesses
• To supplement information from other liver function studies and GI enzyme tests

• To detect skeletal diseases primarily characterized by marked osteoblastic activity
• To assess the effectiveness of vitamin D therapy used for deficiency-induced rickets.

Procedure-related nursing care

Explain the purpose of the test to the patient, and tell him it requires a blood sample. Instruct him to fast for at least 8 hours before the test.

Perform a venipuncture, collecting the sample in a 7-ml red-top tube. Send it to the laboratory at once because ALP activity increases at room temperature from a rise in pH. The sample should be analyzed within 4 hours.

After the venipuncture, tell the patient to resume his normal diet.

Reference values

Benchmark serum ALP levels vary with the laboratory method used. Total serum ALP levels, as measured by chemical inhibition, range from 90 to 239 units/liter for men. For women under age 45, total ALP levels range from 76 to 196 units/liter; for women over age 45, the range widens to 87 to 250 units/liter.

Pregnant women have elevated ALP levels.

Abnormal results

Significant elevations in alkaline phosphatase levels usually indicate skeletal disease or an extrahepatic or intrahepatic biliary obstruction that causes cholestasis. Many acute hepatic diseases also cause alkaline phosphatase levels to rise before serum bilirubin levels change.

A moderate increase may reflect acute biliary obstruction from hepatocellular inflammation in active cirrhosis, mononucleosis, or viral hepatitis. Or it may reflect osteomalacia or deficiency-induced rickets.

A sharp increase in alkaline phosphatase levels may indicate complete biliary obstruction by malignant or infectious infiltrations or fibrosis. Such markedly high levels are most common in Paget's disease and occur occasionally in extensive bone metastasis or hyperparathyroidism.

Rarely, low alkaline phosphatase levels can signal hypophosphatasia or protein or magnesium deficiency.

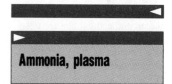

Ammonia, plasma

Used to help determine the severity of hepatocellular damage, this test measures plasma levels of ammonia. Normally, the body uses ammonia to rebuild amino acids. The liver then converts the ammonia to urea for excretion by the kidneys. But in liver diseases, ammonia can bypass the liver and accumulate in the blood.

Purpose

• To help monitor the progression of severe hepatic disease and the effectiveness of therapy
• To recognize impending or established hepatic coma.

Procedure-related nursing care

If the patient is conscious, explain the purpose of the test and tell him it requires a blood sample. Tell him to fast overnight because protein intake may alter the test results.

Before performing the venipuncture, notify laboratory personnel so that they can start their preparations. They'll have only 20 minutes from the time you draw the sample to perform the test.

Perform the venipuncture, collecting the sample in a 10-ml green marble-top tube. Handle the sample gently to prevent hemolysis. Pack the container in ice, and send it to the laboratory immediately. (Don't use a chilled container.)

Before removing pressure from the venipuncture site, make sure the bleeding has stopped. Hepatic disease can prolong bleeding time.

Reference values
Plasma ammonia levels are normally less than 50 µg/dl.

Abnormal results
Severe hepatic disease and hepatic coma caused by cirrhosis or acute hepatic necrosis commonly cause elevated plasma ammonia levels. High levels also occur in Reye's syndrome, GI hemorrhage, severe congestive heart failure, pericarditis, erythroblastosis fetalis, and leukemia.

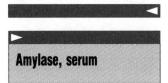

Amylase, serum

An enzyme synthesized primarily in the pancreas and the salivary glands and secreted into the GI tract, amylase helps digest starch and glycogen in the mouth, stomach, and intestines. Changes in serum amylase levels can indicate acute pancreatic disease.

Purpose
• To diagnose acute pancreatitis
• To distinguish acute pancreatitis from causes of abdominal pain that require immediate surgery
• To assess pancreatic injury caused by abdominal trauma or surgery.

Procedure-related nursing care
Explain the purpose of the test to the patient, and tell him you'll need a blood sample. Instruct him to re-

frain from alcohol consumption before the test.

This blood test should be done before other diagnostic or therapeutic interventions. If the patient reports severe pain in his left upper abdominal quadrant, collect the sample in a 7-ml red-top tube immediately.

Reference values
More than 20 methods of measuring serum amylase levels exist, with different ranges of normal values. Test values cannot always be converted to a standard measurement. Serum levels normally range from 30 to 220 units/liter. A general average is less than 300 units/liter.

Abnormal results
The highest serum amylase levels occur 4 to 12 hours after the onset of acute pancreatitis. In 48 to 72 hours, the levels drop to normal. If the doctor suspects pancreatitis but the patient has normal serum levels, a urine test should be ordered.

Moderate serum elevations may result from an obstruction of the common bile duct, the pancreatic duct, or the ampulla of Vater; pancreatic injury from a perforated peptic ulcer; pancreatic cancer; acute salivary gland disease; ectopic pregnancy; peritonitis; ovarian or lung cancer; and impaired renal function.

Slight elevations may occur in an asymptomatic patient. An amylase fractionation test may help determine the source of the amylase and aid in the selection of further tests.

Depressed levels can result from chronic pancreatitis, pancreatic cancer, cirrhosis, hepatitis, and toxemia of pregnancy.

Anion gap

The anion gap test measures the difference between serum levels of two anions, chloride (Cl^-) and bicarbonate (HCO_3^-), on the one hand, and serum levels of two cations, sodium (Na^+) and potassium (K^+), on the other hand. Calculation of the anion gap is based on this physical principle: *Total* concentrations of cations and anions are normally equal, accounting for the electrical neutrality of serum. Thus, any gap between the measured anions and cations reflects the serum concentration of unmeasured anions: sulfates, phosphates, organic acids (such as ketone bodies and lactic acid), and proteins.

An increased anion gap indicates a rise in one or more of these unmeasured anions. This may occur in metabolic acidosis characterized by excessive organic or inorganic acids, including lactic acidosis and ketoacidosis.

A normal anion gap, however, doesn't rule out metabolic acidosis. When acidosis results from a loss of HCO_3^- in urine or other body fluids, renal reabsorption of Na^+ promotes Cl^- retention, and the anion gap remains unchanged. Thus, metabolic acidosis resulting from excessive Cl^- levels is known as normal anion gap acidosis.

Purpose
• To distinguish types of metabolic acidosis
• To monitor renal function in a patient receiving total parenteral nutrition.

Procedure-related nursing care
Explain the purpose of the test to the patient, and tell him the test requires a blood sample. Then perform a venipuncture, and collect the sample in a 10- to 15-ml red-top tube.

Reference values
The anion gap should range from 8 to 14 mEq/liter.

Abnormal results
An anion gap above 14 mEq/liter results from the buildup of metabolic acids and occurs with conditions that cause organic acids, sulfates, or phosphates to accumulate. Such conditions include renal failure; ketoacidosis from starvation, diabetes mellitus, or alcohol ingestion; lactic acidosis; and salicylate, methanol, ethylene glycol (antifreeze), or paraldehyde toxicity.

Although rare, an anion gap below 8 mEq/liter may occur in hypermagnesemia and in paraproteinemic states, such as multiple myeloma and Waldenström's macroglobulinemia.

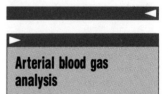

Arterial blood gas analysis

Arterial blood gas (ABG) analysis evaluates gas exchange in the lungs by measuring the partial pressures of oxygen (PaO_2) and carbon dioxide ($PaCO_2$) in arterial blood. PaO_2 indicates how much oxygen the lungs are delivering to the blood. $PaCO_2$ indicates how efficiently the lungs eliminate carbon dioxide.

The test also measures the arterial sample's pH, which indicates the acid-base balance, or the hydrogen ion (H^+) concentration. Acidity indicates an H^+ excess; alkalinity, an H^+ deficit. Other ABG measurements include oxygen (O_2) content, oxygen saturation (SaO_2), and bicarbonate (HCO_3^-) levels.

You may draw blood for ABG analysis by percutaneous arterial puncture or from an arterial line.

Purpose
• To evaluate the efficiency of pulmonary gas exchange
• To determine the blood's acid-base balance
• To monitor respiratory therapy
• To assess the efficiency of mechanical ventilation.

Procedure-related nursing care
Before the procedure. Explain the purpose of the test to the patient, and tell him it requires a blood sample. Instruct him to breathe normally while you draw the sample. If you need to perform an arterial puncture, warn him that he may feel a brief cramping or throbbing pain at the puncture site.

If the patient has just started receiving mechanical ventilation, wait at least 15 minutes before drawing the sample. In that way, you'll get an accurate measurement of the patient's response to mechanical ventilation. If a patient is receiving oxygen therapy, discontinue it for 15 to 20 minutes, if ordered, before drawing a sample. With a patient receiving intermittent positive-pressure breathing, wait at least 20 minutes after treatment stops before drawing a sample; such treatment alters ABG values. For the same reason, don't suction a patient right before drawing an arterial sample.

During the procedure. Perform an arterial puncture or collect the sample from the arterial line, drawing the blood into a heparinized syringe. Put the sample into a bag of ice.

After the procedure. If you performed an arterial puncture, apply

pressure to the puncture site for at least 5 minutes – 10 minutes if you used the femoral artery – and tape a gauze pad firmly over it. Avoid taping around the entire limb.

Note on the laboratory slip whether the patient was receiving oxygen therapy or breathing room air when you drew the sample. If appropriate, note the oxygen flow rate. For a patient receiving mechanical ventilation, note the fraction of inspired oxygen (FIO_2) and tidal volume. For any patient, note the rectal temperature and respiratory rate. Send the sample and the laboratory slip to the laboratory.

Monitor the patient's vital signs. Observe a patient who received an arterial puncture for signs and symptoms of circulatory impairment, including swelling, discoloration, pain, numbness, and tingling in the bandaged arm or leg, and check the puncture site for bleeding.

Reference values
ABG values should fall within these ranges:
• O_2 content: 15% to 23%
• PaO_2: 75 to 100 mm Hg
• $PaCO_2$: 35 to 45 mm Hg
• pH: 7.35 to 7.45
• SaO_2: 94% to 100%
• HCO_3^-: 22 to 26 mEq/liter.

Abnormal results
A PaO_2 level below 50 mm Hg usually indicates hypoxia. A value between 50 and 75 mm Hg may indicate hypoxia, depending on the patient's age and the oxygen concentration he's receiving. After age 60, a patient's normal PaO_2 may fall below 75 mm Hg.

A $PaCO_2$ above 45 mm Hg indicates hypoventilation or hypercapnia; below 35 mm Hg, hyperventilation or hypocapnia. The $PaCO_2$ value can also signal a respiratory acid-base imbalance. A level above 45 mm Hg points to respiratory acidosis; below 35 mm Hg, respiratory alkalosis.

A pH greater than 7.42 indicates alkalosis. A pH less than 7.35 indicates acidosis.

A patient with a PaO_2 between 60 and 100 mm Hg should have an SaO_2 above 85%. If his SaO_2 drops sharply, his PaO_2 has probably fallen below 50 mm Hg.

An HCO_3^- value above 26 mEq/liter points to metabolic, or kidney-related, alkalosis; under 22 mEq/liter, metabolic acidosis. (For more information, see *Recognizing acid-base disorders.*)

Recognizing acid-base disorders

DISORDER	A.B.G. FINDINGS	POSSIBLE CAUSES
Respiratory acidosis (excess CO_2 retention)	• pH <7.35 • HCO_3^- >26 mEq/liter (if compensating) • $PaCO_2$ >45 mm Hg	• Central nervous system depression from drugs, injury, or disease • Hypoventilation from respiratory, cardiac, musculoskeletal, or neuromuscular disease
Respiratory alkalosis (excess CO_2 loss)	• pH >7.45 • HCO_3^- <22 mEq/liter (if compensating) • $PaCO_2$ <35 mm Hg	• Hyperventilation due to anxiety, pain, or improper ventilator settings • Respiratory stimulation from drugs, disease, hypoxia, fever, or high room temperature • Gram-negative bacteremia
Metabolic acidosis (HCO_3^- loss or acid retention)	• pH <7.35 • HCO_3^- <22 mEq/liter • $PaCO_2$ <35 mm Hg (if compensating)	• Depletion of HCO_3^- from renal disease, diarrhea, or small-bowel fistulas • Excessive production of organic acids from hepatic disease; endocrine disorders, such as diabetes mellitus; hypoxia; shock; or drug toxicity • Inadequate excretion of acids due to renal disease
Metabolic alkalosis (HCO_3^- retention or acid loss)	• pH >7.45 • HCO_3^- >26 mEq/liter • PaO_2 >45 mm Hg (if compensating)	• Loss of hydrochloric acid from prolonged vomiting or gastric suctioning • Loss of potassium from increased renal excretion (as in diuretic therapy) or steroid overdose • Excessive alkali ingestion

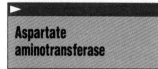

Aspartate aminotransferase

Aspartate aminotransferase (AST) serves as an indicator of hepatic and cardiac diseases. A hepatic enzyme, AST is found in the cytoplasm and mitochondria of many cells—mainly in the liver, heart, skeletal muscles, kidneys, pancreas and, to a lesser extent, the red blood cells. When cellular damage occurs, AST is released into serum. You also may hear this test referred to as aspartate transaminase or serum glutamic-oxaloacetic transaminase (SGOT).

Purpose
• To aid in the detection and differential diagnosis of acute hepatic disease
• To monitor progress in patients with cardiac or hepatic diseases
• To detect a recent myocardial infarction, or MI (together with creatine kinase and lactate dehydrogenase tests).

Procedure-related nursing care
Explain the purpose of the test to the patient. Tell him the test usually requires three venipunctures—one on admission and one each day for the next 2 days.

Perform the venipuncture, collecting the sample in a 7-ml redtop tube. To obtain the most reliable results, draw serum samples at the same time each day.

Reference values
AST levels should range from 8 to 20 units/liter.

Abnormal results
AST levels fluctuate according to the extent of cellular necrosis. Thus, levels may rise slightly and transiently early in the disorder and peak during the most acute phase. Depending on when the initial sample is drawn, subsequent AST levels may rise—indicating increasing tissue damage—or fall—indicating tissue repair. These relative changes provide a reliable way to monitor cellular damage.

Extremely high elevations (more than 20 times normal) may indicate acute viral hepatitis, severe skeletal muscle trauma, extensive surgery, drug-induced hepatic injury, or severe passive hepatic congestion.

High elevations (from 10 to 20 times normal) can result from a severe MI, severe infectious mononucleosis, and alcoholic cirrhosis. Such levels may also occur during the prodromal or resolution stages of conditions that cause extremely high elevations.

Moderate to high elevations (from 5 to 10 times normal) may point to Duchenne's muscular dystrophy, dermatomyositis, or chronic hepatitis. These levels can also occur during the prodromal and resolution stages of diseases that cause high elevations.

Low to moderate elevations (from 2 to 5 times normal) may indicate hemolytic anemia, metastatic hepatic tumors, acute pancreatitis, pulmonary emboli, alcohol withdrawal syndrome, or fatty liver.

AST levels rise slightly after the first few days of a biliary duct obstruction. Relatively low elevations also occur at some time during all of the preceding conditions.

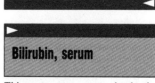

Bilirubin, serum

This test measures serum levels of bilirubin, the predominant pigment in bile. The major product of hemoglobin catabolism, bilirubin is formed in the reticuloendothelial system. It is then bound to albumin, a plasma protein, and transported to the liver as unconjugated (indirect or prehepatic) bilirubin. There it joins with glucuronic acid to form bilirubin glucuronide and bilirubin diglucuronide, and is excreted into bile as conjugated (direct or posthepatic) bilirubin.

Effective bilirubin conjugation and excretion depend on a properly functioning hepatobiliary system and a normal turnover rate of red blood cells (RBCs). Thus, measuring levels of indirect and direct bilirubin can help evaluate hepatobiliary function and RBC production.

Purpose
• To evaluate liver function
• To help detect jaundice and monitor its progression
• To help diagnose biliary obstruction and hemolytic anemia.

Procedure-related nursing care
Explain the purpose of the test to the patient, and tell him you'll need a blood sample. Instruct him to fast for at least 4 hours before the test.

Perform the venipuncture, collecting the sample in a 10- to 15-ml red-top tube. Protect the sample from strong sunlight and ultraviolet light. Tell the patient he can resume his normal diet.

Reference values
Indirect serum bilirubin should measure at or below 1.1 mg/dl; direct serum bilirubin, less than 0.5 mg/dl.

Abnormal results
Elevated indirect serum bilirubin levels can result from hemolysis, a transfusion reaction, hemolytic or pernicious anemia, hemorrhage, and hepatocellular dysfunction (possibly resulting from viral hepatitis or

congenital enzyme deficiencies, such as Gilbert syndrome and Crigler-Najjar syndrome).

Elevated direct serum bilirubin levels usually indicate biliary obstruction. In this disorder, direct bilirubin, blocked from its normal pathway through the liver into the biliary tree, overflows into the bloodstream. Such obstruction may be intrahepatic (from viral hepatitis, cirrhosis, or a chlorpromazine reaction) or extrahepatic (from gallstones or gallbladder or pancreatic cancer). An obstruction also may result from bile duct disease.

If the biliary obstruction continues, indirect bilirubin levels may also rise because of hepatic damage. In severe chronic hepatic damage, direct bilirubin levels may return to normal or near-normal levels eventually, but indirect bilirubin levels remain elevated.

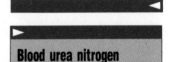

Blood urea nitrogen

This test measures the nitrogen fraction of urea, the chief end product of protein metabolism. Formed in the liver from ammonia and excreted by the kidneys, urea accounts for 40% to 50% of the blood's nonprotein nitrogen.

The blood urea nitrogen (BUN) level reflects protein intake and renal excretory capacity. But the serum creatinine test is a more reliable indicator of uremia.

Purpose
• To evaluate renal function and aid in the diagnosis of renal disease
• To help assess hydration.

Procedure-related nursing care
Explain the purpose of the test to the patient, and tell him you'll need

a blood sample. Then perform a venipuncture, collecting the sample in a 10- to 15-ml red-top tube.

Reference values

BUN levels should range from 8 to 20 mg/dl.

Abnormal results

Elevated BUN levels occur in renal disease, reduced renal blood flow (caused by dehydration, for example), urinary tract obstruction, and conditions that increase protein catabolism (such as burns).

Depressed BUN levels occur in severe hepatic damage, malnutrition, and overhydration.

Calcium, serum

Used to detect several disorders, this test measures serum levels of calcium—a cation that helps regulate and promote neuromuscular and enzyme activity, skeletal development, and blood coagulation. The body absorbs calcium from the GI tract, provided that it contains sufficient vitamin D, and excretes calcium in urine and feces. Over 98% of the body's calcium is found in the bones and teeth. But calcium can shift in and out of these structures. For example, when calcium concentrations in the blood drop below normal, calcium can move out of the bones and teeth to help restore blood levels.

Purpose

• To help diagnose neuromuscular, skeletal, and endocrine disorders; arrhythmias; blood-clotting deficiencies; and acid-base imbalance.

Procedure-related nursing care

Explain the purpose of the test to the patient, and tell him it requires a blood sample. Then perform a venipuncture, collecting the sample in a 10- to 15-ml red-top tube.

Reference values

Serum calcium levels should range from 8.9 to 10.1 mg/dl.

Abnormal results

Abnormally high serum calcium levels (hypercalcemia) may occur in hyperparathyroidism and parathyroid tumors (caused by oversecretion of parathyroid hormone), Paget's disease of the bone, multiple myeloma, metastatic cancer, multiple fractures, or prolonged immobilization. Elevated serum calcium levels may also result from inadequate excretion of calcium, as in adrenal insufficiency and renal disease; excessive calcium ingestion; or overuse of antacids such as calcium carbonate.

Low calcium levels (hypocalcemia) may result from insufficient calcium intake, hypoparathyroidism, total parathyroidectomy, malabsorption, Cushing's syndrome, renal failure, acute pancreatitis, and peritonitis.

Cerebrospinal fluid analysis

A clear substance circulating in the subarachnoid space, cerebrospinal fluid (CSF) has several vital functions. It protects the brain and spinal cord from injury and transports products of neurosecretion, cellular biosynthesis, and cellular metabolism through the central nervous system (CNS).

Most commonly, a doctor obtains three CSF samples by lumbar punc-

LAB TESTS

ture between the third and fourth lumbar vertebrae. If a patient has an infection at this site, lumbar puncture is contraindicated, and the doctor may instead perform a cisternal puncture. If a patient has increased intracranial pressure, the doctor must remove the CSF with extreme caution because the removal of fluid causes a rapid reduction in pressure, which could trigger brain stem herniation. The doctor may instead perform a ventricular puncture on this patient. CSF samples may also be obtained during other neurologic tests—myelography or pneumoencephalography, for instance.

Purpose

• To measure CSF pressure to help detect an obstruction of CSF circulation
• To aid in diagnosing viral or bacterial meningitis, and subarachnoid or intracranial hemorrhage, tumors, and abscesses
• To aid in diagnosing neurosyphilis and chronic CNS infections.

Procedure-related nursing care

Before the procedure. Explain the purpose of the test to the patient and describe the procedure. Make sure the patient has signed a consent form. Tell him to remain still and breathe normally during the procedure because movement and hyperventilation can alter pressure readings and cause injury. Following these instructions will also reduce his risk of developing a headache—the most common adverse effect of a lumbar puncture.

Just before the procedure, obtain a lumbar puncture tray. Place the labeled tubes at the bedside, making sure the labels are numbered sequentially, and include the patient's name, the date, and his room number as well as any laboratory instructions.

During the procedure. If you're assisting with the procedure, position the patient as directed—usually, on his side at the edge of the bed with his knees drawn up as far as possible. This position allows full flexion of the spine and easy access to the lumbar subarachnoid space. Place a small pillow under the patient's head, and bend his head forward so that his chin touches his chest. Help him hold this position during the procedure. Stand in front of him, and place one hand around his neck and the other around his knees.

If the doctor wants the patient sitting, have him sit on the edge of the bed and lower his chest and head toward his knees. Help the patient maintain this position throughout the procedure.

Monitor the patient for signs of adverse reactions, such as elevated pulse rate, pallor, or clammy skin.

Make sure the samples are placed in the appropriately labeled tubes. Record the collection time on the test request form; then send the form and the labeled samples to the laboratory immediately.

After the procedure. After a lumbar puncture, the patient usually lies flat for 8 hours. Some doctors, however, allow a 30-degree elevation of the head of the bed. Encourage the patient to drink plenty of fluids, and remind him that raising his head may cause a headache. If he develops a headache, administer an analgesic as ordered.

Check the puncture site for redness, swelling, drainage, CSF leakage, and hematoma every hour for the first 4 hours, then every 4 hours for the next 20 hours. Monitor the patient's level of consciousness, pupillary reaction, and vital signs. Also observe him for signs and symptoms of complications of the lumbar puncture, such as meningitis, cerebellar tonsillar herniation, and medullary compression.

Reference values

Normal CSF pressure ranges from 50 to 180 mm H_2O. The CSF should appear clear and colorless. Normal protein content ranges between 15 and 45 mg/dl; normal gamma globulin levels, between 3% and 12% of total protein. Glucose levels range between 45 and 85 mg/dl, which is two-thirds of the blood glucose level. CSF should contain 0 to 5 white blood cells per microliter and no red blood cells. All serologic tests should be nonreactive.

The chloride level should be 118 to 130 mEq/liter. And the Gram stain should reveal no organisms.

Abnormal results

For a listing of abnormal results and their possible causes, see *CSF analysis: Abnormal results.*

LAB TESTS

CSF analysis: Abnormal results

ELEMENT	ABNORMAL RESULT	POSSIBLE CAUSES
Cerebrospinal fluid (CSF) pressure	• Increase	• Increased intracranial pressure from hemorrhage, tumor, or edema caused by trauma
	• Decrease	• Spinal subarachnoid obstruction above puncture site
Appearance	• Cloudy	• Infection
	• Xantho- chromic	• Elevated protein level or red blood cell (RBC) breakdown
	• Bloody	• Subarachnoid, intracerebral, or intraventricular hemorrhage; spinal cord obstruction; traumatic puncture
	• Brown	• Meningeal melanoma
	• Orange	• Systemic carotenemia
Protein	• Marked increase	• Tumor, trauma, hemorrhage, diabetes mellitus, polyneuritis, blood in CSF
	• Marked decrease	• Rapid CSF production
Gamma globulin	• Increase	• Demyelinating disease (such as multiple sclerosis), neurosyphilis, Guillain-Barré syndrome

(continued)

CSF analysis: Abnormal results (continued)

ELEMENT	ABNORMAL RESULT	POSSIBLE CAUSES
Glucose	• Increase • Decrease	• Systemic hyperglycemia • Systemic hypoglycemia, bacterial or fungal infection, meningitis, mumps, postsubarachnoid hemorrhage
Cell count	• Increase in white blood cell count • RBCs present	• Meningitis, acute infection, onset of chronic illness, tumor, abscess, infarction, demyelinating disease (such as multiple sclerosis) • Hemorrhage or traumatic puncture
Serologic tests	• Reactive	• Neurosyphilis
Chloride	• Decrease	• Infected meninges (tuberculosis or meningitis)
Gram stain	• Gram-positive or gram-negative organisms	• Bacterial meningitis

---

Chloride, serum

This test measures serum levels of chloride, the major extracellular fluid anion. Interacting with sodium, the major extracellular cation, chloride helps regulate blood volume and arterial pressure by helping to maintain the osmotic pressure of blood.

Chloride levels affect acid-base balance, varying inversely with bicarbonate levels. Excessive chloride loss in gastric juices or other secretions can cause hypochloremic metabolic alkalosis; excessive chloride retention or ingestion can lead to hyperchloremic metabolic acidosis.

Purpose
• To detect acid-base imbalance
• To help evaluate fluid status and extracellular cation-anion balance.

Procedure-related nursing care
Explain the purpose of the test to the patient, and tell him it requires a blood sample. Then perform a venipuncture, collecting the sample in a 10- to 15-ml red-top tube.

Reference values
Serum chloride levels should range from 100 to 108 mEq/liter.

Abnormal results
Elevated chloride levels (hyperchloremia) can result from severe dehydration, complete renal shutdown,

head injury (producing neurogenic hyperventilation), and primary aldosteronism.

Usually associated with low sodium and potassium levels, low chloride levels (hypochloremia) can stem from prolonged vomiting, gastric suctioning, intestinal fistula, chronic renal failure, and Addison's disease. Dilutional hypochloremia can result from congestive heart failure or edema that leads to excess extracellular fluid.

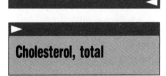

Cholesterol, total

This test measures the circulating levels of free cholesterol and cholesterol esters — the two forms in which this biochemical compound appears in the body.

A structural component in cell membranes and plasma lipoproteins, cholesterol is absorbed from the diet and synthesized in the liver and other body tissues. It helps form adrenocorticoid steroids, bile salts, androgens, and estrogens.

A diet high in saturated fat raises cholesterol levels by stimulating the absorption of lipids, including cholesterol, from the intestine; a diet low in saturated fat lowers cholesterol levels.

Purpose
• To assess the risk of coronary artery disease (CAD)
• To evaluate fat metabolism
• To help diagnose nephrotic syndrome, pancreatitis, hepatic disease, hypothyroidism, and hyperthyroidism.

Procedure-related nursing care
Explain the purpose of the test to the patient, and tell him it requires a blood sample. Make sure he fasts

overnight and refrains from drinking alcohol for 24 hours before the procedure.

Perform a venipuncture, collecting the sample in a 7-ml red-top tube. Send it to the laboratory immediately.

Tell the patient he may resume his normal diet.

Reference values
Total cholesterol concentrations vary with age and sex, normally ranging from 150 to 200 mg/dl.

Abnormal results
Cholesterol levels above 250 mg/dl generally indicate a high risk of CAD and the need for treatment. A patient with a level between 200 and 240 mg/dl has a moderate risk. But if he has other risk factors — if he smokes or has high blood pressure, for instance — his risk of CAD is considered high. Elevated cholesterol levels (hypercholesterolemia) can also indicate incipient hepatitis, lipid disorders, bile duct blockage, nephrotic syndrome, obstructive jaundice, pancreatitis, and hypothyroidism.

Low serum cholesterol levels (hypocholesterolemia) result from malnutrition, cellular necrosis of the liver, and hyperthyroidism.

Complete blood count

A common test, the complete blood count (CBC) provides a fairly comprehensive picture of all the blood's formed elements. Typically, the CBC includes these components: hemoglobin concentration, hematocrit, red blood cell (RBC) and white blood cell (WBC) counts, as well as the WBC differential and stained RBC examination, which are commonly done together.

A CBC is especially useful for evaluating conditions in which the hematocrit doesn't parallel the RBC count, such as microcytic or macrocytic anemia.

After the WBC differential, the same stained slide is evaluated for RBC distribution and morphology—including changes in cell contents, color, size, and shape. This examination provides more information for detecting leukemia, anemia, and thalassemia.

Purpose

• To compare the status of specific blood elements
• To help detect and evaluate anemias
• To indicate the need for further definitive studies.

Procedure-related nursing care

Explain the purpose of the test to the patient, and tell him it requires a blood sample. Then perform a venipuncture, collecting at least a 5-ml sample in a lavender-top tube.

Reference values

(See the entries for the individual tests that make up the CBC.)

Abnormal results

Variations in the size and shape of RBCs are reported as occasional, slight, moderate, marked, or very marked; structural variations are reported as the number of immature or nucleated RBCs per 100 WBCs. Cell inclusions are also noted.

(For implications of specific abnormal results, see the entries for the individual tests that make up the CBC.)

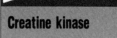

Creatine kinase

An enzyme found mainly in muscle cells and brain tissue, creatine kinase (CK) catalyzes the transfer of a phosphate group from adenosine triphosphate to creatine, releasing energy in the process. Because of this key role in energy production, CK reflects tissue catabolism. An increase in serum CK levels serves as an indicator of cellular trauma.

CK occurs as three distinct isoenzymes: CK-BB, found mainly in brain tissue; CK-MB, located in cardiac muscle (although a small amount also appears in skeletal muscle); and CK-MM, found in skeletal muscle. Because each isoenzyme is associated with a specific location, fractionation and measurement can help pinpoint the site of tissue destruction. Total CK levels help diagnose skeletal muscle disorders, but CK-MM, which constitutes over 99% of the total CK normally present in serum, acts as a more specific indicator.

Purpose

• To diagnose acute myocardial infarction (MI) and reinfarction
• To evaluate possible causes of chest pain and to monitor the severity of myocardial ischemia after cardiac surgery or catheterization or cardioversion
• To detect skeletal muscle disorders that don't have a neurogenic origin, such as Duchenne's muscular dystrophy and early dermatomyositis.

Procedure-related nursing care

Explain the purpose of the test to the patient, and tell him you'll need to collect several blood samples. If he's being tested for a skeletal muscle disorder, instruct him to avoid exercising for 24 hours before the test.

Perform a venipuncture, collecting the sample in a 7-ml red-top tube. If the patient needs an I.M. injection, be sure to draw the sample either before the injection or at least 1 hour after it—otherwise, the test results may be altered. Send the sample to the laboratory at once.

Always collect the sample on schedule, and note the time on the laboratory slip. For a patient with chest pain, note how many hours have elapsed since the pain started.

Reference values

Total CK levels determined by the most commonly performed assay in North America range from 60 to 400 IU/liter for men and from 40 to 150 IU/liter for women. Typical ranges for isoenzyme levels are as follows: CK-BB, 0% of total CK; CK-MB, 0% to 3% of total CK; CK-MM, 97% to 100% of total CK.

Abnormal results

Detectable CK-BB levels may indicate brain tissue injury, certain widespread malignant tumors, severe shock, or renal failure. However, such elevations don't confirm a specific diagnosis.

CK-MB levels above 5% of total CK (more than 10 units/liter) are usually considered positive for MI. With an acute MI or cardiac surgery, CK-MB levels begin rising in 2 to 4 hours, peak in 12 to 24 hours, and return to normal in 24 to 48 hours. Persistent elevations or increasing levels indicate ongoing myocardial damage. Total CK levels follow roughly the same pattern but rise slightly later. Serious skeletal muscle injury, as occurs in certain muscular dystrophies, polymyositis, and severe myoglobinuria, may slightly elevate CK-MB levels.

Rising CK-MM values follow skeletal muscle damage from trauma, such as surgery and I.M. injection. Extremely high levels (50 to 100 times normal) may occur in such diseases as dermatomyositis and muscular dystrophy. Sharp elevations also occur with muscular activity caused by agitation, such as an acute psychotic episode. A moderate rise develops in patients with hypothyroidism.

Elevated total CK levels may occur in patients with severe hypokalemia, carbon monoxide poisoning, malignant hyperthermia, and alcoholic cardiomyopathy. CK levels also increase after seizures. Occasionally, total CK levels rise after a pulmonary or cerebral infarction.

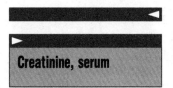

Creatinine, serum

A quantitative analysis of serum creatinine levels, this test provides a more sensitive measure of renal damage than blood urea nitrogen levels do. That's because renal impairment is virtually the only cause of elevated serum creatinine levels.

Creatinine, a nonprotein end product of creatine metabolism, appears in serum in amounts proportional to the body's muscle mass. The kidneys easily excrete creatinine, with little or no tubular reabsorption, so creatinine levels are directly related to the glomerular filtration rate.

Purpose

• To assess renal glomerular filtration
• To screen for renal damage.

Procedure-related nursing care

Explain the purpose of the test to the patient, and tell him you'll need a blood sample. Instruct him to restrict food and fluid intake for about 8 hours before the test.

Perform a venipuncture, using a 10- to 15-ml red-top tube.

Reference values
Serum creatinine levels in men range from 0.8 to 1.2 mg/dl; in women, from 0.6 to 0.9 mg/dl.

Abnormal results
Elevated serum creatinine levels generally indicate renal disease that has damaged at least 50% of the nephrons. Decreased levels may result from a loss of muscle mass in advanced muscular dystrophy.

Creatinine clearance

This test determines how efficiently the kidneys clear creatinine from the blood. The clearance rate is expressed in terms of the volume of blood (in milliliters) that the kidneys can clear of creatinine in 1 minute. The test requires a blood sample and a timed urine specimen.

Creatinine, the chief metabolite of creatine, is produced and excreted in constant amounts that are proportional to total muscle mass. Normal physical activity, diet, and urine volume have little effect on this production, although strenuous exercise and a high-protein diet can affect it.

Purpose
• To assess renal function (primarily glomerular filtration)
• To monitor the progression of renal insufficiency.

Procedure-related nursing care
Explain the purpose of the test to the patient. Tell him that you'll need a timed urine specimen and at least one blood sample. Describe the urine collection procedure. Also, tell him to avoid eating an excessive amount of meat before the procedure and to avoid strenuous exercise during the urine collection period.

Collect a timed urine specimen for a 2-, 6-, 12-, or 24-hour period, as ordered. During the collection period, perform a venipuncture, collecting the blood sample in a 7-ml red-top tube.

Collect the urine specimen in a bottle containing a preservative to prevent creatinine degradation. Refrigerate it or keep it on ice during the collection period. At the end of the period, send the specimen to the laboratory. Then tell the patient he may resume his normal diet and activities.

Reference values
For men, the normal creatinine clearance ranges from 85 to 125 ml/minute. For women, the creatinine clearance ranges from 75 to 115 ml/minute. For older patients, creatinine clearance declines by 6 ml/minute for each succeeding decade of life.

Abnormal results
A low creatinine clearance rate may result from reduced renal blood flow (from shock or renal artery obstruction), acute tubular necrosis, acute or chronic glomerulonephritis, advanced bilateral renal lesions (as occur in polycystic kidney disease, renal tuberculosis, or cancer), or nephrosclerosis. Congestive heart failure and severe dehydration may also cause the creatinine clearance rate to drop.

LAB TESTS

An elevated creatinine clearance rate usually has little diagnostic significance.

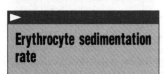

Erythrocyte sedimentation rate

A sensitive but nonspecific test, the erythrocyte sedimentation rate (ESR) measures the time needed for erythrocytes (red blood cells) in a whole blood sample to settle to the bottom of a vertical tube. It commonly provides the earliest indication of disease when other chemical or physical signs are still normal. The rate typically rises significantly in widespread inflammatory disorders caused by infection or autoimmune mechanisms. Localized inflammation and cancer may prolong the ESR elevation.

Purpose
• To aid in diagnosing occult disease, such as tuberculosis, tissue necrosis, and connective tissue disease
• To monitor inflammatory and malignant disease.

Procedure-related nursing care
Explain the purpose of the test to the patient, and tell him you'll need a blood sample. Then perform a venipuncture, collecting the sample in a 7-ml lavender-top, 4.5-ml black-top, or 4.5-ml blue-top tube, depending on laboratory preference.

Examine the sample for clots and clumps; then send it to the laboratory immediately.

Reference values
The ESR normally ranges from 0 to 9 mm/hour in men, and from 0 to 15 mm/hour in women.

Abnormal results
The ESR rises in most anemias, pregnancy, acute or chronic inflammation, tuberculosis, paraproteinemias (especially multiple myeloma and Waldenström's macroglobulinemia), rheumatic fever, rheumatoid arthritis, and some types of cancer.

Polycythemia, sickle cell anemia, hyperviscosity, and low plasma protein levels tend to depress the ESR.

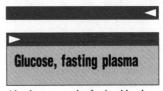

Glucose, fasting plasma

Also known as the fasting blood sugar test, the fasting plasma glucose test measures the patient's plasma glucose levels after a 12- to 14-hour fast.

When a patient fasts, his plasma glucose levels decrease, stimulating the release of the hormone glucagon. This hormone raises plasma glucose levels by accelerating glycogenolysis, stimulating gluconeogenesis, and inhibiting glycogen synthesis. Normally, the secretion of insulin stops the rise in glucose levels. In patients with diabetes, however, the absence or deficiency of insulin allows glucose levels to remain persistently elevated.

Purpose
• To screen for diabetes mellitus and other glucose metabolism disorders
• To monitor drug or dietary therapy in patients with diabetes mellitus
• To help determine the insulin requirements of patients who have uncontrolled diabetes mellitus and those who require parenteral or enteral nutritional support
• To help evaluate patients with known or suspected hypoglycemia.

LAB TESTS

Procedure-related nursing care

Explain the purpose of the test to the patient. Tell him that it requires a blood sample and that he must fast (taking only water) for 12 to 14 hours before the test.

If the patient is known to have diabetes, you should draw his blood before he receives insulin or an oral antidiabetic drug. Tell him to watch for symptoms of hypoglycemia, such as weakness, restlessness, nervousness, hunger, and sweating. Stress that he should report such symptoms immediately.

Prepare the laboratory slip for the blood sample, noting the time of the patient's last pretest meal and pretest medication. Also record the time the sample is collected.

Perform a venipuncture, collecting the sample in a 5-ml gray-top tube. If the sample can't be sent to the laboratory immediately, refrigerate it and transport it as soon as possible.

Give the patient a balanced meal or a snack after the procedure. Assure him that he can now eat and take medications withheld before the procedure.

Reference values

The normal range for fasting plasma glucose levels varies according to the length of the fast. Generally, after a 12- to 14-hour fast, normal values are between 70 and 100 mg/dl.

Abnormal results

Fasting plasma glucose levels greater than 100 mg/dl but less than 140 mg/dl may suggest impaired glucose tolerance. A 2-hour glucose tolerance test that yields a plasma glucose level between 140 and 200 mg/dl, and an intervening oral glucose tolerance test that yields a plasma glucose level greater than or equal to 200 mg/dl confirm the diagnosis.

Levels greater than or equal to 140 mg/dl (obtained on two or more occasions) may indicate diabetes mellitus if other causes of the patient's hyperglycemia have been ruled out. Such a patient will also have a random plasma glucose level greater than or equal to 200 mg/dl along with the classic signs and symptoms of diabetes mellitus — polydipsia, polyuria, ketonuria, polyphagia, and rapid weight loss.

Elevated levels can also result from pancreatitis, recent acute illness (such as myocardial infarction), Cushing's syndrome, pituitary adenoma, pancreatitis, hyperthyroidism, and pheochromocytoma. Hyperglycemia may also stem from chronic hepatic disease, brain trauma, chronic illness, or chronic malnutrition and is typical in eclampsia, anoxia, and seizure disorders.

Depressed plasma glucose levels can result from hyperinsulinism (overdose of insulin being the most common cause), insulinoma, von Gierke's disease, functional or reactive hypoglycemia, hypothyroidism, adrenocortical insufficiency, congenital adrenal hyperplasia, hypopituitarism, islet cell carcinoma of the pancreas, hepatic necrosis, and glycogen storage disease.

Glucose, 2-hour postprandial plasma

This test requires a blood sample drawn 2 hours after the patient eats a meal. The results reflect the metabolic response to a carbohydrate challenge. Normally, the blood glucose level will return to the fasting level within 2 hours.

Purpose

• To monitor the effectiveness of drug or diet therapy in patients with diabetes mellitus
• To identify disorders associated with abnormal glucose metabolism
• To confirm diabetes mellitus in patients with the classic signs and symptoms of the disorder.

Procedure-related nursing care

Explain the purpose of the test to the patient. Tell him it requires a blood sample drawn 2 hours after a meal. Instruct him to fast overnight (except for water) and then to eat a high-carbohydrate breakfast that includes milk, orange juice, cereal with sugar, and toast. Stress that he should avoid smoking and strenuous exercise after the meal.

Prepare the laboratory slip, noting the time of the patient's meal, the sample collection time, and the time the last pretest insulin or antidiabetic dose was given, if appropriate.

Perform a venipuncture, collecting the sample in a 5-ml gray-top tube. If you can't send the sample to the laboratory immediately, place it in the refrigerator and transport it as soon as possible.

Tell the patient he may resume eating and other activities that he discontinued before the test.

Reference values

In a person who doesn't have diabetes, postprandial glucose values usually are less than 145 mg/dl; levels may be slightly higher in older people, increasing an average of 6 mg/dl for each decade.

Abnormal results

Values greater than 140 mg/dl are abnormal in adults under age 50; values greater than 160 mg/dl are abnormal in adults over age 60. A value greater than or equal to 200 mg/dl, along with the classic signs and symptoms of diabetes mellitus, confirms a diagnosis of diabetes mellitus.

Other causes of elevated glucose levels include: pancreatitis, Cushing's syndrome, acromegaly, pheochromocytoma, chronic hepatic disease, nephrotic syndrome, gastrectomy with dumping syndrome, and seizure disorders.

Depressed glucose levels occur in hyperinsulinism, insulinoma, von Gierke's disease, functional or reactive hypoglycemia, hypothyroidism, adrenocortical insufficiency, congenital adrenal hyperplasia, hypopituitarism, islet cell carcinoma of the pancreas, hepatic necrosis, and glycogen storage disease.

LAB TESTS

Glucose tolerance test, oral

The most sensitive method of evaluating borderline diabetes mellitus, the oral glucose tolerance test measures carbohydrate metabolism after ingestion of a challenge dose of glucose.

With this test, the body rapidly absorbs the glucose, causing plasma glucose levels to rise and peak 30 minutes to 1 hour after ingestion. The pancreas responds by secreting more insulin, causing glucose levels to return to normal within 2 hours. During this period, plasma glucose levels are monitored to assess insulin secretion and the body's ability to metabolize glucose. Occasionally, levels are monitored for an additional 2 to 3 hours to aid diagnosis of hypoglycemia and malabsorption syndrome.

If the oral glucose tolerance test is performed on a patient with non-insulin-dependent (Type II) diabetes, his fasting plasma glucose levels may be within the normal range. However, insufficient secretion of insulin after ingestion of carbohydrates will cause his plasma glucose levels to rise sharply and return to normal slowly. This decreased tolerance for glucose helps confirm non-insulin-dependent diabetes.

The oral glucose tolerance test shouldn't be performed on a person who's suspected of having insulinoma because prolonged fasting by such a patient can lead to fainting and coma. It also shouldn't be used for patients with fasting plasma glucose values greater than 140 mg/dl or postprandial plasma glucose values greater than 200 mg/dl.

Purpose
• To confirm diabetes mellitus in selected patients
• To aid in diagnosing hypoglycemia and malabsorption syndrome.

Procedure-related nursing care
Before the procedure. Explain the purpose of the test to the patient, and tell him that it requires several blood samples and a urine specimen. Instruct him to maintain a high-carbohydrate diet, not to smoke, and to avoid caffeine and alcohol for 3 days before the test. Tell him to fast for 10 to 16 hours before the test and to avoid strenuous exercise for 8 hours before and during the test. Suggest that he bring a book or other quiet diversionary material with him because the procedure usually takes several hours.

Alert the patient to the symptoms of hypoglycemia—weakness, restlessness, nervousness, hunger, and sweating—and tell him to report such symptoms immediately.

Prepare the laboratory slip, specifying the time of the patient's last meal and the times of the blood sample collections. Also note the time of the patient's last pretest insulin or oral antidiabetic dose, if appropriate.

During the procedure. Obtain a fasting blood sample by performing a venipuncture—usually between 7 and 9 a.m. Draw the sample into a 7-ml gray-top tube. Collect a urine specimen at the same time, if appropriate.

After collecting these samples, administer the test load of oral glucose. Record the time when the patient starts drinking the solution. Encourage him to drink it all within 5 minutes.

You'll need to draw blood samples 30 minutes, 1 hour, 1½ hours, 2 hours, and 3 hours after the loading dose, as ordered. Use 7-ml gray-top tubes.

Tell the patient to lie down if he feels faint. If he develops severe hypoglycemia, draw a blood sample, record the time on the laboratory slip, and discontinue the test. Administer I.V. glucose or have the patient drink a glass of orange juice to reverse the reaction.

Send all blood and urine samples to the laboratory immediately. If that's not possible, refrigerate them and transport them as soon as possible.

After the procedure. Provide a balanced meal or a snack, observing the patient for signs of a hypoglycemic reaction. Tell the patient to resume his normal diet and activities.

Reference values
Normally, plasma glucose levels peak at 160 to 180 mg/dl 30 minutes to 1 hour after administration of an oral glucose test dose and re-

turn to fasting levels (or lower) within 2 hours. Normal levels are less than 140 mg/dl after 2 hours.

Abnormal results

If the 2-hour sample and at least one other sample (taken up to 2 hours after a 75-g or greater glucose dose) show a glucose level greater than or equal to 200 mg/dl, the test confirms diabetes in a nonpregnant adult.

After an oral glucose dose of 100g, gestational diabetes is confirmed in a pregnant patient if two plasma glucose levels equal or exceed a fasting value of 105 mg/dl, a 1-hour value of 190 mg/dl, a 2-hour value of 165 mg/dl, or a 3-hour value of 145 mg/dl.

Increased glucose levels are associated with other serious conditions, such as Cushing's syndrome, pheochromocytoma, central nervous system lesions, cirrhosis of the liver, myocardial or cerebral infarction, and hyperthyroidism, as well as with anxiety states and pregnancy.

Decreased glucose levels occur in hyperinsulinism, malabsorption syndrome, adrenocortical insufficiency (Addison's disease), hypothyroidism, and hypopituitarism.

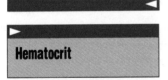

Hematocrit

A common test, hematocrit (HCT) measures the percentage of packed red blood cells (RBCs) in a whole blood sample. Thus, an HCT of 40% means that a 100-ml sample contains 40 ml of packed RBCs. The HCT value depends mainly on the number of RBCs but is also influenced by the size of the average RBC. Therefore, conditions that result in elevated concentrations of blood glucose and sodium (which cause swelling of RBCs) may produce elevated HCT. This test may be automatically performed as part of the complete blood count.

Purpose

• To aid diagnosis of polycythemia, anemia, and abnormal states of hydration
• To aid in calculating RBC indices
• To monitor fluid imbalance
• To monitor blood loss and evaluate blood replacement.

Procedure-related nursing care

Explain the purpose of the test to the patient, and tell him it requires a blood sample drawn from his finger. Then perform a fingerstick on an adult, using a heparinized capillary tube with a red band on the anticoagulant end. Fill the capillary tube from the red-banded end to about two-thirds' capacity, and seal this end with clay.

Reference values

HCT values vary, depending on the patient's sex and age, the type of sample, and the laboratory performing the test. Reference values range from 40% to 54% for men and from 37% to 47% for women.

Abnormal results

High HCT suggests polycythemia or hemoconcentration caused by blood loss; low HCT may indicate anemia or hemodilution.

Hemoglobin, glycosylated

This test measures three minor hemoglobins (Hb): A_{1a}, A_{1b}, and A_{1c}. These three hemoglobins are variants of Hb A formed by glycosylation – a nearly irreversible molecular process in which glucose becomes chemically incorporated in Hb A. Because glycosylation occurs at a constant rate during the 120-day life span of a red blood cell (RBC), glycosylated hemoglobin levels reflect the average blood glucose level during the preceding 6 to 10 weeks. This makes the test most appropriate for evaluating the long-term effectiveness of a patient's diabetes therapy.

Purpose
• To monitor control of diabetes mellitus.

Procedure-related nursing care
Explain the purpose of the test to the patient, and tell him it requires a blood sample. Instruct him to maintain his prescribed medication or diet regimen before the procedure.

Perform a venipuncture, collecting the sample in a 5-ml lavender-top tube. Be sure that you fill the collection tube completely. Then invert it gently several times so that you mix the sample and the anticoagulant adequately.

After the test, schedule the patient for appropriate follow-up testing in 6 to 8 weeks.

Reference values
Glycosylated hemoglobin values are reported as a percentage of the total hemoglobin within an RBC. Because Hb A_{1c} is present in a larger quantity than the other minor hemoglobins, it's the variant commonly measured. Reference values for Hb A_{1c} are usually 6% to 8% of the total hemoglobin within an RBC.

Abnormal results
If Hb A_{1c} accounts for more than 8% of the total hemoglobin within

an RBC, the patient's diabetes mellitus isn't considered under control.

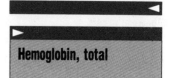

Hemoglobin, total

Usually done as part of the complete blood count, this test measures the grams of hemoglobin (Hb) found in a deciliter (dl, or 100 ml) of whole blood. Hb concentration correlates closely with the red blood cell (RBC) count and is affected by the Hb-RBC ratio and free plasma hemoglobin levels.

Purpose
• To measure the severity of anemia or polycythemia
• To monitor the patient's response to therapy for anemia.

Procedure-related nursing care
Explain the purpose of the test to the patient, and tell him it requires a blood sample. Then perform a venipuncture, collecting the sample in a 7-ml lavender-top tube.

Reference values
Normal Hb concentrations for a man range from 14 to 18 g/dl; for a woman, from 12 to 16 g/dl.

Abnormal results
An elevated total Hb level suggests hemoconcentration from polycythemia or dehydration. A low concentration of Hb may indicate anemia, recent hemorrhage, or fluid retention that is causing hemodilution.

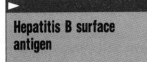

Hepatitis B surface antigen

The earliest and most reliable serologic marker of viral hepatitis infection, the hepatitis B surface antigen (HBsAg) appears in the serum of a patient with hepatitis B virus (HBV) as early as 14 days after exposure and throughout the acute stage of the illness. The antigen can also be detected in a carrier's blood.

After donation, all blood is screened for HBV before it's stored. However, the test doesn't screen for hepatitis A virus.

Purpose
• To screen blood for HBV
• To screen persons at high risk for contracting HBV, such as hemodialysis nurses
• To aid differential diagnosis of viral hepatitis.

Procedure-related nursing care
Explain the purpose of the test to the patient, and tell him that it requires a blood sample. Then perform the venipuncture, using a 10-ml red-top tube to collect the sample. Because HBV is a blood-borne infection, take extra care, following universal precautions. Make sure you wear gloves, avoid accidental needle puncture, wash your hands after the procedure, and properly dispose of the needle.

If you accidentally stick yourself with a used needle, report the incident immediately. Expect to receive gamma globulin to help prevent the disease.

Reference values
Serum is normally negative for HBsAg.

Abnormal results
The presence of HBsAg in a patient with hepatitis confirms hepatitis B. In chronic carriers and persons with chronic active hepatitis, HBsAg may be present in serum several months after the onset of acute infection. HBsAg may also occur in more than 5% of patients with certain diseases other than hepatitis, such as hemophilia, Hodgkin's disease, and leukemia.

HIV antibody: Serum enzyme immunoassay

The enzyme-linked immunosorbent assay (ELISA) detects the antibody to the human immunodeficiency virus (HIV) antigen. The HIV virus causes acquired immunodeficiency syndrome (AIDS). Positive findings are confirmed by the Western blot assay and immunofluorescence. Because this test is highly sensitive and specific, it's used to screen for HIV infection and to test all donated blood.

Purpose
• To aid diagnosis of HIV infection
• To detect exposure to HIV.

Procedure-related nursing care
Explain the purpose of the test to the patient, and tell him it requires a blood sample.

Perform the venipuncture, collecting the sample in a 10-ml red-top barrier tube. Because HIV is a blood-borne infection, take extra care, following universal precautions. Make sure you wear gloves, avoid accidental needle puncture, wash your hands after the procedure, and properly dispose of the needle. If you accidentally stick yourself with a used needle, report the incident immediately.

Reference values

Patients without the antibody will usually test negative.

Abnormal results

A positive test indicates exposure to HIV, but it doesn't necessarily indicate that the patient currently has AIDS. However, the patient will almost certainly develop AIDS within 10 years after being exposed to the virus.

Occasionally, false-positive test results may occur in patients with autoimmune diseases, such as systemic lupus erythematosus, or in patients with antibodies to human leukocyte antigens. Also, a high percentage of false-positive test results may occur in populations with a very low incidence of HIV infection.

Human chorionic gonadotropin, serum

This serum radioimmunoassay provides a quantitative analysis of the human chorionic gonadotropin (HCG) beta-subunit level. Although it's more costly than the routine urine test ordered to confirm pregnancy, it's also much more sensitive.

Purpose

• To detect early pregnancy or to determine the adequacy of hormone production in high-risk pregnancies
• To aid in diagnosing trophoblastic tumors, such as hydatidiform mole or choriocarcinoma, and tumors that secrete HCG ectopically

• To monitor treatment for induction of ovulation and conception.

Procedure-related nursing care

Explain the purpose of the test to the patient, and tell her it requires a blood sample. Then perform a venipuncture, and collect at least a 7-ml sample in a red-top tube.

Reference values

Values for serum HCG should be less than 5 IU/ml.

Abnormal results

Elevated serum HCG levels may indicate pregnancy; sharply elevated levels may indicate a multiple pregnancy. Increased levels may also indicate a tumor. However, the HCG beta-subunit levels can't differentiate between pregnancy and tumor recurrence.

Low serum HCG beta-subunit levels can occur in ectopic pregnancy or pregnancy of less than 9 days.

Human chorionic gonadotropin, urine

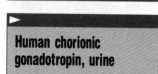

Human chorionic gonadotropin (HCG) is a glycopeptide hormone produced by the trophoblastic cells of the placenta. Although its precise function is unclear, HCG, along with progesterone, apparently maintains the corpus luteum during early pregnancy.

Production of HCG increases steadily during the first trimester, peaking around the 10th week of gestation. Levels then fall to less than 10% of first trimester peak levels.

The qualitative analysis of HCG in the urine can detect pregnancy as early as 10 days after a missed menstrual period. Quantitative measurements may be used to evaluate a suspected hydatidiform mole or HCG-secreting tumors.

Purpose
• To detect and confirm pregnancy
• To aid the diagnosis of hydatidiform mole or HCG-secreting tumors.

Procedure-related nursing care
Explain the purpose of the test to the patient, and inform her that it requires a first-voided morning specimen for a qualitative analysis—or a 24-hour urine collection for a quantitative analysis.

Indicate on the laboratory slip the date of the patient's last menstrual period.

Collect the appropriate urine specimen. If you're collecting a 24-hour specimen, you must either refrigerate it or keep it on ice during the entire collection period.

Reference values
In qualitative analysis, if agglutination fails to occur, test results are positive, indicating that the patient is pregnant.

In quantitative analysis, urine HCG levels in the first trimester of a normal pregnancy may be as high as 500,000 IU/day; in the second trimester, they range from 10,000 to 25,000 IU/day; and in the third trimester, from 5,000 to 15,000 IU/day. After delivery, HCG levels decline rapidly, becoming undetectable within a few days.

You won't normally find measurable levels of HCG in the urine of men or nonpregnant women.

Abnormal results
After the first trimester, elevated urine HCG levels may indicate mul-

tiple pregnancy or erythroblastosis fetalis. Depressed urine HCG levels may indicate threatened spontaneous abortion or ectopic pregnancy.

Measurable levels of HCG in men or nonpregnant women may indicate: choriocarcinoma; testicular or ovarian tumors; melanoma; multiple myeloma; or gastric, hepatic, pancreatic, or breast cancer.

Human leukocyte antigen typing

The human leukocyte antigen (HLA) test identifies a group of antigens present on the surfaces of all nucleated cells but most easily detected on lymphocytes. There are four types of HLA: HLA-A, HLA-B, HLA-C, and HLA-D.

Purpose
• To provide histocompatibility typing of tissue recipients and donors
• To aid genetic counseling
• To aid paternity testing.

Procedure-related nursing care
Explain the purpose of the test to the patient, and tell him it requires a blood sample.

Check the patient's history for recent blood transfusions. HLA testing may be postponed if he has recently received a transfusion.

Perform a venipuncture, and collect the sample in a collection tube containing acid citrate dextrose solution, an anticoagulant.

Reference values
In HLA-A, HLA-B, and HLA-C testing, lymphocytes that react with the test antiserum undergo lysis;

they're detected by phase micros-copy. In HLA-D testing, leukocyte incompatibility is marked by blast formation, DNA synthesis, and pro-liferation.

Abnormal results

Incompatible HLA-A, HLA-B, HLA-C, or HLA-D groups may cause unsuccessful tissue transplan-tation.

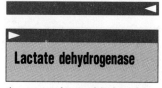

Lactate dehydrogenase

An enzyme, lactate dehydrogenase (LD) catalyzes the reversible con-version of muscle pyruvic acid into lactic acid. Because LD appears in almost all body tissues, cellular damage causes an elevation of total serum LD levels, thus limiting its diagnostic usefulness.

However, five tissue-specific iso-enzymes can be identified and mea-sured: LD_1 and LD_2 appear primar-ily in the heart, red blood cells, and kidneys; LD_3, primarily in the lungs; and LD_4 and LD_5, in the liver and skeletal muscles. This test is widely used to detect myocardial infarction (MI) because LD_1 and LD_2 levels rise 12 to 48 hours after an MI begins, peak in 2 to 5 days, and drop to normal in 7 to 14 days if tissue necrosis doesn't persist.

Purpose

• To aid differential diagnosis of MI, pulmonary infarction, anemias, and hepatic disease
• To support creatine kinase (CK) isoenzyme test results in diagnosing MI or to help in diagnosing MI when CK-MB samples are drawn too late (more than 24 hours after the onset of acute MI)

• To monitor patient response to some forms of chemotherapy.

Procedure-related nursing care

Explain the purpose of the test to the patient, and tell him it requires a blood sample. If the patient is suspected of having experienced an MI, tell him that the test will be repeated on the next two mornings to monitor progressive changes.

Perform a venipuncture, collect-ing the sample in a 7-ml red-top tube. Draw each sample on sched-ule to avoid missing peak levels, and mark the collection time on the laboratory slip.

Send the sample to the labora-tory immediately. If transport is de-layed, keep the sample at room temperature.

Reference values

Total LD levels should range from 45 to 90 units/liter. Distribution of isoenzymes should be as follows:
• LD_1 — 14% to 26% of total
• LD_2 — 29% to 39% of total
• LD_3 — 20% to 26% of total
• LD_4 — 8% to 16% of total
• LD_5 — 6% to 16% of total.

Abnormal results

Because many common disorders raise total LD levels, isoenzyme electrophoresis is usually required for diagnosis. In some disorders, to-tal LD levels may be within normal limits, but abnormal proportions of the isoenzymes indicate specific or-gan tissue damage. For instance, in acute MI the concentration of LD_1 is greater than that of LD_2 within 12 to 48 hours after the onset of symptoms. This reversal of the nor-mal isoenzyme pattern typifies myocardial damage and is referred to as flipped LD.

LD isoenzyme values: Abnormal results

This table shows the correlation between elevated isoenzyme levels (color boxes) and probable diagnoses.

DISEASE	LD_1	LD_2	LD_3	LD_4	LD_5
Cardiopulmonary					
Myocardial infarction	■	■			
Myocardial infarction with hepatic congestion	■	■			■
Rheumatic carditis	■	■			
Myocarditis	■				
Congestive heart failure (decompensated)					■
Shock	■	■	■	■	■
Pulmonary infarction		■	■		

DISEASE	LD_1	LD_2	LD_3	LD_4	LD_5
Hematologic					
Pernicious anemia	■	■			
Hemolytic anemia	■	■			
Sickle cell anemia	■	■			
Gastrointestinal					
Hepatobiliary disorder					■
Hepatitis					■
Active cirrhosis					■
Hepatic congestion					■

LAB TESTS

Lipoprotein-cholesterol fractionation

Cholesterol fractionation tests isolate and measure the cholesterol in serum low-density lipoproteins (LDLs) and high-density lipoproteins (HDLs). LDL and HDL levels are considered significant because the Framingham Heart Study showed that the higher the HDL level, the lower the incidence of coronary artery disease (CAD), and the higher the LDL level, the higher the incidence of CAD.

Purpose
• To assess the risk of CAD.

Procedure-related nursing care
Explain the purpose of the test to the patient, and tell him it requires a blood sample. Tell him to maintain his normal diet for 2 weeks before the test, to abstain from alcohol for 24 hours before the test, and to fast and avoid exercise for 12 to 14 hours before the test.

Perform a venipuncture, collecting the sample in a 7-ml red-top tube. Send the sample to the laboratory immediately, or place it in the refrigerator until you can transport it.

After the test, the patient may resume his diet and any activities restricted by the test.

Reference values

Normal HDL cholesterol levels range from 29 to 77 mg/dl, and normal LDL cholesterol levels range from 62 to 185 mg/dl. These values vary according to age, sex, geographic region, and ethnic group, so check with your laboratory for appropriate normal values.

Abnormal results

High LDL levels increase the risk of CAD. High HDL levels generally reflect a healthy state but also can indicate chronic hepatitis, early-stage primary biliary cirrhosis, or alcohol consumption. Rarely, a sharp rise (one as high as 100 mg/dl) in a second type of HDL (alpha$_2$-HDL) may signal CAD.

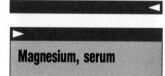

Magnesium, serum

This quantitative analysis measures serum levels of magnesium. Vital to neuromuscular function, this electrolyte helps regulate intracellular metabolism, activates many essential enzymes, and affects the metabolism of nucleic acids and proteins. Magnesium also helps transport sodium and potassium across cell membranes and, through its effect on the secretion of parathyroid hormone, influences intracellular calcium levels.

Most magnesium is found in bone and in intracellular fluid; a small amount is found in extracellular fluid. Absorbed by the small intestine, magnesium is excreted in the urine and feces.

Purpose
• To evaluate electrolyte status
• To assess neuromuscular or renal function.

Procedure-related nursing care

Explain the purpose of the test to the patient, and tell him it requires a blood sample. Then perform a venipuncture, collecting the sample in a 7-ml red-top tube. Handle the sample gently to prevent hemolysis.

Reference values

Serum magnesium levels normally range from 1.7 to 2.1 mg/dl.

Abnormal results

Elevated serum magnesium levels (hypermagnesemia) most commonly occur in renal failure, when the kidneys excrete inadequate amounts of magnesium. Adrenocortical insufficiency (Addison's disease) can also elevate serum magnesium levels.

Decreased serum magnesium levels (hypomagnesemia) most commonly result from chronic alcoholism. Other causes include diarrhea, malabsorption syndrome, faulty absorption after bowel resection, prolonged bowel or gastric aspiration, acute pancreatitis, primary aldosteronism, severe burns, hypercalcemic conditions (including hyperparathyroidism), and certain diuretic therapies.

Occult blood, fecal

Invisible because of its minute quantity, fecal occult blood can be detected by microscopic analysis or by chemical tests for hemoglobin, such as the guaiac or orthotoluidine tests. Small amounts of blood (2 to 2.5 ml/day) normally appear in the feces; these tests are designed to detect greater-than-normal quantities.

Purpose
• To detect GI bleeding
• To aid early diagnosis of colorectal cancer.

Procedure-related nursing care
Explain the purpose of the test to the patient. Tell him it requires three stool specimens. (Occasionally only one random specimen will be used.) Instruct him to avoid contaminating the stool specimen with toilet tissue or urine. Tell him to maintain a high-fiber diet and to avoid eating red meats, poultry, fish, turnips, and horseradish for 48 to 72 hours before the test and throughout the collection period.

Collect three stool specimens or a random specimen, as appropriate. Send the specimen to the laboratory, or perform the test yourself, as ordered.

To perform the test yourself, obtain a small specimen from two different areas of each stool to allow for any variation in the distribution of blood. Use a commercially prepared Hemoccult card and developer. Apply 2 drops of the chemical developer to the paper covering the sample. Note the color after 1 minute. Typically, patients are given the card to take home with instructions to place a stool specimen on the card, close the window, and return the card. Later, the clinician applies the developer and watches for the color reaction.

Tell the patient he may resume his normal diet after the test.

Reference values
Normally, less than 2.5 ml of blood is present, and the test will result in a green reaction.

Abnormal results
A blue reaction that occurs within 30 to 60 seconds is a positive indicator of fecal occult blood. If the blue color appears within this period, consider it strongly positive. However, a faint blue reaction is weakly positive and not necessarily abnormal.

A positive test indicates GI bleeding that can result from several disorders, including varices, peptic ulcer, cancer, ulcerative colitis, dysentery, or hemorrhagic disease.

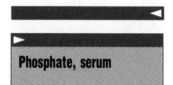

Phosphate, serum

This test measures serum levels of phosphate, the dominant cellular anion. Phosphate helps store and use body energy; helps regulate calcium levels, carbohydrate and lipid metabolism, and acid-base balance; and is essential to bone formation (about 85% of the body's phosphate is found in bone).

Phosphate is absorbed in the small intestine and excreted by the kidneys. Because calcium and phosphate interact in a reciprocal relationship, urinary excretion of phosphate increases or decreases in inverse proportion to serum calcium levels. Abnormal concentrations of phosphate result more often from improper excretion than they do from abnormal ingestion or absorption from dietary sources.

Purpose
• To aid the diagnosis of renal disorders and acid-base imbalance
• To detect endocrine, skeletal, and calcium disorders.

LAB TESTS

Procedure-related nursing care

Explain the purpose of the test to the patient, and tell him it requires a blood sample. Then perform a venipuncture, collecting the sample in a 7-ml red-top tube. Handle the sample gently to prevent hemolysis.

Reference values

Serum phosphate levels normally range from 2.5 to 4.5 mg/dl (or from 1.8 to 2.6 mEq/liter).

Abnormal results

Because serum phosphate levels alone have limited diagnostic value (only a few rare conditions directly affect phosphate metabolism), they should be interpreted in light of serum calcium levels. Although rarely clinically significant, elevated phosphate levels may result from skeletal disease, healing fractures, hypoparathyroidism, acromegaly, diabetic acidosis, high intestinal obstruction, or renal failure. Depressed phosphate levels may result from malnutrition, malabsorption syndrome, hyperparathyroidism, renal tubular acidosis, or treatment of diabetic acidosis.

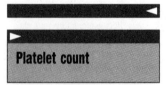

Platelet count

Platelets, or thrombocytes, are the smallest formed elements in the blood. Vital to the formation of the homeostatic plug in vascular injury, platelets promote coagulation by supplying phospholipids to the intrinsic thromboplastin pathway. The platelet count is one of the most important screening tests for platelet function.

Purpose

• To evaluate platelet production
• To assess the effects of chemotherapy or radiation therapy on platelet production
• To aid the diagnosis of thrombocytopenia or thrombocytosis
• To confirm a visual estimate of platelet number and morphology from a stained blood film.

Procedure-related nursing care

Explain the purpose of the test to the patient, and tell him it requires a blood sample. Then perform a venipuncture, collecting the sample in a 7-ml lavender-top tube. Gently mix the sample and the anticoagulant, and send the sample to the laboratory immediately.

Reference values

Normal platelet counts range from 130,000 to 370,000/µl.

Abnormal results

An increased platelet count (thrombocytosis) can result from hemorrhage; infectious disorders; cancer; iron deficiency anemia; recent surgery, pregnancy, or splenectomy; and inflammatory disorders such as collagen vascular disease. In such cases, the platelet count will return to normal after the patient recovers. However, the platelet count will remain elevated in primary thrombocytosis, myelofibrosis with myeloid metaplasia, polycythemia vera, and chronic myelogenous leukemia.

A decreased platelet count (thrombocytopenia) can result from aplastic or hypoplastic bone marrow disease; infiltrative bone marrow disease, such as carcinoma, leukemia, or disseminated infection; megakaryocytic hypoplasia; ineffective thrombopoiesis caused by folic acid or vitamin B_{12} deficiency; pooling of platelets in an enlarged spleen; increased platelet destruction caused by drugs or immune disorders; disseminated intravascular coagulation; Bernard-Soulier syndrome; mechanical injury to platelets; and suppression of bone marrow function caused by chemotherapy or radiation therapy.

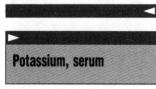

Potassium, serum

This quantitative analysis measures serum levels of potassium. Vital to homeostasis, potassium maintains cellular osmotic equilibrium. It also helps regulate muscle activity by maintaining electrical conduction within the cardiac and skeletal muscles. As well, potassium helps regulate enzyme activity and acid-base balance and influences kidney function.

Potassium levels are affected by variations in the secretion of adrenal steroid hormones and by fluctuations in pH, serum glucose levels, and serum sodium levels. A reciprocal relationship appears to exist between potassium and sodium; a substantial intake of one element causes a corresponding decrease of the other.

Although the body readily conserves sodium, it has no efficient method for conserving potassium. The kidneys excrete daily nearly all the ingested potassium. Even in potassium depletion, potassium excretion continues; therefore, potassium deficiency develops readily and commonly.

Purpose
• To evaluate clinical signs of hyperkalemia or hypokalemia
• To monitor renal function, acid-base balance, and glucose metabolism
• To evaluate neuromuscular and endocrine disorders
• To detect the origin of arrhythmias.

Procedure-related nursing care
Explain the purpose of the test to the patient, and tell him it requires a blood sample. After applying a tourniquet, perform the venipuncture immediately, telling the patient *not* to make a fist. Collect the sample in a 10- to 15-ml red-top tube.

Reference values
Normally, serum potassium levels range from 3.8 to 5 mEq/liter.

Abnormal results
Abnormally high serum potassium levels are common in patients with burns, crushing injuries, diabetic ketoacidosis, and myocardial infarction – conditions in which excessive cellular potassium enters the blood. Hyperkalemia may also indicate reduced sodium excretion, possibly because of renal failure (preventing normal sodium-potassium exchange) or Addison's disease (caused by the absence of aldosterone with consequent potassium buildup and sodium depletion).

Decreased potassium values commonly result from aldosteronism or Cushing's syndrome (marked by hypersecretion of adrenal steroid hormones), loss of body fluids (as in diuretic therapy), or excessive licorice ingestion (because of the aldosterone-like effect of glycyrrhizic acid).

Protein, urine

A quantitative test for proteinuria, a urine protein test aids in the diagnosis of renal disease. Normally, the glomerular capillary membrane allows only proteins of low molecular weight to enter the filtrate. The renal tubules then reabsorb most of these proteins, normally excreting a small amount that's undetectable by a screening test. However, with a damaged glomerular capillary membrane and impaired tubular reabsorption, detectable amounts of proteins will be excreted in the urine.

A qualitative screening test — a simple dipstick test performed on a random urine sample — is commonly done first. If it's positive, the quantitative analysis of a 24-hour urine specimen by acid precipitation will follow. Electrophoresis can detect Bence-Jones protein, hemoglobins, myoglobins, or albumin in the urine.

Purpose
• To aid in the diagnosis of renal disease
• To aid in the diagnosis of preeclampsia in a pregnant patient.

Procedure-related nursing care
Collect a 24-hour urine specimen using a special specimen container obtained from the laboratory. Refrigerate the specimen or place it on ice during the collection period. After collecting the entire specimen, transport it to the laboratory immediately.

Reference values
Normally, up to 150 mg of protein will be excreted in 24 hours.

Abnormal results
Heavy proteinuria (more than 4 g/24 hours) is commonly associated with nephrotic syndrome.

Moderate proteinuria (0.5 to 4 g/24 hours) occurs in several types of renal disease — acute or chronic glomerulonephritis, amyloidosis, toxic nephropathies — and in diseases in which renal failure commonly develops as a late complication of the disease, such as diabetes or heart failure.

Minimal proteinuria is most commonly associated with renal diseases in which glomerular involvement isn't a major factor, such as chronic pyelonephritis.

When accompanied by an elevated white blood cell count, proteinuria indicates urinary tract infection; with hematuria, proteinuria indicates local or diffuse urinary tract disorders.

Not all forms of proteinuria have pathologic significance. Benign proteinuria can result from changes in body position. Functional proteinuria is associated with emotional or physiologic stress and is usually transient.

Protein electrophoresis, serum

This test measures serum levels of albumin and globulins, the major blood proteins, in an electric field by separating the proteins according to their size, shape, and electrical charge at a pH of 8.6. Because each protein fraction moves at a different rate, this movement separates the fractions into recognizable and measurable patterns.

Albumin, which accounts for more than 50% of total serum protein levels, maintains oncotic pressure (preventing capillary plasma leaks) and transports substances that are insoluble in water alone — such as bilirubin, fatty acids, hormones, and drugs.

Four types of globulins exist: $alpha_1$, $alpha_2$, beta, and gamma. The first three types act primarily as carrier proteins that transport lipids, hormones, and metals through the blood. The fourth type, gamma globulin, acts as an important component of the body's immune system.

Although electrophoresis is the most current method for measuring serum protein levels, determinations of total protein and the albumin-globulin (A-G) ratio (normally greater than one) are still commonly performed. No matter which test method is used, a single protein fraction is rarely significant by itself.

Purpose
• To aid the diagnosis of hepatic disease, protein deficiency, blood dyscrasias, renal disorders, and GI and neoplastic diseases.

Procedure-related nursing care
Explain the purpose of the test to the patient, and tell him that it requires a blood sample.

Perform a venipuncture, and collect the sample in a 7-ml red-top tube.

Reference values
Values normally fall in these ranges:
• total serum protein levels, 6.6 to 7.9 g/dl (66 to 79 g/L)
• albumin fraction, 3.3 to 4.5 g/dl (33 to 45 g/L)
• $alpha_1$ globulin, 0.1 to 0.4 g/dl (1 to 4 g/L).
• $alpha_2$ globulin, 0.5 to 1 g/dl (5 to 10 g/L)

• beta globulin, 0.7 to 1.2 g/dl (7 to 12 g/L)
• gamma globulin, 0.5 to 1.6 g/dl (5 to 16 g/L).

Abnormal results
An incease in total protein can indicate chronic inflammatory disease, dehydration, diabetic acidosis, fulminating or chronic infection, monocytic leukemia, or multiple myeloma. A decrease can signal benzene or carbon tetrachloride poisoning, blood dyscrasias, congestive heart failure, essential hypertension, GI disease, hemorrhage, hepatic disease, or Hodgkin's disease. It can also result from hyperthyroidism, malabsorption, nephrosis, a severe burn, surgical or traumatic shock, toxemia of pregnancy, or uncontrolled diabetes mellitus.

An increase in albumin levels results from multiple myeloma. A decrease can stem from acute cholecystitis, collagen disease, essential hypertension, hepatic disease, Hodgkin's disease, hyperthyroidism, or hypogammaglobulinemia. Other possible causes include malnutrition, metastatic cancer, nephritis or nephrosis, peptic ulcer, plasma loss (from burns), rheumatoid arthritis, sarcoidosis, and systemic lupus erythematosus.

An $alpha_1$ globulin level increase can result from an acute infection, cancer, pregnancy, or tissue necrosis. A decrease indicates a genetic deficiency of $alpha_1$-antitrypsin.

An increase in $alpha_2$ globulin may indicate acute infection, an acute myocardial infarction, advanced cancer, nephrotic syndrome, rheumatic fever, rheumatoid arthritis, trauma, or a severe burn. A drop indicates hemolytic anemia or severe liver disease.

Elevated beta globulin levels can result from biliary cirrhosis, Cush-

LAB TESTS

ing's disease, diabetes mellitus, hypothyroidism, malignant hypertension, or nephrotic syndrome. A decrease results from hypocholesterolemia.

A rise in gamma globulin levels can indicate chronic active liver disease, Hodgkin's disease, rheumatoid arthritis, or systemic lupus erythematosus. A decrease can result from lymphocytic leukemia, lymphosarcoma, or nephrotic syndrome.

The A-G ratio is usually evaluated in relation to the total protein level. A low total protein level with a reversed A-G ratio (decreased albumin and elevated globulins) suggests chronic liver disease. A normal total protein level with a reversed A-G ratio suggests myeloproliferative disease (leukemia or Hodgkin's disease) or certain chronic infectious diseases (tuberculosis or chronic hepatitis).

Prothrombin time

This test measures the time required for a fibrin clot to form in a citrated plasma sample after calcium ions and tissue thromboplastin (factor III) have been added. This prothrombin time (PT) is then compared with the fibrin clotting time in a control sample of plasma. The most accurate test results state both the patient's and the control sample's clotting times in seconds.

Because it bypasses the extrinsic coagulation pathway and platelets, the test measures prothrombin activity and evaluates the extrinsic

coagulation system, including factors V and VII, as well as prothrombin and fibrinogen levels.

Purpose
• To monitor a patient's response to oral anticoagulant therapy
• To evaluate the extrinsic coagulation system
• To aid the diagnosis of conditions associated with abnormal bleeding
• To identify patients at risk for excessive bleeding during surgical or other invasive procedures
• To differentiate deficiencies of specific clotting factors
• To monitor the effects of certain diseases (hepatic disease or protein deficiency, for example) on hemostasis.

Procedure-related nursing care
Explain the purpose of the test to the patient, and tell him it requires a blood sample. If the test is being done to monitor the effects of anticoagulant medications, explain that it will be done daily when therapy begins and will be repeated at longer intervals when medication levels stabilize.

Perform a venipuncture, avoiding excessive probing. Collect the sample in a 7-ml blue-top tube and send it to the laboratory promptly.

Reference values
PT values normally range from 9.6 to 11.8 seconds in men and from 9.5 to 11.3 seconds in women. However, values vary, depending on the source of tissue thromboplastin and the type of sensing devices used to measure clot formation.

Abnormal results
Prolonged PT may indicate deficiencies in fibrinogen, prothrombin, or factors V, VII, or X (specific assays can pinpoint such deficiencies);

vitamin K deficiency; and hepatic disease. The prolonged time may also result from oral anticoagulant therapy. A prolonged PT that exceeds 2½ times the control value is commonly associated with abnormal bleeding.

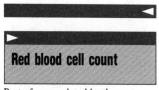

Red blood cell count

Part of a complete blood count, this test determines the number of red blood cells (RBCs) in a cubic millimeter (microliter) of whole blood. The RBC count (also called the erythrocyte count) can be used to calculate two RBC indices, mean corpuscular volume and mean corpuscular hemoglobin. These, in turn, reveal RBC size and hemoglobin concentration and weight.

Purpose
• To supply figures for computing the RBC indices
• To aid in diagnosis of anemia and polycythemia.

Procedure-related nursing care
Explain the purpose of the test to the patient, and tell him you'll need a blood sample. Then draw a venous blood sample, using a 7-ml lavender-top tube. Fill the collection tube completely, and invert it gently several times to mix the sample and the anticoagulant. Handle the sample gently to prevent hemolysis.

Reference values
RBC values vary according to age, sex, the type of blood sample, and altitude. In men, normal RBC counts range from 4.5 to 6.2 million/mm³ (4.5 to 6.2 × 10^{12}/L) of venous blood; in women, from 4.2

to 5.4 million/mm³ (4.2 to 5.4 × 10^{12}/L). People living at high altitudes usually have higher values.

Abnormal results
An elevated RBC count may indicate primary or secondary polycythemia or dehydration. A depressed count may signify anemia, fluid overload, or recent hemorrhage. Further studies, such as stained RBC examination, hematocrit, total hemoglobin levels, RBC indices, and white blood cell counts, confirm a diagnosis.

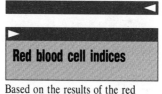

Red blood cell indices

Based on the results of the red blood cell (RBC) count, hematocrit, and total hemoglobin tests, the RBC indices provide important information about the size of RBCs, and the hemoglobin concentration and weight of an average RBC.

The first index, the mean corpuscular volume (MCV) – a ratio of hematocrit, or packed cell volume, to RBC – gives average RBC size. The mean corpuscular hemoglobin (MCH), the ratio of hemoglobin to RBC, expresses the weight of hemoglobin in an average RBC. And the mean corpuscular hemoglobin concentration (MCHC), a ratio of hemoglobin weight to hematocrit, provides the concentration of hemoglobin in 100 ml of packed RBCs.

Purpose
• To help diagnose and classify anemias.

Procedure-related nursing care
Explain the purpose of the test to the patient, and tell him you'll need a blood sample. Draw a venous blood sample, using a 7-ml laven-

der-top tube. Fill the collection tube completely, and invert it gently several times to mix the sample and the anticoagulant. Handle the sample gently to prevent hemolysis.

Check for factors that may alter test results. A high white blood cell count, for instance, will falsely elevate the RBC count when automated or semi-automated counters are used, invalidating all test results.

Reference values
Normal MCV ranges from 84 to 99 μ^3/RBC; normal MCH, from 26 to 34 pg/RBC; and normal MCHC, from 30% to 36%.

Abnormal results
A high MCV suggests macrocytic anemias caused by folic acid or vitamin B_{12} deficiency, inherited disorders of DNA synthesis, or reticulocytosis. Decreased MCV and MCHC indicate microcytic hypochromic anemias caused by iron deficiency, pyridoxine-responsive anemia, or thalassemia.

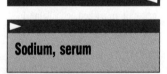

Sodium, serum

This test measures the amount of sodium in the blood. Sodium affects body water distribution, maintains osmotic pressure of extracellular fluid, and helps promote neuromuscular function. It also helps maintain acid-base balance and influences chloride and potassium levels. Sodium is absorbed by the intestines and excreted primarily by the kidneys.

Extracellular sodium concentration helps the kidneys regulate body water. Decreased sodium levels promote water excretion, and in-

creased levels promote retention. For this reason, serum sodium levels are evaluated in relation to the amount of water in the body. Thus, a sodium deficit (hyponatremia) refers to a decreased level of sodium in relation to the body's water level.

The body normally regulates this sodium-water balance through aldosterone, which inhibits sodium excretion and promotes its resorption (with water) by the renal tubules. Decreased sodium levels stimulate aldosterone secretion; elevated levels depress it.

Purpose
• To evaluate fluid-electrolyte and acid-base balance and related neuromuscular, renal, and adrenal functions
• To evaluate the effects of drug therapy (such as diuretics) on serum sodium levels.

Procedure-related nursing care
Explain the purpose of the test to the patient, and tell him it requires a blood sample. Then perform a venipuncture, collecting the sample in a 10- to 15-ml red-top tube. Handle the sample gently to prevent hemolysis.

Reference values
Serum sodium levels normally range from 135 to 145 mEq/liter.

Abnormal results
Elevated serum sodium levels (hypernatremia) may result from inadequate water intake, water loss that exceeds sodium loss (as in diabetes insipidus, impaired renal function, and prolonged hyperventilation), and sodium retention (as in aldosteronism). Hypernatremia can also result from excessive sodium intake.

Hyponatremia may result from inadequate sodium intake or excessive sodium loss caused by profuse

LAB TESTS

sweating, GI suctioning, diuretic therapy, diarrhea, vomiting, adrenal insufficiency, burns, or chronic renal insufficiency with acidosis.

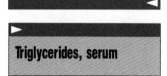

Triglycerides, serum

This test provides a quantitative analysis of triglycerides – the main storage form of lipids. Triglycerides consist of one molecule of glycerol bonded to three molecules of fatty acids. Thus, the degradation of triglycerides leads directly to the production of fatty acids. Together with carbohydrates, triglycerides furnish energy for metabolism.

Triglyceride testing shouldn't be performed while a patient is hospitalized for a myocardial infarction because this condition causes an increase in very-low-density lipoproteins and a decrease in low-density lipoproteins.

Purpose
• To determine the risk of coronary artery disease (CAD)
• To screen for hyperlipidemia
• To identify disorders associated with altered triglyceride levels.

Procedure-related nursing care
Explain the purpose of the test to the patient, and tell him it requires a blood sample. Instruct him to abstain from alcohol for 24 hours before the test and from food for 12 to 14 hours before the test. Also tell him not to take any medications, such as corticosteroids, that may alter his test results.

Perform a venipuncture and collect the sample in a 7-ml lavender-top tube.

After the test, tell the patient he can resume his normal diet.

Reference values
Triglyceride values are age- and sex-related. There is some controversy regarding the most appropriate normal ranges. Nonetheless, serum values of 40 to 160 mg/dl for men and 35 to 135 mg/dl for women are widely accepted.

Abnormal results
Increased or decreased serum triglyceride levels suggest a clinical abnormality that requires additional testing, such as cholesterol measurement, for a definitive diagnosis.

High levels of triglycerides and cholesterol reflect an increased risk of atherosclerosis or CAD.

Markedly increased levels without an identifiable cause reflect congenital hyperlipoproteinemia and require lipoprotein phenotyping to confirm the diagnosis.

A mild-to-moderate increase in serum triglyceride levels indicates biliary obstruction, diabetes mellitus, nephrotic syndrome, endocrinopathies, or excessive consumption of alcohol.

Decreased serum levels are rare, occurring mainly in malnutrition or abetalipoproteinemia.

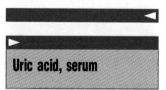

Uric acid, serum

This test measures serum levels of uric acid – the major end metabolite of purine. Large amounts of purine are present in nucleic acids and are derived from dietary and endogenous sources. Uric acid clears the body by glomerular filtration and tubular secretion.

Purpose
• To confirm a diagnosis of gout
• To help detect kidney dysfunction.

Procedure-related nursing care

Explain the purpose of the test to the patient, and tell him it requires a blood sample. Then perform a venipuncture, collecting the sample in a 7-ml red-top tube. Handle the sample gently to prevent hemolysis.

Reference values

Serum uric acid concentrations normally range from 4.3 to 8 mg/dl in men and from 2.3 to 6.6 mg/dl in women.

Abnormal results

Increased serum uric acid levels usually indicate impaired renal function or gout. However, in gout, levels don't correlate with the severity of the disease. Levels also may rise in congestive heart failure, glycogen storage disease (type I, von Gierke's disease), acute infectious diseases (such as infectious mononucleosis), hemolytic or sickle cell anemia, hemoglobinopathies, polycythemia, leukemia, lymphoma, metastatic cancer, and psoriasis.

Depressed serum uric acid levels may indicate defective renal tubular reabsorption (as in Fanconi's syndrome and Wilson's disease) or acute hepatic atrophy.

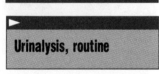

Urinalysis, routine

A common test, routine urinalysis is used to screen for urinary and systemic disorders. Abnormal findings suggest disease and indicate the need for further urine or blood tests to identify the problem.

Laboratory methods used to detect or measure urine components include the evaluation of physical characteristics, such as color, odor, and opacity; screening for pH, protein, sugars, and ketone bodies; refractometry for measuring specific gravity; and microscopic inspection of centrifuged sediment for cells, casts, and crystals.

Purpose

• To screen for renal or urinary tract disease
• To help detect metabolic or systemic disease.

Procedure-related nursing care

Explain the purpose of the test to the patient, and tell him to avoid strenuous exercise before the test. Tell him to avoid excessive amounts of such foods as carrots, rhubarb, and beets, which may cause a change in urine color, and excessive amounts of such foods as meats and cranberry juice, which can lower pH.

Collect a random or clean-catch urine specimen of at least 10 ml. If possible, obtain a first-voided morning specimen. If the urine appears concentrated or diluted, assess the patient's fluid status — dehydration and a decreased or increased fluid intake can affect the urine.

Send the specimen to the laboratory immediately, or refrigerate it if analysis will be delayed longer than 1 hour.

Reference values

Normal urine is clear and straw colored, with a slightly aromatic odor. It has a specific gravity of 1.005 to 1.035 and a pH of 5.0 to 7.0; it contains no protein, glucose, ketones, or other sugars.

On microscopic examination, normal urine contains 0 to 2 red blood cells (RBCs) and 0 to 5 white blood cells (WBCs) per high-power field. It contains few epithelial cells or crystals and no yeast cells, parasites, or casts (except occasional hyaline casts).

Abnormal results

The following abnormal results generally suggest pathologic conditions.

Color. Changes in color can result from diet, drugs, and many metabolic, inflammatory, and infectious diseases.

Odor. In diabetes mellitus, starvation, and dehydration, a fruity odor accompanies formation of ketone bodies. In urinary tract infection (UTI), a fetid odor is common, especially if *Escherichia coli* is present. Maple syrup urine disease and phenylketonuria also cause distinctive odors.

Turbidity. Turbid urine may contain RBCs, WBCs, bacteria, fat, or chyle and may reflect renal infection.

Specific gravity. Low specific gravity (less than 1.005) is characteristic of diabetes insipidus, nephrogenic diabetes insipidus, acute tubular necrosis, and pyelonephritis. Fixed specific gravity, in which values remain 1.010 regardless of fluid intake, occurs in chronic glomerulonephritis with severe renal damage. High specific gravity (greater than 1.020) occurs in nephrotic syndrome, dehydration, acute glomerulonephritis, congestive heart failure, liver failure, and shock.

pH. Alkaline urine pH may result from Fanconi's syndrome, UTI, and metabolic or respiratory alkalosis. Acid urine pH is associated with renal tuberculosis, pyrexia, phenylketonuria, alkaptonuria, and all forms of acidosis.

Protein. Proteinuria suggests renal diseases, such as nephrosis, glomerulosclerosis, glomerulonephritis, nephrolithiasis, polycystic kidney disease, and renal failure. Proteinuria can also result from multiple myeloma.

Sugars. Glycosuria usually indicates diabetes mellitus but may also result from pheochromocytoma, Cushing's syndrome, and increased intracranial pressure. Fructosuria, galactosuria, and pentosuria generally suggest rare hereditary metabolic disorders. However, an alimentary form of pentosuria and fructosuria may follow excessive ingestion of pentose or fructose, resulting in the liver's failure to metabolize the sugar. Because the renal tubules fail to reabsorb pentose or fructose, these sugars spill over into the urine.

Ketones. Ketonuria occurs in diabetes mellitus when cellular energy needs exceed the available cellular glucose. If cells lack glucose, they will metabolize fat, an alternate energy supply. Ketone bodies – the end products of incomplete fat metabolism – accumulate in plasma and are excreted in the urine. Ketonuria may also occur in starvation states and in conditions of acutely increased metabolic demand associated with decreased food intake, such as diarrhea or vomiting.

Cells. Hematuria indicates bleeding within the genitourinary tract and may result from infection, obstruction, inflammation, trauma, tumors, glomerulonephritis, renal hypertension, lupus nephritis, renal tuberculosis, renal vein thrombosis, hydronephrosis, pyelonephritis, scurvy, malaria, parasitic infection of the bladder, subacute bacterial endocarditis, polyarteritis nodosa, and hemorrhagic disorders. Numerous WBCs in urine usually suggest urinary tract inflammation, especially cystitis or pyelonephritis. WBCs and WBC casts in urine suggest renal infection. An excessive num-

LAB TESTS

ber of epithelial cells suggests renal tubular degeneration.

Casts. Plugs of gelled protein, known as casts, form in the renal tubules and collecting ducts by agglutination of protein cells or cellular debris. These casts are flushed loose by urine flow. An excessive number of casts indicates renal disease. Hyaline casts are associated with renal parenchymal disease, inflammation, and trauma to the glomerular capillary membrane; epithelial casts, with renal tubular damage, nephrosis, eclampsia, amyloidosis, and heavy metal poisoning; coarse and fine granular casts, with acute or chronic renal failure, pyelonephritis, and chronic lead intoxication; fatty and waxy casts, with nephrotic syndrome, chronic renal disease, and diabetes mellitus; RBC casts, with renal parenchymal disease (especially glomerulonephritis), renal infarction, subacute bacterial endocarditis, vascular disorders, sickle cell anemia, scurvy, blood dyscrasias, malignant hypertension, collagen disease, and acute inflammation; and WBC casts, with acute pyelonephritis and glomerulonephritis, nephrotic syndrome, pyogenic infection, and lupus nephritis.

Crystals. Some crystals normally appear in urine, but numerous calcium oxalate crystals suggest hypercalcemia. Cystine crystals (cystinuria) reflect an inborn metabolism error.

Other components. Yeast cells and parasites in urine sediment reflect genitourinary tract infection as well as contamination of external genitalia. Yeast cells, which may be mistaken for RBCs, can be identified by their ovoid shape, lack of color, variable size and, in many cases, signs of budding. The most common parasite in sediment is *Trichomonas vaginalis,* a flagellated protozoan that commonly causes vaginitis, urethritis, and prostatovesiculitis.

White blood cell count

Part of the complete blood count, the white blood cell (WBC) count reports the number of WBCs found in a cubic millimeter (microliter) of whole blood. On any given day, the WBC count can vary by as much as 2,000. Such variations may result from strenuous exercise, stress, or digestion. The WBC count can rise or fall significantly in certain diseases, but the count is diagnostically useful only when interpreted in light of the WBC differential and the patient's current clinical status.

Purpose
• To determine the presence of infection or inflammation
• To determine the need for further tests, such as the WBC differential or bone marrow biopsy
• To monitor a patient's response to chemotherapy or radiation therapy.

Procedure-related nursing care
Explain the purpose of the test to the patient. Tell him to avoid strenuous exercise for 24 hours before the test and to avoid eating a heavy meal before the test. If he's receiving treatment for an infection, advise him that this test may be repeated to monitor his progress.

Perform a venipuncture, collecting the sample in a 7-ml lavender-top tube. Handle the sample gently to prevent hemolysis.

After the procedure, tell the patient he may resume normal activities.

Reference values

The WBC count normally ranges from 4,000 to 10,000/µl.

Abnormal results

An elevated WBC count (leukocytosis) usually signals infection, such as abscess, meningitis, or appendicitis. A high count may also result from leukemia or from tissue necrosis caused by burns, myocardial infarction, or gangrene.

A low WBC count (leukopenia) indicates bone marrow depression that can result from viral infections or from toxic reactions after ingestion of mercury or other heavy metals, treatment with antineoplastics, or exposure to benzene or arsenicals. Leukopenia also characteristically accompanies influenza, typhoid fever, measles, infectious hepatitis, mononucleosis, and rubella.

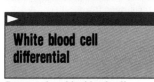

White blood cell differential

Because the white blood cell (WBC) differential evaluates the distribution and morphology of WBCs, it provides more specific information about a patient's immune function than the WBC count. The differential count represents the relative number of each type of WBC in the blood. Multiplying the percentage value of each type by the total WBC count provides the absolute number of each type of WBC.

Purpose

• To evaluate the body's capacity to resist and overcome infection
• To detect and identify various types of leukemia
• To determine the stage and severity of an infection
• To detect allergic reactions
• To assess the severity of allergic reactions (eosinophil count)
• To detect parasitic infections.

Procedure-related nursing care

Explain the purpose of the test to the patient, and tell him it requires a blood sample. Instruct him to avoid strenuous exercise for 24 hours before the test. Then perform a venipuncture, collecting the sample in a 7-ml lavender-top tube.

Reference values

For adults, absolute values and percentages for each of the five WBC differentials are as follows:
• neutrophils – 1,800 to 7,500/µl; 45% to 75%
• eosinophils – 40 to 500/µl; 1% to 5%
• basophils – 0 to 200/µl; 0% to 2%
• lymphocytes – 880 to 4,000/µl; 22% to 40%
• monocytes – 120 to 1,000/µl; 3% to 10%

Abnormal results

Neutrophil levels are increased by:
• infections – osteomyelitis, otitis media, salpingitis, septicemia, gonorrhea, endocarditis, smallpox, chicken pox, herpes, Rocky Mountain spotted fever
• ischemic necrosis from myocardial infarction, burns, or cancer
• metabolic disorders – diabetic acidosis, eclampsia, uremia, thyrotoxicosis
• stress response from acute hemorrhage, surgery, excessive exercise, emotional distress, third trimester of pregnancy, or childbirth
• inflammatory diseases – rheumatic fever, rheumatoid arthritis, acute gout, vasculitis, myositis.
Neutrophil levels are decreased by:
• bone marrow depression from radiation therapy or cytotoxic drugs

• infections – typhoid fever, tularemia, brucellosis, hepatitis, influenza, measles, mumps, rubella, infectious mononucleosis
• hypersplenism – hepatic disease and storage diseases
• collagen vascular diseases – systemic lupus erythematosus, rheumatoid arthritis
• deficiency of folic acid or vitamin B_{12}.

Eosinophil levels are increased by:
• allergic disorders – asthma, hay fever, food or drug sensitivity, serum sickness, angioneurotic edema
• parasitic infections – trichinosis, hookworm, roundworm, amebiasis
• skin diseases – eczema, pemphigus, psoriasis, dermatitis, herpes
• neoplastic diseases – chronic myelocytic leukemia, Hodgkin's disease, metastasis and necrosis of solid tumors
• miscellaneous – collagen vascular disease, adrenocortical hypofunction, ulcerative colitis, polyarteritis nodosa, postsplenectomy, pernicious anemia, scarlet fever, excessive exercise.

Eosinophil levels are decreased by:
• stress response from trauma, shock, burns, surgery, or mental distress
• Cushing's syndrome.

Basophil levels are increased by:
• miscellaneous – chronic myelocytic leukemia, polycythemia vera, some chronic hemolytic anemias, Hodgkin's disease, systemic mastocytosis, myxedema, ulcerative colitis, chronic hypersensitivity states, nephrosis.

Basophil levels are decreased by:
• miscellaneous – hyperthyroidism, ovulation, pregnancy, stress.

Lymphocyte levels are increased by:
• infections – pertussis, brucellosis, syphilis, tuberculosis, hepatitis, infectious mononucleosis, mumps, German measles, cytomegalovirus

• miscellaneous – thyrotoxicosis, hypoadrenalism, ulcerative colitis, immune diseases, lymphocytic leukemia.

Lymphocyte levels are decreased by:
• severe debilitating illness – congestive heart failure, renal failure, advanced tuberculosis
• miscellaneous – defective lymphatic circulation, high levels of adrenal corticosteroids, immunodeficiency due to immunosuppressant therapy.

Monocyte levels are increased by:
• infections – subacute bacterial endocarditis, tuberculosis, hepatitis, malaria, Rocky Mountain spotted fever
• collagen vascular diseases – systemic lupus erythematosus, rheumatoid arthritis, polyarteritis nodosa
• neoplastic diseases – carcinomas, monocytic leukemia, lymphomas.

Monocyte levels are decreased by:
• prednisone treatment
• hairy-cell leukemia.

CHAPTER 5

Nursing diagnoses:
Making selections in common disorders

NANDA Taxonomy

▶

Human response patterns

Pattern 1: Exchanging

1.1.2.1	Altered nutrition: More than body requirements
1.1.2.2	Altered nutrition: Less than body requirements
1.1.2.3	Altered nutrition: Potential for more than body requirements
1.2.1.1	Risk for infection
1.2.2.1	Risk for altered body temperature
1.2.2.2	Hypothermia
1.2.2.3	Hyperthermia
1.2.2.4	Ineffective thermoregulation
1.2.3.1	Dysreflexia
1.3.1.1	Constipation
1.3.1.1.1	Perceived constipation
1.3.1.1.2	Colonic constipation
1.3.1.2	Diarrhea
1.3.1.3	Bowel incontinence
1.3.2	Altered urinary elimination
1.3.2.1.1	Stress incontinence
1.3.2.1.2	Reflex incontinence
1.3.2.1.3	Urge incontinence
1.3.2.1.4	Functional incontinence
1.3.2.1.5	Total incontinence
1.3.2.2	Urinary retention
1.4.1.1	Altered (specify type) tissue perfusion (renal, cerebral, cardiopulmonary, gastrointestinal, peripheral)
1.4.1.2.1	Fluid volume excess
1.4.1.2.2.1	Fluid volume deficit
1.4.1.2.2.2	Risk for fluid volume deficit
1.4.2.1	Decreased cardiac output
1.5.1.1	Impaired gas exchange
1.5.1.2	Ineffective airway clearance
1.5.1.3	Ineffective breathing pattern
1.5.1.3.1	Inability to sustain spontaneous ventilation
1.5.1.3.2	Dysfunctional ventilatory weaning response (DVWR)
1.6.1	Risk for injury
1.6.1.1	Risk for suffocation
1.6.1.2	Risk for poisoning
1.6.1.3	Risk for trauma
1.6.1.4	Risk for aspiration
1.6.1.5	Risk for disuse syndrome
1.6.2	Altered protection
1.6.2.1	Impaired tissue integrity
1.6.2.1.1	Altered oral mucous membrane
1.6.2.1.2.1	Impaired skin integrity
1.6.2.1.2.2	Risk for impaired skin integrity
1.7.1	Decreased adaptive capacity: Intracranial
1.8	Energy field disturbance

Pattern 2: Communicating

2.1.1.1	Impaired verbal communication

Pattern 3: Relating

3.1.1	Impaired social interaction
3.1.2	Social isolation
3.1.3	Risk for loneliness
3.2.1	Altered role performance
3.2.1.1.1	Altered parenting
3.2.1.1.2	Risk for altered parenting
3.2.1.1.2.1	Risk for altered parent/infant/child attachment
3.2.1.2.1	Sexual dysfunction
3.2.2	Altered family processes
3.2.2.1	Caregiver role strain
3.2.2.2	Risk for caregiver role strain
3.2.2.3.1	Altered family process: Alcoholism
3.2.3.1	Parental role conflict
3.3	Altered sexuality patterns

Pattern 4: Valuing

4.1.1	Spiritual distress (distress of the human spirit)
4.2	Potential for enhanced spiritual well-being

Pattern 5: Choosing

5.1.1.1	Ineffective individual coping
5.1.1.1.1	Impaired adjustment
5.1.1.1.2	Defensive coping
5.1.1.1.3	Ineffective denial
5.1.2.1.1	Ineffective family coping: Disabling
5.1.2.1.2	Ineffective family coping: Compromised
5.1.2.2	Family coping: Potential for growth
5.1.3.1	Potential for enhanced community coping
5.1.3.2	Ineffective community coping
5.2.1	Ineffective management of therapeutic regimen (individuals)
5.2.1.1	Noncompliance (specify)
5.2.2	Ineffective management of therapeutic regimen: Families
5.2.3	Ineffective management of therapeutic regimen: Community
5.2.4	Effective management of therapeutic regimen: Individual
5.3.1.1	Decisional conflict (specify)
5.4	Health-seeking behaviors (specify)

Pattern 6: Moving

6.1.1.1	Impaired physical mobility
6.1.1.1.1	Risk for peripheral neurovascular dysfunction
6.1.1.1.2	Risk for perioperative positioning injury
6.1.1.2	Activity intolerance
6.1.1.2.1	Fatigue
6.1.1.3	Risk for activity intolerance
6.2.1	Sleep pattern disturbance
6.3.1.1	Diversional activity deficit
6.4.1.1	Impaired home maintenance management
6.4.2	Altered health maintenance
6.5.1	Feeding self-care deficit
6.5.1.1	Impaired swallowing
6.5.1.2	Ineffective breast-feeding
6.5.1.2.1	Interrupted breast-feeding
6.5.1.3	Effective breast-feeding
6.5.1.4	Ineffective infant feeding pattern
6.5.2	Bathing or hygiene self-care deficit
6.5.3	Dressing or grooming self-care deficit
6.5.4	Toileting self-care deficit
6.6	Altered growth and development
6.7	Relocation stress syndrome
6.8.1	Risk for disorganized infant behavior
6.8.2	Disorganized infant behavior
6.8.3	Potential for enhanced organized infant behavior

Pattern 7: Perceiving

7.1.1	Body image disturbance
7.1.2	Self-esteem disturbance
7.1.2.1	Chronic low self-esteem
7.1.2.2	Situational low self-esteem
7.1.3	Personal identity disturbance
7.2	Sensory or perceptual alterations (specify as visual, auditory, kinesthetic, gustatory, tactile, or olfactory)
7.2.1.1	Unilateral neglect
7.3.1	Hopelessness

NURSING DIAGNOSES

Pattern 8: Knowing

8.1.1	Knowledge deficit (specify)
8.2.1	Impaired environmental interpretation syndrome
8.2.2	Acute confusion
8.2.3	Chronic confusion
8.3	Altered thought processes
8.3.1	Impaired memory

Pattern 9: Feeling

9.1.1	Pain
9.1.1.1	Chronic pain
9.2.1.1	Dysfunctional grieving
9.2.1.2	Anticipatory grieving
9.2.2	Risk for violence: Self-directed or directed at others
9.2.2.1	Risk for self-mutilation
9.2.3	Post-trauma response
9.2.3.1	Rape-trauma syndrome
9.2.3.1.1	Rape-trauma syndrome: Compound reaction
9.2.3.1.2	Rape-trauma syndrome: Silent reaction
9.3.1	Anxiety
9.3.2	Fear

Selecting nursing diagnoses

Cardiovascular disorders

Abdominal aneurysm
- Altered tissue perfusion
- Anxiety
- Decreased cardiac output
- Fluid volume deficit
- Impaired gas exchange
- Impaired physical mobility
- Impaired skin integrity
- Knowledge deficit
- Pain

Arterial occlusive disease
- Activity intolerance
- Altered tissue perfusion
- Diversional activity deficit
- Impaired physical mobility
- Impaired skin integrity
- Ineffective individual coping
- Knowledge deficit
- Pain
- Risk for disuse syndrome
- Risk for infection

Cardiac arrhythmias
- Activity intolerance
- Altered tissue perfusion
- Anxiety
- Decreased cardiac output
- Impaired gas exchange
- Powerlessness

Cardiac tamponade
- Activity intolerance
- Altered tissue perfusion
- Anxiety
- Decreased cardiac output
- Impaired gas exchange
- Pain

Cardiogenic shock
- Altered thought processes
- Altered tissue perfusion
- Anxiety
- Decisional conflict
- Decreased cardiac output
- Dysfunctional grieving
- Fear
- Fluid volume excess
- Hopelessness
- Impaired gas exchange
- Impaired physical mobility
- Risk for injury

Coronary artery disease
- Activity intolerance
- Altered nutrition: More than body requirements
- Altered role performance
- Altered sexuality patterns
- Altered tissue perfusion
- Anxiety

- Decreased cardiac output
- Fluid volume deficit
- Fluid volume excess
- Health-seeking behaviors
- Impaired gas exchange
- Ineffective denial
- Knowledge deficit
- Pain
- Risk for injury

Dilated cardiomyopathy
- Activity intolerance
- Altered family processes
- Altered tissue perfusion
- Anxiety
- Decreased cardiac output
- Fatigue
- Fluid volume excess
- Hopelessness
- Impaired gas exchange
- Impaired physical mobility
- Ineffective breathing pattern
- Knowledge deficit

Endocarditis
- Activity intolerance
- Altered role performance
- Decreased cardiac output
- Diversional activity deficit
- Impaired gas exchange
- Risk for injury

Femoral and popliteal aneurysms
- Activity intolerance
- Altered tissue perfusion
- Defensive coping
- Denial
- Diversional activity deficit
- Impaired physical mobility
- Impaired skin integrity
- Pain
- Risk for infection

Heart failure
- Activity intolerance
- Altered nutrition: Less than body requirements
- Altered tissue perfusion
- Anxiety
- Decreased cardiac output
- Fatigue

- Fluid volume excess
- Ineffective airway clearance
- Ineffective breathing pattern
- Knowledge deficit
- Risk for infection

Hypertension
- Altered tissue perfusion
- Fatigue
- Ineffective individual coping
- Knowledge deficit
- Noncompliance
- Risk for injury

Hypertrophic cardiomyopathy
- Activity intolerance
- Decreased cardiac output
- Fatigue
- Fluid volume excess
- Ineffective individual coping
- Knowledge deficit
- Pain
- Risk for infection

Hypovolemic shock
- Altered thought processes
- Altered tissue perfusion
- Anxiety
- Decreased cardiac output
- Fluid volume deficit
- Risk for injury
- Sensory alteration

Myocardial infarction
- Activity intolerance
- Altered nutrition: Less than body requirements
- Altered sexuality patterns
- Altered tissue perfusion
- Anxiety
- Constipation
- Decreased cardiac output
- Denial
- Fatigue
- Fluid volume excess
- Ineffective individual coping
- Knowledge deficit
- Pain
- Powerlessness
- Risk for injury

NURSING
DIAGNOSES

Myocarditis
- Activity intolerance
- Altered role performance
- Anxiety
- Decreased cardiac output
- Diversional activity deficit
- Impaired gas exchange

Pericarditis
- Altered role performance
- Anxiety
- Decreased cardiac output
- Diversional activity deficit
- Ineffective breathing pattern
- Pain
- Risk for injury

Raynaud's disease
- Altered role performance
- Altered tissue perfusion
- Impaired skin integrity
- Impaired tissue integrity
- Ineffective individual coping
- Ineffective thermoregulation
- Knowledge deficit
- Pain

Rheumatic fever and rheumatic heart disease
- Activity intolerance
- Altered role performance
- Anxiety
- Decreased cardiac output
- Diversional activity deficit
- Fatigue
- Impaired gas exchange
- Knowledge deficit
- Pain
- Risk for infection
- Risk for injury

Septic shock
- Altered thought processes
- Altered tissue perfusion
- Anxiety
- Decreased cardiac output
- Fluid volume deficit
- Impaired gas exchange
- Risk for injury
- Sensory alteration

Thoracic aortic aneurysm
- Anxiety
- Decreased cardiac output
- Hopelessness
- Ineffective breathing pattern
- Knowledge deficit
- Pain

Thrombophlebitis
- Activity intolerance
- Altered tissue perfusion
- Impaired skin integrity
- Pain
- Risk for infection
- Risk for injury

Valvular heart disease
- Activity intolerance
- Altered role performance
- Altered tissue perfusion
- Decreased cardiac output
- Diversional activity deficit
- Fatigue
- Fluid volume excess
- Impaired gas exchange
- Impaired physical mobility
- Ineffective individual coping
- Risk for infection

Varicose veins
- Activity intolerance
- Altered tissue perfusion
- Fatigue
- Impaired skin integrity
- Impaired tissue integrity
- Knowledge deficit
- Pain

Ventricular aneurysm
- Altered tissue perfusion
- Anxiety
- Decreased cardiac output
- Fluid volume excess
- Impaired gas exchange
- Ineffective breathing pattern

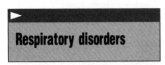

Respiratory disorders

Acute respiratory failure in COPD
• Altered nutrition: Less than body requirements
• Altered tissue perfusion
• Anxiety
• Fatigue
• Fear
• Impaired gas exchange
• Impaired skin integrity
• Impaired verbal communication
• Ineffective airway clearance
• Ineffective breathing pattern
• Sensory or perceptual alterations

Adult respiratory distress syndrome
• Altered nutrition: Less than body requirements
• Altered tissue perfusion
• Anxiety
• Decreased cardiac output
• Fatigue
• Fear
• Impaired gas exchange
• Impaired physical mobility
• Impaired verbal communication
• Risk for impaired skin integrity
• Risk for infection

Asthma
• Anxiety
• Fear
• Impaired gas exchange
• Ineffective airway clearance
• Ineffective breathing pattern
• Knowledge deficit

Atelectasis
• Anxiety
• Fear
• Impaired gas exchange
• Ineffective airway clearance
• Ineffective breathing pattern
• Knowledge deficit
• Risk for infection

Bronchiectasis
• Altered nutrition: Less than body requirements
• Anxiety
• Fatigue
• Impaired gas exchange
• Ineffective airway clearance
• Ineffective breathing pattern

Chronic bronchitis
• Altered family processes
• Altered nutrition: Less than body requirements
• Anxiety
• Fatigue
• Fear
• Impaired gas exchange
• Ineffective breathing pattern
• Knowledge deficit

Cor pulmonale
• Activity intolerance
• Fluid volume excess
• Knowledge deficit
• Risk for injury

Cystic fibrosis
• Altered nutrition: Less than body requirements
• Altered tissue perfusion
• Anxiety
• Fear
• Impaired gas exchange
• Ineffective airway clearance
• Ineffective breathing pattern
• Ineffective family coping

Emphysema
• Activity intolerance
• Altered nutrition: Less than body requirements
• Anxiety
• Fatigue
• Fear
• Impaired gas exchange
• Ineffective airway clearance
• Ineffective breathing pattern
• Knowledge deficit

Hemothorax
• Altered tissue perfusion
• Anxiety

- Fluid volume deficit
- Impaired gas exchange
- Ineffective breathing pattern
- Pain
- Risk for infection

Pleurisy
- Activity intolerance
- Anxiety
- Impaired gas exchange
- Ineffective airway clearance
- Ineffective breathing pattern
- Pain

Pneumonia
- Altered nutrition: Less than body requirements
- Anxiety
- Impaired gas exchange
- Ineffective airway clearance
- Pain
- Risk for fluid volume deficit
- Risk for infection

Pulmonary edema
- Altered tissue perfusion
- Anxiety
- Fear
- Fluid volume excess
- Impaired gas exchange
- Knowledge deficit

Pulmonary embolism
- Altered nutrition: Less than body requirements
- Altered tissue perfusion
- Anxiety
- Decreased cardiac output
- Diversional activity deficit
- Fear
- Impaired gas exchange
- Ineffective airway clearance
- Knowledge deficit
- Pain
- Risk for injury

Pulmonary hypertension
- Activity intolerance
- Anxiety
- Decreased cardiac output
- Fear

- Impaired gas exchange
- Knowledge deficit

Respiratory acidosis
- Decreased cardiac output
- Fear
- Impaired gas exchange
- Ineffective airway clearance
- Risk for fluid volume deficit

Respiratory alkalosis
- Anxiety
- Fatigue
- Fear
- Impaired gas exchange
- Ineffective breathing pattern

Sarcoidosis
- Activity intolerance
- Altered nutrition: Less than body requirements
- Anxiety
- Dysfunctional grieving
- Fear
- Impaired gas exchange
- Knowledge deficit
- Risk for infection

Tuberculosis
- Altered nutrition: Less than body requirements
- Anxiety
- Fear
- Impaired gas exchange
- Ineffective airway clearance
- Knowledge deficit
- Risk for injury

Gastrointestinal disorders

Appendicitis
- Altered GI tissue perfusion
- Altered nutrition: Less than body requirements
- Impaired skin integrity
- Pain
- Risk for fluid volume deficit

Cholelithiasis, cholecystitis, and related disorders
- Altered GI tissue perfusion
- Altered nutrition: Less than body requirements
- Pain
- Risk for fluid volume deficit
- Risk for infection

Cirrhosis
- Activity intolerance
- Altered nutrition: Less than body requirements
- Altered thought processes
- Fluid volume excess
- Hopelessness
- Risk for impaired skin integrity
- Risk for injury

Corrosive esophagitis and stricture
- Altered nutrition: Less than body requirements
- Altered oral mucous membrane
- Anxiety
- Pain
- Risk for infection

Crohn's disease
- Altered nutrition: Less than body requirements
- Body image disturbance
- Chronic low self-esteem
- Diarrhea
- Hopelessness
- Ineffective individual coping
- Pain
- Risk for fluid volume deficit
- Risk for impaired skin integrity

Cryptosporidiosis
- Altered nutrition: Less than body requirements
- Diarrhea
- Fluid volume deficit
- Risk for impaired skin integrity

Diverticular disease
- Altered GI tissue perfusion
- Anxiety
- Constipation

- Diarrhea
- Fluid volume deficit
- Pain

Esophageal diverticula
- Altered nutrition: Less than body requirements
- Anxiety
- Impaired swallowing
- Knowledge deficit
- Pain
- Risk for aspiration

Gastritis
- Altered nutrition: Less than body requirements
- Ineffective individual coping
- Knowledge deficit
- Pain
- Risk for fluid volume deficit

Gastroenteritis
- Altered nutrition: Less than body requirements
- Diarrhea
- Pain
- Risk for fluid volume deficit

Gastroesophageal reflux
- Altered nutrition: Less than body requirements
- Anxiety
- Knowledge deficit
- Pain
- Risk for aspiration

Hemorrhoids
- Constipation
- Knowledge deficit
- Pain
- Risk for infection

Hepatitis
- Activity intolerance
- Altered nutrition: Less than body requirements
- Risk for infection

Hiatal hernia
- Altered nutrition: Less than body requirements

- Impaired swallowing
- Pain
- Risk for aspiration

Inguinal hernia
- Activity intolerance
- Altered GI tissue perfusion
- Pain
- Risk for injury

Intestinal obstruction
- Altered GI tissue perfusion
- Altered nutrition: Less than body requirements
- Constipation
- Fluid volume deficit
- Pain

Intussusception
- Altered GI tissue perfusion
- Anxiety
- Fear
- Knowledge deficit
- Pain
- Risk for fluid volume deficit
- Risk for infection

Irritable bowel syndrome
- Body image disturbance
- Constipation
- Diarrhea
- Ineffective individual coping

Mallory-Weiss syndrome
- Altered nutrition: Less than body requirements
- Anxiety
- Risk for fluid volume deficit

Pancreatitis
- Altered nutrition: Less than body requirements
- Fluid volume deficit
- Hopelessness
- Ineffective breathing pattern
- Pain

Peptic ulcers
- Activity intolerance
- Altered nutrition: Less than body requirements

- Anxiety
- Fluid volume deficit
- Pain
- Sleep pattern disturbance
- Risk for injury

Peritonitis
- Altered GI tissue perfusion
- Altered nutrition: Less than body requirements
- Fear
- Fluid volume deficit
- Pain

Rectal prolapse
- Anxiety
- Constipation
- Knowledge deficit
- Pain
- Risk for infection

Tracheoesophageal fistula
- Altered nutrition: Less than body requirements
- Anxiety (parental)
- Ineffective airway clearance
- Pain
- Risk for aspiration
- Risk for infection

Ulcerative colitis
- Activity intolerance
- Altered nutrition: Less than body requirements
- Body image disturbance
- Diarrhea
- Pain
- Risk for fluid volume deficit
- Risk for impaired skin integrity

Volvulus
- Altered GI tissue perfusion
- Altered nutrition: Less than body requirements
- Pain
- Risk for fluid volume deficit
- Risk for infection

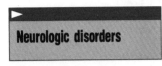

Neurologic disorders

Alzheimer's disease
• Altered nutrition: Less than body requirements
• Altered thought processes
• Bathing or hygiene self-care deficit
• Constipation
• Dressing or grooming self-care deficit
• Feeding self-care deficit
• Impaired verbal communication
• Ineffective family coping
• Knowledge deficit
• Toileting self-care deficit

Amyotrophic lateral sclerosis
• Altered nutrition: Less than body requirements
• Anticipatory grieving
• Anxiety
• Bathing or hygiene self-care deficit
• Dressing or grooming self-care deficit
• Feeding self-care deficit
• Hopelessness
• Impaired physical mobility
• Impaired verbal communication
• Ineffective airway clearance
• Ineffective breathing pattern
• Ineffective family coping
• Knowledge deficit
• Risk for impaired skin integrity
• Risk for infection
• Toileting self-care deficit

Bell's palsy
• Altered nutrition: Less than body requirements
• Anxiety
• Body image disturbance
• Knowledge deficit
• Pain

Cerebral aneurysm
• Altered nutrition: Less than body requirements
• Altered thought processes
• Anxiety
• Impaired gas exchange
• Impaired physical mobility
• Ineffective breathing pattern
• Knowledge deficit
• Pain
• Risk for impaired skin integrity
• Risk for injury
• Sensory or perceptual alterations

Cerebral palsy
• Altered nutrition: Less than body requirements
• Altered thought processes
• Body image disturbance
• Impaired physical mobility
• Knowledge deficit
• Risk for altered parenting
• Risk for impaired skin integrity
• Self-esteem disturbance
• Sensory or perceptual alterations

Cerebrovascular accident
• Altered cerebral tissue perfusion
• Altered nutrition: Less than body requirements
• Anxiety
• Bathing or hygiene self-care deficit
• Dressing or grooming self-care deficit
• Impaired gas exchange
• Impaired physical mobility
• Impaired verbal communication
• Ineffective airway clearance
• Knowledge deficit
• Powerlessness
• Risk for aspiration
• Risk for impaired skin integrity
• Risk for infection
• Risk for injury
• Self-esteem disturbance
• Sensory or perceptual alterations
• Toileting self-care deficit
• Total incontinence

Encephalitis
- Altered nutrition: Less than body requirements
- Altered thought processes
- Anxiety
- Hyperthermia
- Impaired gas exchange
- Impaired physical mobility
- Knowledge deficit
- Pain
- Risk for fluid volume deficit
- Risk for impaired skin integrity

Epilepsy
- Anxiety
- Fear
- Ineffective individual coping
- Knowledge deficit
- Risk for injury
- Social isolation

Guillain-Barré syndrome
- Altered nutrition: Less than body requirements
- Altered urinary elimination
- Anxiety
- Diversional activity deficit
- Fear
- Impaired gas exchange
- Impaired physical mobility
- Impaired verbal communication
- Ineffective breathing pattern

Headache
- Anxiety
- Knowledge deficit
- Pain

Huntington's disease
- Altered health maintenance
- Anxiety
- Chronic low self-esteem
- Impaired physical mobility
- Impaired verbal communication
- Risk for aspiration
- Risk for infection
- Risk for injury
- Self-care deficit
- Total incontinence

Meningitis
- Anxiety
- Hyperthermia
- Impaired gas exchange
- Pain
- Risk for fluid volume deficit
- Risk for impaired skin integrity

Multiple sclerosis
- Activity intolerance
- Altered nutrition: Less than body requirements
- Altered thought processes
- Altered urinary elimination
- Chronic low self-esteem
- Constipation
- Fatigue
- Impaired physical mobility
- Knowledge deficit
- Pain
- Risk for infection
- Risk for injury
- Sensory/perceptual alterations

Myasthenia gravis
- Anxiety
- Bathing or hygiene self-care deficit
- Chronic low self-esteem
- Dressing or grooming self-care deficit
- Fatigue
- Feeding self-care deficit
- Impaired gas exchange
- Impaired physical mobility
- Ineffective airway clearance
- Toileting self-care deficit

Myelitis and acute transverse myelitis
- Anxiety
- Body image disturbance
- Impaired physical mobility
- Knowledge deficit
- Pain
- Risk for infection

Parkinson's disease
- Altered nutrition: Less than body requirements
- Bathing or hygiene self-care deficit
- Body image disturbance
- Chronic low self-esteem
- Constipation
- Dressing or grooming self-care deficit
- Feeding self-care deficit
- Impaired physical mobility
- Impaired social interaction
- Impaired verbal communication
- Risk for injury
- Toileting self-care deficit

Trigeminal neuralgia
- Altered nutrition: Less than body requirements
- Anxiety
- Knowledge deficit
- Pain

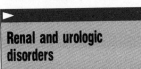

Renal and urologic disorders

Benign prostatic hyperplasia
- Altered urinary elimination
- Pain
- Risk for infection
- Sexual dysfunction

Cystinuria
- Altered urinary elimination
- Knowledge deficit
- Pain
- Risk for infection

Glomerulonephritis, acute poststreptococcal
- Altered nutrition: Less than body requirements
- Altered role performance
- Decreased cardiac output
- Fatigue
- Fluid volume excess

- Impaired gas exchange
- Impaired physical mobility
- Pain
- Risk for infection
- Risk for injury
- Self-care deficit

Glomerulonephritis, chronic
- Altered nutrition: Less than body requirements
- Fatigue
- Fluid volume excess
- Impaired skin integrity
- Risk for infection

Lower urinary tract infection
- Altered urinary elimination
- Pain
- Risk for infection
- Sexual dysfunction
- Sleep pattern disturbance

Medullary sponge disease
- Altered urinary elimination
- Pain
- Risk for infection
- Risk for injury

Nephrotic syndrome
- Altered nutrition: Less than body requirements
- Altered tissue perfusion
- Body image disturbance
- Fluid volume excess
- Risk for infection
- Risk for injury

Neurogenic bladder
- Altered urinary elimination
- Body image disturbance
- Fluid volume deficit
- Impaired skin integrity
- Knowledge deficit
- Risk for infection
- Sensory alteration
- Sexual dysfunction

Polycystic kidney disease
- Altered family processes
- Altered tissue perfusion
- Fatigue
- Fluid volume deficit
- Ineffective individual coping
- Pain
- Risk for infection
- Risk for injury
- Self-care deficit

Prostatitis
- Altered sexuality patterns
- Altered urinary elimination
- Ineffective individual coping
- Knowledge deficit
- Pain
- Risk for infection
- Self-esteem disturbance
- Sexual dysfunction

Pyelonephritis, acute
- Altered tissue perfusion
- Fluid volume excess
- Impaired physical mobility
- Pain
- Risk for infection
- Self-care deficit

Renal calculi
- Altered urinary elimination
- Knowledge deficit
- Pain
- Risk for infection

Renal failure, acute
- Altered family processes
- Altered nutrition: Less than body requirements
- Altered oral mucous membrane
- Decreased cardiac output
- Fear
- Fluid volume deficit
- Fluid volume excess
- Impaired skin integrity
- Risk for infection
- Risk for injury
- Self-care deficit
- Sensory or perceptual alterations

Renal failure, chronic
- Altered family processes
- Altered nutrition: Less than body requirements
- Altered oral mucous membrane
- Altered sexuality patterns
- Altered thought processes
- Altered tissue perfusion
- Decreased cardiac output
- Fluid volume excess
- Impaired gas exchange
- Impaired tissue integrity
- Ineffective family coping
- Pain
- Powerlessness
- Risk for infection
- Risk for injury
- Sexual dysfunction

Renal infarction
- Altered nutrition: Less than body requirements
- Fluid volume excess
- Pain
- Risk for infection

Renal tubular acidosis
- Altered growth and development
- Altered nutrition: Less than body requirements
- Altered parenting
- Altered urinary elimination
- Fluid volume deficit
- Ineffective family coping
- Pain
- Risk for infection

Renal vein thrombosis
- Altered nutrition: Less than body requirements
- Altered tissue perfusion
- Decreased cardiac output
- Fluid volume deficit
- Pain
- Risk for injury

Renovascular hypertension
- Altered nutrition: Less than body requirements
- Altered thought processes
- Altered urinary elimination
- Anxiety

- Decreased cardiac output
- Fluid volume excess
- Pain
- Risk for injury

Tubular necrosis, acute
- Altered nutrition: Less than body requirements
- Altered role performance
- Altered tissue perfusion
- Decreased cardiac output
- Fatigue
- Fluid volume excess
- Impaired gas exchange
- Pain
- Risk for infection
- Risk for injury
- Self-care deficit

Obstetric and gynecologic disorders

Abortion, spontaneous
- Anxiety
- Dysfunctional grieving
- Ineffective family coping
- Ineffective individual coping
- Knowledge deficit
- Risk for infection

Abruptio placentae
- Altered tissue perfusion
- Anxiety
- Dysfunctional grieving
- Fear
- Ineffective family coping
- Ineffective individual coping
- Pain

Ectopic pregnancy
- Anxiety
- Dysfunctional grieving
- Fear
- Fluid volume deficit
- Ineffective individual coping
- Knowledge deficit

Endometriosis
- Anxiety
- Body image disturbance
- Chronic pain
- Ineffective individual coping
- Knowledge deficit
- Sexual dysfunction

Female infertility
- Altered sexuality patterns
- Anxiety
- Body image disturbance
- Dysfunctional grieving
- Hopelessness
- Ineffective family coping
- Ineffective individual coping
- Knowledge deficit
- Powerlessness
- Self-esteem disturbance

Gestational trophoblastic disease
- Anxiety
- Dysfunctional grieving
- Ineffective family coping
- Ineffective individual coping
- Knowledge deficit
- Risk for infection

Mastitis
- Ineffective breast-feeding
- Infection
- Knowledge deficit
- Pain
- Risk for impaired skin integrity

Ovarian cysts
- Altered sexuality patterns
- Anxiety
- Ineffective individual coping
- Knowledge deficit
- Pain

Pelvic inflammatory disease
- Altered sexuality patterns
- Anxiety
- Fluid volume deficit
- Ineffective individual coping
- Knowledge deficit
- Pain

NURSING
DIAGNOSES

Placenta previa
- Anxiety
- Dysfunctional grieving
- Fear
- Fluid volume deficit
- Ineffective family coping
- Ineffective individual coping
- Knowledge deficit
- Pain
- Risk for injury

Pregnancy-induced hypertension
- Activity intolerance
- Altered cerebral or peripheral tissue perfusion
- Altered urinary elimination
- Anxiety
- Fear
- Fluid volume excess
- Ineffective family coping
- Ineffective individual coping
- Knowledge deficit
- Risk for injury
- Sensory or perceptual alterations (visual)

Premature labor
- Altered family processes
- Anxiety
- Dysfunctional grieving
- Fear
- Ineffective breathing pattern
- Ineffective family coping
- Ineffective individual coping
- Pain

Premenstrual syndrome
- Altered family processes
- Altered role performance
- Altered sexuality patterns
- Anxiety
- Body image disturbance
- Fluid volume excess
- Impaired social interaction
- Ineffective individual coping
- Knowledge deficit
- Pain
- Situational low self-esteem

Puerperal infection
- Altered parenting
- Anxiety
- Fluid volume deficit
- Infection
- Knowledge deficit
- Pain
- Risk for impaired skin integrity

Uterine leiomyomas
- Altered sexuality patterns
- Anxiety
- Ineffective individual coping
- Knowledge deficit
- Pain

Vulvovaginitis
- Altered sexuality patterns
- Body image disturbance
- Ineffective individual coping
- Knowledge deficit
- Pain
- Risk for impaired skin integrity
- Risk for infection

Endocrine disorders

Adrenal hypofunction
- Activity intolerance
- Altered nutrition: Less than body requirements
- Altered thought processes
- Body image disturbance
- Fluid volume deficit
- Ineffective individual coping
- Knowledge deficit
- Risk for altered body temperature
- Risk for impaired skin integrity
- Risk for infection
- Sexual dysfunction

Adrenogenital syndrome
• Altered growth and development
• Body image disturbance
• Ineffective family coping
• Ineffective individual coping
• Knowledge deficit
• Risk for fluid volume deficit

Cushing's syndrome
• Activity intolerance
• Altered thought processes
• Body image disturbance
• Fluid volume excess
• Impaired skin integrity
• Ineffective individual coping
• Knowledge deficit
• Risk for infection
• Risk for injury
• Sexual dysfunction

Diabetes insipidus
• Altered growth and development
• Altered oral mucous membrane
• Altered urinary elimination
• Fluid volume deficit
• Hopelessness
• Ineffective family coping
• Ineffective individual coping
• Knowledge deficit
• Sleep pattern disturbance

Diabetes mellitus
• Altered nutrition: More than body requirements
• Altered peripheral tissue perfusion
• Altered urinary elimination
• Anticipatory grieving
• Fluid volume deficit
• Hopelessness
• Impaired adjustment
• Impaired skin integrity
• Ineffective family coping
• Ineffective individual coping
• Knowledge deficit
• Powerlessness
• Risk for infection
• Risk for injury
• Sensory or perceptual alterations (visual)

Goiter, simple
• Altered nutrition: Less than body requirements
• Body image disturbance
• Impaired swallowing
• Ineffective airway clearance
• Ineffective individual coping
• Knowledge deficit

Hyperaldosteronism
• Altered tissue perfusion
• Altered urinary elimination
• Decreased cardiac output
• Ineffective individual coping
• Knowledge deficit
• Pain

Hyperparathyroidism
• Activity intolerance
• Altered nutrition: Less than body requirements
• Altered thought processes
• Anxiety
• Body image disturbance
• Decreased cardiac output
• Fluid volume excess
• Ineffective individual coping
• Knowledge deficit
• Pain
• Risk for injury

Hyperpituitarism
• Activity intolerance
• Altered growth and development
• Altered oral mucous membrane
• Body image disturbance
• Impaired physical mobility
• Ineffective individual coping
• Knowledge deficit
• Pain
• Self-esteem disturbance
• Sensory or perceptual alterations (visual)
• Sexual dysfunction

Hyperthyroidism
• Altered nutrition: Less than body requirements
• Altered thought processes
• Body image disturbance
• Decreased cardiac output
• Diarrhea

- Ineffective individual coping
- Knowledge deficit
- Risk for altered body temperature
- Risk for fluid volume deficit

Hypoparathyroidism

- Altered thought processes
- Anxiety
- Body image disturbance
- Decreased cardiac output
- Impaired skin integrity
- Ineffective breathing pattern
- Ineffective individual coping
- Knowledge deficit
- Risk for injury

Hypopituitarism

- Altered growth and development
- Altered nutrition: Less than body requirements
- Body image disturbance
- Hypothermia
- Ineffective individual coping
- Knowledge deficit
- Risk for infection
- Self-esteem disturbance
- Sensory or perceptual alterations (visual)
- Sexual dysfunction

Hypothyroidism

- Altered cardiopulmonary tissue perfusion
- Altered nutrition: Potential for more than body requirements
- Altered thought processes
- Body image disturbance
- Chronic low self-esteem
- Colonic constipation
- Decreased cardiac output
- Fluid volume excess
- Ineffective individual coping
- Knowledge deficit
- Risk for altered body temperature
- Risk for impaired skin integrity
- Sensory or perceptual alterations (auditory)

Male infertility

- Body image disturbance
- Ineffective family coping
- Ineffective individual coping
- Knowledge deficit
- Self-esteem disturbance

Thyroiditis

- Altered nutrition: Less than body requirements
- Body image disturbance
- Impaired swallowing
- Ineffective airway clearance
- Ineffective individual coping
- Knowledge deficit
- Pain

Neoplastic disorders

Basal or squamous cell carcinoma

- Altered nutrition: Less than body requirements
- Anxiety
- Body image disturbance
- Fear
- Impaired skin integrity
- Ineffective family coping
- Ineffective individual coping
- Knowledge deficit
- Risk for infection
- Self-esteem disturbance

Breast cancer

- Altered nutrition: Less than body requirements
- Anxiety
- Body image disturbance
- Decisional conflict
- Fear
- Impaired physical mobility
- Impaired skin integrity
- Ineffective individual coping
- Knowledge deficit
- Pain

- Risk for infection
- Self-care deficit

Cervical cancer
- Altered sexuality patterns
- Anxiety
- Diversional activity deficit
- Fear
- Impaired physical mobility
- Impaired skin integrity
- Ineffective individual coping
- Pain
- Risk for infection
- Sexual dysfunction

Colorectal cancer
- Altered nutrition: Less than body requirements
- Altered oral mucous membrane
- Anxiety
- Body image disturbance
- Constipation
- Diarrhea
- Fear
- Fluid volume deficit
- Impaired skin integrity
- Ineffective family coping
- Ineffective individual coping
- Knowledge deficit
- Pain
- Risk for infection
- Sexual dysfunction

Esophageal cancer
- Altered nutrition: Less than body requirements
- Anxiety
- Fatigue
- Fear
- Fluid volume deficit
- Impaired swallowing
- Pain
- Risk for aspiration
- Risk for infection

Gastric cancer
- Altered nutrition: Less than body requirements
- Altered oral mucous membrane
- Anxiety
- Diarrhea
- Fatigue

- Fear
- High risk for infection
- Impaired gas exchange
- Impaired skin integrity
- Impaired swallowing
- Knowledge deficit
- Pain

Hodgkin's disease
- Altered nutrition: Less than body requirements
- Altered oral mucous membrane
- Anxiety
- Fatigue
- Fear
- Impaired skin integrity
- Ineffective family coping
- Ineffective individual coping
- Knowledge deficit
- Pain
- Risk for infection

Kaposi's sarcoma
- Altered nutrition: Less than body requirements
- Anticipatory grieving
- Anxiety
- Body image disturbance
- Fatigue
- Fear
- Impaired gas exchange
- Impaired skin integrity
- Ineffective breathing pattern
- Ineffective family coping
- Ineffective individual coping
- Pain
- Risk for infection

Leukemias
- Altered nutrition: Less than body requirements
- Altered protection
- Anticipatory grieving
- Anxiety
- Fatigue
- Fear
- Impaired tissue integrity
- Ineffective family coping
- Ineffective individual coping
- Pain
- Risk for infection
- Risk for injury

For acute leukemia:
- Altered oral mucous membrane
- Altered parenting
- Risk for altered body temperature
  For chronic granulocytic leukemia:
- Altered oral mucous membrane
- Constipation
- Risk for altered body temperature

Lung cancer
- Altered nutrition: Less than body requirements
- Anxiety
- Fatigue
- Fluid volume deficit
- Impaired gas exchange
- Impaired physical mobility
- Impaired skin integrity
- Ineffective airway clearance
- Ineffective breathing pattern
- Knowledge deficit
- Pain
- Risk for infection
- Risk for injury

Malignant brain tumors
- Activity intolerance
- Altered role performance
- Anxiety
- Body image disturbance
- Hopelessness
- Impaired physical mobility
- Impaired skin integrity
- Ineffective breathing pattern
- Ineffective family coping
- Ineffective individual coping
- Ineffective thermoregulation
- Pain
- Powerlessness
- Risk for fluid volume deficit
- Risk for infection
- Risk for injury
- Self-care deficit
- Sensory or perceptual alterations

Malignant melanoma
- Altered nutrition: Less than body requirements
- Anticipatory grieving

- Anxiety
- Body image disturbance
- Fear
- Impaired skin integrity
- Ineffective family coping
- Ineffective individual coping
- Knowledge deficit
- Pain
- Risk for infection

Mesothelioma
- Anxiety
- Fatigue
- Fear
- Fluid volume excess
- Hopelessness
- Impaired gas exchange
- Impaired physical mobility
- Impaired skin integrity
- Ineffective breathing pattern
- Pain
- Risk for infection

Ovarian cancer
- Altered growth and development (in a child)
- Altered nutrition: Less than body requirements
- Anticipatory grieving
- Anxiety
- Fear
- Fluid volume excess
- Hopelessness
- Impaired skin integrity
- Ineffective family coping
- Ineffective individual coping
- Pain
- Risk for infection
- Sexual dysfunction

Pancreatic cancer
- Altered nutrition: Less than body requirements
- Anxiety
- Constipation
- Fluid volume deficit
- Fluid volume excess
- Impaired skin integrity

- Ineffective family coping
- Ineffective individual coping
- Knowledge deficit
- Pain
- Risk for injury

Prostatic cancer
- Altered urinary elimination
- Anxiety
- Fear
- Ineffective family coping
- Ineffective individual coping
- Pain
- Risk for infection
- Sexual dysfunction
- Urinary retention

Thyroid cancer
- Altered nutrition: Less than body requirements
- Anxiety
- Body image disturbance
- Diarrhea
- Impaired gas exchange
- Impaired skin integrity
- Impaired swallowing
- Impaired verbal communication
- Pain

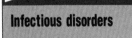

Infectious disorders

Adenoviral infection
- Altered nutrition: Less than body requirements
- Diarrhea
- Fatigue
- Hyperthermia
- Impaired gas exchange
- Impaired skin integrity
- Pain
- Risk for fluid volume deficit
- Risk for infection
- Sensory alteration

Blastomycosis
- Impaired gas exchange
- Impaired physical mobility
- Impaired skin integrity
- Ineffective airway clearance
- Ineffective breathing pattern
- Pain
- Risk for injury

Botulism
- Altered nutrition: Less than body requirements
- Altered oral mucous membrane
- Fear
- Impaired physical mobility
- Impaired swallowing
- Impaired verbal communication
- Ineffective airway clearance
- Ineffective breathing pattern
- Pain
- Self-care deficit
- Sensory alteration

Candidiasis
- Altered oral mucous membrane
- Altered urinary elimination
- Hyperthermia
- Impaired skin integrity
- Impaired swallowing
- Pain
- Risk for aspiration
- Sensory alteration
- Sexual dysfunction

Chancroid
- Altered sexuality patterns
- Body image disturbance
- Impaired skin integrity
- Knowledge deficit
- Pain
- Risk for infection

Chlamydial infections
- Altered sexuality patterns
- Altered urinary elimination
- Impaired skin integrity
- Knowledge deficit
- Pain
- Risk for infection
- Sexual dysfunction

NURSING DIAGNOSES

Chronic fatigue and immune dysfunction syndrome
- Activity intolerance
- Altered role performance
- Altered thought processes
- Fatigue
- Pain
- Powerlessness
- Self-esteem disturbance
- Sleep pattern disturbance

Common cold
- Fatigue
- Impaired skin integrity
- Knowledge deficit
- Pain

Cryptococcosis
- Altered thought processes
- Impaired gas exchange
- Impaired physical mobility
- Pain
- Risk for injury
- Sensory or perceptual alterations

Cytomegalovirus
- Activity intolerance
- Altered nutrition: Less than body requirements
- Altered parenting
- Altered thought processes
- Diarrhea
- Fatigue
- Hyperthermia
- Impaired gas exchange
- Ineffective breathing pattern
- Ineffective family coping
- Pain
- Risk for infection
- Risk for injury
- Sensory or perceptual alterations

Diphtheria
- Altered nutrition: Less than body requirements
- Impaired skin integrity
- Ineffective airway clearance
- Ineffective breathing pattern
- Pain
- Risk for fluid volume deficit

- Risk for infection
- Risk for injury
- Risk for suffocation
- Sensory alteration

Escherichia coli and other enterobacteriaceae infections
- Altered nutrition: Less than body requirements
- Decreased cardiac output
- Diarrhea
- Pain
- Risk for fluid volume deficit
- Risk for impaired skin integrity
- Risk for infection

Enterobiasis
- Impaired skin integrity
- Risk for infection
- Sleep pattern disturbance

Gas gangrene
- Anxiety
- Decreased cardiac output
- Fear
- Impaired skin integrity
- Impaired tissue integrity
- Pain
- Risk for infection

Genital warts
- Altered sexuality patterns
- Body image disturbance
- Knowledge deficit
- Risk for infection
- Risk for injury

Gonorrhea
- Altered sexuality patterns
- Knowledge deficit
- Pain
- Risk for infection

Haemophilus influenzae infection
- Altered nutrition: Less than body requirements
- Altered thought processes
- Anxiety
- Impaired gas exchange
- Impaired swallowing

- Ineffective airway clearance
- Ineffective breathing pattern
- Pain
- Risk for aspiration
- Risk for fluid volume deficit
- Risk for infection
- Sensory alteration

Herpes simplex
- Altered oral mucous membrane
- Altered sexuality patterns
- Altered thought processes
- Impaired skin integrity
- Impaired social interaction
- Knowledge deficit
- Pain
- Powerlessness
- Risk for infection
- Risk for injury
- Sensory alteration
- Social isolation

Herpes zoster
- Altered thought processes
- Body image disturbance
- Diversional activity deficit
- Impaired skin integrity
- Impaired social interaction
- Knowledge deficit
- Pain
- Sensory alteration
- Social isolation

Histoplasmosis
- Activity intolerance
- Altered nutrition: Less than body requirements
- Decreased cardiac output
- Impaired swallowing
- Ineffective breathing pattern
- Pain
- Risk for injury

Infectious mononucleosis
- Activity intolerance
- Altered nutrition: Less than body requirements
- Altered role performance
- Fatigue
- Hyperthermia
- Impaired skin integrity
- Impaired social interaction
- Knowledge deficit
- Pain
- Risk for fluid volume deficit
- Risk for injury

Influenza
- Altered health maintenance
- Fatigue
- Hyperthermia
- Impaired skin integrity
- Ineffective breathing pattern
- Pain
- Risk for fluid volume deficit
- Risk for infection

Legionnaire's disease
- Altered thought processes
- Hyperthermia
- Impaired gas exchange
- Ineffective airway clearance
- Ineffective breathing pattern
- Pain
- Risk for fluid volume deficit
- Risk for injury
- Self-care deficit

Lyme disease
- Altered thought processes
- Decreased cardiac output
- Fatigue
- Hyperthermia
- Impaired physical mobility
- Pain
- Risk for infection

Pneumocystis carinii pneumonia
- Activity intolerance
- Altered nutrition: Less than body requirements
- Anxiety
- Diversional activity deficit
- Fear
- Fluid volume deficit
- Hyperthermia
- Impaired gas exchange
- Impaired social interaction
- Impaired verbal communication
- Ineffective breathing pattern
- Powerlessness
- Risk for infection
- Self-care deficit

Rabies
- Altered nutrition: Less than body requirements
- Anxiety
- Decreased cardiac output
- Hyperthermia
- Impaired swallowing
- Impaired tissue integrity
- Ineffective breathing pattern
- Risk for fluid volume deficit
- Risk for infection
- Sensory alteration

Rubella
- Altered parenting
- Diversional activity deficit
- Hyperthermia
- Impaired skin integrity
- Ineffective family coping (with congenital rubella)
- Pain
- Risk for infection

Rubeola
- Altered nutrition: Less than body requirements
- Altered oral mucous membrane
- Fatigue
- Hyperthermia
- Impaired skin integrity
- Risk for infection
- Sensory or perceptual alterations (visual)

Salmonella infection
- Activity intolerance
- Altered nutrition: Less than body requirements
- Diarrhea
- Hyperthermia
- Pain
- Risk for fluid volume deficit
- Risk for infection
- Self-care deficit

Scarlet fever
- Activity intolerance
- Altered oral mucous membrane
- Hyperthermia
- Impaired skin integrity
- Pain
- Risk for infection

Syphilis
- Altered sexuality patterns
- Altered thought processes
- Body image disturbance
- Impaired physical mobility
- Impaired skin integrity
- Knowledge deficit
- Risk for infection
- Risk for injury
- Sexual dysfunction

Tetanus
- Altered nutrition: Less than body requirements
- Altered urinary elimination
- Impaired physical mobility
- Ineffective airway clearance
- Ineffective breathing pattern
- Pain
- Risk for disuse syndrome
- Risk for injury
- Self-care deficit

Toxic shock syndrome
- Altered thought processes
- Diarrhea
- Fluid volume deficit
- Hyperthermia
- Pain

Toxoplasmosis
- Activity intolerance
- Fatigue
- Fluid volume deficit
- Hyperthermia
- Impaired skin integrity
- Ineffective breathing pattern
- Pain
- Risk for injury
- Sensory or perceptual alterations

Trichomoniasis
- Altered sexuality patterns
- Altered urinary elimination
- Impaired skin integrity
- Knowledge deficit
- Pain
- Risk for infection
- Sexual dysfunction

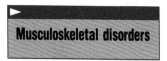

Musculoskeletal disorders

Carpal tunnel syndrome
• Altered role performance
• Anxiety
• Impaired physical mobility
• Pain
• Self-care deficit

Gout
• Anxiety
• Impaired physical mobility
• Ineffective individual coping
• Knowledge deficit
• Pain
• Risk for injury
• Sleep pattern disturbance

Herniated disk
• Activity intolerance
• Anxiety
• Fear
• Impaired physical mobility
• Pain
• Risk for injury
• Self-care deficit

Muscular dystrophy
• Activity intolerance
• Altered nutrition: More than body requirements
• Body image disturbance
• Constipation
• Impaired physical mobility
• Ineffective breathing pattern
• Ineffective family coping
• Ineffective individual coping
• Self-care deficit

Osteoarthritis
• Anxiety
• Body image disturbance
• Impaired physical mobility
• Ineffective individual coping
• Pain
• Self-care deficit
• Sleep pattern disturbance

Osteogenesis imperfecta
• Altered growth and development
• Impaired physical mobility
• Knowledge deficit
• Pain
• Risk for infection
• Risk for injury
• Self-esteem disturbance
• Sensory alteration

Osteomyelitis
• Activity intolerance
• Anxiety
• Fear
• Fluid volume excess
• Impaired physical mobility
• Impaired tissue integrity
• Knowledge deficit
• Pain
• Risk for infection
• Risk for injury

Osteoporosis
• Altered nutrition: Less than body requirements
• Body image disturbance
• Impaired physical mobility
• Knowledge deficit
• Pain
• Risk for impaired skin integrity
• Risk for injury
• Self-care deficit

Paget's disease
• Impaired home maintenance management
• Impaired physical mobility
• Knowledge deficit
• Pain
• Risk for impaired skin integrity
• Risk for injury

Scoliosis
• Anxiety
• Body image disturbance
• Fear
• Impaired physical mobility
• Knowledge deficit
• Pain
• Risk for injury

Septic arthritis
- Anxiety
- Fear
- Impaired physical mobility
- Knowledge deficit
- Pain
- Risk for infection
- Self-care deficit

Tendinitis and bursitis
- Anxiety
- Impaired physical mobility
- Knowledge deficit
- Pain
- Self-care deficit

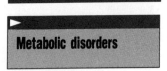

Metabolic disorders

Calcium imbalance
For hypercalcemia:
- Altered urinary elimination
- Decreased cardiac output
- Knowledge deficit
- Risk for injury
  For hypocalcemia:
- Decreased cardiac output
- Impaired gas exchange
- Knowledge deficit
- Risk for injury

Chloride imbalance
For hyperchloremia:
- Altered thought processes
- Fluid volume excess
- Ineffective breathing pattern
- Risk for injury
  For hypochloremia:
- Ineffective breathing pattern
- Knowledge deficit
- Risk for injury

Gaucher's disease
- Altered parenting
- Chronic pain
- Impaired gas exchange
- Knowledge deficit

- Risk for infection
- Risk for injury

Glycogen storage disease
- Activity intolerance
- Body image disturbance
- Decreased cardiac output
- Knowledge deficit
- Risk for infection

Hypoglycemia
- Anxiety
- Knowledge deficit
- Noncompliance
- Risk for injury

Lactose intolerance
- Altered nutrition: Less than body requirements
- Diarrhea
- Impaired skin integrity
- Knowledge deficit
- Pain
- Risk for fluid volume deficit

Magnesium imbalance
For hypermagnesemia:
- Altered nutrition: More than body requirements
- Impaired gas exchange
- Knowledge deficit
- Risk for injury
  For hypomagnesemia:
- Altered nutrition: Less than body requirements
- Impaired swallowing
- Knowledge deficit
- Risk for injury

Metabolic acidosis
- Altered oral mucous membrane
- Altered thought processes
- Ineffective breathing pattern
- Knowledge deficit
- Risk for injury

Metabolic alkalosis
- Altered thought processes
- Decreased cardiac output
- Ineffective breathing pattern
- Knowledge deficit
- Risk for injury

Phosphate imbalance

For hyperphosphatemia:
- Knowledge deficit
- Risk for injury
  For hypophosphatemia:
- Impaired gas exchange
- Knowledge deficit
- Pain
- Risk for injury

Porphyrias

- Constipation
- Impaired gas exchange
- Impaired skin integrity
- Knowledge deficit
- Pain
- Risk for injury

Potassium imbalance

- Constipation
- Decreased cardiac output
- Diarrhea
- Knowledge deficit
- Risk for injury

Sodium imbalance

For hypernatremia:
- Altered oral mucous membrane
- Altered thought processes
- Knowledge deficit
- Risk for injury
  For hyponatremia:
- Altered thought processes
- Fatigue
- Knowledge deficit
- Risk for injury

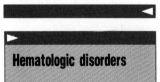

Hematologic disorders

Anemias

- Fatigue
- Knowledge deficit
- Pain
- Risk for infection

For pernicious anemia:
- Activity intolerance
- Altered nutrition: Less than body requirements
- Altered oral mucous membrane
- Altered tissue perfusion
- Impaired gas exchange
- Impaired physical mobility
- Impaired swallowing
- Risk for injury
- Self-care deficit
- Sensory alteration
  For aplastic or hypoplastic anemia:
- Activity intolerance
- Altered oral mucous membrane
- Altered thought processes
- Altered tissue perfusion
- Decreased cardiac output
- Hypothermia
- Impaired gas exchange
- Impaired physical mobility
- Risk for injury
  For sideroblastic anemia:
- Altered oral mucous membrane
- Decreased cardiac output
- Impaired skin integrity
- Risk for injury
  For iron deficiency anemia:
- Activity intolerance
- Altered growth and development
- Altered nutrition: Less than body requirements
- Altered thought processes
- Altered tissue perfusion
- Impaired gas exchange
- Risk for poisoning
  For sickle cell anemia:
- Altered growth and development
- Altered tissue perfusion
- Anxiety
- Body image disturbance
- Hyperthermia
- Impaired gas exchange
- Impaired tissue integrity
- Risk for fluid volume deficit
- Risk for injury

Disseminated intravascular coagulation
- Activity intolerance
- Altered tissue perfusion
- Anxiety
- Fatigue
- Fear
- Impaired gas exchange
- Impaired physical mobility
- Impaired skin integrity
- Impaired tissue integrity
- Pain
- Risk for fluid volume deficit
- Risk for injury

Hemophilia
- Activity intolerance
- Altered tissue perfusion
- Anxiety
- Impaired adjustment
- Impaired physical mobility
- Ineffective individual coping
- Knowledge deficit
- Pain
- Powerlessness
- Risk for fluid volume deficit
- Risk for injury
- Social isolation

Polycythemias
- Activity intolerance
- Anxiety
- Fatigue
- Knowledge deficit
- Risk for infection
- Risk for injury
  For secondary polycythemia:
- Altered protection
- Fear
- Impaired gas exchange
- Risk for fluid volume deficit
  For polycythemia vera:
- Altered nutrition: Less than body requirements
- Altered tissue perfusion
- Risk for impaired skin integrity

Thrombocytopenia
- Activity intolerance
- Altered protection
- Anxiety
- Body image disturbance
- Fatigue
- Impaired skin integrity
- Knowledge deficit
- Risk for infection
- Risk for injury

von Willebrand's disease
- Activity intolerance
- Altered tissue perfusion
- Anxiety
- Fatigue
- Ineffective family coping
- Ineffective individual coping
- Knowledge deficit
- Risk for fluid volume deficit
- Risk for injury

Immune disorders

Acquired immunodeficiency syndrome
- Activity intolerance
- Altered family processes
- Altered health maintenance
- Altered nutrition: Less than body requirements
- Altered oral mucous membrane
- Altered protection
- Altered sexuality patterns
- Altered thought processes
- Anticipatory grieving
- Anxiety
- Body image disturbance
- Defensive coping
- Denial
- Fatigue
- Fear
- Hopelessness
- Hyperthermia
- Impaired skin integrity
- Impaired tissue integrity
- Ineffective individual coping

- Knowledge deficit
- Parental role conflict
- Powerlessness
- Risk for fluid volume deficit
- Risk for infection
- Social isolation

Allergic rhinitis
- Altered health maintenance
- Impaired skin integrity
- Knowledge deficit
- Pain

Anaphylaxis
- Altered thought processes
- Anxiety
- Decreased cardiac output
- Fear
- Impaired gas exchange
- Impaired skin integrity
- Ineffective breathing pattern
- Knowledge deficit
- Pain
- Risk for suffocation

Atopic dermatitis
- Body image disturbance
- Impaired skin integrity
- Impaired social interaction
- Knowledge deficit
- Risk for infection

Lupus erythematosus
- Altered nutrition: Less than body requirements
- Altered oral mucous membrane
- Altered protection
- Altered urinary elimination
- Body image disturbance
- Constipation
- Decreased cardiac output
- Diarrhea
- Fatigue
- Impaired physical mobility
- Impaired skin integrity
- Impaired tissue integrity
- Impaired verbal communication
- Ineffective breathing pattern
- Knowledge deficit
- Pain
- Risk for infection
- Sensory or perceptual alterations

Psoriatic arthritis
- Altered protection
- Altered role performance
- Body image disturbance
- Fatigue
- Impaired physical mobility
- Impaired skin integrity
- Ineffective individual coping
- Pain

Rheumatoid arthritis
- Activity intolerance
- Altered health maintenance
- Altered nutrition: Less than body requirements
- Altered peripheral tissue perfusion
- Altered protection
- Altered role performance
- Anticipatory grieving
- Fatigue
- Fear
- Hopelessness
- Impaired physical mobility
- Knowledge deficit
- Pain
- Powerlessness
- Risk for impaired skin integrity
- Risk for infection
- Self-care deficit
- Sexual dysfunction

Selective IgA deficiency
- Altered health maintenance
- Altered nutrition: Less than body requirements
- Altered protection
- Diarrhea
- Risk for infection

Sjögren's syndrome
- Altered oral mucous membrane
- Altered sexuality patterns
- Fatigue
- Impaired skin integrity
- Impaired swallowing
- Impaired tissue integrity
- Pain
- Risk for infection
- Risk for injury
- Sensory alteration
- Sexual dysfunction

NURSING
DIAGNOSES

Urticaria and angioedema
- Altered nutrition: Less than body requirements
- Altered oral mucous membrane
- Impaired skin integrity
- Knowledge deficit
- Risk for infection
- Risk for suffocation

Vasculitis
- Activity intolerance
- Altered nutrition: Less than body requirements
- Altered oral mucous membrane
- Altered tissue perfusion
- Body image disturbance
- Decreased cardiac output
- Hyperthermia
- Impaired gas exchange
- Impaired physical mobility
- Impaired skin integrity
- Ineffective breathing pattern
- Pain
- Risk for infection
- Risk for injury
- Sensory alteration

Eye, ear, nose, and throat disorders

Adenoid hyperplasia
- Anxiety
- Fear
- Ineffective breathing pattern
- Knowledge deficit
- Pain
- Risk for aspiration

Blepharitis
- Altered health maintenance
- Body image disturbance
- Impaired skin integrity
- Risk for injury

Cataract
- Anxiety
- Risk for infection
- Risk for injury
- Sensory or perceptual alterations (visual)

Conjunctivitis
- Altered health maintenance
- Anxiety
- Risk for infection
- Sensory or perceptual alterations (visual)

Glaucoma
- Anxiety
- Fear
- Knowledge deficit
- Pain
- Risk for injury
- Sensory or perceptual alterations (visual)

Hearing loss
- Altered nutrition: More than body requirements
- Anxiety
- Fear
- Impaired verbal communication
- Knowledge deficit
- Risk for injury
- Self-esteem disturbance
- Sensory alteration (auditory)

Laryngitis
- Fear
- Impaired verbal communication
- Ineffective breathing pattern
- Knowledge deficit

Macular degeneration, age-related
- Fear
- Risk for injury
- Sensory or perceptual alterations (visual)
- Social isolation

Ménière's disease
- Altered nutrition: More than body requirements
- Anxiety
- Fear
- Fluid volume deficit
- Knowledge deficit
- Risk for injury
- Sensory alteration (auditory)

Nasal polyps
- Ineffective breathing pattern
- Knowledge deficit
- Pain
- Risk for injury

Otitis media
- Impaired verbal communication
- Knowledge deficit
- Pain
- Risk for infection
- Sensory alteration (auditory)

Otosclerosis
- Anxiety
- Fear
- Impaired verbal communication
- Knowledge deficit
- Risk for infection
- Sensory alteration (auditory)

Pharyngitis
- Altered nutrition: Less than body requirements
- Altered oral mucous membrane
- Fatigue
- Knowledge deficit
- Pain
- Risk for fluid volume deficit

Ptosis
- Altered health maintenance
- Risk for infection
- Risk for injury
- Sensory or perceptual alterations (visual)

Retinitis pigmentosa
- Body image disturbance
- Dysfunctional grieving
- Fear

- Powerlessness
- Risk for injury
- Sensory or perceptual alterations (visual)

Septal perforation and deviation
- Altered oral mucous membrane
- Anxiety
- Ineffective airway clearance
- Knowledge deficit
- Risk for infection

Sinusitis
- Altered oral mucous membrane
- Anxiety
- Fear
- Ineffective breathing pattern
- Knowledge deficit
- Pain
- Risk for infection

Stye
- Altered health maintenance
- Impaired skin integrity
- Pain
- Risk for infection
- Risk for injury
- Sensory or perceptual alterations (visual)

Tonsillitis
- Anxiety
- Fear
- Ineffective breathing pattern
- Knowledge deficit
- Risk for aspiration
- Risk for fluid volume deficit

Vocal cord paralysis
- Anxiety
- Fear
- Impaired verbal communication
- Ineffective breathing pattern
- Knowledge deficit
- Risk for aspiration

NURSING DIAGNOSES

Vocal cord polyps and nodules
- Anxiety
- Fear
- Impaired verbal communication
- Knowledge deficit
- Risk for injury

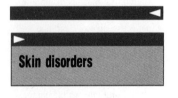

Skin disorders

Acne vulgaris
- Body image disturbance
- Impaired skin integrity
- Knowledge deficit
- Risk for infection
- Situational low self-esteem

Albinism
- Body image disturbance
- Defensive coping
- Knowledge deficit
- Risk for impaired skin integrity
- Situational low self-esteem

Alopecia
- Body image disturbance
- Risk for impaired skin integrity
- Risk for infection
- Situational low self-esteem

Dermatitis
- Altered oral mucous membrane
- Body image disturbance
- Impaired skin integrity
- Knowledge deficit
- Risk for infection

Dermatophytosis
- Body image disturbance
- Impaired skin integrity
- Pain
- Risk for infection

Impetigo
- Body image disturbance
- Impaired skin integrity
- Impaired tissue integrity
- Risk for infection

Pediculosis
- Body image disturbance
- Impaired skin integrity
- Risk for impaired skin integrity
- Risk for infection
- Situational low self-esteem

Photosensitivity reactions
- Body image disturbance
- Knowledge deficit
- Risk for fluid volume deficit
- Risk for impaired skin integrity
- Risk for infection

Pressure ulcers
- Altered nutrition: Less than body requirements
- Altered protection
- Impaired physical mobility
- Impaired skin integrity
- Risk for impaired tissue integrity
- Risk for infection

Psoriasis
- Body image disturbance
- Impaired skin integrity
- Knowledge deficit
- Pain
- Powerlessness
- Social isolation

Rosacea
- Body image disturbance
- Impaired skin integrity
- Knowledge deficit
- Risk for infection
- Situational low self-esteem

Scabies
- Body image disturbance
- Impaired skin integrity
- Risk for infection
- Situational low self-esteem

Tinea versicolor
- Body image disturbance
- Impaired skin integrity
- Risk for infection

Vitiligo
- Body image disturbance
- Knowledge deficit
- Risk for impaired skin integrity
- Situational low self-esteem

Warts
- Body image disturbance
- Impaired skin integrity
- Pain
- Risk for infection

Mental and emotional disorders

Alcoholism
- Altered family process: Alcoholism
- Altered protection
- Altered role performance
- Altered thought processes
- Anxiety
- Defensive coping
- Denial
- Hopelessness
- Impaired physical mobility
- Impaired social interaction
- Impaired tissue integrity
- Ineffective family coping
- Ineffective individual coping
- Noncompliance
- Personal identity disturbance
- Powerlessness
- Risk for injury
- Risk for violence
- Self-care deficit
- Sensory or perceptual alterations
- Sleep pattern disturbance
- Spiritual distress

Bipolar disorder
For the manic phase:
- Altered health maintenance
- Altered nutrition: Less than body requirements
- Altered thought processes
- Chronic low self-esteem
- Denial
- Impaired home maintenance management
- Impaired physical mobility
- Impaired verbal communication
- Ineffective individual coping
- Risk for violence: Self-directed or directed at others
- Self-care deficit
- Sensory or perceptual alterations
- Sexual dysfunction
- Sleep pattern disturbance
- Social isolation

For the depressive phase:
- Altered health maintenance
- Altered nutrition: Less than body requirements
- Altered thought processes
- Altered urinary elimination
- Chronic low self-esteem
- Constipation
- Denial
- Hopelessness
- Impaired home maintenance management
- Impaired physical mobility
- Impaired verbal communication
- Ineffective individual coping
- Powerlessness
- Risk for violence: Self-directed or directed at others
- Self-care deficit
- Sensory or perceptual alterations
- Sexual dysfunction
- Sleep pattern disturbance
- Social isolation

Dyspareunia
- Altered family processes
- Altered sexuality patterns
- Anxiety
- Knowledge deficit
- Sexual dysfunction

Erectile dysfunction
- Altered family processes
- Altered sexuality patterns
- Anxiety
- Ineffective individual coping
- Knowledge deficit
- Self-esteem disturbance
- Sexual dysfunction

Gender identification disorders
- Altered family processes
- Altered growth and development
- Altered role performance
- Anxiety
- Body image disturbance
- Chronic low self-esteem
- Impaired social interaction
- Ineffective family coping
- Ineffective individual coping
- Personal identity disturbance
- Powerlessness
- Risk for injury
- Sexual dysfunction
- Social isolation

Generalized anxiety disorder
- Altered nutrition: Less than body requirements
- Anxiety
- Chronic low self-esteem
- Constipation
- Defensive coping
- Denial
- Diarrhea
- Impaired home maintenance management
- Ineffective individual coping
- Powerlessness
- Self-esteem disturbance
- Sensory or perceptual alterations
- Sleep pattern disturbance

Major depression
- Altered nutrition: Less than body requirements
- Altered nutrition: More than body requirements
- Altered parenting
- Altered thought processes
- Anxiety
- Chronic low self-esteem
- Constipation

- Denial
- Diversional activity deficit
- Dysfunctional grieving
- Fatigue
- Hopelessness
- Impaired home maintenance management
- Impaired social interaction
- Ineffective individual coping
- Personal identity disturbance
- Powerlessness
- Risk for injury
- Risk for violence: Self-directed or directed at others
- Self-care deficit
- Sensory or perceptual alterations
- Sexual dysfunction
- Sleep pattern disturbance
- Social isolation
- Spiritual distress

Paraphilias
- Altered role performance
- Altered sexuality patterns
- Anxiety
- Chronic low self-esteem
- Impaired social interaction
- Personal identity disturbance
- Risk for injury
- Risk for violence: Directed at others
- Self-esteem disturbance
- Sexual dysfunction

Personality disorders
- Altered parenting
- Altered role performance
- Altered sexuality patterns
- Altered thought processes
- Anxiety
- Chronic low self-esteem
- Fear
- Impaired adjustment
- Impaired social interaction
- Ineffective individual coping
- Powerlessness
- Sexual dysfunction
- Social isolation

Phobias
- Altered thought processes
- Anxiety
- Fear
- Impaired social interaction
- Impaired verbal communication
- Ineffective family coping
- Ineffective individual coping
- Pain
- Personal identity disturbance
- Powerlessness
- Social isolation

Posttraumatic stress disorder
- Altered health maintenance
- Altered role performance
- Altered thought processes
- Anxiety
- Chronic low self-esteem
- Fear
- Hopelessness
- Impaired adjustment
- Impaired social interaction
- Ineffective family coping
- Ineffective individual coping
- Pain
- Personal identity disturbance
- Post-trauma response
- Powerlessness
- Rape-trauma syndrome
- Risk for violence: Self-directed or directed at others
- Sensory or perceptual alterations
- Sexual dysfunction
- Sleep pattern disturbance
- Social isolation
- Spiritual distress

Premature ejaculation
- Altered family processes
- Altered sexuality patterns
- Anxiety
- Knowledge deficit
- Self-esteem disturbance
- Sexual dysfunction

Psychoactive drug abuse and dependence
- Altered protection
- Altered role performance
- Altered thought processes

- Anxiety
- Defensive coping
- Denial
- Functional incontinence
- Hopelessness
- Impaired physical mobility
- Impaired social interaction
- Impaired tissue integrity
- Ineffective family coping
- Ineffective individual coping
- Noncompliance
- Personal identity disturbance
- Powerlessness
- Risk for injury
- Risk for violence: Self-directed or directed at others
- Self-care deficit
- Sensory or perceptual alterations
- Sleep pattern disturbance
- Spiritual distress

Schizophrenia
- Altered nutrition: Less than body requirements
- Altered role performance
- Altered thought processes
- Anxiety
- Body image disturbance
- Fear
- Fluid volume deficit
- Hopelessness
- Impaired home maintenance management
- Impaired social interaction
- Impaired verbal communication
- Ineffective family coping
- Ineffective individual coping
- Personal identity disturbance
- Powerlessness
- Risk for injury
- Risk for violence: Self-directed or directed at others
- Self-care deficit
- Sensory or perceptual alterations
- Sleep pattern disturbance
- Social isolation

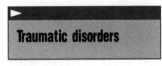

Traumatic disorders

Asphyxia
• Anxiety
• Decreased cardiac output
• Impaired gas exchange
• Ineffective airway clearance
• Ineffective breathing pattern
• Ineffective individual coping
• Risk for aspiration
• Risk for suffocation

Burns
• Altered nutrition: Less than body requirements
• Altered peripheral tissue perfusion
• Altered protection
• Anxiety
• Body image disturbance
• Decreased cardiac output
• Fluid volume deficit
• Hypothermia
• Impaired gas exchange
• Impaired physical mobility
• Impaired skin integrity
• Ineffective airway clearance
• Ineffective individual coping
• Knowledge deficit
• Pain
• Risk for infection
• Sensory or perceptual alterations

Cold injuries
• Altered health maintenance
• Altered tissue perfusion
• Anxiety
• Decreased cardiac output
• Hypothermia
• Impaired gas exchange
• Impaired physical mobility
• Impaired skin integrity
• Risk for disuse syndrome
• Risk for infection

Electric shock
• Altered tissue perfusion
• Anxiety
• Decreased cardiac output
• Impaired skin integrity
• Ineffective breathing pattern
• Pain
• Risk for injury
• Sensory alteration

Extremity injuries
• Impaired physical mobility
• Knowledge deficit
• Pain
   For amputation:
• Altered peripheral tissue perfusion
• Altered role performance
• Body image disturbance
• Fear
• Fluid volume deficit
• Impaired skin integrity
• Ineffective individual coping
• Risk for infection
   For arm or leg fracture:
• Altered tissue perfusion
• Anxiety
• Decreased cardiac output
• Diversional activity deficit
• Fear
• Impaired skin integrity
• Ineffective individual coping
• Risk for disuse syndrome
• Risk for fluid volume deficit
• Risk for infection
• Risk for injury
• Self-care deficit
   For dislocation or subluxation:
• Altered peripheral tissue perfusion
• Impaired skin integrity
• Risk for disuse syndrome
• Self-care deficit
   For sprain or strain:
• Impaired physical mobility
• Pain
• Risk for injury

Head injuries
- Pain
  For cerebral contusion:
- Altered thought processes
- Anxiety
- Impaired verbal communication
- Risk for fluid volume deficit
- Risk for infection
- Risk for injury
- Sensory or perceptual alterations
- Sleep pattern disturbance
  For concussion:
- Anxiety
- Risk for fluid volume deficit
- Risk for injury
- Sleep pattern disturbance
  For jaw dislocation or fracture:
- Altered nutrition: Less than body requirements
- Anxiety
- Impaired verbal communication
- Ineffective airway clearance
- Risk for aspiration
- Risk for fluid volume deficit
- Risk for infection
- Sensory or perceptual alterations
  For nose fracture:
- Body image disturbance
- Impaired tissue integrity
- Ineffective airway clearance
- Risk for infection
  For skull fracture:
- Altered nutrition: Less than body requirements
- Altered thought processes
- Anxiety
- Impaired skin integrity
- Ineffective breathing pattern
- Ineffective family coping
- Risk for infection
- Risk for injury
- Sensory or perceptual alterations

Heat syndrome
- Altered thought processes
- Decreased cardiac output
- Fluid volume deficit
- Hyperthermia
- Impaired gas exchange
- Impaired home maintenance management

- Knowledge deficit
- Sensory or perceptual alterations

Near drowning
- Decreased cardiac output
- Fluid volume deficit
- Hypothermia
- Impaired gas exchange
- Ineffective airway clearance
- Ineffective breathing pattern
- Risk for aspiration
- Risk for infection

Neck and spinal injuries
- Anxiety
- Impaired physical mobility
- Knowledge deficit
- Pain
  For spinal injury:
- Diversional activity deficit
- Ineffective breathing pattern
- Risk for aspiration
- Risk for disuse syndrome
- Risk for impaired skin integrity
- Risk for infection
- Self-care deficit
- Sensory alteration

Open wounds
- Anxiety
- Decreased cardiac output
- Fluid volume deficit
- Impaired gas exchange
- Impaired physical mobility
- Impaired skin integrity
- Pain
- Risk for infection

Poisoning
- Altered thought processes
- Anxiety
- Diarrhea
- Fluid volume deficit
- Impaired skin integrity
- Ineffective breathing pattern
- Knowledge deficit
- Pain
- Risk for aspiration
- Risk for injury
- Sensory or perceptual alterations

Radiation exposure
- Altered nutrition: Less than body requirements
- Altered oral mucous membrane
- Altered thought processes
- Anxiety
- Fluid volume deficit
- Impaired skin integrity
- Risk for infection

Rape-trauma syndrome
- Altered oral mucous membrane
- Anxiety
- Ineffective individual coping
- Pain
- Powerlessness
- Rape-trauma syndrome
- Risk for infection
- Self-esteem disturbance
- Sleep pattern disturbance

Thoracic and abdominal injuries
- Anxiety
- Fluid volume deficit
- Impaired gas exchange
- Pain
- Risk for infection
  For blunt chest injury:
- Impaired physical mobility
- Ineffective airway clearance
- Ineffective breathing pattern
- Knowledge deficit
- Risk for impaired skin integrity
  For blunt or penetrating abdominal injury:
- Altered tissue perfusion
- Decreased cardiac output
- Impaired skin integrity
  For penetrating chest injury:
- Altered tissue perfusion
- Decreased cardiac output
- Impaired skin integrity
- Ineffective breathing pattern

CHAPTER 6

Surgical patient care:
Reviewing the techniques

Preoperative care

▶

Assessing the preoperative patient

A thorough preoperative assessment is the foundation of good surgical care, providing a baseline for comparison throughout a patient's treatment and recovery. This assessment also helps identify conditions that impair the patient's ability to tolerate the stress of surgery or to comply with postoperative routines.

Initial steps

Begin your preoperative assessment by focusing on problem areas suggested by the patient's history and on any body system directly affected by the surgical procedure.

• Note your patient's general appearance. Does he look healthy and well-nourished, or does he appear ill?

• Record height, weight, and vital signs. Compare blood pressure bilaterally, using a cuff two-thirds the length of the patient's arm. Document the patient's position during this procedure.

• Update vital sign measurements at least twice a day throughout the preoperative period. Use these measurements to establish a baseline.

Systematic examination

Examine your patient thoroughly from head to toe, using these procedures as a guide.

Head and neck

• Check the patient's scalp for lesions or parasitic infection.

• Check the jugular veins for distention.

• Note the color of the sclerae. A yellowish color suggests jaundice.

• Evert the lower eyelid and note the color of the conjunctivae. Pale tissue suggests anemia.

• Check the nose and throat for signs of respiratory infection.

• Assess the mouth for sores, ulcerations, or bleeding of tongue, gums, and cheeks. Check the lips for a bluish or gray color, which may suggest cyanosis.

• Check the neck for stiffness or cervical node enlargement.

Neurologic system

• Assess the patient's level of conber that anxiety may make him slightly disoriented. Note whether his pupils are uniform in size and shape.

• Assess gross motor movements while the patient stands or walks as well as fine motor movements (for example, while he writes). Look for any neurologic changes, such as slurred speech.

• Inform the doctor of any behavioral changes (for instance, from lethargy to agitation), which may indicate increased intracranial pressure.

• If you know or suspect that your patient has a neurologic problem, conduct a complete neurologic examination.

Extremities and skin

• Look for changes in the skin color or temperature that suggest impaired circulation. Check for cyanotic nail beds and finger clubbing.

• Note any skin lesions.

• Assess skin turgor for signs of dehydration.

• Check extremities for edema. Ask the patient if his feet, ankles, or fingers ever swell.

• Note hair distribution on the patient's extremities. Uneven hair distribution suggests poor peripheral circulation.
• Carefully palpate leg veins for varicosity.
• Check all peripheral pulses (radial, pedal, femoral, and popliteal) bilaterally. Note any differences in quality, rate, or rhythm.

Respiratory system

• Document the patient's respiratory rate and pattern. A patient with questionable pulmonary status may require an alternative to inhalation anesthesia, such as a spinal block.
• Assess breathing pattern. Check for asymmetrical chest expansion and accessory muscle use.
• Auscultate the anterior and posterior chest for breath sounds. Listen for wheezing, coughing, and crackles. Note dyspnea.
• Ask the patient whether he smokes. If he does, ask how many packs per day and whether he's recently quit or cut down in anticipation of surgery. His doctor should have advised him to stop 4 to 6 weeks before surgery.

Cardiovascular system

• Inspect the patient's chest for abnormal pulsations. Auscultate at the fifth intercostal space over the left midclavicular line. If you can't hear an apical pulse, ask the patient to turn onto his left side; the heart may shift closer to the chest wall. Note the rate and quality of the apical pulse.
• Auscultate heart sounds. If you hear thrills, suspect mitral valve regurgitation or stenosis. Remember that murmurs you hear on the right side of the heart are more likely to change with respiration than left-sided murmurs.
• Palpate the chest to find the point of maximal impulse.

GI system

• Note the contour and symmetry of the abdomen; check for distention.
• Note the position and color of the umbilicus; look for herniation.
• Auscultate bowel sounds in each quadrant. Ask the patient if his bowel movements are regular.
• Percuss the abdomen for air and fluid.
• Palpate the abdomen for softness, firmness, and bladder height. Note any tenderness.
• Assess the six Fs: fat, fluid, flatus, feces, fetus (possibility of pregnancy), and fibroid tissue (or any unusual mass).

Genitourinary system

• Obtain a urine sample, if ordered; note color and clarity.
• Ask the patient if he ever experiences any pain, burning, or bleeding during urination.
• Also ask about urinary frequency and incontinence. Is he able to empty his bladder completely? Does he awaken at night to urinate?
• If indicated, monitor urine output and try to correlate any excess or deficit with blood urea nitrogen or creatinine levels. If urine output falls, first assess catheter patency and urinary drainage system patency, if applicable. Compare intake and output over the last several days as well as daily weights.
• Note the general appearance of the patient's genitalia.
• If your patient is female, ask when her last menstrual period occurred, and find out if her cycle is regular. In addition, ask if she could possibly be pregnant.

Psychological status

• Set aside time to allow the patient to discuss any feelings about the impending surgery. This is important because depression and anxiety can significantly impact recovery. Offer the patient the option of seeing a clergyman.

• Be understanding of the patient's fears and regressive behavior, regardless of age.

• Expect some anxiety. If the patient seems inappropriately relaxed or unconcerned, consider whether he's suppressing his fears. Such a patient may cope poorly with surgical stress, and it is important to encourage him to seek support from family or friends. If possible, allow them to visit with the patient preoperatively. Also, include them in your nursing care plan.

Teaching the preoperative patient

Your teaching can help the patient cope with the physical and psychological stress of surgery. Because of the rising number of shorter hospital stays and same-day surgeries, preadmission and preoperative teaching has become more important than ever.

Explaining preoperative measures

Include in your teaching strategy an evaluation of the patient's understanding of his upcoming surgery so you can correct any misconceptions. Structure the teaching to accommodate a short time period, and use the following teaching tips as a guide.

• Urge the patient to read the surgical consent form carefully and to ask questions before signing.

• Explain that the results of chest X-rays, a complete blood count (CBC), urine studies, an electrocardiogram (ECG), and other preoperative tests will determine readiness for surgery.

• Discuss the rationale behind hair removal (if ordered) — to prevent surgical wound infection by cleaning the skin of microorganisms found in body hair.

• Stress the importance of withholding food and fluids for a specified time before surgery.

• Inform the patient that after he has completed all preoperative routines, including dressing in a surgical cap and gown, he'll receive preanesthetic medication. Tell the patient that this medication will help him relax, although he probably won't fall asleep. His mouth will feel dry, because the medication helps dry up secretions.

• Tell the patient that he will receive an I.V. line either before he goes to surgery or after he gets to the operating room.

• Help the patient deal with fears about anesthesia. Assure him that the anesthesiologist will monitor his condition throughout surgery and provide the right amount of anesthetic.

• Show the patient's family where they can wait during the operation. If they want to visit preoperatively, tell them to arrive 2 hours before surgery is scheduled.

AGE ALERT When the patient is a child, you can help make the surgical experience less threatening by using therapeutic play. Follow these guidelines:

• Allow the child to choose play articles.

• Provide materials specific to the

child's experiences, such as nasogastric tube, syringe, or bandages.
• Allow play to be unstructured.
• Provide supervision to prevent accidental injury.

Previewing operating room procedures

Counsel the patient on operating room (OR) procedures.
• Warn the patient that he may have to wait a short time in the holding area, an area allocated to patients awaiting surgery. Explain that the doctors and nurses will wear surgical dress and that even though they'll be observing him closely, they probably won't talk to him. Tell him that this will allow the medication to take effect.
• When discussing transfer procedures and techniques, describe sensations the patient will experience. Advise the patient that he'll be taken to the operating room on a stretcher and then transferred from the stretcher to the operating table. For his own safety, he'll be strapped securely to the table. The operating room nurses will check his vital signs frequently.
• Warn the patient that the operating room may feel cool. Electrodes may be put on his chest to monitor his heart rate during surgery.
• Describe the drowsy, floating sensation he'll feel as the anesthetic takes effect. Tell him it's important that he relax at this time.

Getting ready for recovery

Prepare the patient for his stay in the recovery room. Briefly describe the sensations the patient will experience when the anesthetic wears off. Tell him that the recovery room nurse will call his name, then ask him to answer questions and follow simple commands, such as wiggling his toes. He may feel pain at the surgical site, but the nurse will try to minimize it.

• Describe the oxygen delivery device, such as the nasal cannula, that he'll need after surgery.
• Tell the patient that once he's recovered from the anesthesia, he'll return to his room. He'll be able to see his family, but will probably feel drowsy and wish to nap.
• Make sure he's aware that you'll be taking his blood pressure and pulse frequently. That way, he won't be alarmed by these routine procedures.
• Reduce the patient's anxiety about postoperative pain by advising him of pain-control measures that you'll be using. Explain that the doctor will order pain medication to be given every 3 to 4 hours or according to the patient's needs.
• Instruct the patient to describe pain in terms of its quality, severity, and location. Encourage him to let you know as soon as he feels any pain instead of waiting until it becomes intense.
• Discuss the type of medication he'll receive, how it works, and the route of administration. Also describe measures you'll take to relieve pain and promote patient comfort, such as positioning, diversionary activities, and splinting.
• Teach the patient coughing exercises, unless he's scheduled for neurosurgery or eye surgery. If he's scheduled for chest or abdominal surgery, teach him how to splint his incision before he coughs. Instruct the patient to take a slow, deep breath, then breathe out through his mouth. Have him take a second breath in the same manner. Next, tell him to take a third deep breath and hold it. He should then cough two or three times to clear his breathing passages. Have him take three to five normal breaths, exhaling slowly and relaxing after each breath.

SURGICAL
PATIENTS

• Also teach deep-breathing exercises. Have the patient lie on his back in a comfortable position with one hand placed on his chest and the other over his upper abdomen. Instruct him to exhale normally, close his mouth, and inhale deeply through his nose. His chest should not expand. Have him hold his breath and slowly count to five. Next, have him purse his lips and exhale completely through his mouth without letting his cheeks expand. Tell the patient to repeat the exercise 5 to 10 times.

• Teach the patient the techniques of early mobility and ambulation. Explain that postoperative exercises help to prevent complications, such as atelectasis, thrombophlebitis, constipation, and loss of muscle tone.

• Demonstrate and have the patient use an incentive spirometer, and explain that this device will provide feedback when he's doing deep-breathing exercises. Explain how simple leg exercises, such as alternately contracting the calf muscles, will prevent venous pooling after surgery.

Identifying hazardous drugs

Some drugs may cause hazardous complications or interactions during or after surgery. So always review your patient's medication record carefully before he undergoes surgery. Use this chart to identify common drugs that can be hazardous to surgical patients.

DRUG	POSSIBLE EFFECTS
Antianxiety drugs	
Diazepam Valium	• Excessive sedation • Preoperative or postoperative nausea and vomiting • Local tissue irritation (with I.V. administration)
Hydroxyzine hydrochloride Vistaril	• Drowsiness and dry mouth
Midazolam hydrochloride Versed	• Respiratory depression (with high doses)
Antiarrhythmics	
All types	• Laryngospasm • Intensified cardiac depression, reduced cardiac output

Identifying hazardous drugs *(continued)*

DRUG	POSSIBLE EFFECTS
Antiarrhythmics *(continued)*	
Procainamide Pronestyl	• Prolonged or enhanced effects of neuro-muscular blockers • Hypotension
Propranolol Inderal	• Prolonged or enhanced effects of neuro-muscular blockers • Depressed myocardial function • Hypotension • Laryngospasm
Antibiotics	
All types	• Masked symptoms of infection
Aminoglycosides Amikacin, Gentamicin, Kanamycin, Neomycin, Netilmicin, Streptomycin, Tobramycin	• Increased risk of neuromuscular block-ade and respiratory paralysis
Erythromycin Erythrocin, E-Mycin	• Prolonged action of opiates
Anticholinergics	
Atropine sulfate	• Excessive dryness of the mouth, tachy-cardia, flushing, depressed sweating • Increased intraocular pressure, blurred vision, dilated pupils • Urine retention • Agitation and delirium (in elderly)
Glycopyrrolate Robinul	• Excessive dryness of the mouth, tachy-cardia, flushing, depressed sweating • Increased intraocular pressure, blurred vision, dilated pupils • Urine retention
Scopolamine hydrobromide Triptone, Isopto-Hyoscine	• Excessive dryness of the mouth, tachy-cardia, flushing • Increased intraocular pressure, blurred vision, dilated pupils • Urine retention • Excessive drowsiness • Agitation and delirium (in elderly)

(continued)

SURGICAL PATIENTS

Identifying hazardous drugs *(continued)*

DRUG	POSSIBLE EFFECTS
Anticoagulants	
Heparin Liquaemin **Warfarin** Coumadin	• Increased risk of hemorrhage
Anticonvulsants	
Magnesium sulfate	• Increased risk of neuromuscular blockade
Antidiabetics	
Insulin	• Increased insulin requirement during stress and healing • Diminished insulin requirement during fasting
Antihypertensives	
All types	• Worsened hypotension
Central nervous system depressants	
Alcohol, sedative hypnotics	• If given with general anesthetics: increased risk of respiratory depression, apnea, or hypotension
Corticosteroids	
Betamethasone, cortisone, dexamethasone, hydrocortisone, methylprednisolone, paramethasone, prednisolone, prednisone, triamcinolone	• Delayed wound healing • Risk of acute adrenal insufficiency • Increased risk of infection • Masked symptoms of infection • Increased risk of hemorrhage
Diuretics	
Furosemide Lasix **Potassium-depleting diuretics**	• If given with certain anesthetics: increased risk of hypotension • Increased risk of complications associated with hypokalemia

SURGICAL
PATIENTS

Identifying hazardous drugs *(continued)*

DRUG	POSSIBLE EFFECTS
Histamine₂-receptor antagonists	
Cimetidine Tagamet **Ranitidine** Zantac	• Decreased clearance of diazepam, lidocaine, propranolol, and all other drugs
Miotics	
Demecarium, echothiophate, isoflurophate	• If given with succinylcholine: increased risk of neuromuscular blockade, cardiovascular collapse, prolonged respiratory depression, or apnea. Effect may occur up to a few months after the patient stops the drug.
Narcotics	
Meperidine hydrochloride Demerol **Morphine sulfate**	• Depressed respiration, circulation, and gastric motility • Dizziness, tachycardia, and sweating • Hypotension, restlessness, and excitement • Preoperative or postoperative nausea and vomiting
Opiates	
All types	• If given with certain I.V. anesthetics (such as midazolam, propofol, thiopental, and droperidol): increased risk of respiratory depression, apnea, or hypotension
Sedative-hypnotics	
Pentobarbital sodium Nembutal Sodium	• Confusion or excitement, especially in the elderly or in patients with severe pain
Thyroid hormones	
All types	• If given with ketamine: increased risk of hypertension and tachycardia
Tranquilizers	
Promethazine hydrochloride Phenergan	• Postoperative hypotension

SURGICAL
PATIENTS

Reviewing care on the day of surgery

Early on the day of surgery, follow these procedures.

• Verify that the patient has had nothing by mouth since midnight.

• Be sure diagnostic test results appear on the chart.

• Ask the patient to remove jewelry, makeup, or nail polish; to shower with antimicrobial soap, if ordered; and to perform mouth care. Warn him against swallowing water.

• Instruct the patient to remove any dentures or partial plates. Note on the chart if he has dental crowns, caps, or braces. Also have him remove any contact lenses, glasses, prostheses, and hearing aids. If the patient wishes to keep his hearing aid in place, inform operating room and postanesthesia care unit staff of this decision.

• Tell the patient to void and to put on a surgical cap and gown.

• Take and record vital signs.

• Give preoperative medication 45 to 75 minutes before starting anesthesia.

Preparing the bowel for surgery

The extent of bowel preparation depends on the type and site of surgery. For example, a patient scheduled for several days of postoperative bed rest who hasn't had a recent bowel movement may receive a mild laxative or enema. But a patient slated for GI, pelvic, perianal, or rectal surgery will undergo more extensive intestinal preparation.

Preoperative enemas or an osmotic cathartic solution such as magnesium citrate may help empty the intestine, thereby minimizing injury to the colon and improving visualization of the operative site.

Expect to perform extensive intestinal preparation for patients undergoing elective colon surgery. During surgical opening of the colon, escaping bacteria may invade adjacent tissue, leading to infection. Perform a mechanical prep and administer antimicrobial agents as ordered. Mechanical bowel prep removes gross stool; oral antimicrobials suppress potent microflora without encouraging resistant strains.

If enemas are ordered to clear the bowel and the third enema still hasn't removed all stool, notify the doctor. Repeated enemas may cause fluid and electrolyte imbalances. Elderly patients and those who are allowed nothing by mouth and haven't received I.V. fluids are at high risk.

Preparing the skin for surgery

Before surgery, the patient's skin must be as free as possible from microorganisms to reduce the risk of infection at the incision site. This involves cleaning the area with an antiseptic detergent solution and, if hospital policy directs, removing hair.

Hair removal should be done as close to the time of surgery as possible, such as in the holding area. Because depilatories reduce infection risk from skin injury, they're preferred over shaving if the patient is not allergic to them. However, shaving is sometimes required.

Equipment

• Antiseptic soap solution • tap water • bath blanket • two clean basins • linen-saver pad • adjustable light • sterile razor with new blade, if needed • scissors • gloves.
Optional: 4″ × 4″ gauze pads, cotton-tipped applicators, nail polish remover, orangewood stick, trash bag, towel.

Implementation

• Dilute the antiseptic detergent solution with warm tap water in one basin for washing, and pour plain warm water into the second basin for rinsing.
• Explain the procedure to the patient. Provide privacy, wash your hands, and put on gloves.
• Position the patient comfortably, drape him with the bath blanket, and place a linen-saver pad beneath him. Expose a small portion of the preparation area. Usually, this area extends 12″ (30 cm) in each direction from the expected incision site.
• Assess skin condition and report skin breaks to the doctor. (Skin breaks increase risk of infection and can cause cancellation of surgery.)
• Make sure that you remove jewelry from the operative site.
• As ordered, clip any long hairs from the area with scissors; shave remaining hair to remove microorganisms.
• Use a gauze pad to spread liquid soap over the site to be shaved.
• Pull the skin taut in the direction opposite that of hair growth because this makes the hair rise and facilitates shaving.
• Holding the razor at a 45-degree angle, shave with short strokes in the direction of hair growth to avoid skin irritation.
• Rinse the razor and reapply liquid soap to the skin as needed to keep the area moist.

• Change the rinse water if necessary. Rinse and inspect the preparation area. Notify the doctor of any new nicks or abrasions. File a report, if required.
• Proceed with a 10-minute scrub. Wash the area with a gauze pad dipped in antiseptic soap solution. Using a circular motion, start at the expected incision site and work outward to avoid recontamination. Apply light friction while washing to improve the antiseptic effect of the solution. Replace the gauze pad as necessary.
• Clean skin folds because they harbor microorganisms. Scrub the perineal area last, if appropriate. Pull loose skin taut. Use cotton-tipped applicators to clean the umbilicus and an orangewood stick to clean under fingernails and toenails, as appropriate.
• Dry the area with a towel. Remove linen-saver pad.
• Dispose of soiled supplies according to hospital policy.
• Shave facial or neck hair on women and children only if ordered.

Where to remove hair

Specific instructions for hair removal depend on the surgical site.

Shoulder and upper arm

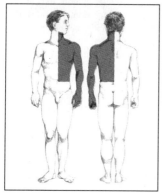

On the operative side, remove hair from fingertips to hairline and from center chest to center spine, extending to iliac crest and including the axilla.

Forearm, elbow, and hand

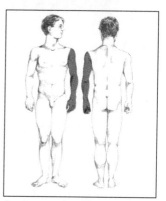

On the operative side, remove hair from fingertips to shoulder. Include the axilla, unless surgery is for hand. Trim and clean fingernails.

Knee and lower leg

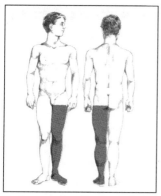

On the operative side, remove hair from toes to just below the groin. Clean and trim toenails.

Ankle and foot

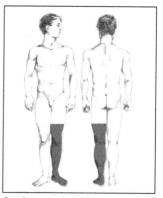

On the operative side, remove hair from toes to 3″ (8 cm) above the knee. Clean and trim toenails.

Hip

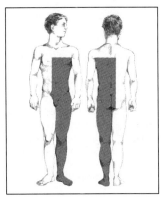

On the operative side, remove hair from toes to nipple line and at least 3″ (8 cm) beyond midline back and front, including the pubis. Clean and trim toenails.

Thigh

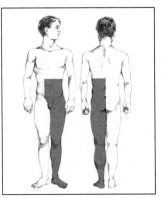

On the operative side, remove hair from toes to 3″ (8 cm) above the umbilicus and from midline front to midline back, including the pubis. Clean and trim toenails.

Chest

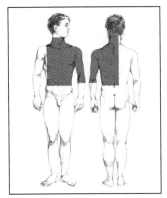

Remove hair from chin to iliac crests. On the unaffected side, prep over to nipple line; on affected side (operative side), to midline of back, and include axilla and arm to elbow. (For thoracotomy, prep 2″ [5 cm] beyond midline of back).

Abdomen

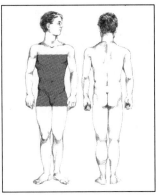

Remove hair from 3″ (8 cm) above the nipple to upper thighs, including the pubis.

(continued)

SURGICAL
PATIENTS

Lower abdomen

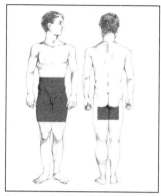

Remove hair from 2″ (5 cm) above the umbilicus to midthighs, including the pubic area. For femoral ligation, remove hair to midline of thighs in back. For hernia and embolectomy, remove hair to costal margin and down to knees, as ordered.

Flank

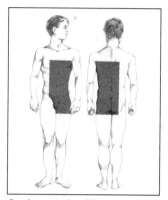

On the operative side, remove hair from nipple line to pubis, 3″ (8 cm) beyond the midline in back, and 2″ (5 cm) past the abdominal midline. Include pubic area and, on affected side, the upper thigh.

Reviewing common general anesthetics

DRUG	INDICATIONS	ADVANTAGES
Inhalation agents		
Nitrous oxide	Maintains anesthesia; may provide an adjunct for inducing general anesthesia	• Has little effect on heart rate, myocardial contractility, respiration, blood pressure, liver, kidneys or metabolism in absence of hypoxia • Produces excellent analgesia • Allows for rapid induction and recovery • Doesn't increase capillary bleeding • Doesn't sensitize myocardium to epinephrine

Perineum

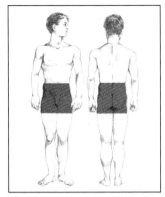

Remove hair from the pubis, perineum, and perianal area—from the waist to at least 3″ (8 cm) below the groin in front and at least 3″ below the buttocks in back.

Spine

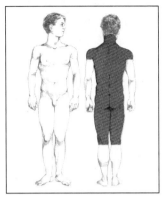

Remove hair from the entire back, including shoulders and neck to hairline, and down to both knees.

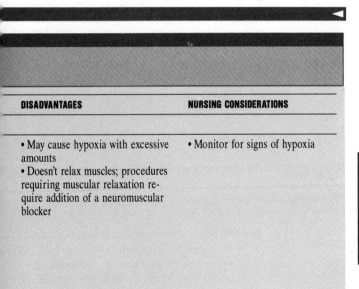

DISADVANTAGES	NURSING CONSIDERATIONS
• May cause hypoxia with excessive amounts • Doesn't relax muscles; procedures requiring muscular relaxation require addition of a neuromuscular blocker	• Monitor for signs of hypoxia

SURGICAL
PATIENTS

(continued)

Reviewing common general anesthetics (continued)

DRUG	INDICATIONS	ADVANTAGES
Inhalation agents (continued)		
Halothane Fluothane	Maintains general anesthesia	• Is easy to administer • Allows for rapid, smooth induction and recovery • Has a relatively pleasant odor; is nonirritating • Depresses salivary and bronchial secretions • Causes bronchodilation • Easily suppresses pharyngeal and laryngeal reflexes
Enflurane Ethrane	Maintains anesthesia; occasionally is used to induce anesthesia	• Allows for rapid induction and recovery • Is nonirritating and eliminates secretions • Causes bronchodilation • Provides good muscle relaxation • Allows cardiac rhythm to remain stable
Isoflurane Forane	Maintains general anesthesia; occasionally is used to induce general anesthesia	• Allows for rapid induction and recovery • Causes bronchodilation • Provides excellent muscle relaxation • Allows for extremely stable cardiac rhythm
I.V. barbiturates		
Thiopental sodium Pentothal	Is used primarily to induce general anesthesia	• Promotes rapid, smooth, and pleasant induction and quick recovery • Infrequently causes complications • Doesn't sensitize autonomic tissues of heart to catecholamines

DISADVANTAGES	NURSING CONSIDERATIONS
• May cause myocardial depression leading to arrhythmias • Sensitizes heart to action of catecholamine • May cause circulatory or respiratory depression, depending on the dose • Has no analgesic property	• Watch for arrhythmias, hypotension, respiratory depression • Monitor for fall in body temperature; patient may shiver after prolonged use. Shivering increases oxygen consumption.
• Causes myocardial depression • Lowers seizure threshold • Increases hypotension as depth of anesthesia increases • May cause shivering during recovery • May cause circulatory or respiratory depression, depending on the dose	• Monitor patient for decreased heart and respiratory rates, and hypotension • Watch for shivering that may lead to increased oxygen consumption
• May cause circulatory or respiratory depression, depending on dose • Potentiates the action of nondepolarizing muscular relaxants • May cause patient to shiver • Tends to lower blood pressure as depth of anesthesia increases; pulse remains somewhat elevated	• Watch for respiratory depression and hypotension • Watch for shivering that may lead to increased oxygen consumption
• Is associated with airway obstruction, respiratory depression, and laryngospasm, possibly leading to hypoxia • Doesn't provide muscle relaxation and produces little analgesia • May cause cardiovascular depression, especially in hypovolemic or debilitated patients	• Watch for signs and symptoms of hypoxia, airway obstruction, and cardiovascular and respiratory depression

(continued)

Reviewing common general anesthetics *(continued)*

DRUG	INDICATIONS	ADVANTAGES
I.V. benzodiazepines		
Diazepam Valium	Induces general anesthesia; provides amnesia during balanced anesthesia	• Minimally affects the cardiovascular system • Acts as a potent anticonvulsant • Produces amnesia
Midazolam Versed	Induces general anesthesia; provides amnesia during balanced anesthesia	• Minimally affects the cardiovascular system • Acts as a potent anticonvulsant • Produces amnesia
I.V. nonbarbiturate drugs		
Ketamine hydrochloride Ketalar	Produces a dissociative state of consciousness; induces anesthesia when a barbiturate is contraindicated. Sole anesthetic agent for short diagnostic and surgical procedures not requiring skeletal muscle relaxation	• Produces rapid anesthesia and profound analgesia • Does not irritate veins or tissues • Maintains a patent airway without endotracheal intubation because it suppresses laryngeal and pharyngeal reflexes
Propofol Diprivan	Is used for induction and maintenance of anesthesia; is particularly useful for short procedures and outpatient surgery	• Allows for quick, smooth induction • Permits rapid awakening and recovery • Causes less vomiting
I.V. tranquilizer		
Droperidol Inapsine	Is used preoperatively and during induction and maintenance of anesthesia as an adjunct to general or regional anesthesia	• Allows for rapid, smooth induction and recovery • Produces sleepiness and mental detachment for several hours

DISADVANTAGES	NURSING CONSIDERATIONS
• May cause irritation when injected into a peripheral vein • Has a long elimination half-life	• Monitor patient's vital signs
• Can cause respiratory depression	• Monitor patient's vital signs, respiratory rate, and volume
• May cause unpleasant dreams, hallucinations, and delirium during recovery • Increases heart rate, blood pressure, and intraocular pressure • Preserves muscle tone, leading to poor relaxation during surgery	• Protect patient from visual, tactile, and auditory stimuli during recovery • Monitor patient's vital signs
• Can cause hypotension • Can cause pain if injected into small veins • May cause clonic or myoclonic movements upon emergence • May interact with benzodiazepines, increasing propofol's effects • Does not cause profound analgesia	• Monitor patient for hypotension • Prepare for rapid emergence
• May cause hypotension because it's a peripheral vasodilator	• Monitor patient for increased pulse rate and hypotension

SURGICAL
PATIENTS

(continued)

Reviewing common general anesthetics *(continued)*

DRUG	INDICATIONS	ADVANTAGES
Narcotics		
Fentanyl citrate Sublimaze	Is used preoperatively for minor and major surgery, urologic procedures, and gastroscopy; also used as an adjunct to regional anesthesia and for inducing and maintaining general anesthesia	• Promotes rapid, smooth induction and recovery • Doesn't cause histamine release • Minimally affects cardiovascular system • Can be reversed by a narcotic antagonist (naloxone)
Neuroleptics		
Droperidol and fentanyl Innovar	Is used for short procedures during which the patient must remain conscious; also used as a premedication and as an adjunct for inducing and maintaining general anesthesia	• Allows for rapid, smooth induction and recovery • Produces somnolence and psychological indifference to the environment without total unconsciousness • Eliminates voluntary movement • Makes it possible to use less analgesia postoperatively • Produces satisfactory amnesia

DISADVANTAGES	NURSING CONSIDERATIONS
• May cause respiratory depression, euphoria, bradycardia, bronchoconstriction, nausea, vomiting, and miosis • May cause skeletal-muscle and chest-wall rigidity	• Observe for respiratory depression • Watch for nausea and vomiting. If vomiting occurs, position the patient to prevent aspiration • Monitor blood pressure • Decrease postoperative narcotics to one-third to one-fourth of usual dose
• May cause respiratory depression, extrapyramidal symptoms, apnea, laryngospasm, bronchospasm, bradycardia, and hallucinations	• Closely monitor patient's vital signs • Decrease postoperative narcotic to one-third to one-fourth usual dose for first 8 hours

Reviewing common neuromuscular blockers

DRUG	ADVERSE EFFECTS	NURSING CONSIDERATIONS
Nondepolarizing neuromuscular blockers		
Atracurium besylate Tracrium	• Slight hypotension in a few patients	• Acts for 20 to 30 minutes • May cause slight histamine release • Won't accumulate with repeated doses • Is useful in underlying hepatic, renal, and cardiac disease
Gallamine triethiodide Flaxedil	• Tachycardia and hypertension • Allergic reaction in patients sensitive to iodine	• Acts for 15 to 35 minutes • May cause tachycardia after doses of 0.5 mg/kg; avoid using in cardiac disease • Doesn't cause bronchospasm • Accumulates; don't administer to patients with impaired renal function
Metocurine iodide Metubine	• Hypotension • Bronchospasm	• Acts for 25 to 90 minutes; 60 minutes is average; depends on the dose and general anesthetic • May cause histamine release
Pancuronium bromide Pavulon	• Tachycardia • Transient skin rashes and a burning sensation at injection site	• Acts for 35 to 45 minutes • Is five times more potent than curare • Doesn't cause ganglion blockage, so it doesn't usually lead to hypotension • Has a vagolytic action that increases heart rate
Tubocurarine chloride Tubarine	• Hypotension • Bronchospasm	• Acts for 25 to 90 minutes with single large dose or multiple single doses: may last 24 hours • Causes histamine release; in higher doses, causes sympathetic ganglion blockade • May have prolonged action in elderly or debilitated patients and in those with renal or liver disease

Reviewing common neuromuscular blockers *(continued)*

DRUG	ADVERSE EFFECTS	NURSING CONSIDERATIONS
Nondepolarizing neuromuscular blockers *(continued)*		
Vecuronium bromide Norcuron	• Minimal and transient cardiovascular effects • Skeletal muscle weakness or paralysis; respiratory insufficiency; respiratory paralysis; prolonged, dose-related apnea	• Acts for 25 to 40 minutes • Probably metabolized mostly in liver • Has a short duration of action and causes fewer cardiovascular effects than other nondepolarizing neuromuscular blockers
Depolarizing neuromuscular blockers		
Succinylcholine chloride (suxamethonium chloride) Anectine, Quelicin, Sucostrin	• Respiratory depression • Bradycardia • Excessive salivation • Hypotension • Arrhythmias • Tachycardia • Hypertension • Increased intraocular and intragastric pressure • Fasciculations • Muscle pain • Malignant hyperthermia	• Acts for 5 to 10 minutes • Is metabolized mostly in plasma by pseudocholinesterase; therefore, it's contraindicated in patients with a deficiency of plasma cholinesterase due to a genetic variant defect, liver disease, uremia, or malnutrition • Use cautiously in patients with glaucoma or penetrating wounds of the eye; those undergoing eye surgery; or those with burns, severe trauma, spinal cord injuries, muscular dystrophy, or cardiovascular, hepatic, pulmonary, metabolic, or renal disorders. Succinylcholine may cause sudden hyperkalemia and consequent cardiac arrest. • Can cause pregnant patients who also receive magnesium sulfate to experience increased neuromuscular blockade because of decreased pseudocholinesterase levels

SURGICAL PATIENTS

Postoperative care

▶
Monitoring the postoperative patient

This phase of care aims at minimizing complications through early detection and prompt treatment.

Equipment
Thermometer • watch with second hand • stethoscope • sphygmomanometer • postoperative flowchart or other documentation tool.

Implementation
• Obtain the patient's record from the postanesthesia care unit (PACU) nurse.
• Transfer the patient from the PACU stretcher to the bed. Position him properly. Keep transfer movements smooth to minimize pain and complications.
• If the patient has had orthopedic surgery, have a coworker move the affected extremity as you transfer the patient.
• If the patient is in skeletal traction, have a coworker move the weights as you and another coworker transfer the patient.
• Ensure the patient's comfort, and raise the side rails of the bed to ensure his safety.
• Assess the patient's level of consciousness, skin color, and mucous membranes. Monitor respiratory status by assessing his airway. Note breathing rate and depth; auscultate breath sounds. If ordered, administer oxygen and initiate oximetry.
• Monitor the patient's postoperative pulse rate, which should be within 20% of the preoperative rate.
• Compare postoperative blood pressure to preoperative blood pressure. It should be within 20% of the

preoperative level unless the patient suffered a hypotensive episode during surgery.
• Assess the patient's body temperature. If it's lower than 95° F (35° C), apply blankets.
• Assess the patient's infusion sites for redness, pain, swelling, or drainage.
• Assess surgical wound dressings. If they're soiled, assess the drainage and outline the soiled area. Note the date and time of assessment on the dressing. Check the soiled area often; if it enlarges, reinforce the dressing and alert the doctor.
• Note the presence and condition of any drains and tubes. Note the color, type, odor, and amount of drainage. Make sure all drains are properly connected and free of kinks and obstructions.
• If the patient has had vascular or orthopedic surgery, assess the appropriate extremities. Notify the doctor of abnormalities.
• As the patient recovers from anesthesia, monitor his respiratory and cardiovascular status closely. Be alert for airway obstruction and hypoventilation caused by laryngospasm, or for sedation, which can lead to hypoxemia.
• Encourage coughing and deep-breathing exercises unless the patient has had nasal, ophthalmic, or neurologic surgery.
• Administer postoperative medications, as ordered.
• Remove all fluids from the patient's bedside until he is alert enough to eat and drink. Before giving liquids, assess his gag reflex.

Special considerations
• If the patient received spinal anesthesia, keep him supine with the bed adjusted to between 0 degrees and 20 degrees for at least 6 hours to reduce the risk of spinal headache from CSF leakage.

• If the patient has had epidural anesthesia, monitor his respiratory status closely. Respiratory arrest may result from paralysis of the diaphragm caused by the anesthetic.

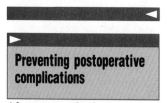

Preventing postoperative complications

After surgery, take these steps to avoid complications.

Turn and reposition the patient

Performed every 2 hours, turning and repositioning promotes circulation, thereby reducing the risk of skin breakdown – especially over bony prominences. When the patient is in a lateral recumbent position, tuck pillows under bony prominences to reduce friction and promote comfort. Each time you turn the patient, carefully inspect the skin to detect redness or other signs of breakdown.

Keep in mind that turning and repositioning may be contraindicated in some patients, such as those who have undergone neurologic or musculoskeletal surgery that demands immobilization postoperatively.

Encourage coughing and deep breathing

Deep breathing promotes lung expansion, which helps clear anesthetics from the body. Coughing and deep breathing also lower the risk of pulmonary and fat emboli and of hypostatic pneumonia associated with secretion buildup in the airways.

Encourage the patient to deep breathe at least every 2 hours and to cough. To reduce pain, show the patient how to splint his incision with his hands or a pillow. Also show him how to use an incentive spirometer. Because deep breathing does not increase intracranial pressure, it's safe to do after a variety of neurosurgical procedures.

Monitor nutrition and fluids

Adequate nutrition and fluid intake is essential to ensure proper hydration, promote healing, and provide energy to match the increased basal metabolism associated with surgery. If the patient has a protein deficiency or compromised immune function preoperatively, expect to deliver supplemental protein via parenteral nutrition to promote healing. If he has renal failure, this treatment would be contraindicated because his inability to break down protein could lead to dangerously high blood nitrogen levels.

Promote exercise and ambulation

Early postoperative exercise and ambulation can significantly reduce the risk of thromboembolism as well as improve ventilation and brighten the patient's outlook.

Perform passive range-of-motion exercises – or better yet, encourage active range-of-motion exercises – to prevent joint contractures and muscle atrophy and to promote circulation. These exercises can also help you assess the patient's strength and tolerance.

Before encouraging ambulation, have the patient dangle his legs over the side of the bed and perform deep-breathing exercises. How well the patient tolerates this step is often a key predictor of out-of-bed tolerance.

Begin ambulation by helping the patient walk a few feet from his bed to a sturdy chair. Then have him gradually progress each day from ambulating in his room to ambulating in the hallway, with or without assistance, as necessary.

Document frequency of ambulation and patient tolerance, including use of analgesics.

Managing postoperative complications

Despite your best efforts, complications sometimes occur. By knowing how to recognize and manage them, you can limit their effects.

Abdominal distention, paralytic ileus, and constipation
Sluggish peristalsis and paralytic ileus usually last 24 to 72 hours postoperatively and cause abdominal distention. Paralytic ileus occurs whenever autonomic innervation of the gastrointestinal tract becomes disrupted. Causes include intraoperative manipulation of intestinal organs; hypokalemia; wound infection; and use of codeine, morphine, and atropine. Postoperative constipation usually stems from colonic ileus caused by diminished GI motility and impaired perception of rectal fullness.

Assessment
• To detect abdominal distention, monitor abdominal girth and ask the patient if he feels bloated.
• To assess for paralytic ileus, auscultate for bowel sounds in all four quadrants.
• Monitor flatus or stool passage and abdominal distention.
• Ask about feelings of abdominal fullness or nausea.

Interventions
• To treat abdominal distention, encourage ambulation and give nothing by mouth until bowel sounds return.

• Insert a rectal tube or a nasogastric tube, as ordered. Keep the nasogastric tube patent and functioning properly.
• To treat paralytic ileus, encourage ambulation and administer medications such as dexpanthenol, as ordered. If the ileus does not resolve within 24 to 48 hours, insert a nasogastric tube, as ordered. Keep the nasogastric tube patent and functioning properly.
• To treat constipation, encourage ambulation and administer stool softeners, laxatives, and nonnarcotic analgesics, as ordered.

Atelectasis and pneumonia
After surgery, atelectasis may result from hypoventilation and excessive retained secretions. This provides a medium for bacterial growth and sets the stage for stasis pneumonia.

Assessment
• To detect atelectasis, auscultate for diminished or absent breath sounds over the affected area and note dullness on percussion.
• Assess for decreased chest expansion; mediastinal shift toward the side of collapse; fever; restlessness or confusion; worsening dyspnea; and elevated blood pressure, pulse rate, and respiratory rate.
• To detect pneumonia, watch for sudden onset of shaking chills with high fever and headache.
• Auscultate for diminished breath sounds or for telltale crackles over the affected lung area.
• Assess for dyspnea, tachypnea, sharp chest pain exacerbated by inspiration, productive cough with pinkish or rust-colored sputum, and cyanosis with hypoxemia that is confirmed by arterial blood gas measurement.
• Chest X-rays show patchy infiltrates or consolidation areas.

Interventions
• Encourage the patient to deep-breathe and cough every hour while he's awake. *Note:* Coughing is contraindicated in patients who have undergone neurosurgery and eye surgery.
• Demonstrate incentive spirometer use.
• As ordered, perform chest physiotherapy, give antibiotics, and administer humidified air or oxygen.
• Reposition the patient every 2 hours. Elevate the head of the bed.

Hypovolemia
A total blood volume loss of 15% to 25% may result from blood loss and severe dehydration, third-space fluid sequestration (as in burns, peritonitis, intestinal obstruction, or acute pancreatitis), and fluid loss (as in excessive vomiting or diarrhea).

Assessment
• Check for hypotension and a rapid, weak pulse.
• Note cool, clammy and, perhaps, mottled skin.
• Check for rapid, shallow respirations.
• Assess for oliguria or anuria, and lethargy.

Interventions
• To increase blood pressure, administer I.V. crystalloids, such as 0.9% sodium chloride or lactated Ringer's solutions.
• To restore urine output and fluid volume, give colloids, such as plasma, albumin, or dextran.

Pericarditis
This acute or chronic inflammation affects the pericardium, the fibroserous sac that envelops, supports, and protects the heart. After surgery, pericarditis may result from bacterial, fungal, or viral infection, or from postcardiac injury that leaves the pericardium intact but causes blood to leak into the pericardial cavity.

Assessment
• To detect pericarditis, assess for sharp, sudden pain, starting over the sternum and radiating to the neck, shoulders, back, and arms.
• Ask the patient to take a deep breath, then to sit up and lean forward. Pericardial pain is often pleuritic, increasing with deep inspiration and decreasing when the patient sits up and leans forward. You also may hear a pericardial friction rub.

Interventions
• Keep the patient on complete bed rest in an upright position.
• Provide analgesics and oxygen, as ordered.
• Assess pain in relation to respiration and body position to distinguish pericardial pain from myocardial ischemia pain.
• Monitor for signs of cardiac compression or cardiac tamponade. Signs include decreased blood pressure, increased central venous pressure, and pulsus paradoxus. Because cardiac tamponade requires immediate treatment, keep a pericardiocentesis set at bedside whenever pericardial effusion is suspected.

Postoperative psychosis
Mental aberrations may stem from physiologic causes (cerebral anoxia, fluid and electrolyte imbalance, malnutrition, and drugs such as tranquilizers, sedatives, and narcotics) or psychological causes (fear, pain, and disorientation).

Assessment
• Assess the patient's mental status and compare it with the preoperative baseline.

Interventions

• Reorient the patient frequently to person, place, and time. Call him by his preferred name and encourage him to move about.
• Provide clean eyeglasses and a working hearing aid, if appropriate. Use sedatives and restraints only if needed.

Septicemia and septic shock

Septicemia may stem from a break in asepsis during surgery or wound care, or from peritonitis (as in ruptured appendix or ectopic pregnancy). The most common cause of postoperative septicemia is *Escherichia coli*. Septic shock occurs when bacteria release endotoxins into the bloodstream, decreasing vascular resistance and resulting in dramatic hypotension.

Assessment

• To detect septicemia, check for fever, chills, rash, abdominal distention, prostration, pain, headache, nausea, or diarrhea.
• Early indicators of septic shock include fever and chills; warm, dry, flushed skin; slightly altered mental status; increased pulse and respiratory rates; decreased or normal blood pressure; and reduced urine output.
• Late indicators include pale, moist, cold skin and decreased mentation, pulse and respiratory rates, blood pressure, and urine output.

Interventions

• To treat septicemia, obtain specimens (blood, wound, and urine) for culture and sensitivity tests.
• Administer antibiotics, as ordered.
• Monitor vital signs and level of consciousness.
• To treat septic shock, administer I.V. antibiotics, as ordered.
• Monitor serum peak and trough levels.

• Give I.V. fluids and blood or blood products to restore circulating blood volume.

Thrombophlebitis and pulmonary embolism

Postoperative venous stasis associated with immobility may lead to thrombophlebitis—an inflammation of a vein, usually in the leg, accompanied by clot formation. If a clot breaks away, it may become lodged in the lung, causing a pulmonary embolism.

Assessment

• To detect thrombophlebitis, ask high-risk patients about leg pain, functional impairment, or edema.
• Inspect legs from feet to groin and record calf circumference. Note any engorgement of the cavity behind the medial malleolus and increased temperature in the affected leg. Identify areas of cordlike venous segments.
• To detect a pulmonary embolism, assess for sudden anginal or pleuritic chest pain; dyspnea; rapid, shallow respirations; cyanosis; restlessness; and possibly a thready pulse.
• Auscultate for fine-to-coarse crackles over the affected lung.

Interventions

• To treat thrombophlebitis, elevate the affected leg and apply warm compresses.
• As ordered, administer analgesics and I.V. heparin.
• Monitor prothrombin and partial thromboplastin times daily.
• To treat a pulmonary embolism, administer oxygen, analgesics, and I.V. heparin, as ordered. Elevate the head of the bed.

Urine retention

The patient may not be able to void spontaneously within 12 hours after surgery. Retention is usually transient and reversible.

Assessment
• Monitor intake and output for the absence of voided urine.
• Assess for bladder distention above the level of the symphysis pubis, discomfort, or pain. Also note restlessness, anxiety, diaphoresis, and hypertension.

Interventions
• To treat urinary retention, help the patient ambulate as soon as possible after surgery, unless contraindicated.
• Assist him to a normal voiding position and, if possible, leave him alone.
• Turn the water on so the patient can hear it, and pour warm water over his perineum.
• Stroke the inner aspect of the thigh.

Wound infection
The most common wound complication, wound infection is also a major factor in wound dehiscence. Complete dehiscence leads to evisceration.

Assessment
• To detect infection, assess surgical wounds for increased tenderness, deep pain, and edema, especially from the third to fifth days after the operation.
• Monitor for increased pulse rate and temperature, and an elevated white blood cell count.
• Note a temperature pattern of spikes in the afternoon or evening, returning to normal by morning.

Interventions
• As ordered, obtain a wound culture and sensitivity test, administer antibiotics, and irrigate the wound with an appropriate solution.
• Monitor wound drainage.

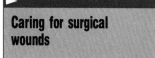

Caring for surgical wounds

Proper care of surgical wounds helps prevent infection, protects the skin from maceration and excoriation, allows removal and measurement of wound drainage, and promotes comfort.

Managing a draining wound involves two techniques: dressing and pouching. Dressing is indicated when drainage doesn't compromise skin integrity. Lightly seeping wounds with drains, as well as wounds with minimal purulent drainage, usually can be managed with packing and gauze dressings.

Wounds draining more than 100 ml in 24 hours or those with excoriating drainage require pouching.

Equipment and preparation
Waterproof trash bag • clean gloves • sterile gloves • gown, if indicated • sterile 4″ × 4″ gauze pads • abdominal bandage dressing (ABD) pads, if needed • sterile cotton-tipped applicators • topical medication, if ordered • adhesive or other tape • soap and water. Optional: skin protectant, nonadherent pads, acetone-free adhesive remover or baby oil, 0.9% sodium chloride solution, a graduated container, and Montgomery straps or a T-binder.

For a wound with a drain: sterile scissors • sterile 4″ × 4″ gauze pads without cotton lining • sump drain • ostomy pouch or other collection bag • precut drain dressings • adhesive tape.

For pouching: pouch with or without drainage port • skin protectant • sterile gauze pads.

Determine the type of dressing needed. Assemble all equipment in the patient's room. Check the expiration date on each sterile package, and inspect for tears. Place the trash bag where you can avoid reaching across the sterile field or the wound when disposing articles.

Implementation

• Check the doctor's order for wound care instructions. Note location of drains to avoid dislodging them during the procedure.
• Explain the procedure to the patient and position him properly. Expose only the wound site.
• Wash your hands. Put on a gown, if necessary, and clean gloves.

Removing the old dressing

• Hold the skin and pull the tape or dressing toward the wound. This protects newly formed tissue. Use adhesive remover or baby oil, if needed. Don't apply solvents to the incision.
• Remove the soiled dressing. If needed, loosen gauze with sterile 0.9% sodium chloride solution.
• Check the dressing for the amount, type, color, and odor of drainage. Discard the dressing and gloves in the waterproof trash bag.
• If ordered, obtain a wound culture.

Caring for the wound

• Establish a sterile field for equipment and supplies. Squeeze the needed amount of ordered ointment onto the sterile field. Pour antiseptic from a nonsterile bottle into a sterile container. Put on sterile gloves.
• If you aren't using prepackaged swabs, saturate sterile gauze pads with the prescribed cleaning agent. Avoid using cotton balls because these may shed particles in the wound.
• Squeeze excess solution from the pad or swab. Wipe once from the top to the bottom of the incision; discard. With a second pad, wipe

from top to bottom in a vertical path next to the incision; discard.
• Continue to work outward from the incision in lines running parallel to it. Always wipe from the clean area toward the less clean area. Use each pad or swab for only one stroke. Use sterile cotton-tipped applicators to clean tight-fitting wire sutures, deep wounds, or wounds with pockets.
• If the patient has a surgical drain, clean the drain's surface last. Clean the surrounding skin by wiping in half or full circles from the drain site outward.
• Clean to at least 1″ (2.5 cm) beyond the new dressing or 2″ (5 cm) beyond the incision.
• Check for signs of infection, dehiscence, or evisceration. If you observe such signs or the patient reports pain, notify the doctor.
• Wash the surrounding skin with soap and water and pat dry. Apply prescribed topical medication and a skin protectant, if warranted.
• If ordered, pack the wound with gauze pads or folded strips, using the wet-to-damp method. Avoid using cotton-lined gauze pads.

Applying a fresh gauze dressing

• Place sterile 4″ × 4″ gauze pads at the wound center and move pads outward to the edges of the wound site. Extend the gauze at least 1″ (2.5 cm) beyond the incision in each direction. Use enough sterile dressings to absorb all drainage until the next dressing change.
• When the dressing is in place, remove and discard gloves. Secure the dressing with strips of tape, a T-binder, or Montgomery straps.
• For the recently postoperative patient or a patient with complications, check the dressing every 30 minutes or as ordered. If the wound is healing properly, check it at least every 8 hours.

Dressing a wound with a drain
• Using sterile scissors, cut a slit in a sterile 4″ × 4″ gauze pad. Fold the pad in half, and cut inward from the center of the folded edge. Don't use a cotton-lined gauze pad. Prepare a second pad the same way.
• Press one folded pad close to the skin around the drain so that the tubing fits into the slit. Press the second folded pad around the drain from the opposite direction to encircle the tubing.
• Layer as many uncut sterile pads around the tubing as needed to absorb drainage. Secure the dressing with tape, a T-binder, or Montgomery straps.

Pouching a wound
• To create a pouch, first measure the wound, and cut an opening in the collection pouch's facing ⅛″ (0.3 cm) larger than the wound.
• Apply a skin protectant as needed.
• Make sure the drainage port at the bottom of the pouch is closed. Then press the contoured pouch opening around the wound, beginning at its lower edge.
• To empty the pouch, put on gloves, insert bottom half of the pouch into a graduated collection container, and open the drainage port. Note the color, consistency, odor, and amount of fluid.
• Wipe the bottom of the pouch and the drainage port with a gauze pad; reseal the port. Change the pouch if it leaks or comes loose.

Special considerations
• Because many doctors prefer to change the first postoperative dressing, avoid changing it unless ordered. If you have no such order and drainage comes through the dressing, reinforce the dressing with fresh sterile gauze. To prevent bacterial growth, don't allow a rein-

forced dressing to remain in place longer than 24 hours. Replace any dressing that becomes wet from the outside as soon as possible.
• Consider all dressings and drains infectious.
• If the patient has two wounds in the same area, cover each separately with layers of sterile 4″ × 4″ gauze pads. Then cover both sites with an ABD pad secured to the skin with tape.

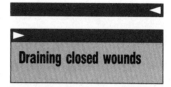

Draining closed wounds

Inserted during surgery, a closed-wound drain promotes healing and prevents swelling by suctioning serosanguineous fluid at the wound site. By removing this fluid, the drain helps reduce the risk of infection and skin breakdown as well as the number of dressing changes.

A closed-wound drain consists of perforated tubing connected to a portable vacuum unit. The distal end of the tubing lies within the wound and usually leaves the body from a site other than the primary suture line to preserve the integrity of the surgical wound. The tubing exit site is treated as an additional surgical wound; the drain is usually sutured to the skin. The drain may be left in place for longer than 1 week to accommodate heavy drainage.

Equipment
Graduated cylinder • sterile laboratory container, if needed • alcohol sponges • sterile gloves • clean gloves • sterile gauze pads • antiseptic cleaning agent • prepackaged povidone-iodine swabs • waterproof trash bag.

Implementation

• Check the doctor's order and assess the patient's condition. Explain the procedure to the patient. Provide privacy. Wash your hands and put on gloves.
• Unclip the vacuum unit. Using aseptic technique, remove the spout plug to release the vacuum.
• Empty the unit's contents into a graduated cylinder. Note the amount and appearance of the drainage. If ordered, empty the drainage into a sterile laboratory container and send it to the laboratory for diagnostic testing.
• Maintaining aseptic technique, clean the unit's spout and plug with an alcohol sponge.
• To reestablish the vacuum that creates the drain's suction power, fully compress the vacuum unit. Keep the unit compressed as you replace the spout plug.
• Check the patency of the equipment. Make sure the tubing is free of twists, kinks, and leaks because the drainage system must be airtight to work properly. Keep the vacuum unit compressed when you release manual pressure; rapid reinflation indicates an air leak. If this occurs, recompress the unit and secure the spout plug.
• Secure the vacuum unit to the patient's bedding or, if he is ambulatory, to his gown. Fasten it below wound level to promote drainage. To prevent possible dislodgment, do not apply tension on drainage tubing. Remove and discard gloves, and wash hands thoroughly.
• Put on sterile gloves. Check sutures for signs of pulling or tearing, and for swelling or infection of surrounding skin. Gently clean with sterile gauze pads soaked in an antiseptic cleaning agent or with a povidone-iodine swab.

• Properly dispose of drainage, solutions, and trash bag, and clean or dispose soiled equipment and supplies.

Special considerations

• Empty the system and measure its contents once during each shift if drainage has accumulated; do so more often if drainage is excessive.
• If the patient has more than one closed drain, number the drains so you can record drainage from each site.

Note: Be careful not to mistake chest tubes for closed-wound drains because the vacuum of a chest tube should never be released.

Managing dehiscence and evisceration

Occasionally the edges of a wound may fail to join, or may separate after they seem to be healing normally. Called wound dehiscence, this abnormality may lead to a more serious complication: evisceration, where a portion of the viscera protrudes through the incision. In turn, this can lead to peritonitis and septic shock.

Equipment

Two sterile towels • 1 liter of sterile 0.9% sodium chloride solution • sterile irrigation set, including a basin, a solution container, and a 50-ml catheter-tip syringe • several large abdominal dressings • sterile, waterproof drape • linen-saver pads • sterile gloves • waterproof trash bag.

If the patient will return to the operating room, gather: I.V. administration set and I.V. fluids • nasogastric intubation equipment • sedative, as ordered • suction apparatus.

Implementation

• Tell the patient to stay in bed. If possible, stay with him while someone else notifies the doctor and collects the equipment.

• Place a linen-saver pad under the patient and create a sterile field. Place the basin, solution container, and 50-ml syringe on the sterile field.

• Open the bottle of 0.9% sodium chloride solution and pour 400 ml into the solution container and 200 ml into the sterile basin.

• Place several abdominal dressings on the sterile field. Wearing sterile gloves, place one or two dressings into the basin.

• Place the moistened dressings over the exposed viscera. Cover with a sterile, waterproof drape.

• Keep the dressings moist by gently moistening with saline solution frequently. If the viscera appears dusky or black, notify the doctor immediately. Interrupted blood supply may cause a protruding organ to become ischemic and necrotic.

• Keep the patient on strict bed rest in low Fowler's position (no more than 20 degrees' elevation) with his knees flexed.

• Monitor vital signs every 15 minutes to detect shock. Prepare to return to the operating room.

• Prepare for nasogastric tube insertion, as ordered. Nasogastric intubation may make the patient gag, causing further evisceration. For this reason, the tube may be inserted in the operating room.

• Administer preoperative medications, as ordered.

Special considerations

• To help prevent dehiscence and evisceration, inspect the incision with each dressing change. By day 5 to 9 postoperatively, feel for a healing ridge which forms directly under the suture line. A lack of a healing ridge may indicate that the patient is at risk for dehiscence and evisceration. Treat early signs of infection immediately. Make sure bandages aren't so tight that they limit blood supply to the wound.

• If the patient has weak abdominal walls, apply an abdominal binder. Encourage the high-risk patient to splint his abdomen with a pillow during straining, coughing, or sneezing.

• If a postoperative patient detects a sudden gush of pinkish serous drainage on his wound dressing, inspect the incision for dehiscence. If the wound seems to be separating slowly and evisceration hasn't developed, place the patient in a supine position and call the doctor.

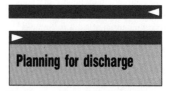

Planning for discharge

Begin planning for discharge during your first contact with the patient. The initial nursing history and preoperative assessment, as well as subsequent assessments, can provide useful information.

Recognizing potential problems early will help your discharge plan succeed. Assess the strengths and limitations of the patient and family. Consider physiologic factors (such as general physical and functional abilities, current medications, and general nutritional status), psychological factors (such as self-concept, motivation, and learning abilities), and social factors (such as duration of care needed, types of services available, and the family's involvement in the patient's care).

Medications

Explain the purpose of drug therapy, the proper dosages and routes, any special instructions, how long the regimen will last, any potential adverse effects, and when to notify the doctor. Try to establish a medication schedule that fits the patient's life-style.

Diet

Discuss dietary restrictions with both the patient and, if appropriate, the person who will prepare his meals. Assess the patient's usual dietary intake. If appropriate, discuss the cost of the diet and how restrictions may affect other family members. Recommend a good diet book. Refer the patient to a dietitian, if appropriate.

Activity

After surgery, patients are often advised not to lift heavy objects. Restrictions usually last 4 to 6 weeks after surgery. Discuss how limitations will affect the patient's daily routine. Let him know when he can return to work, drive, and resume sexual activity. If the patient seems unlikely to comply, discuss compromises.

Home care procedures

Use nontechnical language and include caretakers when teaching about home care. After the patient watches you demonstrate a procedure, have him repeat the procedure.

Explain to the patient that he may not have to use the same equipment he used in the hospital; discuss what's available to him at home. If the patient needs to rent or purchase equipment, such as a hospital bed or walker, give him a list of suppliers.

Wound care

Teach the patient about changing his wound dressing. Tell him to keep the incision clean and dry, and teach proper hand-washing technique. Specify whether (and when) he should shower or bathe.

Potential complications

Teach the patient to recognize wound infection and other potential complications. Provide written instructions about reportable signs and symptoms, such as incisional bleeding or discharge, or acute pain. Advise the patient to call the doctor with any questions.

Return appointments

Stress the importance of scheduling and keeping checkup appointments, and make sure the patient has the doctor's office telephone number. If the patient has no transportation, refer him to an appropriate community resource.

Referrals

Reassess whether the patient needs referral to a home care agency or other community resource. Discuss with the family how they will handle the patient's return home. In some hospitals, the responsibility for making referrals falls to a home care coordinator or discharge planning nurse.

CHAPTER 7

Bedside care:
Performing common procedures safely and correctly

Common procedures

Common procedures

Arterial pressure monitoring

An invasive technique, arterial pressure monitoring provides continuous and accurate arterial pressure readings through a transducer that converts blood pressure into electrical impulses. These impulses are displayed on a monitor screen and recorded on paper tape. A visible and audible alarm sounds when the pressure exceeds preset limits.

Equipment and preparation
• Preassembled arterial pressure monitoring setup, as shown below
• monitoring equipment • gloves
• hypoallergenic tape • antimicrobial ointment • dry, sterile dressing.

If you'll need to obtain a blood sample from an arterial line, also

assemble: • 5-ml syringe • 5- to 10-ml syringe • two sterile 4″ × 4″ gauze pads. Optional: blood collection tubes.

Implementation
Describe the procedure to the patient.

To calibrate an arterial line
• Level transducer at fifth intercostal space in midanterior-posterior line. Zero equipment according to manufacturer's directions.
• Obtain pressure readings. Set alarms between 10 and 20 mm Hg above and below the reading.

To change tubing
• Prepare a new arterial pressure monitoring setup, including flush solution. Activate the flush device to clear all air from the line. Wash your hands, and put on gloves.
• Turn the alarms off. Clamp the tubing before disconnecting it. Disconnect the old segment of tubing,

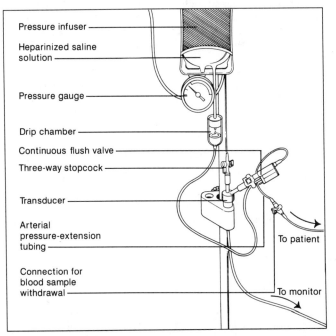

Pressure infuser

Heparinized saline solution

Pressure gauge

Drip chamber

Continuous flush valve

Three-way stopcock

Transducer

Arterial pressure-extension tubing

Connection for blood sample withdrawal

To patient

To monitor

BEDSIDE CARE

and immediately replace it with new tubing.

• Activate the flush device to clear blood from the line and catheter.

• Apply a sterile dressing if the tubing to the catheter was changed.

• Level the transducer, zero the equipment, and set the alarms.

To obtain a blood sample from an arterial line

• Wash your hands, put on gloves, and turn off the alarms.

• Open a package of sterile 4″ × 4″ gauze pads. Remove the dead-end cap from the stopcock closest to the patient and place it on a sterile 4″ × 4″ gauze pad.

• Insert the 5-ml syringe into the stopcock. Turn off the stopcock to the flush solution. Slowly withdraw 3 to 5 ml of blood from the line.

• Turn the stopcock halfway back to the open position, and remove and discard the syringe. Replace it with the 5- to 10-ml specimen syringe.

• Turn off the stopcock to the flush solution. Using the new syringe, slowly withdraw the required amount of blood. Turn the stopcock to the original position. Remove the syringe.

• Activate the flush device. Turn off the stopcock to the patient, and flush the stopcock port. Return the stopcock to the original position. Turn on the alarms. Transfer the blood to the appropriate tubes, and send the specimens to the laboratory.

Special considerations

• Always use sterile technique, and maintain electrical safety when working with arterial lines.

• Many factors can alter pressure readings and waveforms, including air in the tubing, in the transducer, or in both; an inappropriate transducer level; loose connections; cracks or leaks in the system; a clot in the catheter; and the catheter tip resting against the vessel wall.

• Level and zero the system at the beginning of each shift and after any manipulation of the patient or system.

• Check the patient's cuff blood pressure for comparison every 4 to 8 hours, depending on hospital policy. Change the dressing and tubing every 24 to 72 hours.

• Monitor the patient frequently. Considerable blood can be lost quickly if the system becomes disconnected. Keep alarms on at all times, except when replacing tubing, as noted.

Arterial puncture for blood gas analysis

Obtaining an arterial blood sample requires percutaneous puncture of the brachial, radial, or femoral artery or withdrawal of a sample from an arterial line. Once drawn, the sample can be analyzed for arterial blood gases (ABG) to evaluate ventilation.

Equipment and preparation

Many hospitals use a commercial ABG kit that contains all the equipment listed below (except the adhesive bandage and ice). If your hospital does not, collect these items.

• 10-ml glass syringe or plastic luer-lock syringe specially made for drawing blood gases • 1-ml ampule of aqueous heparin (1:1,000) • 20G 1¼″ needle • 22G 1″ needle • alcohol sponge • povidone-iodine sponge • two 2″ × 2″ gauze pads • gloves • rubber cap for syringe hub or rubber stopper for needle • ice-filled plastic bag or emesis basin label • laboratory request form • adhesive bandage.

Prepare collection equipment before entering the patient's room. Wash your hands; open the ABG kit, and remove the specimen label and plastic bag. Record pertinent information on the label, and fill the plastic bag with ice.

To heparinize the syringe, attach the 20G needle to the syringe. Open the ampule of heparin. Draw all the heparin into the syringe. Hold the syringe upright, and pull the plunger back to the 7-ml mark. Slowly force the heparin toward the hub of the syringe and expel all but about 0.1 ml.

To heparinize the needle, replace the 20G needle with the 22G needle. Hold the syringe upright, tilt it slightly, and eject the remaining heparin.

Before attempting a radial puncture, perform Allen's test to assess the adequacy of the blood supply to the patient's hand. To do this test, rest the patient's arm on the mattress or bedside stand, and support his wrist with a rolled towel. Have him clench his fist. Then, using your index and middle fingers, press on the radial and ulnar arteries. Hold this position for a few seconds.

Without removing your fingers from the patient's arteries, have him unclench his fist and relax his hand. The palm will be blanched because your fingers have impaired normal blood flow.

Release pressure on the ulnar artery. If the hand becomes flushed, which indicates blood filling the vessels, you can safely proceed with the radial artery puncture. If the hand doesn't flush, perform the test on the other arm.

Implementation

• Explain the procedure to the patient, wash your hands, and put on gloves.

• Place a rolled towel under the patient's wrist. Locate the artery and palpate it for a strong pulse.

• Using a povidone-iodine or alcohol sponge, use a circular motion to clean the puncture site, starting in the center of the site and spiraling outward. If you use alcohol, apply it with friction for 30 seconds or until the final sponge comes away clean. If using a povidone-iodine sponge, allow the skin to dry.

• Palpate the artery with the index and middle fingers of one hand while holding the syringe over the puncture site with the other hand.

• Hold the needle bevel up at a 30- to 45-degree angle. When puncturing the brachial artery, hold the needle at a 60-degree angle.

• Puncture the skin and arterial wall in one motion, following the path of the artery. Watch for blood backflow, but don't pull on the plunger because arterial blood should enter the syringe automatically. Fill the syringe to the 5-ml mark.

• After collecting the sample, press a gauze pad firmly over the puncture site until bleeding stops – for at least 5 minutes. Apply a small adhesive bandage to the site.

• Check the syringe for air bubbles. Remove any bubbles by holding the syringe upright and slowly ejecting some of the blood onto a 2″ × 2″ gauze pad.

• Insert the needle into a rubber stopper, or remove the needle and place a rubber cap directly on the needle hub. Put the labeled sample in the ice-filled plastic bag or emesis basin, and send the sample to the laboratory immediately.

• Monitor the patient's vital signs, and observe for signs of circulatory impairment or bleeding.

Special considerations

• If the patient is receiving oxygen, make sure that his therapy has been

BEDSIDE CARE

under way for at least 15 minutes before drawing arterial blood.
• If the patient has just received a breathing treatment, nebulizer treatment, or suctioning, wait about 20 minutes before drawing the blood sample.

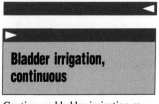

Bladder irrigation, continuous

Continuous bladder irrigation requires placement of a triple-lumen catheter. One lumen controls balloon inflation, one allows irrigant inflow, and one allows irrigant outflow, as shown below. The continuous flow of irrigating solution through the bladder also creates a mild tamponade that may help prevent venous hemorrhage.

Equipment and preparation
• One 4-liter container or two 2-liter containers of irrigating solution (usually 0.9% sodium chloride solution) or the prescribed amount of medicated solution • Y-type tubing made specifically for bladder irrigation • alcohol or povidone-iodine sponge.

Before starting continuous bladder irrigation, double-check the irrigating solution against the doctor's order. If the solution contains an antibiotic, check the patient's chart to make sure he's not allergic to the drug.

Implementation
• Wash your hands. Assemble all equipment at the patient's bedside.

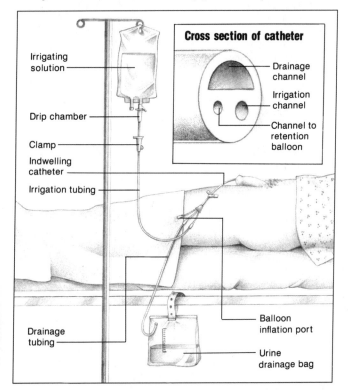

Irrigating solution

Drip chamber

Clamp

Indwelling catheter

Irrigation tubing

Drainage tubing

Cross section of catheter

Drainage channel

Irrigation channel

Channel to retention balloon

Balloon inflation port

Urine drainage bag

• Explain the procedure, and provide privacy.

• Insert the spike of the Y-type tubing into the container of irrigating solution. (If you have a two-container system, insert one spike into each container.)

• Squeeze the drip chamber on the spike of the tubing.

• Open the flow clamp, and flush the tubing to remove air, which could cause bladder distention. Then close the clamp.

• Hang the irrigating solution on the I.V. pole.

• Clean the opening to the inflow lumen of the catheter with alcohol or a povidone-iodine sponge. Insert the distal end of the Y-type tubing securely into the inflow lumen (third port) of the catheter.

• Make sure the catheter's outflow lumen is securely attached to the drainage bag tubing.

• Open the flow clamp under the container of irrigating solution, and set the drip rate as ordered.

• To prevent air from entering the system, don't allow the primary container to empty completely before replacing it.

• If you have a two-container system, simultaneously close the flow clamp under the nearly empty container and open the flow clamp under the reserve container. This prevents reflux of irrigating solution from the reserve container into the nearly empty one.

• Hang a new reserve container on the I.V. pole, and insert the tubing, maintaining asepsis.

• Empty the drainage bag about every 4 hours or as often as needed. Use sterile technique.

Special considerations

• Check the inflow and outflow lines periodically for kinks to make sure the solution is running freely.

• Measure the outflow volume accurately. It should equal or, allowing for urine production, slightly exceed inflow volume. If inflow volume exceeds outflow volume postoperatively, notify the doctor immediately.

• Also assess outflow for changes in appearance and for blood clots, especially if irrigation is being performed postoperatively to control bleeding. If drainage is bright red, irrigating solution should usually be infused rapidly until drainage clears. Notify the doctor immediately if you suspect hemorrhage. If drainage is clear, the solution is usually given at a rate of 40 to 60 drops/minute. The doctor typically specifies the rate for antibiotic solutions.

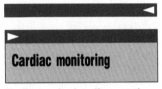

Cardiac monitoring

Cardiac monitoring allows continuous observation of the heart's electrical activity. Cardiac monitors can display the patient's rhythm and heart rate, produce a printed record of cardiac rhythm, and sound an alarm if the patient's heart rate rises above or falls below specified limits. Some can also recognize abnormal heartbeats and trigger an alarm if the heartbeats exceed a set limit.

Equipment and preparation

• Cardiac monitor • leadwires • patient cable • disposable pregelled electrodes • alcohol sponges • 4″ × 4″ gauze pads. Optional: shaving supplies, washcloth.

Plug the monitor into an electrical outlet and turn it on to warm up the unit. Insert the cable into the appropriate socket in the monitor.

Connect the leadwires to the cable. You may be using a 3-, 4-, or 5-

leadwire system. Each leadwire should be labeled: right arm (RA), left arm (LA), right leg (RL), left leg (LL), and (in a 5-leadwire system) a chest lead (C or V). Connect an electrode to each of the leadwires.

Implementation

• Explain the procedure to the patient, provide privacy, and ask him to expose his chest. Wash your hands.

• Determine electrode positions on the patient's chest, based on the system and lead you're using. With single-lead monitoring, you place the lead electrodes on the chest.

• If the leadwires and patient cable aren't permanently attached, verify that the electrode placement corresponds to the label on the cable.

• If necessary, clip or shave an area about 4″ (10 cm) in diameter around each electrode site. Clean the area with an alcohol sponge and dry it to remove skin secretions that may interfere with electrode function.

• Gently abrade the dried area by rubbing it briskly until it reddens to remove dead skin cells and to promote better electrical contact. (Some electrodes have a small, rough patch for abrading the skin; otherwise, use a dry washcloth or a gauze pad.)

• Remove the backing from the pregelled electrode, making sure that the gel is moist.

• Apply the electrode to the site, and press firmly to ensure a tight seal. Repeat with the remaining electrodes.

• When the electrodes are in place, check for a tracing on the cardiac monitor. Assess the quality of the electrocardiogram. To verify that each beat is being detected, compare the digital heart rate display with your count of the patient's heart rate.

• If necessary, use the gain control to adjust the size of the rhythm tracing and the position control to adjust the waveform position on the recording paper.

• Set the upper and lower limits of the heart rate alarm, based on unit policy. Turn the alarm on.

Special considerations

• Make sure all electrical equipment and outlets are grounded to avoid electric shock and interference. Also ensure that the patient is dry to prevent electric shock.

• Avoid opening the electrode packages until just before using to prevent the gel from drying out.

• Avoid placing the electrodes on bony prominences, hairy areas, areas where defibrillator pads will be placed, or areas for chest compression.

• If the patient's skin is exceptionally oily, scaly, or diaphoretic, rub the electrode site with a dry 4″ × 4″ gauze pad before applying the electrode to help reduce interference in the tracing.

• Assess skin integrity, and reposition the electrodes either every 24 hours or as necessary.

Cardiac output measurement

Measuring cardiac output—the amount of blood ejected from the heart—helps evaluate cardiac function. Measurement is done indirectly by the thermodilution method. This involves inserting a balloon-tipped, flow-directed catheter into a large vein, advancing it to the right side of the heart, and positioning it in the pulmonary artery. A solution is injected into the proximal or right atrium port of the pulmonary artery catheter. A computer calculates the cardiac output from temperature changes in the injected solution in the proximal lumen and from the temperature of the pulmonary artery.

Equipment

• Cardiac output computer setup, as shown below • 500-ml bag of dextrose 5% in water (D_5W) • closed injection system • 10-ml syringe • stopcocks.

Implementation

• Wash your hands. Explain the procedure to the patient. Assure him that he won't feel any discomfort.
• Place the patient in the supine position (his head may be slightly elevated).
• Attach the thermistor tubing from the cardiac output machine to the thermistor port on the pulmonary artery catheter in order to accurately measure the patient's core temperature.
• Attach the temperature probe from the cardiac output machine to the appropriate area on the proximal port to measure the temperature of the injectant.
• Before injecting the ordered solution, ensure that the catheter is not in the wedge position because this can trigger a false-high reading and damage the pulmonary artery.
• Remove the stopcock cap, and connect the syringe to the stopcock on the proximal lumen so that the syringe and the catheter lumen are in a straight line. Open the stopcock to instill the injectant as described below. Using aseptic technique, replace the syringe after each injection.
• If using a closed system, spike the 500-ml bag of D_5W, and prime the system. Connect the luer-lock end of the system to the proximal lumen of the pulmonary artery catheter so that the syringe and the catheter lumen are in a straight line. The closed system should remain in place at all times to reduce the risk of contamination. One or more stopcocks may be used between the catheter and the closed system.
• Turn on the computer and calibrate it, if necessary.

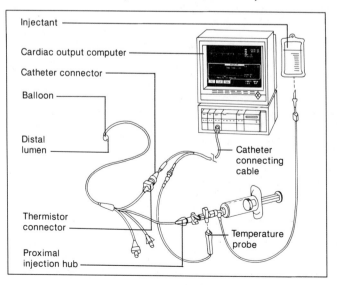

Injectant

Cardiac output computer

Catheter connector

Balloon

Distal lumen

Catheter connecting cable

Thermistor connector

Temperature probe

Proximal injection hub

• Open the clamp on the closed system, and fill the syringe from the bag of D_5W.
• Open the stopcock to the patient and verify that READY appears on the computer. Depress the start button. Inject the solution with one smooth, rapid motion (within 4 seconds). Inject 5 to 10 ml for an adult and 3 ml for a child. Cardiac output values will be displayed on the computer screen. Repeat the procedure two more times, waiting 1 minute between each injection.
• Calculate the average of the three measurements to determine cardiac output.
• Return all stopcocks to the original positions. With the system closed, verify that the clamp on the injection system is also closed.

Special considerations

• If ordered, calculate the cardiac index—cardiac output divided by body surface area. The normal range is 2.5 to 4.2 liters/minute.
• Although many hospitals ice the injectant before injection, this is usually not necessary if there is a 10° F (-12.2° C) difference between the patient's temperature and that of the room air or injectant.

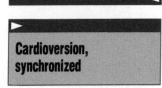

Cardioversion, synchronized

Like defibrillation, synchronized cardioversion delivers an electric current to the heart to correct an arrhythmia. With cardioversion, however, much lower energy levels are used, and the burst of electricity is timed to coincide with the peak of the R wave.

Equipment

• Defibrillator • conductive gel pads
• sedative crash cart containing emergency resuscitation equipment
• oxygen • pulse oximeter.

Implementation

• If the situation is not an emergency, explain the procedure to the patient.
• Connect monitoring leads from the defibrillator unit in the crash cart to the patient. Remove telemetry and bedside monitors to prevent damage to those units. Assess the patient's cardiac rhythm.
• Turn the defibrillator on, and make sure it's set for the synchronous mode so that the electric current can be delivered with the peak of the R wave. Administer sedatives as ordered. If necessary, administer oxygen and monitor arterial oxygen saturation with a pulse oximeter.
• Expose the patient's chest and apply the conductive pads, or apply conductive gel to one paddle and rub the two paddles together to distribute the gel. Make sure that no excess gel drips off the paddles; excess gel can cause arcing of current.
• Place one pad to the right of the sternum, just below the clavicle; the other, at the fifth or sixth intercostal space in the left anterior axillary line.
• Set the machine to the appropriate energy level, usually between 25 and 100 joules. This will vary, depending on the cardiac rhythm.
• If not already done, activate the synchronized mode by depressing the synch button. When synchronized, an indicator should recognize each QRS complex.
• Press the charge button on the machine or on the paddles. A blinking light or constant hissing noise signals that the paddles are charging. When fully charged, the light will remain on, the hissing

will cease, and the machine may show a digital display of the energy level.
• Reassess the patient's rhythm and pulse to determine the need for cardioversion.
• Press the paddles firmly on the chest over the conductive pads.
• Instruct personnel to stand clear of the patient and bed to avoid electric shock.
• Discharge the current by pushing both paddle discharge buttons simultaneously. There will be a slight delay while the defibrillator synchronizes with the R wave.
• If cardioversion is unsuccessful, repeat the procedure two or three more times as ordered, gradually increasing the energy level with each additional countershock. Make sure the synchronization indicator remains on.
• If normal rhythm is restored, continue to monitor the patient, and supplement ventilation, as needed.

Note: If cardioversion results in ventricular fibrillation or ventricular tachycardia with no pulse, turn the synchronization switch off and defibrillate the patient. Have emergency medications available.
• If the paddles have been recharged but are not used again, clear the charge by turning the machine off, adjusting the energy selector dial, or placing the paddles in their protective housing and discharging them into the machine.

Special considerations
Defibrillators vary, so familiarize yourself with your hospital's equipment.

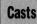

Casts

A cast is a hard mold that encases a body part to provide immobilization without discomfort. Casts may be constructed of plaster, fiberglass, or synthetic materials.

Equipment and preparation
• Tubular stockinette • casting material • plaster rolls • plaster splints (if necessary) • bucket of water • sink equipped with plaster trap • linen-saver pad • sheet wadding • sponge or felt padding (if necessary). Optional: rubber gloves, cast stand.

Gently squeeze the packaged casting material to make sure the envelopes don't have any air leaks. Follow the manufacturer's directions for water temperature when preparing plaster.

Implementation
• Explain the procedure to the patient. If using plaster, warn him that heat will build under the cast because of a chemical reaction between the water and plaster.
• Cover the appropriate parts of the patient's bedding and gown with a linen-saver pad. If the cast is applied to the wrist or arm, remove rings that may interfere with circulation.
• Assess the skin in the affected area, noting any redness, contusions, or open wounds. Assess neurovascular status to serve as a baseline.
• Support the limb in the prescribed position while the doctor applies the tubular stockinette and sheet wadding. He then wraps the limb in sheet wadding, starting at the distal end. As he applies the sheet wadding, check for wrinkles.

BEDSIDE CARE

To prepare plaster casting

• Immerse a roll of plaster casting on its end in the bucket of water. When air bubbles stop rising from the roll, remove it, gently squeeze out excess water, and hand it to the doctor. As he applies the first roll, prepare a second roll.

• After applying each roll, the doctor will smooth it to remove wrinkles, spread plaster into the cloth webbing, and empty air pockets. If using plaster splints, he'll apply them in the middle layers. Before wrapping the last roll, he'll pull the ends of the tubular stockinette over the cast edges and use the final roll to keep the ends of the stockinette in place.

To prepare cotton and polyester casting

• Open materials one roll at a time because cotton and polyester casting must be applied within 3 minutes.

• Immerse the roll in cold water, and squeeze it four times to ensure uniform wetness. Then remove it for immediate application.

To prepare fiberglass casting

If using water-activated fiberglass, immerse the tape rolls in tepid water for 10 to 15 minutes. Open one roll at a time. Avoid squeezing out excess water before application. If using light-cured fiberglass, you can unroll the material more slowly because it remains soft until it's exposed to ultraviolet light.

To complete casting

• As necessary, petal the cast's edges to reduce roughness. Use a cast stand or the palm of your hand to support the cast until it becomes firm. Evaluate circulation and neurologic status in the affected and unaffected extremities.

• Elevate the limb above heart level to facilitate venous return and reduce edema.

• Pour water from the plaster bucket only into a sink with a plaster trap.

Special considerations

A fiberglass cast dries immediately after application. A plaster extremity cast dries in 24 to 48 hours; a plaster spica or body cast, in 48 to 72 hours. During drying, the cast must be positioned to prevent a surface depression that could cause pressure areas or dependent edema. Neurovascular status must be assessed, drainage monitored, and the condition of the cast checked periodically.

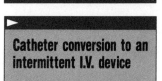

Catheter conversion to an intermittent I.V. device

The patient who doesn't require continuous I.V. infusion may require I.V. solutions and medications administered intermittently. To accommodate this, the doctor may order an existing I.V. line converted to a heparin lock. A male adapter plug allows for easy conversion. This venipuncture device may be referred to as a heparin lock, a p.r.n. adapter, an intermittent, or an INT.

Equipment

• Male adapter plugs, long or short, with a luer or slip design, as shown at the top of the next page • dilute heparin or 0.9% sodium chloride solution • I.V. line with clamp • 20G 1″ needle; alternately, a recessed needle or needleless system • alcohol pad.

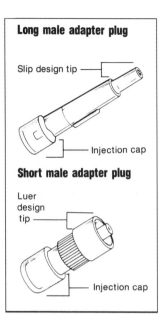

Long male adapter plug

Slip design tip

Injection cap

Short male adapter plug

Luer design tip

Injection cap

Implementation

• Explain the procedure to the patient.
• Wash your hands. Wear gloves when in direct patient contact.
• Prime the male adapter plug with dilute heparin. Then clamp the I.V. tubing, remove the I.V. administration set from the catheter or needle hub, and insert the male adapter plug as shown.
• Next, inject the remaining dilute heparin to fill the line and prevent clot formation.
• Refer to your hospital's policy on maintaining heparin-lock patency because these procedures vary among hospitals.

To administer medication

• To administer the prescribed medication or solution, attach a 20G 1″ needle, a recessed needle, or a needleless system to the end of the I.V. tubing (any regular I.V. tubing can be used).
• Carefully clean the injection cap system with an alcohol pad. Then

insert the needle into the injection cap.
• Be sure to secure the needle or needleless system with tape to prevent dislodgement of the heparin lock.
• Now adjust the flow rate to administer the medication over the specified infusion time. Remember to carefully inspect the venipuncture site for evidence of infiltration.
• When the infusion is completed, remove the needle or needleless system from the heparin lock. Remove the needle or needleless system from the I.V. tubing and discard it appropriately.
• Attach a new sterile needle with cap or a new needleless system to the end of the I.V. tubing.
• Flush the injection cap according to your hospital's policy. You may use 0.9% sodium chloride solution, dilute heparin, or both to flush the system. The flushing procedure will keep the I.V. catheter patent and will prepare the heparin lock for reuse.

Central venous line maintenance

After insertion, a central venous (CV) line must be carefully maintained. This includes regularly flushing the catheter to maintain patency and periodically changing the injection cap.

Equipment

For flushing a catheter

• 0.9% sodium chloride solution or heparinized saline flush solution
• alcohol sponge • gauze pad.

For changing an injection cap
• Alcohol sponge or povidone-iodine sponge • injection cap • padded clamp.

Implementation
To flush the catheter
• Flush the catheter routinely according to your hospital's policy. (This varies from once every 12 hours to once weekly. Most clinicians agree that flushing should be done twice daily for 3 to 4 days after insertion and from once daily to three times a week thereafter.)
• Typically, a CV catheter with a two-way valve (Groshong catheter) must be flushed with 0.9% sodium chloride solution weekly. All lumens of a multilumen catheter (except the Groshong) must be flushed regularly. (No flushing is needed with a continuous infusion through a single-lumen catheter.) Many hospitals use a heparinized saline flush solution available in premixed 10-ml multidose vials, but others use 3 to 5 ml.
• To flush the catheter, start by cleaning the cap with an alcohol sponge (or gauze pad saturated with 70% alcohol solution). Allow it to dry.
• Inject the recommended amount of flush solution.
• After flushing the catheter, maintain positive pressure by keeping your thumb on the plunger of the syringe while withdrawing the needle. This prevents blood backflow and potential clotting in the line.
• CV catheters used for intermittent infusions have injection caps. But unlike heparin lock adapters, these caps contain a small amount of empty space, so you don't have to preflush the cap before connecting it.

To change the injection cap
• The frequency of cap changes varies according to hospital policy and the number of times that the cap is used. Use strict aseptic technique when changing the cap. Repeated punctures of the injection port increase the risk of infection. Also, pieces of the rubber stopper may break off after repeated punctures, increasing the risk of embolism.
• Clean the connection site with an alcohol sponge or a povidone-iodine sponge.
• Instruct the patient to perform Valsalva's maneuver while you quickly disconnect the old cap and connect the new cap using aseptic technique. If he can't perform Valsalva's maneuver, use a padded clamp to prevent air from entering the catheter.

Special considerations
• Change the dressing at least once a week, according to hospital policy, or if it becomes moist, soiled, or nonocclusive.
• Change tubing and solution every 24 to 48 hours, or according to hospital policy, while the CV line is in place. Use sterile technique for all dressing, tubing, and solution changes. Assess the site for signs of infection, such as discharge, inflammation, and tenderness.

Central venous pressure monitoring

Measurements of central venous pressure (CVP) are made with a manometer connected to a catheter that's usually threaded through the subclavian or jugular vein and placed in or near the right atrium.

Equipment and preparation
• Disposable CVP manometer set with stopcock, extension tubing, and leveling rod or yardstick • I.V.

pole • I.V. solution, as ordered • I.V. tubing • tape.

Gather the appropriate equipment, and wash your hands. Clamp the manometer to the I.V. pole, spike the I.V. container, and hang it 30″ to 36″ (76 to 91 cm) above the insertion site to prevent blood from backing up in the catheter.

Next, insert the distal end of the tubing into the left side of the stopcock. Turn the stopcock to the container-to-patient position, open the flow clamp, and flush the tubing. Then turn the stopcock to the container-to-manometer position. Make sure the tubing doesn't contain an in-line filter, which can distort pressure readings. Fill the manometer column with I.V. solution (20 to 25 cm H_2O or about 10 cm H_2O higher than the expected CVP reading). Then close the flow clamp on the tubing.

Avoid overfilling the manometer to prevent inactivation of the filter and increased risk of contamination; also, if a small plastic ball is used to indicate fluid level in the manometer, it may be forced from the tube and rendered useless.

Implementation

• Explain the procedure to the patient. Then loosen the cover on the distal end of the extension tubing (from the stopcock to the patient), and ask him to perform Valsalva's maneuver to avoid formation of an air embolus. Quickly disconnect the existing I.V. tubing, remove the covering from the new tubing, and connect it to his catheter.

• If the patient is unconscious, wait until he inhales fully, then quickly connect the tubing. Lowering the head of the bed also helps prevent an air embolus. If he's intubated, maintain full inflation as you connect the tubing. Finally, adjust the flow clamp to the desired infusion rate.

• Place the patient in a supine position (his head can be slightly raised).

• Adjust the manometer so that the stopcock aligns horizontally with the right atrium.

• To find the position of the right atrium, locate the fourth intercostal space at the midaxillary line. This site becomes the zero reference point — the location for all subsequent readings.

• If the manometer has a leveling rod, extend it between the zero reference point and the zero mark at the bottom of the manometer scale. If the rod has a small viewing window, a bubble will appear between two lines in the window when the rod is horizontal.

• When the stopcock of the manometer is level with the right atrium, tape the manometer set to the I.V. pole to secure its position. Recheck the level before each pressure reading. If an adjustment is required, first raise or lower the bed and then readjust the manometer on the I.V. pole.

• Check the patency of the line by briefly increasing the infusion rate. If the line is not patent, notify the doctor. Never irrigate a clogged CVP line. This avoids possible release of a thrombus. If the line is patent, proceed.

• As before, turn the stopcock to the container-to-manometer position to fill the manometer with I.V. solution.

• Then turn the stopcock to the manometer-to-patient position; the fluid level then falls with inspiration, as intrathoracic pressure decreases, and rises slightly with expiration.

• When the fluid column stabilizes, tap the manometer lightly to dislodge air bubbles that may distort pressure readings. Then position yourself so that the top of the fluid column is at eye level. Note the lowest level the fluid reaches, and take your reading from the base of the meniscus. If the manometer has a small ball floating on the fluid surface, take the reading from the ball's midline.

• If the fluid fails to fluctuate during breathing, the end of the catheter may be pressed against the vein wall. Ask the patient to cough to change its position slightly.

• Maintain catheter patency by returning the stopcock to the container-to-patient position after you take the reading. Check for blood backflow.

• Readjust the infusion rate, and check all connections to help prevent an embolus or bleeding.

• Return the patient to a comfortable position.

Special considerations

• If the patient is connected to a ventilator and is receiving positive end-expiratory pressure, you may obtain variable CVP readings. For example, when the stopcock is turned to the manometer-to-patient position, the fluid level may not fall with inspiration and rise slightly with expiration because intrathoracic pressure doesn't change.

• To detect significant changes, record all pressure readings while the patient is connected to the ventilator, and take readings at end-expiration before the next inspiration begins.

• Report any deviations from the prescribed CVP range to the doctor. Avoid making pressure observations when the patient is sitting up because this position causes false-low measurements if the patient has been put in a sitting position within 3 minutes of the manometer reading.

▶ **Chest physiotherapy**

This procedure includes postural drainage, chest percussion and vibration, and coughing and deep-breathing exercises.

Equipment

• Stethoscope • pillows • tilt or postural drainage table (if available) or adjustable hospital bed • emesis basin • facial tissues • suction equipment, as needed • equipment for oral care • trash bag. Optional: sterile specimen container, mechanical ventilator, supplemental oxygen.

Implementation

• Explain the procedure to the patient.

• Wash your hands; then auscultate the patient's lungs to determine baseline respiratory status.

• For generalized disease, postural drainage usually begins with the lower lobes, continues with the middle lobes, and ends with the upper lobes. For localized disease, drainage begins with the affected lobes and proceeds to the other lobes to avoid spreading the disease to uninvolved areas.

• Position the patient as ordered. The illustrations below show the various postural drainage positions and the specific lung areas affected. Instruct the patient to remain in each position for 10 to 15 minutes. During this time, perform percussion and vibration, as ordered.

Lower lobes: Posterior basal segments

Elevate the foot of the bed 30 degrees. Have the patient lie prone with his head lowered. Position pillows under his chest and abdomen, as shown below. Percuss his lower ribs on both sides of his spine.

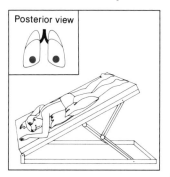

Lower lobes: Lateral basal segments
Elevate the foot of the bed 30 degrees. Instruct the patient to lie on his abdomen with his head lowered and his upper leg flexed over a pillow for support. Then have him rotate a quarter turn upward, as shown below. Percuss his lower ribs on the uppermost portion of his lateral chest wall.

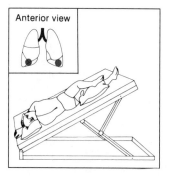

Lower lobes: Anterior basal segments
Elevate the foot of the bed 30 degrees. Instruct the patient to lie on his side with his head lowered.

Then place pillows as shown below. Percuss with a slightly cupped hand over his lower ribs just beneath the axilla. If an acutely ill patient has trouble breathing in this position, adjust the bed to an angle he can tolerate. Then begin percussion.

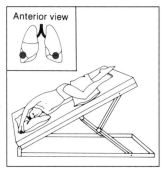

Lower lobes: Superior segments
With the bed flat, have the patient lie on his abdomen. Place two pillows under his hips, as shown below. Percuss on both sides of his spine at the lower tip of his scapulae.

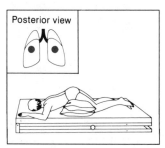

Right middle lobe: Medial and lateral segments
Elevate the foot of the bed 15 degrees. Have the patient lie on his left side with his head down and his knees flexed. Then have him rotate a quarter turn backward. Place a pillow behind him, from shoulders to hips, as shown at the top of page 280. Percuss with your hand moderately cupped over the right

nipple. For a woman, cup your hand so that its heel is under the armpit and your fingers extend forward beneath the breast.

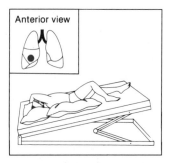

Left upper lobe: Superior and inferior segments, lingular portion

Elevate the foot of the bed 15 degrees. Have the patient lie on his right side with his head down and knees flexed. Then have him rotate a quarter turn backward. Place a pillow behind him, from shoulders to hips, as shown below. Percuss with your hand moderately cupped over his left nipple. For a woman, cup your hand so that its heel is beneath the armpit and your fingers extend forward beneath the breast.

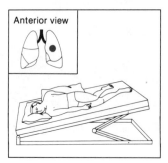

Upper lobes: Anterior segments

Make sure the bed is flat. Have the patient lie on his back with a pillow under his knees, as shown below. Then have him rotate slightly away from the side being drained. Percuss between his clavicle and nipple.

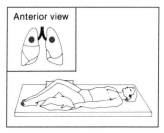

Upper lobes: Apical segments

Keep the bed flat. Have the patient lean back at a 30-degree angle against you and a pillow, as shown below. Percuss with a cupped hand between his clavicles and the top of each scapula.

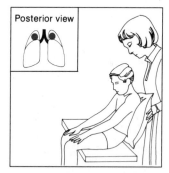

Upper lobes: Posterior segments

Keep the bed flat. Have the patient lean over a pillow at a 30-degree angle, as shown at the top of the next page. With cupped hands, percuss his upper back on each side.

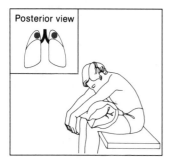

Posterior view

• After postural drainage, percussion, or vibration, instruct the patient to cough to remove loosened secretions. First, tell him to inhale deeply through his nose and then exhale in three short huffs. Then have him inhale deeply again and cough through a slightly open mouth. Three consecutive coughs are highly effective. An effective cough sounds deep, low, and hollow; an ineffective one, high-pitched. Have the patient perform exercises for about 1 minute and then rest for 2 minutes. Gradually progress to a 10-minute exercise period four times daily.

• Provide oral hygiene because secretions may taste foul or have a stale odor.

• Auscultate the patient's lungs to evaluate the effectiveness of this therapy.

Special considerations

• Modify chest physiotherapy according to the patient's condition. If he tires quickly during therapy, shorten the sessions because fatigue leads to shallow respirations and increased hypoxia.

• Maintain adequate hydration to prevent mucus dehydration and promote easier mobilization. Avoid performing postural drainage immediately before or within 1½ hours after meals to avoid nausea and possible aspiration of food or vomitus.

• Because chest percussion can induce bronchospasm, adjunct treatment such as nebulizer therapy should precede chest physiotherapy.

• Refrain from percussing over the spine, liver, kidneys, or spleen to avoid internal injury. Also avoid performing percussion on bare skin or the female patient's breasts. Percuss over soft clothing or place a thin towel over the chest wall.

• Explain coughing and deep-breathing exercises preoperatively, so the patient can practice them. Postoperatively, splint the incision using your hands or, if possible, teach the patient to splint it himself to minimize pain during coughing.

Colostomy and ileostomy care

A patient with an ascending or transverse colostomy or an ileostomy may wear an external pouch to collect fecal matter. Most disposable systems can be used from 2 to 7 days. A pouching system needs changing if a leak develops, and needs emptying when it's one-third to one-half full. The best time to change the system is 2 to 4 hours after meals.

Equipment

• Pouching system (drainable or closed-bottomed, disposable or reusable, one-piece or two-piece) • stoma measuring guide • washcloth and towel • closure clamp • toilet or bedpan • water or pouch cleaning solution • gloves • facial tissues. Optional: ostomy belt, paper tape, mild nonmoisturizing soap, skin shaving equipment.

Implementation

Provide privacy and emotional support.

To fit the pouch and skin barrier

• For a pouch with an attached skin barrier, measure the stoma with the measuring guide, as shown below. Select the opening size that matches the stoma.

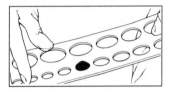

• For an adhesive-backed pouch with a separate skin barrier, measure the stoma, and trace the selected size opening onto the paper back of the skin barrier's adhesive side, as shown below. Cut out the opening so that it is ⅛″ (0.3 cm) larger than the stoma.

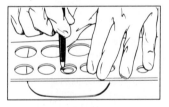

• Avoid fitting the pouch too tightly to prevent injuring the stoma or skin. Avoid cutting the opening too big because it may expose the skin to fecal matter and moisture. The pouch opening should closely match the stoma size.
• Between 6 weeks and 1 year after surgery, the stoma will shrink to its permanent size, making pattern-making unnecessary unless the patient gains weight, has additional surgery, or injures the stoma.

To apply or change the pouch

• Put on gloves; then remove and discard the old pouch. Wipe the stoma and skin with a facial tissue. Wash the peristomal skin with soap and water, rinse well, and pat dry. Inspect the skin and stoma. Shave surrounding hair, if necessary.
• If applying a separate skin barrier, peel off the backing, center the barrier over the stoma, and press down to secure.
• Remove the paper backing from the adhesive side of the pouching system, center the pouch opening over the stoma, and press gently to secure, as shown below.

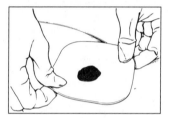

• For a system with flanges, align the lip of the pouch flange with the bottom edge of the skin barrier flange. Then apply pressure to the pouch flange, beginning at the bottom, until the pouch adheres to the barrier flange.
• Encourage the patient to remain still for about 5 minutes to improve adherence.
• Attach an ostomy belt for further security, if desired. Apply a closure clamp to the drainge end of the pouch, if necessary. If desired, apply paper tape to the pouch edges.

To empty the pouch

• Tilt the bottom of the pouch upward, and remove the closure clamp. Turn up a cuff on the lower end of the pouch and allow it to drain into the toilet or bedpan. Wipe the bottom of the pouch, and reapply the closure clamp.
• To empty a two-piece flanged system, unsnap the pouch. Let the drainage flow into the toilet.

• Release flatus through the gas release valve, if present, or by tilting the pouch bottom upward and releasing the clamp. In a flanged system, loosen the seal between the flanges. Never make a pinhole in a pouch to release gas. This destroys the odor-proof seal.

Special considerations
• Use adhesive solvents and removers only after patch-testing the patient's skin for hypersensitivity.
• Remove the pouching system if the patient reports burning or itching beneath it or purulent drainage around the stoma.

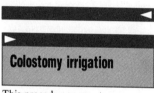

Colostomy irrigation

This procedure serves two purposes: it allows a patient with a descending or sigmoid colostomy to regulate bowel function, and it cleans the large bowel before and after tests, surgery, or other procedures.

Equipment and preparation
• Colostomy irrigation set (contains an irrigation drain or sleeve, an ostomy belt [if needed] to secure the drain or sleeve, water-soluble lubricant, drainage pouch clamp, and irrigation bag with clamp, tubing, and cone tip) • 1,000 ml (about 30 oz or 1 qt) of tap water irrigant warmed to about 100° F (37.8° C) • 0.9% sodium chloride solution (for cleaning enemas) • I.V. pole or wall hook • washcloth and towel • water • ostomy pouching system • linen-saver pad • gloves. Optional: bedpan or chair, mild nonmoisturizing soap, rubber band or clip, small dressing or bandage, stoma cap.

When performing colostomy irrigation in the bathroom, have the patient sit on the toilet or a chair facing the toilet. If it's done in bed, place the bedpan beside the bed.

Fill the irrigation bag with warmed tap water or 0.9% sodium chloride solution to perform bowel cleaning. Hang the bag on the I.V. pole or wall hook. The bottom of the bag should be at the patient's shoulder level to prevent the fluid from entering the bowel too quickly.

Prime the tubing with irrigant to prevent air from entering the colon, possibly causing cramps.

Implementation
• Explain the procedure, provide privacy, and wash your hands.
• If the patient is in bed, place a linen-saver pad under him to protect the sheets.
• Put on gloves. Then remove the ostomy pouch if the patient uses one.
• Place the irrigation sleeve over the stoma. If the sleeve doesn't have an adhesive backing, secure it with an ostomy belt. If the patient has a two-piece pouching system with flanges, snap off the pouch and save it. Snap on the irrigation sleeve.
• Place the open-ended bottom of the irrigation sleeve into a bedpan or toilet to promote drainage by gravity.
• Lubricate your gloved small finger with water-soluble lubricant and insert the finger into the stoma. If you're teaching the patient, have him do this to determine the bowel angle at which to insert the cone safely.
• Lubricate the cone with water-soluble lubricant to prevent it from irritating the mucosa.
• Insert the cone into the top opening of the irrigation sleeve, then into the stoma. Angle the cone to match the bowel angle; insert it gently.
• Unclamp the irrigation tubing and

allow the water to flow slowly. If no clamp is present, pinch the tubing to control flow. The water should enter the colon over 10 to 15 minutes. (If the patient reports cramping, slow or stop the flow, keep the cone in place, and have him take a few deep breaths.)

• Have the patient remain stationary for 15 to 20 minutes so that the initial effluent can drain.

• Wait about 45 minutes for the bowel to finish eliminating the irrigant and effluent. Then remove the irrigation sleeve. To clean the bowel, repeat the procedure with warmed 0.9% sodium chloride solution until the return solution is clear.

• Using a washcloth, mild soap, and water, clean the area around the stoma; then rinse and dry with a clean towel. Notify the doctor of marked stoma color changes because a pale hue may result from anemia, and substantial darkening suggests a change in blood flow to the stoma.

• Apply a clean pouch. If the patient has a regular bowel elimination pattern, he may prefer a small dressing, bandage, or commercial stoma cap.

• Discard a disposable irrigation sleeve. Rinse a reusable irrigation sleeve and hang it to dry.

Special considerations

Don't force the catheter into the stoma because bowel perforation may result. Avoid using too much irrigant, which may cause fluid and electrolyte imbalances.

Defibrillation

During defibrillation, an electric current passes through the patient's heart via two electrode paddles positioned on his chest. This current depolarizes the myocardium, usually allowing the sinoatrial node to resume control of the heart. Defibrillation is most effective when it's initiated as soon as possible after the onset of ventricular fibrillation or pulseless ventricular tachycardia. Specially trained nurses, often the first to recognize the need for defibrillation, can perform the procedure in many hospitals.

Equipment

• Defibrillator conductive gel or gel pads • crash cart with emergency resuscitation equipment.

Defibrillation paddles are available in both adult size (13 cm in diameter) and pediatric size (8 cm in diameter), as well as in anterolateral and anteroposterior types.

Implementation

• Assess the patient to determine the lack of a pulse. Call for help, and perform cardiopulmonary resuscitation (CPR) until the defibrillator and crash cart arrive.

• Connect the monitoring leads from the defibrillator unit to the patient. Be sure to remove any telemetry or bedside monitors to prevent damage to those units.

• Assess the patient's cardiac rhythm for ventricular fibrillation or pulseless ventricular tachycardia.

• Turn on the defibrillator. If you're using a unit that can also be used for synchronized cardioversion, make sure that it's set on the asynchronous mode.

• Expose the patient's chest.

• Apply conductive gel to the paddles. Make sure no excess gel is dripping from the paddles; excess gel will cause arcing of current.

• If you're using gel pads, place them where the paddles will be located. To avoid possible electric shock, do not cover any of the electrocardiogram leadwires or electrodes.

• For anterolateral paddle placement, position one paddle to the right of the upper sternum, just below the right clavicle, and the other at the fifth or sixth intercostal space in the left anterior axillary line.

• For anteroposterior placement, position the anterior paddle directly over the heart at the precordium, to the left of the lower sternal border. Place the flat posterior paddle under the patient's body beneath the heart and immediately below the scapulae (but not under the vertebral column).

• Set the machine at the energy level for initial defibrillation (200 joules for adults and 2 joules/kg for infants and children).

• Charge the paddles by pressing the charge button on the machine or on the paddles themselves. A blinking light or a constant hissing noise will signal that the paddles are charging. When they're fully charged, the light will stop blinking, the hissing will cease, and the machine may show a digital display of the energy level.

• Apply the paddles to the patient's chest. Press them firmly against the skin. Reassess the patient's cardiac rhythm, pulse, and level of consciousness to determine the need for defibrillation.

• Instruct personnel to stand clear of the patient and bed to avoid risk of shock.

• Discharge the current by pressing both of the paddle discharge buttons simultaneously.

• If defibrillation is unsuccessful, repeat the procedure two more times. Increase the energy level as ordered. (For adults, the American Heart Association recommends 200 joules for the first attempt, 200 to 300 joules for the second, and no more than 360 joules for the third.)

• Perform the three countershocks in rapid succession; it's unnecessary to resume CPR between each one.

• If the patient remains without a pulse after the three initial countershocks, resume CPR, and give supplemental oxygen to ensure maximum oxygenation and perfusion of vital organs. Begin administering medication.

• If normal rhythm is restored, continue to monitor the patient, and provide supplemental oxygen and ventilation as needed.

• If the paddles have been recharged but are not used again, clear the charge by turning off the machine, adjusting the energy selector dial, or placing the paddles into their protective housing and discharging them into the machine. Do not discharge the paddles against each other or into the air.

• Prepare the defibrillator for immediate reuse by cleaning and restocking any used equipment and medications.

Special considerations

• Defibrillators vary among manufacturers, so familiarize yourself with your hospital's equipment.

• The unit's operation should be checked at least every 8 hours and after each use.

Defibrillation using an automated external defibrillator

The automated external defibrillator (AED) is commonly used for early defibrillation. The AED is equipped with a microcomputer that senses and analyzes a patient's heart rhythm at the push of a button. Then it audibly or visually prompts you to deliver a shock.

Equipment
• AED • prepackaged electrodes.

Implementation
• After discovering that the patient is unresponsive to your questions, pulseless, and apneic, follow Basic Life Support and Advanced Cardiac Life Support protocols.
• Open the electrode packets and attach the electrodes to the AED. Then expose the patient's chest. Remove the backing film from the pads. Place the pad attached to the white cable connector on the right upper portion of the patient's chest, just beneath his clavicle. Place the pad attached to the red cable connector to the left of the heart's apex.
• Press the AED's ON button. The machine will perform a brief self-test. When the machine is ready, ask everyone to stand clear, and press the ANALYZE button. Be careful not to touch or move the patient while the AED is in analysis mode (15 to 30 seconds).
• When the patient needs a shock, the AED will display a "Stand clear" message amd emit a beep that changes into a steady tone as it's charging.
• When the AED is fully charged and ready to deliver a shock, it will prompt you to press the SHOCK button. (Some AED models automatically deliver a shock within 15 seconds after analyzing the patient's rhythm. If a shock weren't needed, the AED would display "No shock indicated" and prompt you to "Check patient.")
• Make sure no one is touching the patient or his bed, and call out "Stand clear." Then press the

SHOCK button on the AED.
• After the first shock, the AED will automatically reanalyze the patient's rhythm. If no additional shock is needed, the machine will prompt you to check the patient. However, if the patient is still in ventricular fibrillation, the AED will automatically begin recharging at a higher joule level to prepare for a second shock. Repeat the steps you performed before shocking the patient. According to the AED algorithm, the patient can be shocked up to three times at increasing joule levels (200, 200 to 300, and 360 joules).
• If the patient is still in ventricular fibrillation after three shocks, resume cardiopulmonary resuscitation for 1 minute. Then press the ANALYZE button on the AED to identify the heart rhythm. If the patient is still in ventricular fibrillation, continue the algorithm sequence until the code team leader arrives.
• After the code, remove and transcribe the AED's computer memory module or tape, or prompt the AED to print a rhythm strip with code data. Follow hospital policy for analyzing and storing code data.

Special considerations
After using an AED, give a synopsis to the code team leader, and document your actions.

Duodenal or jejunal feeding

This procedure involves delivery of a liquid feeding formula, usually in the form of a continuous drip, directly to the duodenum or jejunum.

Equipment and preparation

• Feeding formula • enteral administration set containing a gavage container, drip chamber, roller clamp or flow regulator, and tube connector • I.V. pole • 60-ml syringe with adapter tip • water. Optional: pump administration set (for an enteral infusion pump), Y-connector, antidiarrheal medication.

Be sure to refrigerate formulas prepared in the dietary department or pharmacy. Refrigerate commercial formulas only after opening them.

Check the date on all formula containers. Use powdered formula within 24 hours of mixing. Always shake the container well.

Allow the formula to warm to room temperature before administration, but never warm it over direct heat.

After closing the flow clamp on the administration set, pour the appropriate amount of formula into the gavage bag. Hang no more than a 4- to 6-hour supply at one time to prevent bacterial growth.

Open the flow clamp on the administration set to remove air from the lines and prevent air from entering the patient's stomach.

Implementation

• Provide privacy, wash your hands, and explain the procedure.
• Place the patient in low Fowler's position, and assess the abdomen for bowel sounds and distention.
• Aspirate for residual formula prior to intermittent feedings and every 4 to 6 hours for continuous feedings.
• Open the enteral administration set, and hang the gavage container on the I.V. pole.
• Open the flow clamp and regulate the flow to the desired rate. To regulate the rate using a volumetric infusion pump, follow the manufacturer's directions. Most patients receive small amounts initially, with volumes increasing gradually after tolerance is established.
• Flush the tube every 4 hours with water. A needle catheter jejunostomy tube may require flushing every 2 hours to prevent formula buildup. A Y-connector may be useful for frequent flushing.

Special considerations

• Small-bore feeding tubes may kink, making instillation impossible. If this occurs, try changing the patient's position, or withdraw the tube a few inches and restart. Never use a guide wire to reposition the tube.
• Constantly monitor the flow rate of a blended or high-residue formula to determine if the formula is clogging the tubing. To prevent this, squeeze the bag frequently.
• Glycosuria, hyperglycemia, and diuresis can indicate an excessive carbohydrate level, leading to hyperosmotic dehydration, which can be fatal. Monitor urine and blood glucose levels to assess glucose tolerance. Perform fingerstick blood glucose determinations every 6 hours or as ordered. Also monitor serum electrolytes, blood urea nitrogen, serum glucose, serum osmolality, and other pertinent parameters to determine the patient's response to therapy and assess his hydration status.
• Check the flow rate hourly to ensure correct infusion.
• Most patients tolerate continuous drip duodenal and jejunal feedings better than bolus feedings. Bolus feedings can cause such complications as hyperglycemia, glycosuria, and diarrhea.
• Until the patient acquires a tolerance for the formula, you may need to dilute it to one-half or three-quarters strength to start and increase it gradually.

▶

Enema administration

This procedure involves instilling a solution into the rectum and colon. If using a retention enema, the patient holds the solution within the rectum or colon for 30 minutes to 1 hour. If using an irrigating enema, he expels it almost completely within 15 minutes.

Equipment and preparation

• Prescribed solution • bath thermometer • enema administration bag with attached rectal tube and clamp • I.V. pole • gloves • linen-saver pads • bath blanket • bedpan with cover, or bedside commode • water-soluble lubricant • toilet tissue • bulb syringe or funnel • plastic bag for equipment • water • gown • washcloth • soap and water • if observing enteric precautions: plastic trash bags, labels. Optional (for patients who can't retain solution): plastic rectal tube guard, indwelling urinary catheter or Verden rectal catheter with 30-ml balloon and syringe.

Prepare the prescribed type and amount of solution as indicated. Because some ingredients may be mucosal irritants, be sure the proportions are correct and the agents are thoroughly mixed to avoid localized irritation.

Warm the solution to reduce patient discomfort. Clamp the tubing, and fill the solution bag with the prescribed solution. Unclamp the tubing, flush the solution through the tubing, then reclamp it.

Hang the solution container on the I.V. pole, and take all the supplies to the patient's room. If you're using an indwelling urinary catheter or a Verden catheter, fill the syringe with 30 ml of water.

Implementation

• Assess the patient's condition, provide privacy, and explain the procedure.
• Ask the patient if he's had previous difficulty retaining an enema to determine whether you'll need to use a rectal tube guard or a catheter.
• Wash your hands, and put on gloves.
• Help the patient put on a hospital gown, and assist him into the left-lateral Sims' position to facilitate the solution's flow into the descending colon.
• Place linen-saver pads under the patient's buttocks to prevent soiling the linens.
• Replace the top bed linens with a bath blanket.
• Make sure a bedpan, commode, or bathroom, as indicated, is readily available.
• Lubricate the distal tip of the rectal catheter with water-soluble lubricant to facilitate rectal insertion.
• Separate the patient's buttocks, and touch the anal sphincter with the rectal tube to stimulate contraction. As the sphincter relaxes, tell the patient to breathe deeply through the mouth as you advance the tube. If he feels pain or the tube meets continued resistance, notify the doctor. This may signal an unknown stricture or abscess.
• If using an indwelling urinary catheter or a Verden catheter as a rectal tube, insert the lubricated catheter as you would a rectal tube. Then gently inflate the catheter's balloon with 20 to 30 ml of water. Pull the catheter back against the patient's internal anal sphincter to seal off the rectum. When using either catheter, avoid inflating the balloon above 45 ml because over-inflation can compromise blood flow to rectal tissues and cause possible necrosis.
• When using a rectal tube, hold it

in place throughout the procedure because bowel contractions and the pressure of the tube against the anal sphincter can promote tube displacement.

• Hold the solution container slightly above bed level, and release the tubing clamp. Then raise the container gradually to start the flow—usually at a rate of 75 to 100 ml/minute for an irrigating enema, but at the slowest possible rate for a retention enema to avoid stimulating peristalsis and to promote retention.

• Adjust the flow rate of an irrigating enema by raising or lowering the solution container. However, be sure not to raise it higher than 18″ (46 cm) for an adult, 12″ (31 cm) for a child, and 6″ to 8″ (15 to 20 cm) for an infant, because excessive pressure can force colon bacteria into the small intestine or rupture the colon.

• Assess the patient's tolerance frequently during instillation. If he's uncomfortable, clamp the tubing to stop the flow. Then hold his buttocks together or firmly press toilet tissue against the anus. Instruct him to gently massage his abdomen and breathe slowly and deeply through his mouth to relax abdominal muscles and promote retention. Resume administration at a slower flow rate when discomfort passes, but interrupt flow any time he feels discomfort.

• If the flow slows or stops, the catheter tip may be clogged or lodged against the rectal wall. Turn the catheter slightly to free it without stimulating defecation. If it remains clogged, withdraw the catheter, flush it with solution, and reinsert.

• After administering most of the prescribed solution, clamp the tubing. Stop the flow before the container empties completely to avoid introducing air into the bowel.

• For a flush enema, stop the flow by lowering the solution container below bed level and allowing gravity to siphon the enema from the colon. Continue to raise and lower the container until gas bubbles cease or the patient feels more comfortable and abdominal distention subsides. Don't allow the solution container to empty completely before lowering it because this may introduce air into the bowel.

• For an irrigating enema, instruct the patient to retain the solution for 15 minutes if possible.

• For a retention enema, instruct the patient to avoid defecation for the prescribed time. If you're using an indwelling urinary catheter, leave the catheter in place to promote retention. When the solution has remained in the colon for the recommended time or for as long as the patient can tolerate it, assist him onto a bedpan or to the commode or bathroom, as required.

• If you've used a rectal tube, remove it when you have completed the procedure.

• Provide privacy while the patient expels the solution. Tell him not to flush the toilet. Cover the bedpan or commode, and take it to the utility room for observation, or observe the contents of the toilet if applicable. Carefully note fecal color, consistency, amount, and foreign matter. Send ordered specimens to the laboratory.

• Properly dispose of gloves and enema equipment. Wash your hands. Ventilate the room or use air freshener.

Special considerations

• Because patients with salt-retention disorders may absorb sodium from the saline enema solution, administer the solution cautiously to such patients and monitor their electrolyte status.

• Schedule a retention enema before

BEDSIDE CARE

meals because a full stomach may make retention difficult.

• If the patient fails to expel the solution within 1 hour because of diminished neuromuscular response, you may need to remove the enema solution. Review your hospital's policy because you may need a doctor's order. Inform the doctor when a patient can't expel an enema spontaneously because of possible bowel perforation or electrolyte imbalance.

• If the doctor orders enemas until returns are clear, give no more than three to avoid excessive irritation of the rectal mucosa. Notify the doctor if the returned fluid isn't clear after three admininstrations.

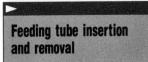

Feeding tube insertion and removal

Inserting a feeding tube nasally or, sometimes, orally into the stomach or duodenum allows a patient who can't or won't eat to receive nourishment. The feeding tube also permits supplemental feedings in a patient with exceptionally high nutritional requirements — an unconscious patient or one with extensive burns, for example. The preferred feeding tube route is nasal, but the oral route may be used for patients with such conditions as a deviated septum or a head or nose injury.

Equipment and preparation
For insertion
• Feeding tube (#6 to #18 French, with or without guide) • linen-saver pad • gloves • hypoallergenic tape • water-soluble lubricant • cotton-tipped applicators • skin preparation (such as tincture of benzoin) • facial tissues • penlight • small cup of water with straw, or ice chips

• emesis basin • 60-ml syringe • stethoscope.

During use
• Mouthwash or saltwater solution • toothbrush.

For removal
• Linen-saver pad • tube clamp • bulb syringe.

Have the proper size tube available. Usually, the doctor orders the smallest-bore tube that will allow free passage of the liquid feeding formula. Read the instructions on the tubing package carefully because tube characteristics vary among manufacturers.

Examine the tube to make sure it's free of defects such as cracks or rough or sharp edges. Next, run water through the tube to check for patency, activate the coating, and allow for easier removal of the guide.

Implementation
• Explain the procedure to the patient, and provide privacy. Wash your hands, and put on gloves.
• Assist the patient into semi-Fowler's (or high Fowler's) position, and place a linen-saver pad across his chest to protect him from spills.
• To determine the tube length needed to reach the stomach, first extend the distal end of the tube from the tip of the patient's nose to his earlobe. Coil this portion of the tube around your fingers so that the end will remain curved as you insert it. Then extend the uncoiled portion from the earlobe to the xiphoid process. Use a small piece of hypoallergenic tape to mark the total length of these two portions.

To insert the tube nasally
• Using the penlight, assess nasal patency. Inspect nasal passages for a deviated septum, polyps, or other obstructions. As the patient

breathes through his nose, occlude one nostril and then the other to determine which has the better airflow. Assess the patient's history of nasal injury or surgery.

• Lubricate the curved tip of the tube (and the feeding tube guide, if appropriate) with a small amount of water-soluble lubricant to ease insertion and prevent tissue injury.

• Ask the patient to hold the emesis basin and facial tissues in case he needs them.

• To advance the tube, insert the curved, lubricated tip into the more patent nostril and direct it along the nasal passage toward the ear on the same side. When it passes the nasopharyngeal junction, turn the tube 180 degrees to aim it downward into the esophagus and advance it. Then give him a small cup of water with a straw, or ice chips. Direct him to sip the water or suck on the ice and to swallow frequently without clamping his teeth down on the tube. This will ease the tube's passage. Advance the tube as he swallows.

To insert the tube orally

• Have the patient lower his chin to close his trachea, and ask him to open his mouth.

• Place the tip of the tube at the back of the patient's tongue, give him water, and instruct him to swallow as above.

To position the tube

• Keep passing the tube until the tape marking the appropriate length reaches the patient's nostril or lips.

• To check tube placement, attach the syringe filled with 10 cc of air to the end of the tube. Gently inject the air into the tube as you auscultate the patient's abdomen with the stethoscope about 3″ (8 cm) below the sternum. Listen for a whoosing sound, which signals that the tube reached its target in the stomach. If the tube remains coiled in the esophagus, you'll feel resistance when you inject the air, or the patient may belch.

• If you hear the whooshing sound, gently try to aspirate gastric secretions. Successful aspiration confirms correct tube placement. If no gastric secretions return, the tube may be in the esophagus. You'll need to advance the tube or reinsert it before proceeding.

• After confirming proper tube placement, remove the tape marking the tube length.

• Tape the tube to the patient's nose, and remove the guide wire. *Note:* In some cases, X-rays may be ordered to verify tube placement.

• To advance the tube to the duodenum, especially a tungsten-weighted tube, position the patient on his right side. This lets gravity assist tube passage through the pylorus. Move the tube forward 2″ to 3″ (5 to 8 cm) hourly until X-ray studies confirm duodenal placement. (An X-ray film must confirm placement before feeding begins because duodenal feeding can cause nausea and vomiting if accidentally delivered to the stomach.)

• Apply skin preparation to the patient's cheek before securing the tube with tape. This helps the tube adhere to the skin and also prevents irritation.

• Tape the tube securely to the patient's cheek to avoid excessive pressure on his nostrils.

To remove the tube

• Protect the patient's chest with a linen-saver pad.

• Flush the tube with air, clamp or pinch it to prevent fluid aspiration during withdrawal, and withdraw it gently but quickly.

• Promptly cover and discard the used tube.

BEDSIDE CARE

Special considerations

• Flush the feeding tube every 8 hours with up to 60 ml of 0.9% sodium chloride solution or water to maintain patency.

• Retape the tube at least daily and as needed. Alternate taping the tube toward the inner and outer side of the nose to avoid constant pressure on the same nasal area. Inspect the skin for redness and breakdown.

• Provide nasal hygiene daily using cotton-tipped applicators and water-soluble lubricant to remove crusted secretions. Assist the patient with oral hygiene at least twice daily. Help him brush his teeth, gums, and tongue with mouthwash or a mild saltwater solution.

• If the patient can't swallow the feeding tube, use a guide to aid insertion.

• Precise feeding tube placement is especially important because small-bore feeding tubes may slide into the trachea without causing immediate signs or symptoms of respiratory distress, such as coughing, choking, gasping, or cyanosis. However, the patient will usually cough if the tube enters the larynx. To be sure that the tube clears the larynx, ask the patient to speak. If he can't, the tube is in the larynx. Withdraw the tube at once and reinsert.

• When aspirating gastric contents to check tube placement, pull gently on the syringe plunger because negative pressure may collapse a small-bore feeding tube or traumatize the stomach lining or bowel. If you meet resistance during aspiration, stop the procedure because resistance may result simply from the tube lying against the stomach wall. If the tube coils above the stomach, you'll be unable to aspirate stomach contents. To rectify this, change the patient's position or withdraw the tube a few inches, readvance it, and try to aspirate again. If the tube was inserted with a guide wire, do not use the guide wire to reposition the tube. The doctor may do so, using fluoroscopic guidance.

• If the patient will use a feeding tube at home, make appropriate home care nursing referrals, and teach him and his caregivers how to use and care for a feeding tube.

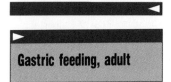

Gastric feeding, adult

Delivery of a liquid feeding formula directly to the stomach is indicated when a patient can't eat normally, as in dysphagia, oral or esophageal obstruction or injury, or unconsciousness.

Equipment and preparation

• Feeding formula • graduated container • 120 ml of water • gavage bag with tubing and flow regulator clamp • towel or linen-saver pad • 60-ml syringe • stethoscope. Optional: infusion controller and tubing set, adapter to connect gavage tubing to feeding tube.

A bulb syringe or large catheter-tip syringe may be substituted for a gavage bag. Refrigerate formulas prepared in the dietary department or pharmacy as well as commercial formulas that have been opened. Use powdered formula within 24 hours of mixing. Allow the formula to warm to room temperature before administration.

After closing the flow clamp, pour the appropriate amount of formula into the gavage bag. Hang no more than a 4- to 6-hour supply at one time to prevent bacterial overgrowth. Open the flow clamp to remove air from the lines.

Implementation

• Provide privacy, and wash your hands.
• If the patient has a nasal or oral tube, cover his chest with a towel or linen-saver pad to protect against spills.
• Assess the patient's abdomen for bowel sounds and distention. Elevate the bed to semi-Fowler's or high Fowler's position.
• Check placement of the feeding tube. To do so, remove the cap or plug from the tube, and inject 5 to 10 cc of air. At the same time, auscultate the patient's stomach with the stethoscope. Listen for a whooshing sound to confirm tube positioning in the stomach. Aspirate stomach contents to confirm tube patency and placement and to assess gastric emptying. Reinstill any aspirate obtained.
• Connect the gavage bag tubing to the feeding tube. If using a bulb or catheter-tip syringe, remove the bulb or plunger, and attach the syringe to the pinched-off feeding tube to prevent excess air from entering the patient's stomach.
• If using an infusion controller, thread the tube from the formula container through the controller according to the manufacturer's directions. Purge the tubing of air and attach it to the feeding tube.
• Open the regulator clamp on the gavage bag tubing, and adjust the flow rate. When using a bulb syringe, fill the syringe with formula, and release the feeding tube to allow formula to flow through it. The height at which you hold the syringe will determine the flow rate. When the syringe is three-quarters empty, pour in more formula.
• After administering the proper amount of formula, flush the tubing with 60 ml of water.
• If administering a continuous feeding, flush the feeding tube, and aspirate for residual formula every 4 hours.
• To discontinue gastric feeding, close the regulator clamp on the gavage bag tubing, and disconnect the syringe from the feeding tube; if using an infusion controller, turn it off. Cover the end of the feeding tube with its plug or cap.
• Leave the patient in semi-Fowler's or high Fowler's position for at least 30 minutes.
• Rinse all reusable equipment with warm water. Change equipment every 24 hours or according to the hospital's policy.

Special considerations

• If the patient becomes nauseated or vomits, stop the feeding immediately.
• If the patient develops diarrhea, administer small, frequent, less concentrated feedings, or administer bolus feedings over a longer time. Make sure that the formula isn't cold and that proper storage and sanitation practices have been followed.
• Glycosuria, hyperglycemia, and diuresis can indicate an excessive carbohydrate level, leading to hyperosmotic dehydration, which can be fatal. Monitor urine and blood glucose levels. Perform fingerstick blood glucose determinations every 6 hours or as ordered.

Gastric lavage

After poisoning or a drug overdose, gastric lavage flushes the stomach and removes ingested substances through a nasogastric (NG) tube. For patients with gastric or esophageal bleeding, lavage with tepid or iced water or 0.9% sodium chloride solution may be used to stop bleeding.

Equipment and preparation

• Lavage setup (two graduated containers for drainage, three pieces of large-lumen rubber tubing, Y-connector, and clamp or hemostat)
• 2 or 3 liters of 0.9% sodium chloride solution or tap water • basin of ice, if ordered • Ewald tube or any large-lumen gastric tube, typically #20 French or greater • water-soluble lubricant or anesthetic ointment • stethoscope • ½" hypoallergenic tape • 50-ml bulb syringe or catheter-tip syringe • gloves • linen-saver pad or towel • Yankauer or tonsil-tip suction device • suction apparatus. Optional: patient restraints.

Set up lavage equipment. If iced lavage is ordered, chill the desired irrigant in a basin of ice. Lubricate the end of the NG tube with water-soluble lubricant or anesthetic ointment.

Implementation

• Explain the procedure to the patient, provide privacy, and wash your hands.
• Put on gloves, and drape the towel or linen-saver pad over the patient's chest.
• The doctor inserts the NG tube orally or nasally and advances it slowly and gently. He then checks the tube's placement by injecting 30 cc of air into the tube and auscultating the patient's abdomen with a stethoscope. If the tube is in place, he'll hear air entering the stomach.
• Because the patient may vomit during insertion, be prepared to suction the airway with a Yankauer or tonsil-tip suction device. To prevent aspiration, place the patient in semi-Fowler's position.
• After securing the NG tube and making sure the irrigant inflow tube on the lavage setup is clamped, connect the unattached

end of this tube to the NG tube, as shown on page 295.
• Aspirate or allow stomach contents to empty into the drainage container before instilling irrigant. If you're using a syringe irrigation set, aspirate stomach contents with a 50-ml bulb syringe or catheter-tip syringe before instillation.
• After you confirm proper tube placement, assist the patient into the left lateral position to instill solution. Positioning the patient's head slightly lower than the stomach will speed removal of lavage solution and will minimize passage of gastric contents into the duodenum.
• Begin gastric lavage by instilling 250 ml of irrigant to assess the patient's tolerance and prevent vomiting. If you're using a syringe, instill about 50 ml of solution at a time until you've instilled between 250 and 500 ml.
• Clamp the inflow tube, and unclamp the outflow tube to allow the irrigant to flow out. If you're using the syringe irrigation kit, aspirate the irrigant with the syringe, and empty it into a calibrated container. Measure the outflow amount to be sure that it at least equals the amount of irrigant instilled.
• If the drainage amount falls significantly short, reposition the tube and gently massage the abdomen to promote outflow.
• Repeat the inflow-outflow cycle until returned fluids appear clear.
• Assess the patient's vital signs, urine output, and level of consciousness (LOC) every 15 minutes. Notify the doctor of any changes.

Special considerations

• Never leave a patient alone during gastric lavage. Observe continuously for any changes in his LOC, and monitor vital signs frequently because vagal response to intubation can depress heart rate.

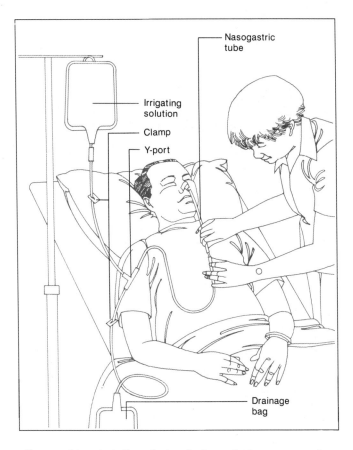

Nasogastric tube

Irrigating solution

Clamp

Y-port

Drainage bag

• If you need to restrain the patient, secure restraints on the same side of the bed so that you can free them quickly. Avoid restraining the patient in a "spread eagle" position, which would prevent him from turning and leave him at risk for aspirating vomitus.

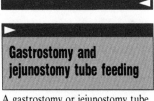

Gastrostomy and jejunostomy tube feeding

A gastrostomy or jejunostomy tube usually is sutured in place during surgery and used for postoperative feeding or for long-term enteral access. A percutaneous endoscopic gastrostomy (PEG) or jejunostomy (PEJ) tube is inserted endoscopically for nutrition, drainage, and decompression.

With either tube type, feedings may begin when peristalsis resumes (usually about 24 hours).

Equipment
• For feeding: room temperature formula • large-bulb or catheter-tip syringe • 120 ml of water • 4″ × 4″ gauze pads • skin protectant • soap • antibacterial ointment • gravity-drip feeding bags • hypoallergenic tape • gloves • enteral infusion pump.

BEDSIDE CARE

For decompression
• Suction setup with tubing and straight drainage collection set.

Implementation
• Provide privacy, and wash your hands. Explain the procedure to the patient. Assess for bowel sounds, and monitor for abdominal distention.
• Have the patient sit or assume semi-Fowler's position to help prevent esophageal reflux and aspiration. Have the patient maintain this position for 1 hour after an intermittent feeding.
• Put on gloves. Measure residual gastric contents by aspirating with a syringe every 4 hours for continuous feedings or prior to the next intermittent feeding. Return the residual aspirate to prevent acid-base and electrolyte imbalances. If the residual aspirate is more than twice the hourly rate or if more than 75 ml of undigested formula remains, withhold the feeding and recheck in 1 hour. Notify the doctor if contents are still too high.
• Allow 30 ml of water to flow into the feeding tube to establish patency.

Intermittent feedings
• Allow gravity to help the formula flow over 30 to 45 minutes. Faster infusions may cause bloating, cramps, or diarrhea.
• Start slowly (200 ml daily) and increase as tolerated to reach the desired intake.
• After feeding, flush the tube with 30 to 60 ml of water to ensure patency. Cap the tube to avoid leaks.
• Rinse the feeding set with hot water to avoid contaminating subsequent feedings. Allow the tube to dry between feedings.

Continuous feedings
• Measure gastric contents every 4 hours.

• If using a pump, set up the equipment according to directions and fill the feeding bag. If feeding by gravity, fill the container with formula, and purge air from the tubing.
• Monitor the drip or infusion rate frequently to ensure accurate delivery.
• Flush the tube with 30 to 60 ml of water every 4 hours to ensure patency. Monitor intake and output to detect fluid or electrolyte imbalances.

Decompression
• Connect the PEG port to the suction device. Jejunostomy feeding may be given simultaneously via the PEJ port of the double-lumen tube.

Tube exit site care
• Gently remove the dressing by hand. Never cut it, because you may cut the tube or sutures.
• At least daily, clean the skin around the tube's exit site with a 4″ × 4″ gauze pad soaked in the ordered cleaning solution. When healed, wash the site daily with soap. Rinse with water and pat dry. Apply skin protectant, if needed, and antibacterial ointment to reduce maceration.
• Coil the tube, if necessary, and tape it to the abdomen to prevent pulling and contamination. PEG and PEJ tubes have internal and external bumpers that make tape anchors unnecessary.

Special considerations
• Don't use formula that has passed its expiration date or been open for longer than 1 day.
• If the patient vomits or complains of nausea or satiety, stop immediately. Aspirate for residual gastric secretions, flush the tube, and try again in 1 hour. The volume or rate may need to be decreased.

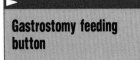

Gastrostomy feeding button

An alternative feeding device to a gastrostomy tube for ambulatory patients receiving long-term enteral feedings, the gastrostomy feeding button has a mushroom dome at one end and two wing tabs and a flexible safety plug at the other. When inserted into an established stoma, the button lies almost flush with the skin, with only the top of the safety plug visible. A one-way antireflux valve mounted just inside the mushroom dome prevents accidental leakage of gastric contents.

Equipment

• Gastrostomy feeding button of the correct size (#18, #22, #24, or #28 French) • obturator • water-soluble lubricant • gloves • feeding accessories, including adapter, feeding catheter, food syringe or bag, and formula • catheter clamp • cleaning equipment, including water, a syringe, cotton-tipped applicator, pipe cleaner, and mild soap or povidone-iodine solution. Optional: pump to provide continuous infusion over several hours.

Implementation

Explain the insertion, reinsertion, and feeding procedure to the patient. Tell him the doctor will perform the initial insertion.

To feed

• Wash your hands, and put on gloves.
• Attach the adapter and feeding catheter to the syringe or feeding bag. Clamp the catheter, and fill the syringe or bag and catheter with formula. Refill the syringe before it's empty. These steps prevent

air from entering the stomach and distending the abdomen.
• Open the safety plug, and attach the adapter and feeding catheter to the button. Elevate the syringe or feeding bag above stomach level, and gravity-feed the formula for 15 to 30 minutes, varying the height as needed to alter the flow rate. Use a pump for continuous infusion or for feedings lasting several hours.

After feeding

• Flush the button with 10 ml of water, and clean the inside of the feeding catheter with a cotton-tipped applicator and water to preserve patency and to dislodge formula or food particles. Lower the syringe or bag below stomach level to allow burping.

Remove the adapter and feeding catheter. The antireflux valve should prevent gastric reflux.

Snap the safety plug in place to keep the lumen clean and prevent leakage if the antireflux valve fails.

If the patient feels nauseated or vomits after feeding, vent the button with the adapter to control emesis or allow for burping.
• Wash the catheter and syringe or feeding bag in warm soapy water, and rinse thoroughly. Clean the catheter and adapter with a pipe cleaner, and rinse well before using for the next feeding. Soak the equipment once a week according to manufacturer's recommendations.

Special considerations

• The gastrostomy feeding button does not allow for aspiration of gastric material.
• Once daily, clean the peristomal skin with mild soap and water or povidone-iodine solution, and let the skin air-dry for 20 minutes to avoid skin irritation. Also clean the

site whenever spillage from the feeding bag occurs.
• Keep intake and output records.
• Note the appearance of the stoma and skin.
• Before discharge, be sure the patient can insert and care for the gastrostomy feeding button.

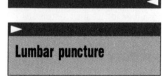

Lumbar puncture

This procedure involves insertion of a sterile needle into the subarachnoid space of the spinal canal, usually between the third and fourth lumbar vertebrae. A lumbar puncture may be used to detect increased intracranial pressure (ICP) or blood in cerebrospinal fluid (CSF); to obtain CSF for laboratory analysis; to inject dyes or gases for contrast studies of the brain and spinal cord; to administer drugs or anesthetics; and to relieve ICP. It is contraindicated in papilledema and suspected brain tumors.

Equipment
• Overbed table • one or two pairs of sterile gloves for the doctor • sterile gloves for the nurse • povidone-iodine solution • sterile gauze pads • alcohol sponges • sterile fenestrated drape • 3-ml syringe for local anesthetic • 25G ¾" sterile needle for injecting local anesthetic (usually 1% lidocaine) • 18G or 20G 3¾" spinal needle with stylet (22G needle for children) • three-way stopcock, manometer (optional) • small adhesive bandage • three sterile collection tubes with stoppers • laboratory request forms • labels • light source, such as a gooseneck lamp.

Disposable lumbar puncture trays containing most of the sterile equipment needed are available.

Implementation
• Explain the procedure to the patient to ease his anxiety, and be sure he has signed a consent form.
• Inform him that he may experience headache after lumbar puncture; however, cooperation during the procedure minimizes the effect.
• Provide privacy, and have the patient void.
• Wash your hands thoroughly.
• Open the equipment tray on an overbed table; avoid contaminating the sterile field.
• Illuminate the puncture site, and adjust the height of the patient's bed to allow the doctor to perform the procedure comfortably.
• Place the patient on his side at the edge of the bed, with his chin to his chest and his knees to his abdomen. Place one hand behind his head and the other hand behind his knees to keep him in position, as shown below. Tell him to stay as still as possible to minimize discomfort and trauma.
• The doctor cleans the puncture site with three different sterile gauze pads soaked in povidone-io-

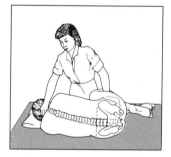

dine solution. Next, he drapes the area with the fenestrated drape to provide a sterile field. (He may replace his sterile gloves to avoid introducing povidone-iodine.)
• If the equipment tray lacks an am-

pule of anesthetic, clean the injection port of a multidose vial with an alcohol sponge. Then invert it 45 degrees so that the doctor can insert a 25G needle and syringe and withdraw the anesthetic.

• Before injection of the anesthetic, tell the patient that he'll experience transient burning and local pain. Ask him to report any other persistent pain or sensations because they may indicate that the needle should be repositioned.

• When the doctor inserts the spinal needle, have the patient remain still and breathe normally. Hold him firmly to prevent movement.

• When the needle is in place, the doctor injects contrast media or anesthetic, or he attaches a manometer with a three-way stopcock to the needle hub to read CSF pressure. If ordered, help the patient extend his legs to provide a more accurate pressure reading.

• The doctor then detaches the manometer and allows 2 or 3 ml of fluid to drain from the needle hub into each tube. Mark the tubes in sequence, stopper and label them, and send them to the lab.

• After the doctor removes the spinal needle, clean the puncture site with povidone-iodine solution, and apply a small adhesive bandage.

Special considerations

• During the puncture, watch closely for adverse reactions: elevated pulse rate, pallor, or clammy skin. Alert the doctor immediately if any of these occur.

• The patient may be ordered to lie flat for 8 to 12 hours after the procedure.

• Do not refrigerate CSF before transport.

Manual ventilation

An inflatable device that can be attached to a face mask or directly to an endotracheal or tracheostomy tube, a hand-held resuscitation bag allows manual delivery of oxygen or room air to the lungs of a patient who can't breathe by himself.

Equipment and preparation

• Resuscitation bag • mask • oxygen source • oxygen tubing • nipple adapter and oxygen flowmeter. Optional: positive end-expiratory pressure valve, oxygen accumulator.

Unless the patient is intubated or has a tracheostomy, select a mask that fits snugly over the mouth and nose, and attach it to the bag.

If oxygen is readily available, connect the hand-held resuscitation bag to the oxygen. Attach one end of the tubing to the bottom of the bag and the other end to the nipple adapter on the flowmeter of the oxygen source. Turn on the oxygen, and adjust the flow rate to the patient's condition. If necessary, use an oxygen accumulator to increase the oxygen concentration.

Set up suction equipment if time allows.

Implementation

• Before using the hand-held resuscitation bag, make sure the patient's upper airway is free of foreign objects. Suction the patient to remove any secretions that may obstruct the airway. If necessary, insert an oropharyngeal or nasopharyngeal airway to maintain airway patency. If the patient has a tracheostomy or endotracheal tube in place, suction the tube.

• If appropriate, remove the bed's headboard, and stand at the head of the bed to help keep the patient's neck extended and to free space at the side of the bed for other activities, such as cardiopulmonary resuscitation.

• Tilt the patient's head backward, if not contraindicated, and pull his jaw forward to move the tongue away from the base of the pharynx and prevent obstruction of the airway.

• Keeping your nondominant hand on the mask, press downward to seal the mask against the face. For an adult patient, use your dominant hand to compress the bag every 5 seconds to deliver about 1 liter of air. For a child, compress it every 4 seconds (15 breaths/minute); for an infant, compress it every 3 seconds (20 breaths/minute). Infants and children should receive 250 to 500 cc of air in each breath.

• Deliver breaths with the patient's own inspiratory effort, if any is present. Don't attempt to deliver a breath as the patient exhales.

• Observe the patient's chest to ensure that it rises and falls with each compression. If ventilation fails to occur, check the fit of the mask and the patency of the patient's airway; if necessary, reposition the patient's head and insert an oral airway.

Special considerations

• Avoid neck hyperextension if the patient has a possible cervical injury; instead, use the jaw-thrust technique to open the airway. If you need both hands to keep the patient's mask in place and maintain hyperextension, use your lower arm to compress the bag against your side.

• Watch through the clear part of the mask for vomiting. If it occurs, stop immediately, lift the mask, wipe and suction, and resume compressions.

• Underventilation commonly occurs because the bag is difficult to keep tightly on the patient's face

while ensuring an open airway. What's more, the volume of air delivered to the patient varies with the type of bag used and the hand size of the person compressing the bag. An adult with a small or medium-sized hand may not consistently deliver 1 liter of air. For these reasons, have someone assist with the procedure, if possible.

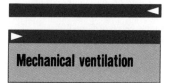

Mechanical ventilation

A mechanical ventilator moves air in and out of a patient's lungs. It does not ensure adequate gas exchange. Positive-pressure ventilators exert positive pressure on the airway, which causes inspiration and, at the same time, increases the patient's tidal volume. Negative-pressure ventilators create negative pressure, which pulls the patient's thorax outward and allows air to flow into the lungs.

Equipment and preparation

• Oxygen source • air source that can supply a 50-psi mechanical ventilator • humidifier • ventilator circuit tubing, connectors, and adapters • condensation collection trap • spirometer, respirometer, or electronic device to measure flow and volume • in-line thermometer • probe for gas sampling and measuring airway pressure • bacterial filter • gloves • hand-held resuscitation bag with reservoir • suction equipment • sterile distilled water • equipment for arterial blood gas (ABG) analysis • soft restraints, if indicated.

In most hospitals, a respiratory therapist sets up the ventilator. In most cases, you'll need to add sterile distilled water to the humidifier and connect the ventilator to the gas source.

Implementation

• Verify the doctor's order for ventilator support. Prepare for intubation, if necessary.
• Explain the procedure to the patient and his family to ease anxiety.
• Perform a physical assessment, and draw blood for ABG analysis to find a baseline.
• Suction the patient, if necessary.
• Plug in the ventilator, adjust the settings, make sure alarms are set, and fill the humidifier with sterile distilled water.
• Put on gloves. Connect the endotracheal tube to the ventilator. Observe for chest expansion, and auscultate for bilateral breath sounds to verify that the patient is being ventilated.
• To assess adequate ventilation and to avoid oxygen toxicity, monitor the patient's ABG values after completing initial ventilator setup (usually 20 to 30 minutes later), after changing ventilator settings, and as the patient's clinical condition indicates. Be prepared to adjust ventilator settings, depending on ABG values.
• Check the ventilator tubing frequently for condensation, which can cause resistance to airflow and be aspirated by the patient. As needed, drain condensate into a collection trap, or briefly disconnect the patient from the ventilator (ventilating him with a hand-held resuscitation bag if necessary) and empty the water. Do not drain condensate into the humidifier because it may be contaminated.
• Check the in-line thermometer to see that delivered air is near body temperature.
• Monitor vital signs and pulse oximetry; count spontaneous breaths and ventilator-delivered breaths.
• To reduce the risk of contamination, change, clean, or dispose of ventilator tubing and equipment according to hospital policy. Typically, ventilator tubing should be changed every 24 to 48 hours, sometimes more often.
• As ordered, wean the patient.

Special considerations

• Ventilator alarms should always be on.
• Provide emotional support during all phases of ventilation to ease anxiety. Explain procedures even if the patient is unresponsive.
• Unless contraindicated, turn the patient every 1 to 2 hours, perform active or passive range-of-motion exercises, and place him upright regularly.
• Assess peripheral circulation, and watch for fluid volume excess or dehydration.
• Place the call light within the patient's reach, and find a way to communicate because the patient will have difficulty speaking.
• Administer a neuromuscular blocker and sedative, as ordered, to relax the patient or eliminate breathing efforts. Observe closely.
• Ensure that the patient gets adequate rest because fatigue can delay weaning.
• When weaning, observe for signs of hypoxia. Schedule weaning around the patient's routine.

Nasogastric tube insertion

Usually inserted to decompress the stomach, a nasogastric (NG) tube can prevent vomiting after surgery until peristalsis resumes. It may also be used to assess and treat upper GI bleeding, aspirate gastric secretions, perform gastric lavage, and administer medications and nutrients.

Equipment and preparation
• Tube (usually #14, #16, or #18 French for an adult) • towel or linen-saver pad • facial tissues • emesis basin • penlight • 1″ or 2″ hypoallergenic tape • gloves • water-soluble lubricant • cup of water with straw • stethoscope • catheter-tip or bulb syringe or irrigation set • ordered suction equipment.

Inspect the NG tube for defects and for patency by flushing it with water.

To ease insertion, increase a stiff tube's flexibility by coiling it around your gloved fingers or by dipping it into warm water. Stiffen a limp tube by chilling it in ice.

Implementation
• Provide privacy. Wash and glove your hands. Explain the procedure, and emphasize that swallowing will ease the tube's advancement.
• Help the patient into high Fowler's position unless contraindicated. Stand at the patient's right side if you're right-handed or at her left side if you're left-handed.
• Drape the towel or linen-saver pad over the patient's chest to protect against spills. Have the patient gently blow his nose to clear his nostrils.
• Place the facial tissues and emesis basin within the patient's reach. Help the patient face forward with his neck in a neutral position.
• To determine how long the tube must be to reach the stomach, hold the end of it at the tip of the patient's nose. Extend the tube to the earlobe and down to the xiphoid process. Mark this distance on the tube with tape.
• Use a penlight to inspect each nostril for a deviated septum or other abnormalities. Ask the patient

if he has ever had a nasal injury or nasal surgery. Assess airflow in both nostrils and choose the nostril with the better airflow.
• Lubricate the first 3″ (8 cm) of the tube with a water-soluble lubricant. Instruct the patient to hold his head straight and upright.
• Grasp the tube with the end pointing downward and insert it into the more patent nostril. Aim downward and toward the ear closer to the chosen nostril. When the tube reaches the nasopharynx, you'll feel resistance. Instruct the patient to lower his head slightly to close the trachea and open the esophagus.
• Rotate the tube 180 degrees toward the opposite nostril.
• Unless contraindicated, direct the patient to sip water from a straw and swallow as you slowly advance the tube. Watch for signs of respiratory distress, which may mean that the tube is in the bronchus and must be removed immediately.
• Stop advancing the tube when the tape mark reaches the patient's nostril.
• Examine his mouth and throat for a coiled section of tubing, which indicates an obstruction.
• Attach a catheter-tip or bulb syringe to the tube, and try to aspirate stomach contents. If unsuccessful, position the patient on the left side and aspirate again. If you still can't aspirate stomach contents, advance the tube 1″ or 2″ (2.5 to 5 cm). Inject 10 cc of air into the tube while you auscultate for air sounds over the epigastric region. If these tests don't confirm tube placement, you'll need X-ray verification.
• Secure the NG tube to the patient's nose with hypoallergenic tape or a designated tube holder. If using tape, you will need 4″ (10 cm) of 1″ tape. Split one end of the tape up the center about 1½″ (4 cm).

Make tabs on the split ends (by folding sticky sides together). Stick the uncut tape end on the patient's nose so that the split in the tape starts about ½″ (1 cm) to 1½″ from the tip of the nose. Crisscross the tabbed ends around the tube. Apply another piece of tape over the bridge of the nose to secure.
• To reduce discomfort from the weight of the tube, tie a slip knot around the tube with a rubber band or wrap a piece of tape around the end of the tube and leave a tab. Fasten the tape tab or rubber band to the patient's gown with a safety pin.
• Attach the tube to suction equipment, if ordered, and set the designated suction pressure.

Special considerations
• If the patient has a condition that prevents nasal insertion, pass the tube orally after removing any dentures. Sliding the tube over the tongue, proceed as you would for nasal insertion.
• When confirming placement, never place the tube's end in a container of water. If the tube is in the trachea, the patient may aspirate water.
• If the patient is unconscious, tilt his chin toward his chest to close the trachea. Then advance the tube between respirations to ensure that it doesn't enter the trachea. While advancing the tube, stroke the patient's neck to encourage swallowing and facilitate passage down the esophagus.
• Irrigate the NG tube attached to suction with 20 to 30 ml of saline solution to ensure patency.
• Vomiting after tube placement suggests tubal obstruction or incorrect position. Assess immediately to determine the cause.

Oxygen administration, adult

A patient needs oxygen therapy when hypoxemia results from a respiratory or cardiac emergency or from increased or impaired metabolic function.

Equipment and preparation
The equipment needed depends on the type of delivery system ordered and includes selections from the following list: • oxygen source (wall unit, cylinder, liquid tank, or concentrator) • flowmeter • adapter, if using a wall unit, or a pressure-reduction gauge, if using a cylinder • sterile humidity bottle and adapters • OXYGEN PRECAUTION and NO SMOKING signs • sterile distilled water • appropriate oxygen delivery system (nasal cannula, simple mask, partial rebreather mask, nonrebreather mask, Venturi mask, aerosol mask, tracheostomy collar, T-tube, tent, or oxygen hood) • small- and large-diameter connection tubing • jet adapter for Venturi mask (if adding humidity).

Although a respiratory therapist typically sets up, maintains, and manages the equipment, you need a working knowledge of the oxygen system being used.

Check the oxygen outlet port to verify flow.

Implementation
• Assess the patient's condition. Obtain baseline vital signs and laboratory data to support findings. In an emergency, verify that the patient has an open airway.
• Explain the procedure to the patient, and let him know why he needs oxygen.
• Check the patient's room to make sure it's safe for oxygen administra-

tion. Whenever possible, replace electrical devices with nonelectrical ones, and post a NO SMOKING sign. If the patient smokes, make sure that all cigarettes and matches are removed. Oxygen supports combustion, and the smallest spark can cause a fire.
• Place an OXYGEN PRECAUTION sign over the patient's bed and on the door to his room.
• Help place the oxygen delivery device on the patient. Make sure it fits properly and is stable.
• Monitor the patient's response to oxygen therapy. Check his arterial blood gas (ABG) values during initial adjustments of oxygen flow. After the patient is stabilized, pulse oximetry may be used instead. Check the patient frequently for signs of hypoxia, such as decreased level of consciousness, increased heart rate, arrhythmias, restlessness, perspiration, dyspnea, use of accessory muscles, yawning or flared nostrils, and cyanosis.
• Observe the patient's skin integrity to prevent skin breakdown on pressure points from the oxygen delivery device. Wipe moisture from the patient's face and the mask, as needed.
• If the patient will be receiving oxygen at a concentration above 60% for more than 24 hours, watch for signs of oxygen toxicity. Remind the patient to cough and deep-breathe to prevent atelectasis. Measure ABG values repeatedly to determine whether high oxygen concentrations are still necessary.

Special considerations
• Never administer oxygen at more than 2 liters/minute by nasal cannula to a patient with chronic lung disease, unless otherwise ordered. This is because some patients with chronic lung disease have become dependent on a state of hypercapnia and hypoxia to stimulate respi-

rations; supplemental oxygen could cause them to stop breathing.
• When monitoring a patient's response to a change in oxygen flow, check the pulse oximetry monitor or measure ABG values 20 to 30 minutes after adjusting the flow.

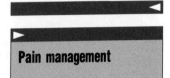

Pain management

To assess and manage pain, the nurse must depend on the patient's subjective description in addition to objective tools. The goal of pain management is to keep the pain at a level acceptable to the patient.

Equipment
• Oral hygiene supplies • water
• nonnarcotic analgesic (such as aspirin or acetaminophen). Optional: patient-controlled analgesia (PCA) device, mild narcotic (such as oxycodone or codeine), strong narcotic (such as levorphanol, meperidine, morphine, fentanyl, or hydromorphone).

Implementation
• Explain to the patient how pain medications work with other pain management therapies to provide relief.
• Ask the patient to describe the duration, severity, and source of pain. Observe the patient for physiologic or behavioral clues to the pain's severity.
• Use the nursing process to provide patient care.

To give medications
• If the patient is allowed oral intake, begin with a nonnarcotic analgesic every 4 to 6 hours, as ordered. If the patient needs more relief, administer a mild narcotic, as ordered.

• If he needs still more relief, administer a strong narcotic (orally, if possible), as ordered. Teach the patient to use a PCA device, if ordered.
• In PCA, the patient controls I.V. delivery of an analgesic (usually morphine) by pressing the button on a delivery device. This provides analgesia at the level the patient needs and when he needs it. The device prevents accidental overdosing by imposing a lockout time between doses—usually 6 to 10 minutes—during which the patient receives no analgesic, even if he pushes the button.
• To receive PCA therapy, a patient must be able to understand and comply with instructions and procedures, and have no history of allergy to the analgesic. PCA is contraindicated in patients with limited respiratory reserve, a history of drug abuse or chronic sedative or tranquilizer use, or a psychiatric disorder.
• During PCA therapy, monitor and record the amount of analgesic infused and the patient's respiratory rate. Also, check for infiltration into subcutaneous tissues and for catheter occlusion, which may cause the drug to back up in the primary I.V. tubing. If the analgesic nauseates your patient, you may need to administer an antiemetic drug.

To provide emotional support
• Spend time talking with the patient. Because of his pain, he may be anxious and frustrated. Such feelings exacerbate pain.

To perform comfort measures
• Periodically reposition the patient to reduce muscle spasms and tension. Support his body in a neutral position with the aid of pillows.
• Give the patient a back massage to help relax tense muscles. Perform passive range-of-motion exer-

cises. Provide for adequate sleep.
• Provide oral hygiene. Many medications tend to dry the mouth.

To use cognitive therapy
• Help the patient enhance the effect of analgesics by using distraction, guided imagery, deep breathing, and relaxation. Start these techniques when the patient feels little or no pain. Or, if he feels persistent pain, begin with short, simple exercises.

Special considerations
Evaluate your patient's response to pain management. If he's still in pain, reassess him and alter your plan of care as appropriate. Less medication is often required to achieve pain relief if analgesics are given before, rather than after, the onset of severe pain. Using an around-the-clock or fixed schedule is often effective with trauma, postoperative, and cancer patients.

AGE ALERT Be aware that an elderly patient's pain may be difficult to assess because he may have cognitive impairment and be fearful of possible adverse effects.

Passive range-of-motion exercises

Used to move the patient's joints through as full a range of motion (ROM) as possible, passive ROM exercises improve or maintain joint mobility and help prevent contractures. These exercises are indicated for the patient with temporary or permanent loss of mobility, sensation, or consciousness. Passive ROM exercises require recognition of the patient's limits of motion and support of all joints during movement.

BEDSIDE CARE

Implementation

Determine the joints that need ROM exercises, and consult the doctor or physical therapist about limitations or precautions for specific exercises. Perform all exercises slowly, gently, and to the end of normal range of motion or to the point of pain, but no further.

Raise the bed to a comfortable working height.

To exercise the neck

• Support the patient's head with your hands and extend his neck, flex his chin to the chest, and tilt his head laterally toward each shoulder.
• Rotate his head from right to left.

To exercise the shoulder

• Support the patient's arm in an extended, neutral position; then extend his forearm and flex it back. Abduct his arm outward from the side of his body, as shown below, and adduct it back to his side.

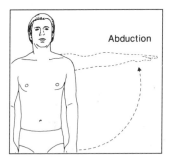

Abduction

• Rotate the shoulder so that his arm crosses the midline, and bend his elbow so that his hand touches his opposite shoulder, then touches the mattress for complete internal rotation.
• Return his shoulder to a neutral position and, with his elbow bent, push his arm backward so that the back of his hand touches the mattress for complete external rotation.

To exercise the elbow

• Place the patient's arm at his side, palm upward. Flex and extend his arm at the elbow.

To exercise the forearm

• Twist his hand to bring the palm up (supination); then twist it back to bring the palm down (pronation), as shown below.

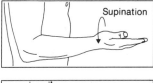

Supination

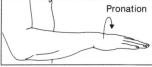

Pronation

To exercise the wrist

• Stabilize his forearm and flex and extend his wrist, as shown below.

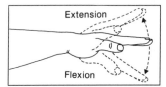

Extension

Flexion

• Rock his hand sideways for lateral flexion, and rotate his hand in a circular motion.

To exercise the fingers and thumb

• Extend the patient's fingers, and then flex his hand into a fist; repeat extension and flexion of each joint of each finger and thumb separately.
• Spread two adjoining fingers apart (abduction), and then bring them together (adduction).
• Oppose each fingertip to his thumb, and rotate his thumb and each finger in a circle.

To exercise the hip and knee

• Fully extend the patient's leg, and then bend his hip and knee toward his chest, allowing full joint flexion.
• Next, move his straight leg sideways, out and away from the other leg (abduction), and then back, over, and across it (adduction).
• Rotate his straight leg internally toward the midline, and then externally away from the midline.

To exercise the ankle

• Bend the patient's foot so that his toes point upward (dorsiflexion); then bend his foot so that his toes point downward (plantar flexion), as shown below.

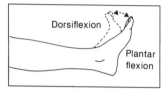

Dorsiflexion

Plantar flexion

• Rotate his ankle in a circular motion.
• Invert his ankle so that the sole of his foot faces the midline, and evert his ankle so that the sole faces away from the midline.

To exercise the toes

• Flex the patient's toes toward the sole of his foot, and then extend them back toward the top of his foot.
• Spread two adjoining toes apart (abduction), and bring them together (adduction).

Special considerations

Joints begin to stiffen within 24 hours of disuse, so start passive ROM exercises as soon as possible, and perform them at least once a shift. Repeat each exercise at least three times.

Peripheral line insertion

This procedure involves selecting a venipuncture device and insertion site, applying a tourniquet, preparing the site, and performing the venipuncture. Common insertion sites include the cephalic and basilic veins in the lower arm and the veins in the dorsum of the hand.

Equipment and preparation

Alcohol sponges • povidone-iodine sponges • antimicrobial ointment • gloves • tourniquet • two I.V. needles or I.V. catheter devices • sterile 2″ × 2″ gauze pads or a transparent semipermeable dressing • 1″ hypoallergenic tape • I.V. solution with attached and primed administration set • I.V. pole. Optional: armboard, roller gauze, warm packs, antimicrobial solution, local anesthetic, U-100 insulin syringe with 27G needle.

Select the smallest gauge needle or catheter device available for the infusion unless subsequent therapy will require a larger one. If you're using a winged infusion set, connect the adapter to the administration set, and prime the needle with fluid. Then place the needle on a sterile surface. If you're using a catheter device, open the package.

Implementation

• Hang the I.V. solution with attached primed administration set on the I.V. pole near the patient's bed. Wash your hands, and explain the procedure to the patient.
• Choose a small vein unless a large vein will be needed for subsequent therapy. Start with a vein at the most distal site so that you can

move proximally for subsequent I.V. infusions. For infusion of an irritating medication, choose a large vein distal to any nearby joint.

• Place the patient's arm in a dependent position to increase capillary fill. If necessary, warm the skin by rubbing, or cover the arm with warm packs for 5 to 10 minutes.

• Apply a tourniquet about 6″ (15 cm) above the intended puncture site. Check for a distal pulse. If it is not present, release the tourniquet, and reapply it with less tension.

• Palpate the vein with your index and middle fingers, while stretching it to prevent rolling.

• If necessary, raise the vein further by flicking the skin over the vein, placing the extremity in a dependent position for several seconds and rubbing the skin upward toward the tourniquet. Or tell the patient to open and close his fist several times.

• Leave the tourniquet in place for no more than 2 minutes.

• Put on gloves. Clip the hair around the insertion site, if necessary, and clean the site with an antimicrobial solution. Using a circular motion, work outward 2″ to 4″ (5 to 10 cm). Allow the antimicrobial solution to dry. If ordered, administer a local anesthetic.

• Grasp the needle or catheter. If you're using a winged infusion set, hold the short edges of the wings (with the needle's bevel facing upward) between the thumb and forefinger of your dominant hand. Squeeze the wings together. If using an over-the-needle catheter, grasp the plastic hub with your dominant hand, remove the cover, and examine the catheter tip. If the edge isn't smooth, replace the device.

• If using a through-the-needle

catheter, grasp the needle hub with one hand, and unsnap the needle cover. Rotate it until the bevel faces upward.

• Using the thumb of your opposite hand, stretch the skin taut below the puncture site to stabilize the vein.

• Lightly press the vein with your thumb about 1½″ (4 cm) from the intended insertion site.

• For the direct approach, hold the needle bevel up and enter the skin over the vein at a 30- to 45-degree angle. For the indirect approach, enter the skin slightly adjacent to the vein. Direct the device into the side of the vein wall.

• Advance the device until you meet resistance. Lower the needle to a 15- to 20-degree angle and slowly pierce the vein, as shown below.

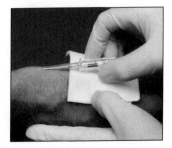

When you observe blood backflow behind the hub, tilt the needle slightly upward and advance it farther into the vein.

• If you're using a winged infusion set, advance the needle fully, if possible, and hold it in place. Release the tourniquet, open the administration set clamp slightly, and check for free flow or infiltration.

• If using an over-the-needle catheter, advance the device to at least half of its length. Then remove the tourniquet.

• Grasp the catheter hub and withdraw the needle while pressing lightly on the catheter tip to prevent bleeding, as shown below.

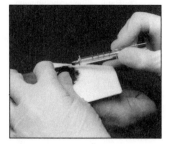

• Advance the catheter up to the hub or until you meet resistance.
• To advance the catheter while infusing I.V. solution, release the tourniquet, and remove the inner needle. Attach the I.V. tubing and begin the infusion. While stabilizing the vein with one hand, use the other hand to advance the catheter. Then decrease the I.V. flow rate.
• To advance the catheter before starting the infusion, first release the tourniquet. While stabilizing the vein with one hand, use the other to advance the catheter up to the hub. Remove the inner needle, and attach the I.V. tubing.
• If using a through-the-needle catheter, remove the tourniquet, hold the needle in place with one hand, and, with the other, grasp the catheter through the protective sleeve. Thread the catheter through the needle until the hub is within the needle collar. Never pull back on the catheter without pulling back on the needle to avoid severing and releasing the catheter into the circulation.
• If you feel resistance, withdraw the catheter and needle slightly and reinsert them, rotating the catheter as you pass the valve. Then withdraw the metal needle and cover it with the protector. Remove the stylet and protective sleeve, and attach the administration set to the catheter hub. Open the administration

set clamp slightly, and check for free flow or infiltration.
• Apply a transparent semipermeable dressing to secure the device. Or apply antiseptic ointment at the insertion site and cover it with a sterile gauze pad or small adhesive bandage.
• Loop the I.V. tubing on the patient's limb, and secure with tape. Label the last piece of tape with the type and gauge of needle or catheter, the date and time of insertion, and your initials. Adjust the flow rate, as ordered.
• If the puncture site is near a movable joint, secure the armboard with roller gauze or tape to provide stability.

Special considerations
• Change a gauze or transparent dressing when you change the administration set.
• Rotate the I.V. site every 48 to 72 hours or according to your hospital policy.

Peripheral line maintenance

Routine maintenance of I.V. sites and systems includes regular assessment and rotation of the site and periodic changes of the dressing, tubing, and solution. Typically, I.V. dressings are changed every 48 hours or whenever the dressing becomes wet, soiled, or nonocclusive. I.V. tubing is changed every 48 to 72 hours or according to hospital policy, and I.V. solution is changed every 24 hours or as needed. Assess the site every 2 hours if a transparent semipermeable dressing is used (otherwise with every dressing change), and rotate it every 48 to 72 hours.

BEDSIDE CARE

Equipment and preparation
For dressing changes
• Sterile gloves • povidone-iodine or alcohol sponges • povidone-iodine or other antimicrobial ointment, according to hospital policy • adhesive bandage, sterile 2″ × 2″ gauze pad, or transparent semipermeable dressing • 1″ adhesive tape.

For solution changes
• Solution container • alcohol sponge.

For tubing changes
• I.V. administration set • sterile 2″ × 2″ gauze pad • adhesive tape for labeling • sterile gloves. Optional: hemostats.

Commercial kits containing the equipment for dressing changes are available.

If your hospital keeps I.V. equipment and dressings in a tray or cart, have it nearby, if possible, because you may have to use a new venipuncture site, depending on the current site's condition.

If you're changing the solution and tubing, attach and prime the I.V. administration set before entering the patient's room.

Implementation
Wash your hands, and wear sterile gloves when working near the venipuncture site.

Explain the procedure to the patient to allay his fears and ensure cooperation.

To change the dressing
• Remove the old dressing, open all supply packages, and put on sterile gloves.
• Hold the needle or catheter in place with your nondominant hand to prevent accidental movement or dislodgement, which could puncture the vein and cause infiltration.
• Assess the site for signs of infection, infiltration, and thrombophle-

bitis. If any of these is present, apply pressure to the area with a sterile 2″ × 2″ gauze pad, and remove the catheter or needle. Maintain pressure on the area until the bleeding stops, and apply an adhesive bandage. Start the I.V. in another site (preferably the other extremity) using fresh equipment and solution.
• If the venipuncture site is intact, hold the needle or catheter, and carefully clean around it with a povidone-iodine or alcohol sponge. Work in a circular motion outward from the site to avoid introducing bacteria into the clean area. Allow the area to dry completely.
• Apply povidone-iodine or other antimicrobial ointment, and cover with an adhesive bandage or sterile 2″ × 2″ gauze pad and retape. When using a transparent semipermeable dressing, you may omit the povidone-iodine ointment. The transparent dressing allows visualization of the site. It maintains sterility and is placed over the site to halfway up the catheter or needle hub.

To change the solution
• Wash your hands. Inspect the new solution container for cracks, leaks, and other damage. Check the solution for discoloration, turbidity, and particulates. Note the date and time the solution was mixed and its expiration date.
• Clamp the tubing when inverting it to prevent air from entering the tubing. Keep the drip chamber half full.
• If you're replacing a bag, remove the seal or tab from the new bag, and remove the old bag from the pole. Remove the spike, insert it into the new bag, and adjust the flow rate.
• If you're replacing a bottle, remove the cap and seal from the new bottle and wipe the rubber port with

an alcohol sponge. Clamp the line, remove the spike from the old bottle, and insert the spike into the new bottle. Then hang the new bottle, and adjust the flow rate.

To change tubing
• Reduce the I.V. flow rate, remove the old spike from the container, and hang it on the I.V. pole. Place the cover of the new spike loosely over the old one.
• Keeping the old spike in an upright position above the patient's heart level, insert the new spike into the I.V. container.
• Prime the system. Hang the new I.V. container and primed set on the pole, and grasp the new adapter in one hand. Then stop the flow rate in the old tubing.
• Put on sterile gloves.
• Place a sterile gauze pad under the needle or catheter hub to create a sterile field. Press one of your fingers over the catheter to prevent bleeding, as shown below.

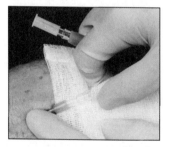

• Gently disconnect the old tubing, being careful not to dislodge or move the I.V. device. (If you have trouble disconnecting the old tubing, use a hemostat to hold the hub securely while twisting the tubing to remove it. Or use one hemostat on the venipuncture device and another on the hard plastic end of the tubing. Don't clamp the hemostats shut; this may crack the tubing adapter or the venipuncture device.)

• Remove the protective cap from the new tubing, and connect the new adapter to the needle or catheter. Hold the hub securely to prevent dislodging the needle or catheter tip, as shown below.

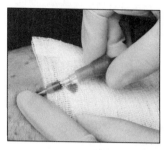

• Observe for blood backflow into the new tubing to verify that the needle or catheter is still in place. (You may not be able to do this with small-gauge catheters.)
• Adjust the clamp to maintain the flow rate.
• Retape and recheck the flow rate because taping may alter it.
• Label the tubing and container with the date and time, and the solution with a time strip.

Special considerations
• Check the prescribed I.V. flow rate before each solution change to prevent errors. If you crack the adapter or hub (or if you accidentally dislodge the needle or catheter from the vein), remove it. Apply pressure and an adhesive bandage to stop bleeding. Perform a venipuncture at another site, and restart the I.V. infusion.
• Flow rates may change 20% to 40% during an infusion. If you're not using an infusion pump, check the flow rate every hour.

BEDSIDE CARE

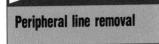

Peripheral line removal

Peripheral I.V. lines need to be removed after the completion of therapy, for needle or catheter changes, and for suspected infection or infiltration.

Equipment
• Alcohol sponges • sterile gauze pad • antiseptic ointment • adhesive bandage.

Implementation
• To remove the I.V. line, first clamp the I.V. tubing to stop the flow of solution. Then gently remove all tape from the skin.
• Using aseptic technique, open the gauze pad and adhesive bandage, and place them within reach. Put on gloves.
• Hold the sterile gauze pad over the puncture site, and use your other hand to withdraw the needle or catheter slowly and smoothly, keeping it parallel to the skin.
• With the gauze pad, apply firm pressure over the puncture site for 1 or 2 minutes after the device has been removed or until bleeding has stopped.
• Clean the site, and apply the adhesive bandage. Or if blood oozes from the site, apply a pressure bandage.
• If drainage appears at the puncture site, send the tip of the device and a sample of the drainage to the laboratory to be cultured according to hospital policy. (A draining site may or may not be infected.)
• Clean the area, and apply antiseptic ointment and a sterile dressing.
• Place the needle or catheter in a puncture-resistant container. Be sure to avoid recapping the needle. Remove and discard gloves.
• Instruct the patient to restrict activity for about 10 minutes and leave the dressing in place for at least 8 hours. Periodically return and inspect the site for bleeding or bruising. If the patient feels lingering tenderness at the site, apply warm packs.

Special considerations
• Upon removal of the I.V. line, inspect the catheter tip. If it's not smooth, assess the patient immediately, and notify the doctor.
• Also check the length of the catheter, comparing it to the length of the catheter when it was inserted, to assess for catheter breakage.

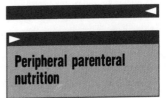

Peripheral parenteral nutrition

Using a solution that combines amino acids, dextrose in water, and a lipid emulsion, peripheral parenteral nutrition (PPN) can satisfy caloric needs without the risks associated with a central venous line. It's used to maintain or restore fluid and electrolyte balance, to maintain homeostasis before and after surgery, and to help a patient meet minimum calorie and protein requirements. PPN also may be used as an adjunct to oral or enteral feedings for a patient who needs to supplement his low-calorie intake. Alternately, it can be given to a patient who is unable to absorb enteral therapy.

Equipment and preparation
• Amino acid–dextrose solution at room temperature (dextrose should not exceed 12.5%) • lipid emulsion • two controllers • Y-type non-phthalate administration set • alcohol sponges • I.V. pole and veni-

puncture equipment, if necessary
• sterile gloves.

Inspect the lipid emulsion. If it looks frothy or oily, contains particles, or is of questionable stability or sterility, return it to the pharmacy. Avoid shaking the bottle. Inspect the amino acid–dextrose solution for cloudiness, turbidity, and particles, and the bottle for cracks; if any of these is present, return the bottle to the pharmacy.

Using aseptic technique, close the flow clamp on the nonphthalate tubing. Remove the cap from the lipid bottle, and wipe the stopper with an alcohol sponge. Hold the bottle upright, and insert the vented spike. Invert the bottle, and squeeze the drip chamber until it fills to the desired level. Open the flow clamp, allow fluid to flow to the Y-connector, and close the clamp.

Remove the cap from the amino acid–dextrose solution, and wipe the stopper with an alcohol sponge. Hold the bottle upright, and insert the nonvented spike. Squeeze the drip chamber to eliminate dripping, invert the bottle, and squeeze the drip chamber until fluid reaches the desired level. With the Y-connector facing upward and the air vent downward, open the clamp. Purge the filter and line, and close the clamp.

Hang the lipid emulsion higher than the amino acid–dextrose so that the lipid emulsion doesn't flow back into the amino acid set. Attach the controllers to the I.V. pole, and prepare according to manufacturer's instructions.

Implementation

Explain the procedure to the patient.

If necessary, perform a venipuncture, selecting the largest available vein.

To start the infusion

• Connect the administration set to the I.V. needle or catheter hub. Turn on the controllers and set them to the desired flow rate. Open the flow clamps to allow the controllers to regulate flow.
• Monitor vital signs every 10 minutes for the first 30 minutes and every hour thereafter.

To change the solutions

• Remove the protective caps, and wipe the stoppers with alcohol sponges. Turn off the controllers, and close the flow clamps. Using strict aseptic technique, remove each spike, and insert it in the new container.
• Hang the containers, turn on the controllers, and set the flow rate. Open the flow clamps.

To change the solutions and tubing

• Hang the new solution container and tubing alongside the old ones. Put on sterile gloves.
• Examine the skin above the insertion site for signs of phlebitis. If present, start a new line.
• Turn off the controllers, and close the flow clamps on the old tubing. Disconnect the tubing from the needle or catheter hub, and connect the new tubing. Open the flow clamps on the new containers to equal slow flow rates.
• Replace the old tubing in the controllers with the new tubing. Turn on the controllers, set them to the desired flow rate, and open the flow clamps.

To change a dressing and needle or catheter

• Change the dressing according to hospital policy, and inspect the site for signs of phlebitis. Change the catheter according to hospital policy or at the onset of signs of phlebitis.

Special considerations
• Never reuse a partially empty bottle of lipid emulsion. All bottles, bags, tubing, and filters should be changed every 24 hours.
• Because lipase synthesis increases insulin requirements, increase the insulin dosage of the patient with diabetes, as ordered. For the patient with hypothyroidism, administer thyroid-stimulating hormone — which affects lipase activity — as ordered, to prevent intravascular accumulations of triglycerides.
• Observe the patient's reaction to the lipid emulsion. Because of possible hypersensitivity reactions, the lipid emulsion infusion should be started at no more than 20 ml/hour. Check serum triglyceride levels; these should return to normal within 18 hours after infusion of a bottle of lipid emulsion.

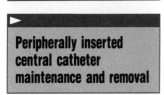

Peripherally inserted central catheter maintenance and removal

For a patient who needs central venous (CV) therapy for 5 days to several months or who requires repeated venous access, a peripherally inserted central catheter (PICC) line may be the best option. The doctor may order a PICC line if your patient has suffered trauma or burns resulting in chest injury or if he has respiratory compromise resulting from chronic obstructive pulmonary disease, a mediastinal mass, cystic fibrosis, or pneumothorax. With any of these conditions, a PICC line helps avoid complications that may occur with a CV line.

Made of silicone or polyurethane, a PICC is soft and flexible, with increased biocompatibility. It may range from 16G to 23G in diameter and from 16″ to 24″ (40.5 to 61 cm) in length. PICCs are available in single- and double-lumen versions, with or without guide wires. A guide wire stiffens the catheter, easing its advancement through the vein, but it can damage the vessel if used improperly.

A PICC line is used increasingly for patients receiving home care. The device is easier to insert than other CV devices and provides safe, reliable access for drugs and blood sampling. A single catheter may be used for the entire course of therapy (approximately 1 to 140 days), with greater convenience and at reduced cost.

Infusions commonly given by PICC include total parenteral nutrition, chemotherapy, antibiotics, narcotics, analgesics, and blood products. PICC therapy works best when introduced early in treatment; it shouldn't be considered a last resort for patients with sclerotic or repeatedly punctured veins.

The patient receiving PICC therapy must have a peripheral vein large enough to accept a 14G or 16G introducer needle and a 3.8G to 4.8G catheter. The doctor or a specially trained nurse inserts the PICC via the basilic, median basilic, or cephalic veins. He then threads it to the superior vena cava or subclavian vein, as shown opposite, or to a noncentral site, such as the axillary vein.

PICC therapy causes fewer and less severe complications than conventionally placed CV lines. Phlebitis, perhaps the most common complication, may occur during the first 48 to 72 hours after PICC insertion. It's more common in left-sided insertions and when a large-gauge catheter is used. Air embolism, always a potential risk of venipuncture, poses less danger in PICC therapy than in traditional CV lines because the line is inserted below heart level.

Some patients complain of pain at the catheter insertion site, usually from chemical properties of the infused drug or fluid.

Catheter tip migration may occur with vigorous flushing. Patients receiving chemotherapy are most vulnerable to this complication because of frequent nausea and vomiting and subsequent changes in intrathoracic pressure.

Catheter occlusion is a relatively common complication.

Equipment

• Normal saline solution • clamp • prescribed drug • dressings • tape • sterile gloves • sterile mask • alcohol swabs • povidone-iodine swabs and ointment • linen-saver pad • sterile gauze pads • clean gloves.

Implementation

• Explain the procedure to the patient and answer any questions.

To administer drugs

• As with any CV line, be sure to check for blood return and flush with normal saline solution before administering a drug through a PICC line.

• Clamp the 7″ (17.5 cm) extension tubing, and connect the empty syringe to the tubing. Release the clamp and aspirate slowly to verify blood return. Flush with 3 ml of normal saline solution; then administer the drug.

• After giving the drug, flush again with 3 ml of normal saline solution. (And remember to flush with the same solution between infusions of incompatible drugs or fluids.)

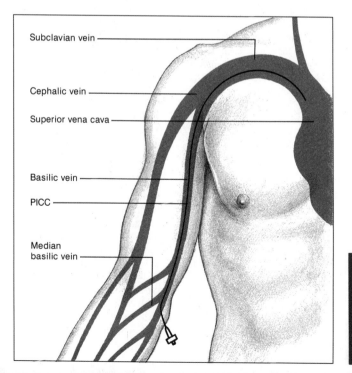

Subclavian vein

Cephalic vein

Superior vena cava

Basilic vein

PICC

Median basilic vein

To change the dressing

• Change the dressing every 4 days for an inpatient and every 5 to 7 days for a home care patient. If possible, choose a transparent semipermeable dressing, which has a high moisture-vapor transmission rate. Use aseptic technique.

• Wash your hands and assemble the necessary supplies. Position the patient with his arm extended away from the body at a 45- to 90-degree angle. Put on a sterile mask.

• Open a package of sterile gloves and use the inside of the package as a sterile field. Then open the transparent semipermeable dressing and drop it onto the field. Remove the old dressing by holding your left thumb on the catheter and stretching the dressing parallel to the skin. Repeat this last step with your right thumb holding the catheter. Free the remaining section of the dressing from the catheter by peeling toward the insertion site from the distal end to the proximal end to prevent catheter dislodgment.

• Put on the sterile gloves. Clean the area thoroughly with three alcohol swabs, starting at the insertion site and working outward from the site. Repeat this step three times with povidone-iodine swabs and pat dry.

• Apply the dressing carefully. Secure the tubing to the edge of the dressing over the tape with ¼″ adhesive tape.

To remove a PICC

• You'll remove a PICC when therapy is complete, if the catheter becomes damaged or broken and can't be repaired or, possibly, if the line becomes occluded. Measure the catheter after you remove it to ensure that the line has been removed intact and thus help prevent formation of emboli in the catheter.

• Assemble the necessary equipment at the patient's bedside.

• Explain the procedure to the patient. Wash your hands. Then place a linen-saver pad under the patient's arm.

• Remove the tape holding the extension tubing. Open two sterile gauze pads on a clean, flat surface. Put on clean gloves. Stabilize the catheter at the hub with one hand. Without dislodging the catheter, use your other hand to gently remove the dressing by pulling it toward the insertion site.

• Next, gently tug on the PICC. It should come out easily. If you feel resistance, apply tension to the line by taping it down. Then try removing it again in a few minutes.

• Once you successfully remove the catheter, apply manual pressure to the site with a sterile gauze pad for 1 minute.

• Cover the site with the povidone-iodine ointment, and tape a new folded gauze pad in place. Dispose of used items properly, and wash your hands.

• Measure and inspect the catheter. If any part has broken off during removal, notify the doctor immediately, and monitor the patient for signs of distress.

Special considerations

• Be aware that the doctor or a specially trained nurse probably will place the PICC in the superior vena cava if the patient will receive therapy in the hospital.

• For a hospital patient receiving intermittent PICC therapy, flush the catheter with 6 ml of normal saline solution and 6 ml of heparin (10 units/ml) after each use. For catheters that aren't being used, a weekly flush of 2 ml (1,000 units/ml) of heparin will maintain patency.

• You can use a declotting agent, such as urokinase, to clear a clotted PICC line, but make sure you read the manufacturer's recommendations first.

• Remember to add an extension set to all PICC lines so you can start and stop an infusion away from the insertion site. An extension set will also make using a PICC line easier for the patient who will be administering infusions himself. Use sterile tape or Steri-Strips to secure the hub and extension set away from the insertion site.

• If a patient will be receiving blood or blood products through the PICC line, you should use at least an 18G catheter.

• Assess the catheter insertion site through the transparent semipermeable dressing every 24 hours. Look at the catheter and check for any bleeding, redness, drainage, and swelling. Ask your patient if he's having any pain associated with therapy. Although bleeding is common for the first 24 hours after insertion, excessive bleeding after that period of time must be evaluated.

• Monitor the catheter length outside the body; document the measurement in the patient's chart and assess at least every 8 hours.

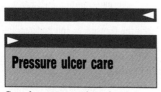

Pressure ulcer care

Care for pressure ulcers involves cleaning and dressing.

Equipment and preparation

• Hypoallergenic tape or elastic netting • overbed table • sterile irrigation set with bulb syringe • two pairs of gloves • 0.9% sodium chloride or other cleaning solution, as ordered • sterile 4″ × 4″ gauze pads • selected topical dressing • linen-saver pads • impervious plastic trash bag • disposable wound-measuring device • sterile cotton-

tipped applicators. Optional: skin sealant.

Assemble equipment. Cut tape into strips for securing dressings. Loosen existing dressing edges and tapes before putting on gloves. Attach an impervious plastic trash bag to the overbed table.

Implementation

Before any dressing change, wash your hands. Observe principles of universal precautions.

To clean the pressure ulcer

• Provide privacy, and explain the procedure to the patient. Position him for comfort and to allow easy access to the pressure ulcer site.

• Cover the bed linens with a linen-saver pad to prevent soiling. Open the sterile irrigation set. Pour 0.9% sodium chloride solution into the irrigation container carefully to avoid splashing. Put the bulb syringe into the opening in the irrigation container.

• Open packages of sterile supplies and arrange them on a sterile field in order of use.

• Put on gloves to remove the old dressing, and discard it in the impervious plastic trash bag.

• Inspect the wound, and measure its perimeter with the disposable wound-measuring device.

• Using the bulb syringe, gently irrigate the pressure ulcer.

• Remove soiled gloves, and put on a fresh pair.

• Insert a sterile cotton-tipped applicator into the wound to assess wound tunneling.

• Using the gauze pads, blot dry the skin around the ulcer. Reassess the condition of the skin and ulcer.

• Apply the appropriate topical dressing.

To apply a hydrocolloid dressing

• Choose a presized dressing or cut one to overlap the pressure ulcer by about 1″ (2.5 cm). Remove the dressing from its package, and apply it to the wound. To minimize irritation, smooth out wrinkles as you apply the dressing.

• If you need to secure the dressing with tape, first apply a skin sealant to the skin around the ulcer. After the area dries, tape the dressing to the skin. The sealant protects the skin and helps the tape adhere.

• Remove your gloves, and discard them in the impervious trash bag. Dispose of refuse according to your hospital's policy, and wash your hands.

• Change a hydrocolloid dressing every 1 to 7 days as needed.

To apply a transparent dressing

• Clean and dry the wound as described above.

• Select a dressing to overlap the ulcer by 2″ (5 cm). Lay the dressing over the ulcer. Press on the edges of the dressing to promote adherence.

• If necessary, aspirate accumulated fluid with an 18G to 20G needle and syringe using aseptic technique to preserve dressing integrity. Then clean the aspiration site with an alcohol sponge, and cover it with a transparent dressing.

• Change the dressing every 3 to 7 days.

To apply a calcium alginate dressing

• Irrigate the pressure ulcer with 0.9% sodium chloride solution. Blot the surrounding skin dry.

• Apply the calcium alginate to the ulcer surface. Cover the area with a second dressing, as ordered. Secure it with hypoallergenic tape or elastic netting.

• If the wound is draining heavily, change the dressing once or twice daily for the first 3 to 5 days. As drainage decreases, change the dressing less frequently — every 2 to 4 days, or as ordered.

Special considerations

As a rule, avoid using tincture of benzoin compound as a skin sealant. This agent triggers an allergic reaction in some patients.

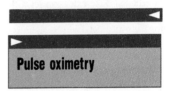

Pulse oximetry

Performed intermittently or continuously, pulse oximetry using the finger or ear is used to monitor arterial oxygen saturation (SpO_2).

Equipment

• Oximeter • finger or ear probe • alcohol sponges • nail polish remover, if necessary.

Implementation

Explain the procedure to the patient.

To perform pulse oximetry using the finger

• Select a finger for the test, either the index finger or a smaller finger. Make sure the patient isn't wearing false fingernails, and remove any nail polish from the test finger. Place the transducer (photodetector) probe over the patient's finger so that light beams and sensors oppose each other.

• Assess the finger for skin integrity every 4 to 8 hours. Move the probe to a new location as needed to prevent tissue trauma.

• For a neonate or a small infant, wrap the probe around the foot so that light beams and detectors oppose each other. For a large infant, use a probe that fits on the big toe, and secure it to the foot.

• Turn on the power switch. If the device is working properly, a beep will sound, a display will light momentarily, and the pulse searchlight will flash. The SpO_2 and pulse rate

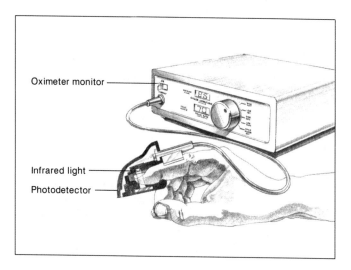

Oximeter monitor

Infrared light

Photodetector

displays will show stationary zeros. After four to six heartbeats, the SpO_2 and pulse rate displays will supply information with each beat, and the pulse amplitude indicator will begin tracking the pulse.

To perform pulse oximetry using the ear

• Using an alcohol sponge, massage the patient's earlobe for 10 to 20 seconds. Mild erythema indicates adequate vascularization. Following the manufacturer's instructions, attach the ear probe to the earlobe or pinna. Use the ear probe stabilizer for prolonged or exercise testing. Be sure to establish good contact.
• After a few seconds, a saturation reading and a pulse waveform will appear on the oximeter's screen. Leave the ear probe in place for 3 or more minutes until the readings stabilize at the highest point, or take three separate readings and average them. Revascularize the patient's earlobe each time.

Special considerations

• Normal SpO_2 levels for pulse oximetry using the finger and ear are 95% to 100% for adults, and 93.8% to 100% by 1 hour after birth for healthy, full-term neonates. Lower levels may signal hypoxemia. Notify the doctor of any significant change in the patient's condition.

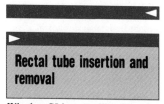

Rectal tube insertion and removal

Whether GI hypomotility slows the normal release of gas and feces or results in paralytic ileus, inserting a rectal tube may relieve the discomfort of distention and flatus.

Equipment

• Stethoscope • linen-saver pads
• drape • water-soluble lubricant
• commercial kit or #22 to #32 French rectal tube made of soft rubber or plastic • container (emesis basin, plastic bag, or water bottle with vent) • tape • gloves.

BEDSIDE CARE

Implementation

• Take all equipment to the patient's bedside, provide privacy, and wash your hands.
• Explain the procedure, and encourage the patient to relax.
• Check for abdominal distention. Using the stethoscope, auscultate for bowel sounds.
• Place the linen-saver pads under the patient's buttocks to absorb any drainage that may leak from the tube.
• Position the patient in left-lateral Sims' position to facilitate rectal tube insertion.
• Put on gloves.
• Drape the patient's exposed buttocks.
• Lubricate the rectal tube tip with water-soluble lubricant to ease insertion and prevent rectal irritation.
• Lift the patient's right buttock to expose the anus.
• Insert the rectal tube tip into the anus, advancing the tube 2″ to 4″ (5 to 10 cm) into the rectum. Direct the tube toward the umbilicus along the anatomic course of the large intestine.
• As you insert the tube, tell the patient to breathe slowly and deeply, or suggest that he bear down as he would for a bowel movement to relax the anal sphincter and ease insertion.
• Using tape, secure the rectal tube to the buttocks. Then attach the tube to the container to collect possible leakage.
• Remove the tube after 15 to 20 minutes. If the patient reports continued discomfort or if gas wasn't expelled, you can repeat the procedure in 2 or 3 hours, if ordered.
• Clean the patient, and replace soiled linens and the linen-saver pad. Be sure the patient feels as comfortable as possible. Again, check for abdominal distention, and listen for bowel sounds.

• If you will reuse the equipment, clean it and store it in the bedside cabinet; otherwise, discard the tube.

Special considerations

• Do not use a rectal tube on a patient with recent rectal or prostatic surgery, recent myocardial infarction, or a disease of the rectal mucosa.
• Fastening a plastic bag (like a balloon) to the external end of the tube lets you observe gas expulsion. Leaving a rectal tube in place indefinitely does little to promote peristalsis, can reduce sphincter responsiveness, and may lead to permanent sphincter damage or pressure necrosis of the mucosa.
• Repeat insertion periodically to stimulate GI activity. If the tube fails to relieve distention, notify the doctor.

Restraints, leather

When soft restraints aren't sufficient and sedation is dangerous or ineffective, leather restraints prevent the confused, disoriented, or combative patient from injuring himself or others. Depending on the patient's behavior, leather restraints may be applied to all limbs (four-point restraint) or to one arm and one leg (two-point restraint). The duration of such restraint is governed by state law and by hospital policy.

Equipment and preparation

• Two wrist and two ankle leather restraints • four straps • key • large gauze pads to cushion each extremity.

Before entering the patient's room, make sure that the restraints are the correct size. Use the patient's build and weight as a guide. Be sure the straps of leather restraints are unlocked and the key fits the locks.

Implementation

• Obtain a doctor's order for the restraint, if required. However, never leave a confused or combative patient unattended or unrestrained while attempting to secure the order.

• Tell the patient what you're about to do, and describe the restraints to him. Assure him that they are being used to protect him from injury rather than to punish him.

• Before entering the patient's room, obtain adequate assistance to restrain him, if necessary. Enlist the aid of several coworkers, and organize their efforts, giving each person a specific task; for example, one person explains the procedure to the patient and applies the restraints while the others immobilize his arms and legs.

• Place the patient in a supine position on the bed, with each arm and leg securely held down to minimize combative behavior and to prevent injury to the patient and others. Immobilize the patient's arms and legs at the joints — knee, ankle, shoulder, and wrist — to minimize his movement without exerting excessive force.

• Apply pads to the patient's wrists and ankles to reduce friction between his skin and the leather, thereby preventing skin irritation and breakdown.

• Wrap the restraint around the gauze pads. Then insert the metal loop through the hole that gives the best fit. Apply the restraints securely but not too tightly. You should be able to slip one or two fingers between the restraint and the patient's skin. A tight restraint can compromise circulation; a loose one can slip off or move up the patient's arm or leg, causing skin irritation and breakdown.

• Thread the strap through the metal loop on the restraint, close the metal loop, and secure the strap to the bed frame, out of the patient's reach.

• Lock the restraint by pushing in the button on the side of the metal loop, and tug it gently to be sure it's secure. After the restraint is secure, a coworker can release the arm or leg. Flex the patient's arm or leg slightly before locking the strap to allow room for movement and to prevent frozen joints and dislocations.

• Place the key in an accessible location at the nurse's station.

• After applying leather restraints, observe the patient regularly to give emotional support and to reassess the need for continued use of the restraint. Check his pulse rate and vital signs at least every 2 hours. Remove or loosen the restraints one at a time, every 2 hours, and perform passive range-of-motion exercises, if possible. Watch for signs of impaired peripheral circulation, such as cool, cyanotic skin.

• To unlock the restraint, insert the key into the metal loop opposite the locking button. This releases the lock, and the metal loop can be opened.

Special considerations

• Because the authority to use restraints varies among hospitals, you should know your hospital's policy.

• Remember to offer food and fluids, and the use of a bedpan and a urinal.

• You may be able to apply restraints without a doctor's order in an emergency. Also, be sure to know your state's regulations governing such restraints. For example, some states prohibit the use of four-point restraints.

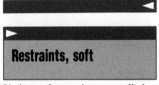

Restraints, soft

Various soft restraints—vest, limb, mitt, belt, or body—limit movement to prevent the confused, disoriented, or combative patient from injuring himself or others.

Equipment and preparation
• Restraint • gauze pads, if needed.
Make sure the restraints are the correct size. Use the patient's build and weight as a guide. If necessary, use gauze pads or washcloths to build up restraints that are too loose; tape them down securely.

Implementation
Obtain a doctor's order for the restraint, if required. If necessary, obtain adequate assistance to restrain the patient before entering his room.
Assure the patient that the restraints are being used to protect, not punish, him.

To apply a vest restraint
• Help the patient to sit if possible. Slip the vest over his gown. Crisscross the cloth flaps in front, placing the opening at his throat. Never crisscross the flaps in the back because he may choke if he tries to squirm out of the vest.
• Pass the tab on one flap through the slot on the opposite flap. Adjust the vest for comfort. You should be able to slip your fist between the vest and the patient. Avoid wrapping too tightly because it may restrict respiration.
• Tie all restraints to the bed frame or chair, out of the patient's reach.

Use a bow or a knot that can be released quickly in an emergency. Leave 1″ to 2″ (2.5 to 5 cm) of slack in the straps to allow room for movement and to allow the patient to stretch and breathe deeply.

To apply a limb restraint
• Wrap the patient's wrist or ankle with gauze to help prevent skin irritation. Wrap the restraint around the gauze pads.
• Pass the strap on the narrow end of the restraint through the slot in the broad end, and adjust. You should be able to slip one or two fingers between the restraint and the patient's skin.
• Tie the restraint as above.
• After applying the restraint, monitor for impaired circulation in the extremity distal to the restraint. If necessary, loosen the restraint. Perform range-of-motion (ROM) exercises regularly to stimulate circulation and prevent contractures.

To apply a mitt restraint
• Roll up a washcloth or gauze pad, and place it in the patient's palm. Have him form a loose fist; then pull the mitt over it, and secure the closure.
• If using transparent mesh mitts, check hand movement and skin color often to assess circulation. Remove the mitts regularly, and perform passive ROM exercises.

To apply a belt restraint
• Center the flannel pad of the belt on the bed. Then wrap the short strap of the belt around the bed frame and fasten it under the bed.
• Position the patient on the pad. Then have him roll to one side while you guide the long strap around his waist and through the slot in the pad.
• Wrap the long strap around the bed frame and fasten it under the bed. After applying the belt, slip

your hand between it and the patient to ensure a secure but comfortable fit.

To apply a body restraint

• Place the restraint flat on the bed, with arm and wrist cuffs facing down and the V at the head of the bed. Then place the patient in the prone position on top of the restraint.
• Lift the V over the patient's head. Thread the chest belt through one of the loops in the V to ensure a snug fit. Secure the straps around his chest, thighs, and legs. Turn him on his back.
• Secure the straps to the bed frame to anchor the restraint. Then secure the straps around the patient's arms and wrists.

Special considerations

• Because the authority to use restraints varies among hospitals, be sure you know your hospital's policy. Also become familiar with your state's regulations on the use of restraints.

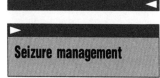

Seizure management

When a patient has a generalized seizure, nursing care aims to prevent injury and serious complications. It also includes observation of seizure characteristics to help determine the area of the brain involved. Prolonged seizure activity requires emergency medical intervention.

Equipment

• Oral airway • suction equipment • equipment for I.V. line insertion • 1 liter of 0.9% sodium chloride solution • anticonvulsant, such as diazepam, phenytoin, or phenobarbital, as ordered • emergency resuscitation equipment • 50-ml bolus of dextrose 50% in water, as ordered • 100-mg bolus of thiamine, as ordered • pillows, side-rail pads, blankets, or other soft material. Optional: endotracheal intubation set.

Implementation

• If you're with a patient when he experiences an aura — a peculiar sensation preceding the onset of a seizure — help him into bed, raise the side rails, and adjust the bed so that it's flat. If he's away from his room, lower him to the floor. Put a pillow under his head to keep it from hitting the floor.
• Stay with the patient, and be ready to intervene if complications develop. If necessary, have another staff member gather equipment and call the doctor.
• If the patient is in the beginning of the tonic phase and if hospital protocol permits, you may insert an oral airway into his mouth so his tongue doesn't block his airway. If an oral airway isn't available, don't hold his mouth open or place your hands inside because you may be bitten. Once the patient's jaw becomes rigid, don't try to force the airway into place because you may break his teeth or cause other injury.
• Move sharp or hard objects out of the patient's way, and loosen his clothing.
• Don't forcibly restrain the patient or restrict his movements during the seizure because the force of his tonic-clonic movements may cause muscle strain or even joint dislocation.
• Continually assess the patient during the seizure. Observe the earliest symptoms, how the seizure progresses, its form, and its duration. This may help determine the seizure's type and cause.
• After the tonic-clonic phase,

maintain a patent airway by turning the patient on his side and applying suction if necessary.
• If ordered, establish an I.V. line, and infuse 0.9% sodium chloride solution at a keep-vein-open rate.
• If the seizure lasts longer than 10 minutes, administer an anticonvulsant, as ordered.
• For a diabetic patient, administer 50 ml of dextrose 50% in water by I.V. push, as ordered. For an alcoholic patient, a 100-mg bolus of thiamine may stop the seizure.
• If the seizure is prolonged and the patient becomes hypoxemic, prepare for intubation.
• If the seizure continues despite medical treatment, you may need to prepare the patient for general anesthesia or neuromuscular blockade to stop seizure activity. If these procedures are used, continuous EEG monitoring should be performed to determine when the seizure activity stops.

Special considerations
• After the seizure, monitor vital signs and mental status every 15 to 30 minutes for 2 hours. If the patient remains obtunded for more than 2 hours, notify the doctor. When he awakens, reorient and reassure him. Ask him about his aura or activities preceding the seizure. The type of aura helps pinpoint the site in the brain where the seizure originated.
• Because a seizure commonly indicates an underlying disorder, a complete diagnostic workup will be ordered if the cause isn't evident.
• If you suspect that the patient has sustained a serious injury from the seizure, notify the doctor, and arrange for evaluation and treatment.
• Expect most patients to experience a postictal period of decreased mental status lasting 30 minutes to

24 hours. Reassure your patient that this does not indicate incipient brain damage.

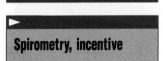

Spirometry, incentive

In this procedure, a breathing device helps the patient achieve maximal ventilation. The device measures respiratory flow or respiratory volume and induces the patient to take a deep breath and hold it for several seconds. Incentive spirometry benefits the patient on prolonged bed rest.

Equipment and preparation
• Flow or volume incentive spirometer, as indicated, with sterile disposable tube and mouthpiece
• stethoscope • watch • tape.
    The tube and mouthpiece are sterile on first use and should be cleaned after each use.
    Assemble the ordered equipment at the patient's bedside. Remove the sterile flow tube and mouthpiece from the package, and attach them to the device. Set the flow rate or volume goal, as determined by the doctor or respiratory therapist and based on the patient's preoperative performance.

Implementation
• Assess the patient's condition. Explain the procedure, emphasizing the need to perform it regularly to maintain alveolar inflation.
• Wash your hands.
• Assist the patient to a comfortable sitting or semi-Fowler's position to promote optimal lung expansion. If you're using a flow incentive spirometer and the patient is unable to assume or maintain the desired position, he can perform the procedure in any position as

long as the device remains upright. Tilting a flow incentive spirometer decreases the required patient effort and reduces the exercise's effectiveness.

• Auscultate the patient's lungs to provide a baseline for comparison with posttreatment auscultation.

• Instruct the patient to insert the mouthpiece and close his lips tightly around it because a weak seal may alter flow or volume readings.

• Instruct the patient to exhale normally and then inhale as slowly and as deeply as possible. If he has difficulty with this step, tell him to suck as he would through a straw, but more slowly. Ask him to retain the entire volume of air he inhaled for 3 seconds or, if you're using a device with a light indicator, until the light turns off.

• Tell the patient to remove the mouthpiece and exhale normally. Allow him to relax and take several normal breaths before attempting another breath with the spirometer. Repeat this sequence 5 to 10 times during every waking hour. Note tidal volumes.

• Evaluate the patient's ability to cough effectively, and encourage him to cough after each effort because deep lung inflation may loosen secretions and facilitate their removal. Observe any expectorated secretions.

• Auscultate the patient's lungs, and compare findings with the first auscultation.

• Instruct the patient to remove the mouthpiece. Wash the device in warm water, and shake it dry. Avoid immersing the spirometer itself because this enhances bacterial growth and impairs the internal filter's effectiveness in preventing inhalation of extraneous material.

• Place the mouthpiece in a plastic storage bag between exercises, and label it and the spirometer, if applicable, with the patient's name to avoid inadvertent use by another patient.

Special considerations

• If the patient is scheduled for surgery, make a preoperative assessment of his respiratory pattern and capability so that you can set appropriate postoperative goals. Then teach him to use the spirometer before surgery so that he can practice the exercise.

• Avoid exercising at mealtime to prevent nausea. If the patient has difficulty breathing only through his mouth, provide a noseclip to fully measure each breath. Provide paper and pencil so the patient can note exercise times. Exercise frequency varies with condition and ability.

• Immediately after surgery, monitor the exercise frequently to ensure compliance and assess achievement.

Suture removal

The goal of this procedure is to remove skin sutures from a healed wound without damaging newly formed tissue. For a sufficiently healed wound, sutures are usually removed 7 to 10 days after insertion. Techniques for removal depend on the method of suturing, but all require sterile procedure to prevent contamination.

Equipment and preparation

• Waterproof trash bag • adjustable light • clean gloves, if the wound is dressed • sterile gloves • sterile forceps or sterile hemostat • 0.9% sodium chloride solution • sterile gauze pads • antiseptic cleaning agent • sterile curve-tipped suture scissors • povidone-iodine sponges. Optional: adhesive butterfly strips or Steri-Strips, compound benzoin tincture or other skin protectant.

Prepackaged, sterile suture-removal trays are available. Check the expiration date on each sterile package, and inspect for tears. Open the waterproof trash bag, and place it near the patient's bed. Position the bag properly to avoid reaching across the sterile field or the suture line when disposing of soiled articles.

Implementation

• If your hospital allows you to remove sutures, check the doctor's order to confirm the exact time and details of this procedure.
• Check for patient allergies, especially to adhesive tape and topical medications.
• Tell the patient that you're going to remove the stitches from his wound. Assure him that this procedure usually is painless, but may tickle.
• Provide privacy, and position the patient so he's comfortable without placing undue tension on the suture line. Because some patients experience nausea or dizziness during the procedure, have him recline, if possible. Adjust the light so that it shines directly on the suture line.
• Wash your hands. If the wound has a dressing, put on gloves, and carefully remove it. Discard the dressing and gloves in the waterproof trash bag.
• Observe the patient's wound for gaping, signs of infection, or embedded sutures. Notify the doctor if the wound has failed to heal properly.
• Establish a sterile work area that includes all the supplies you'll need for suture removal and wound care. Put on sterile gloves. Open the sterile suture removal tray, if used.
• Observing sterile technique, clean the suture line to reduce microorganisms and the risk of infection. Cleaning should also moisten the sutures sufficiently to ease removal.
• Proceed according to the type of suture you're removing. Because the visible part of a suture is exposed to skin bacteria, be sure to cut sutures at the skin surface on one side of the visible part of the suture. Remove the suture by lifting and pulling the visible end off the skin to avoid drawing this contaminated portion back through subcutaneous tissue.

To remove plain interrupted sutures

• Using sterile forceps, grasp the knot of the first suture and raise it off the skin. This will expose a small portion of the suture that was below skin level.
• Place the rounded tip of sterile curved-tip suture scissors against the skin, and cut through the exposed portion of the suture.
• Then, still holding the knot with the forceps, pull the cut suture up and out of the skin in the direction shown below. Pull in a smooth continuous motion to avoid causing the patient pain. Discard the suture.

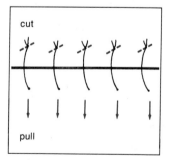

• Repeat the process, removing every other suture initially; if the wound doesn't gape, you can then remove the remaining sutures as ordered.

To remove plain continuous sutures

• Cut the first suture on the side opposite the knot.
• Next, cut the same side of the next suture in line.
• Then lift the first suture out in the direction shown below.

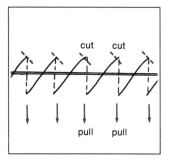

• Proceed along the suture line, grasping each suture where you grasped the knot on the first one.

To remove mattress interrupted sutures

• If possible, remove the small visible portion of the suture opposite the knot by cutting it at each visible end and lifting the small piece away from the skin to prevent pulling it through and contaminating subcutaneous tissue.
• Then remove the rest of the suture by pulling it out in the direction shown below.

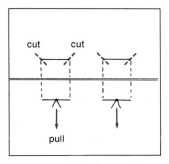

• If the visible portion is too small to cut twice, cut it once, and pull the entire suture out in the opposite direction.
• Repeat for the remaining sutures, and monitor the incision carefully for infection.

To remove mattress continuous sutures

• Follow the procedure for removing mattress interrupted sutures, first removing the small visible portion of the suture, if possible, to prevent pulling it through and contaminating subcutaneous tissue.
• Then extract the rest of the suture in the direction shown below.

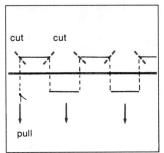

• If ordered, remove only every other suture to maintain some support for the incision. Then go back and remove the remaining sutures.

After removing sutures

• Wipe the incision gently with gauze pads soaked in an antiseptic cleaning agent or with a povidone-iodine sponge.
• Apply a light sterile gauze dressing, if needed, to prevent infection and irritation from clothing. Then discard your gloves.
• Tell the patient that he may shower in 1 or 2 days if the incision heals well and his doctor permits it.

Special considerations

• If the wound dehisces during suture removal, apply butterfly adhesive strips or Steri-Strips to support and approximate the edges, and call the doctor immediately to repair the wound.

• Apply butterfly adhesive strips or Steri-Strips after any suture removal, if desired, to give added support to the incision line. Use a small amount of compound benzoin tincture or other skin protectant to ensure adherence.

• Before discharge, teach the patient how to remove the dressing and care for the wound. Instruct him to call the doctor immediately if he observes wound discharge or any other abnormal change.

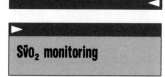

Sv̄O₂ monitoring

This procedure uses a fiber-optic thermodilution pulmonary artery (PA) catheter to continuously monitor oxygen delivery to tissues and oxygen consumption by tissues. Monitoring mixed venous oxygen saturation (Sv̄O₂) allows rapid detection of impaired oxygen delivery and helps evaluate a patient's response to drug administration, endotracheal tube suctioning, ventilator setting changes, positive endexpiratory pressure, and fraction of inspired oxygen.

Equipment and prepration

• Fiber-optic PA catheter • CO-oximeter (monitor) • optical module and cable • gloves.

Review the manufacturer's instructions for assembly and use of the fiber-optic PA catheter. Connect the optical module and cable to the monitor.

Next, peel back the wrapping covering the catheter just enough to uncover the fiber-optic connector. Attach the fiber-optic connector to the optical module while allowing the rest of the catheter to remain in its sterile wrapping. Calibrate the fiber-optic catheter by following the manufacturer's instructions.

Implementation

• Wash your hands, and put on gloves.

• Explain the procedure to the patient to allay his fears and promote cooperation.

• Assist with the insertion of the fiber-optic catheter just as you would for a regular PA catheter.

• After the catheter is inserted, confirm that the light intensity tracing on the graphic printout is within normal range to ensure correct positioning and function of the catheter.

• Observe the digital readout and record the Sv̄O₂ on graph paper. Repeat readings at least once each hour to monitor and document trends.

• Set the machine alarms 10% above and 10% below the patient's current Sv̄O₂ reading.

To recalibrate the monitor

• Draw a mixed venous blood sample from the distal port of the PA catheter. Send it to the laboratory for analysis to compare the laboratory's Sv̄O₂ measurement with the measurement indicated by the fiberoptic catheter.

• If the catheter values and the laboratory values differ by more than 4%, follow the manufacturer's instructions to enter the Sv̄O₂ value obtained by the laboratory into the oximeter.

• Recalibrate the monitor every 24 hours, or whenever the catheter has been disconnected from the optical module.

Special considerations

• Sv̄O₂ usually ranges from 60% to 80%, with the normal value around 75%. If the patient's Sv̄O₂ drops below 60%, or if it varies by more than 10% for 3 minutes or longer, reassess the patient. If the S̄v̄O₂ does not return to the baseline value after appropriate nursing interventions, notify the doctor. A decreasing S̄v̄O₂ or a value less than 60% indicates impaired oxygen delivery, as occurs during hemorrhage, hypoxia, shock, arrhythmias, or suctioning. S̄v̄O₂ may also decrease as a result of increased oxygen demand from hyperthermia, shivering, or seizures.

• If the intensity of the tracing is low, ensure that all connections between the catheter and oximeter are secure and that the catheter is patent and not kinked.

• If the tracing is damped or erratic, try to aspirate blood from the catheter to check for patency. If you can't aspirate blood, notify the patient's doctor so that he can replace the catheter.

• Also check the PA waveform to determine whether the catheter has wedged. If the catheter has wedged, attempt to flush the line. Also turn the patient from side to side and instruct him to cough. If the catheter remains wedged, notify the patient's doctor immediately.

• If the tracing shows a high intensity, the catheter may be pressing against a vessel wall. Flush the line. If the tracing doesn't return to normal, notify the doctor so he can reposition the catheter.

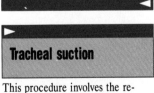

Tracheal suction

This procedure involves the removal of secretions from the trachea or bronchi by means of a catheter inserted through the mouth, nose, tracheal stoma, tracheostomy tube, or endotracheal tube. This procedure helps maintain a patent airway to promote optimal gas exchange and to prevent pneumonia from pooled secretions.

Equipment and preparation

• Oxygen source (wall or portable unit) • hand-held resuscitation bag with 15-mm adapter or with positive end-expiratory pressure (PEEP) valve, if indicated • wall or portable suction apparatus • collection container • connecting tube • suction catheter kit, or a sterile suction catheter, one sterile glove, one clean glove, and a disposable sterile solution container • 1-liter bottle of sterile water or 0.9% sodium chloride solution • sterile water-soluble lubricant (for nasal insertion) • syringe for deflating cuff of endotracheal or tracheostomy tube • waterproof trash bag.

Choose a suction catheter with a diameter no larger than half the inside diameter of the tracheostomy or endotracheal tube. Place the suction apparatus at the preferred side of the bed to facilitate suctioning. Attach the collection container to the suction unit and the connecting tube to the collection container. Label and date the 0.9% sodium chloride solution or sterile water. Open the waterproof trash bag.

Implementation

• Before suctioning, determine whether your hospital requires a doctor's order, and obtain one if necessary.

• Assess the patient's vital signs, breath sounds, and general appearance, and review blood gas values, if available. Evaluate the patient's ability to cough and deep breathe. If you'll be performing nasotracheal suctioning, check the patient's history for nasal obstruction or nasal trauma.

• Wash your hands. Explain the procedure to the patient. Unless contra-

BEDSIDE CARE

indicated, place him in semi-Fowler's or high Fowler's position.

• Remove the top from the 0.9% sodium chloride solution or water bottle, and open the package containing the sterile solution container.

• Using strict aseptic technique, open the suction catheter kit, and put on the gloves. If using individual supplies, open the suction catheter and gloves, placing the sterile glove on your dominant hand and the nonsterile glove on your nondominant hand.

• Using your nondominant hand, pour 0.9% sodium chloride solution or sterile water into the solution container. Place a small amount of water-soluble ointment on the sterile work area.

• Using your dominant hand, remove the catheter from its wrapper. Keep it coiled so it can't touch a nonsterile object. Use your other hand to attach the connecting tubing to the catheter.

• Occlude the suction port to assess suction pressure. Set the suction pressure according to hospital policy.

• Dip the catheter tip in the 0.9% sodium chloride solution to lubricate the outside of the catheter. Then occlude the control valve with the thumb of your nondominant hand, and suction a small amount of solution through the catheter. This lubricates the inside of the catheter to facilitate passage of secretions. For nasal insertion, lubricate the tip of the catheter with the water-soluble lubricant.

• If the patient is not intubated or is intubated but not receiving supplemental oxygen or aerosol, instruct him to take three to six deep breaths to help prevent hypoxia during suctioning. If the patient is not intubated but is receiving oxygen, instruct him to take three to six deep breaths while using his supplemental oxygen, if indicated.

• If the patient is being mechani-

cally ventilated, preoxygenate him by delivering three to six breaths with a resuscitation bag with the oxygen flowmeter set at 15 liters/minute. If the patient is being maintained on PEEP, evaluate the need to use a resuscitation bag with a PEEP valve.

• Alternatively, preoxygenate the mechanically ventilated patient by delivering three to six breaths using the sigh mode on the ventilator after adjusting the fraction of inspired oxygen (FIO_2) and tidal volume according to hospital policy and patient need.

Nasotracheal insertion in a nonintubated patient

• Disconnect the oxygen from the patient, if applicable. Using your nondominant hand, raise the tip of the patient's nose, and insert the catheter into the patient's nostril while rolling it between your fingers.

• As the patient inhales, advance the catheter as far as possible. Don't apply suction during insertion. If the patient coughs, pause briefly, and resume advancement when he inhales.

Insertion in an intubated patient

• Using your nonsterile hand, disconnect the patient from the ventilator.

• Using your sterile hand, insert the catheter into the artificial airway. Advance the catheter, without applying suction, until you meet resistance. If the patient coughs, pause briefly, and then resume advancement.

Suctioning the patient

• After inserting the catheter, apply suction intermittently by removing and replacing the thumb of your nondominant hand over the control valve. Simultaneously use your dominant hand to withdraw the catheter as you roll it between your thumb and forefinger. Never suction for

more than 10 seconds at a time.
• If needed, resume oxygen delivery, and hyperoxygenate the patient's lungs before continuing. Observe the patient, and allow him to rest for a few minutes before the next suctioning.

After suctioning

• Hyperoxygenate the patient being maintained on a ventilator with a hand-held resuscitation bag or ventilator with 100% FIO_2. Then readjust FIO_2 and tidal volume to ordered settings.
• Assess the need for upper airway suctioning. If the cuff on the endotracheal or tracheostomy tube is inflated, suction the upper airway before deflating the cuff. Be sure to change the catheter and sterile glove before suctioning the lower airway.
• Discard gloves and catheter in the waterproof trash bag. Clear the connecting tubing by aspirating the remaining 0.9% sodium chloride solution or water. Discard and replace suction equipment and supplies according to hospital policy. Wash your hands.

Special considerations

• Because of tracheobronchial anatomy, the catheter tends to enter the right mainstem bronchus.
• Instillation of 0.9% sodium chloride solution into the trachea before suctioning may stimulate a cough but does not liquefy secretions. Adequate hydration and bronchial hygiene techniques have a greater effect on mobilizing secretions.
• Because oxygen is removed along with secretions, the patient may experience hypoxemia and dyspnea. Anxiety may alter respiratory patterns. Cardiac arrhythmias can result from hypoxia and stimulation of the vagus nerve in the tracheobronchial tree. In addition, tracheal

or bronchial trauma can result from traumatic or prolonged suctioning.
• Patients with compromised cardiovascular or pulmonary status are at risk for hypoxemia, arrhythmias, hypertension, or hypotension. Patients with a history of nasopharyngeal bleeding who are taking anticoagulants, who've had a recent tracheostomy, or who have a blood dyscrasia incur an increased risk of bleeding as a result of suctioning. Use caution when suctioning patients who have increased intracranial pressure because it may increase pressure further. When doing so, closely monitor the patient for signs and symptoms of increased intracranial pressure.
• If the patient experiences laryngospasm or bronchospasm (rare complications) during suctioning, discuss with the patient's doctor the use of bronchodilators or lidocaine to reduce the risk of this complication.

Urinary catheter maintenance

Performed daily after the patient's bath and immediately after perineal care, routine indwelling catheter care aims to prevent infection and other complications by keeping the catheter insertion site clean. Because some studies suggest that catheter care increases the risk of infection rather than lowers it, hospital policy dictates whether or not a patient receives daily catheter care. Regardless of the catheter care policy, the equipment and the patient's genitalia require twice-daily inspection.

Equipment and preparation
For catheter care
• Povidone-iodine solution (or other antiseptic cleaning agent) • sterile gloves • basin • eight sterile 4″ × 4″ gauze pads • sterile absorbent cotton balls or cotton-tipped applicators • collection bag • adhesive tape • waste receptacle. Optional: safety pin, rubber band, gooseneck lamp, antibiotic ointment, specimen container.

For perineal cleaning
• Washcloth • additional basin • soap and water or institution's specified cleansing agent.

Wash your hands, and take all equipment to the patient's bedside. Open the gauze pads, place several in the first basin, and pour some povidone-iodine solution or other cleaning agent over them.

Some hospitals specify that, after wiping the urinary meatus with cleaning solution, you should wipe it off with wet, sterile gauze pads to prevent possible irritation from the cleaning solution. If this is your hospital's policy, pour water into the second basin, and moisten three more gauze pads.

Implementation
• Explain the procedure to the patient, and provide privacy. Place a gooseneck lamp at the bedside if additional light is needed.
• Inspect the catheter for any problems, and check the urine drainage for mucus, blood clots, sediment, and turbidity. If you notice any of these conditions, obtain a urine specimen, and notify the doctor.
• Inspect the outside of the catheter where it enters the urinary meatus for encrusted material and suppurative drainage. Also inspect the tissue around the meatus for irritation or swelling.
• Remove any adhesive tape securing the catheter to the patient's

thigh or abdomen. Inspect the area for signs of adhesive burns.
• Put on the sterile gloves. Use a saturated, sterile gauze pad or cotton-tipped applicator to clean the outside of the catheter and the tissue around the meatus. To avoid contaminating the urinary tract, always clean by wiping away from the urinary meatus. Use a dry gauze pad to remove encrusted material.
   Note: Don't pull on the catheter during cleaning. This can injure the urethra and bladder wall. It can also expose a section of the catheter that was inside the urethra so that when you release the catheter, the newly contaminated section will reenter the urethra, possibly introducing infectious organisms.
• Remove your gloves, and tear off a piece of adhesive tape. Retape the catheter to the other thigh or opposite side of the abdomen.
   Note: Provide enough slack before securing the catheter to prevent tension on the tubing. This helps avoid injuring the urethral lumen or bladder wall.
• Attach the tubing to the sheet with the plastic clamp provided. Attach the collection bag, below bladder level, to the bed frame.

Special considerations
• Your hospital may require the use of specific cleaning agents for catheter care, so check the policy manual before beginning this procedure. A doctor's order will be needed to apply antibiotic ointments in the urinary meatus.
• Avoid raising the drainage bag above bladder level to prevent reflux of urine, which may contain bacteria. Make sure to keep the drainage bag off the floor to prevent possible contamination. When moving a patient to a stretcher or wheelchair, attach the drainage bag to the frame below bladder level. To prevent traumatic injury to the urethral

lumen or bladder wall, disconnect the drainage bag and tubing from the bed linen and bed frame before helping the patient out of bed.

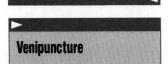

Venipuncture

Performed to obtain a blood sample, venipuncture involves piercing a vein with a needle and collecting blood in a syringe or evacuated tube. Venipuncture is usually performed using the antecubital fossa, but it can also be performed on a vein in the wrist, the dorsum of the hand or foot, or another accessible location.

Equipment and preparation
• Tourniquet • gloves • syringe or evacuated tubes and needle holder • 70% ethyl alcohol or povidone-iodine sponges • 20G or 21G needle for the forearm or 25G for the wrist, hand, or ankle, or for children • color-coded tubes containing appropriate additives • labels • laboratory request form • 2″ × 2″ gauze pads • adhesive bandage.

If you're using evacuated tubes, open the needle packet, attach the needle to its holder, and select the appropriate tubes. If you're using a syringe, attach the appropriate needle to it. Label all collection tubes with the patient's name and room number, the doctor's name, and the date and time of collection.

Implementation
• Wash your hands, and put on gloves. Explain the procedure to the patient. If the patient is on bed rest, ask him to lie supine with his arms at his sides. Ask the ambulatory patient to sit in a chair and support his arm on an armrest or table.

• Assess the patient's veins to determine the best puncture site. Observe the skin for the vein's blue color, or palpate the vein for a firm rebound sensation.
• Tie a tourniquet 2″ (5 cm) proximal to the area chosen. By impeding venous return while allowing arterial flow, a tourniquet produces venous dilation. If arterial perfusion remains adequate, you'll be able to feel the radial pulse.
• Clean the venipuncture site with a povidone-iodine sponge or an alcohol sponge. Don't wipe off the povidone-iodine with alcohol because alcohol cancels the effect of povidone-iodine. Wipe in a circular motion from the site outward. If you use alcohol, apply it with friction for 30 seconds, or until the sponge comes away clean. If you use povidone-iodine, allow the skin to dry.
• To immobilize the vein, press just below the site with your thumb, and draw the skin taut.
• Position the needle with the bevel up, the shaft parallel to the path of the vein, and at a 30-degree angle to the arm. Insert the needle into the vein. If you're using a syringe, venous blood will appear in the hub; pull the plunger of the syringe gently until you obtain the required sample. Pulling too forcibly may collapse the vein.
• If you're using a needle holder and evacuated tube, a drop of blood will appear inside the needle holder. Grasp the holder firmly, and push down on the collection tube until the needle punctures the rubber stopper. Blood will flow into the tube automatically.
• Remove the tourniquet as soon as blood flows adequately to prevent stasis and hemoconcentration, which can impair test results. If flow is sluggish, leave the tourniquet in place longer, but remove it before withdrawing the needle.

• After you've drawn the sample, place a gauze pad over the puncture site, and remove the needle from the vein. When using an evacuated tube, remove it from the needle holder to release the vacuum before withdrawing the needle from the vein.
• Apply gentle pressure to the puncture site for 2 or 3 minutes or until bleeding stops.
• If you've used a syringe, detach the needle from the syringe, open the collection tube, and empty the sample into the tube, being careful to avoid foaming, which may cause hemolysis.
• Check the venipuncture site to make sure a hematoma hasn't developed. If it has, apply warm soaks.

Special considerations
• Never draw a venous sample from an arm or leg being used for I.V. therapy or blood administration because this may affect test results. Don't draw a venous sample from an infection site because this could introduce pathogens into the vascular system. Also avoid edematous areas, arteriovenous shunts, or sites of previous hematoma or vascular injury.

CHAPTER 8

Precautions:
Preventing the spread of contagious disease

Precaution principles

What is an infectious substance?

The Occupational Safety and Health Administration (OSHA) and the Centers for Disease Control and Prevention (CDC) define the following materials as infectious, requiring you to observe universal precautions:
• blood
• semen
• vaginal secretions
• cerebrospinal fluid
• synovial fluid
• pericardial fluid
• pleural fluid
• peritoneal fluid
• amniotic fluid
• saliva (in dental procedures)
• any body fluid visibly contaminated with blood
• any unidentified body fluid
• any unfixed tissue or organ other than intact skin
• cell, tissue, or organ culture containing human immunodeficiency virus (HIV)
• culture medium or other solution containing hepatitis B virus (HBV).

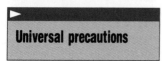

Universal precautions

This system of precautions and procedures was developed by the Centers for Disease Control and Prevention (CDC) in response to the increasing incidence of human immunodeficiency virus (HIV), hepatitis B virus (HBV), and other blood-borne diseases. The CDC recommends that caregivers handle all blood and potentially bloody body substances and tissues as if they're infectious, regardless of the patient's diagnosis.

Universal precautions encompass most of the individual blood and body fluid isolation precautions previously recommended by the CDC for patients with known or suspected blood-borne pathogens. Universal precautions are meant to be combined with other category- or disease-specific isolation precautions.

Universal precautions apply to the specific materials designated as infectious by the Occupational Safety and Health Administration (OSHA) and the CDC. They don't apply to feces, saliva, nasal secretions, sputum, sweat, tears, vomitus, or urine unless visible traces of blood are present.

Body substance isolation (BSI) is an extension of the CDC guidelines for universal precautions, first implemented at Harborview Medical Center in Seattle. BSI considers all body substances potentially infectious, regardless of the patient's diagnosis. It advocates the consistent use of barriers whenever contact with moist body substances, mucous membranes, and nonintact skin is possible. Its precautions extend beyond blood and blood-tinged fluids to include feces, urine, wound drainage, oral secretions, vomitus, and any other body substance.

Implementation
• Wash your hands immediately if they become contaminated with blood or body fluids. Also wash them before and after patient care and after removing gloves.

• Wear gloves if you will or may potentially come in contact with blood, specimens, tissue, body fluids or excretions, or contaminated surfaces or objects.

• Change your gloves between patient contacts to avoid cross-contamination.

• Wear a gown, face shield, goggles, and a mask during procedures likely to generate droplets of blood or body fluids, such as surgery, endoscopic procedures, or dialysis.

• Handle used needles or other sharp implements carefully. Do not bend, break, reinsert them into their original sheaths, or unnecessarily handle them. Discard them intact, immediately after use, into an impervious disposal box. These measures reduce the risk of accidental injury or infection.

• Immediately notify your employee health provider of all needle-stick accidents, mucosal splashes, or contamination of open wounds with blood or body fluids to allow investigation of the incident and appropriate care and documentation.

• Properly label all specimens collected from patients, and place them in plastic bags at the collection site.

• Promptly clean all blood and body fluid spills with a 1:10 dilution of bleach to water (mixed daily) or with an approved hospital-strength disinfectant effective against HBV and HIV.

• Disposable food trays and dishes aren't necessary.

• If you have an exudative lesion, avoid all direct patient contact until the condition has resolved and you've been cleared by the employee health provider.

Special considerations

• Keep mouthpieces, resuscitation bags, and other ventilation devices nearby to minimize the need for emergency mouth-to-mouth resuscitation, thus reducing the risk of exposure to body fluids.

• Because precautions can't be specified for every clinical situation, you must use your judgment in individual cases. What's more, if occupational exposure to blood is likely, you should receive an HBV vaccine.

Recommended barriers to infection

The list below presents the minimum requirements for using gloves, gowns, masks, and eye protection to avoid contacting and spreading pathogens. It assumes that you wash your hands thoroughly in all cases. Refer to your hospital's guidelines and use your own judgment when assessing the need for barrier protection in specific situations.

Key

 Gloves

 Gown

 Mask

 Eye wear

Bathing, for patient with open lesions

 if soiling likely

Bedding, changing visibly soiled

 if soiling likely

Bleeding or pressure application to control it

 if soiling likely

 if splattering likely

 if splattering likely

Blood glucose (capillary) testing

Cardiopulmonary resuscitation

 if splattering likely

 if splattering likely

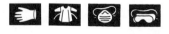 if splattering likely

---

Central venous line insertion and venesection

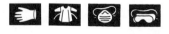

Central venous pressure measurement

Chest drainage system change

 if splattering likely

 if splattering likely

 if splattering likely

Chest tube insertion or removal

 if soiling likely

 if splattering likely

 if splattering likely

Cleaning (feces, spilled blood or body substances, or surfaces contaminated by blood or body fluids)

 if soiling likely

Colonoscopy, flexible sigmoido-
scope

Coughing, frequent and forceful by
patient; direct contact with secretions

Dialysis, peritoneal (collecting a
specimen)

Dialysis, peritoneal (initiating acute
treatment, performing an exchange,
terminating acute treatment, dis-
mantling tubing from cycler, discarding peritoneal drainage, irrigating peritoneal catheter, changing
tubing, or assisting with insertion
of acute peritoneal catheter outside
sterile field)

 if splattering likely

 if splattering likely

Dialysis, peritoneal (skin care at
catheter site)

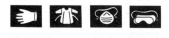

Dressing change for burns

Dressing removal or change for
wounds with little or no drainage

Dressing removal or change for
wounds with large amount of drainage

 if soiling likely

Emptying drainage receptacles, including suction containers, urine
receptacles, bedpans, emesis basins

 if soiling likely

 if splattering likely

 if splattering likely

Enema

 if soiling likely

Fecal impaction, removal of

Fecal incontinence, placement of indwelling urinary catheter for, and emptying bag of

 if splattering likely

Gastric lavage

 if soiling likely

Incision and drainage of abscess

 if splattering likely

Intravenous or intra-arterial line (insertion, removal, tubing change at catheter hub)

Intubation or extubation

 if splattering likely

 if splattering likely

 if splattering likely

Invasive procedures (lumbar puncture, bone marrow aspiration, paracentesis, liver biopsy) outside sterile field

Irrigation, indwelling urinary catheter

Irrigation, vaginal

 if soiling likely

Irrigation, wound

 if soiling likely

 if splattering likely

 if splattering likely

Joint or nerve injection

Lesion biopsy or removal

Medication administration (eye, ear, or nose drops; I.M. or S.C.; I.V. directly into or indirectly into hub of catheter or heparin lock; oral; rectal or vaginal suppository; topical for lesion)

Nasogastric tube, insertion or irrigation

 if soiling likely

 if splattering likely

 if splattering likely

Oral and nasal care

Ostomy care, irrigation, and teaching

 if soiling likely

Oxygen tubing, drainage of condensate

Pelvic exam and Papanicolaou (Pap) test

Perineal cleaning

Postmortem care

 if soiling likely

Pressure ulcer care

Shaving

Specimen collection (blood, stool, urine, sputum, wound)

Suctioning, nasotracheal or endotracheal

 if soiling likely

 if splattering likely

 if splattering likely

Suctioning, oral or nasal

PRECAUTIONS

Temperature, rectal

Tracheostomy suctioning and cannula cleaning

 if soiling likely

if splattering likely

if splattering likely

Tracheostomy tube change

if splattering likely

if splattering likely

Urine and stool testing

Wound packing

 if soiling likely

Checklist of reportable diseases

Certain contagious diseases must be reported to local and state public health officials and, ultimately, to the Centers for Disease and Prevention Control (CDC). Typically, these diseases fit one of two categories: those reported individually on definitive or suspected diagnosis, and those reported by the number of cases per week. The most commonly reported diseases include hepatitis, measles, viral meningitis, salmonellosis, shigellosis, syphilis, and gonorrhea.

In most states, the patient's doctor must report communicable diseases to health officials. In hospitals, the infection-control practitioner or epidemiologist reports them. However, you should know the reporting requirements and procedure. Fast, accurate reporting helps to identify and control infection sources, prevent epidemics, and guide public health policy.

The following list notes reportable diseases and conditions. Because disease reporting laws vary among states, the list isn't conclusive.

• Acquired immunodeficiency syndrome (AIDS)
• Amebiasis
• Animal bites
• Anthrax (cutaneous or pulmonary)
• Aseptic meningitis
• Botulism (food-borne, infant)
• Brucellosis
• Cholera
• Diphtheria (cutaneous or pharyngeal)
• Encephalitis (postinfectious or primary)
• Gastroenteritis (hospital outbreaks)

- Gonorrhea
- Group A beta-hemolytic strepto-coccal infections (including scarlet fever)
- Guillain-Barré syndrome
- Hepatitis A (include suspected source)
- Hepatitis B (include suspected source)
- Hepatitis C, formerly called non-A, non-B (include suspected source)
- Hepatitis, unspecified (include suspected source)
- Influenza
- Legionellosis (Legionnaires' disease)
- Leprosy
- Leptospirosis
- Malaria
- Measles (rubeola)
- Meningitis (specify etiology)
- Meningococcal disease
- Mumps
- Pertussis
- Plague (bubonic or pneumonic)
- Poliomyelitis (spinal paralytic)
- Psittacosis
- Rabies
- Reye's syndrome
- Rheumatic fever
- Rocky Mountain spotted fever
- Rubella (congenital syndrome)
- Rubella (German measles)
- Salmonellosis (excluding typhoid fever)
- Shigellosis
- Smallpox
- Staphylococcal infections (neonatal)
- Syphilis (congenital < 1 year)
- Syphilis (primary or secondary)
- Tetanus
- Toxic shock syndrome
- Trichinosis
- Tuberculosis
- Tularemia
- Typhoid fever
- Typhus (flea- and tick-borne)
- Varicella (chicken pox)
- Yellow fever

Basic procedures

Putting on and removing a gown and cap

Handling isolation garb properly is important for protecting yourself and avoiding contamination. Follow these steps when using a gown and cap.

Implementation
- Put the gown on and wrap it around the back of your uniform. Tie the strings or fasten the snaps or pressure-sensitive tabs at the neck. Make sure your uniform is completely covered, and secure the gown at the waist.
- Put on the cap so it covers all of your hair.
- When you want to remove your gown, remember that the outside surfaces of this barrier clothing are contaminated.
- With gloves on, untie the waist strings of the gown, which are also considered contaminated.
- Untie the neck straps of your gown. Grasp the outside at the back of the shoulders and pull it down over your arms, turning it inside out to contain pathogens as you remove it.
- Holding the gown well away from you, fold it inside out. Discard a cloth gown in the laundry and a paper gown in a trash container.

Putting on sterile gloves

Properly putting on sterile gloves helps prevent the spread of pathogens between your hands and any surface you touch. Most important, don't allow the outer surface of either glove to touch any nonsterile surface, including your hands, as you put them on.

Implementation

• Make sure that the opening of each glove is cuffed, which will allow you to handle the nonsterile inside of the glove rather than the sterile outside.

• Using your nondominant hand, pick up the opposite glove by grasping the exposed inside of the cuff, as shown below.

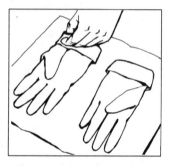

• Pull the glove onto your dominant hand. Be sure to keep your dominant thumb folded inward against your palm to avoid touching the sterile outside of the glove as you pull it on, as shown below.

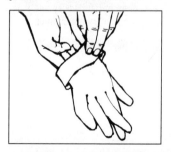

• Allow the glove to come uncuffed as you finish inserting your hand, but don't touch the outside of the glove with your nondominant hand.

• Slip your gloved dominant fingers under the loose glove's cuff to pick it up, as shown below. This way, your sterile dominant fingers touch only the sterile outside of the nondominant glove.

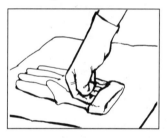

• Slide your nondominant hand into the glove, holding your sterile dominant thumb away from your nonsterile arm, as shown below.

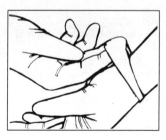

Allow the glove to come uncuffed as you finish putting it on, but don't touch the skin side of the cuff with your sterile dominant hand.

Removing contaminated gloves

To prevent the spread of pathogens from contaminated gloves to your skin surface, follow these steps carefully.

Implementation

• Using your nondominant hand, pinch the glove of the dominant hand near the top, as shown below. Avoid allowing the glove's outer surface to buckle inward against your skin.

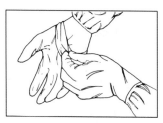

• Pull downward, allowing the glove to turn inside out as it comes off, as shown below. Keep the glove from your dominant hand in your nondominant hand after removing it.

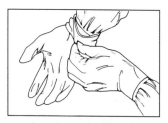

• Now insert the first two fingers of your ungloved dominant hand under the edge of the nondominant glove, as shown at the top of the right column. Avoid touching the glove's outer surface or folding it against the wrist of your nondominant hand.

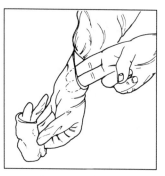

• Pull downward, so the glove turns inside out as it comes off, as shown below. Continue pulling until the glove completely encloses the glove from your dominant hand and has its uncontaminated inner surface facing out.

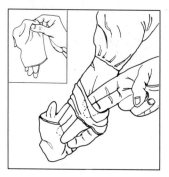

• Discard your gloves in the appropriate trash container.

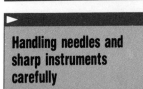

Putting on and removing a mask

Wear a face mask to avoid spreading or inhaling airborne particles.

Implementation
• Place the mask snugly over your nose and mouth. Secure the ear loops or tie the strings behind your head high enough so the mask won't slip off.
• If the mask has a metal strip, squeeze it to fit your nose firmly but comfortably. If you wear eyeglasses, tuck the mask under their lower edge.
• To remove your mask, untie it, holding it by the strings. Discard it and the cap in the trash container. If the patient's disease is spread by airborne pathogens, consider removing the mask and cap last.

Handling needles and sharp instruments carefully

To prevent accidents—especially needle sticks—handle needles and other sharp instruments with caution after a procedure and also when cleaning and disposing of them. In recent years, manufacturers have developed new equipment, such as retractable needle sheath covers and blunt-ended needles, to help minimize the risk of needle-stick injuries.

Implementation
• Do not recap used needles by hand.
• Do not remove used needles from disposable syringes by hand.
• Do not bend, break, or otherwise manipulate used needles by hand.
• Place used needles into a puncture-resistant container. (To avoid being forced to recap a needle, remember to locate the needle container as close to the area of use as possible and replace the puncture-resistant needle container before it becomes full.) If the container is more than three-fourths full, close it securely and dispose of it according to the institution's policy. Do not put more used needles into it.
• Never attempt to push a needle into a bulging container.

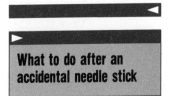

What to do after an accidental needle stick

If you sustain a needle-stick injury, follow these guidelines for your protection.

Implementation
• *Immediately* clean the puncture site, and express blood from the wound.
• Report the incident by contacting your employee health department and describing the incident.
• Then follow these further precautions.

Needle contaminated by human immunodeficiency virus (HIV)
• Obtain medical counseling.
• Arrange for HIV testing at regular intervals (typically, 6 weeks, 3 months, 6 months, and 1 year) after the injury. If test findings are normal after 1 year, no further follow-up is necessary.

Needle contaminated by hepatitis B
• If you've been vaccinated against hepatitis B, be tested to measure your level of hepatitis B antibodies. If your antibody level is low, consider having a booster vaccine. Also arrange for follow-up testing.
• If you haven't been vaccinated against hepatitis B, or if you're a nonresponder to the vaccine, discuss immune globulin therapy with your doctor.
• Get regular checkups for clinical evidence of hepatitis. If the results are positive, seek treatment, but if results are negative for 1 year, you'll need no further follow-up.

Needle contaminated by blood-borne infection
• Get a tetanus shot, if appropriate.
• As needed, obtain antibiotic or other treatment.

Needle contamination unknown
• Get tested for HIV and hepatitis B. Also get a tetanus shot, if necessary, and consult your doctor about your health risks.

Discarding contaminated equipment

To protect yourself and your patients from infection, observe precautions to dispose of soiled linens or dressings, used disposable equipment, and contaminated reusable equipment. As needed, be sure to have a biohazard container available to dispose of contaminated waste. Also as needed, replace the red biohazard bags that line the container.

Keep in mind that regulations for contaminated-waste disposal vary from state to state and may change periodically.

Removing soiled linens
• According to universal precautions, all linens used in patient care settings should be considered soiled. Wearing gloves when changing bed linens is also recommended. If the bed linens are saturated with blood, feces, urine, or other body fluids, you may need to put on a gown as well as gloves.
• Handle linens as little as possible and with minimum agitation to prevent contaminating yourself. If certain areas of the linens are heavily soiled, fold the fabric so that the soiled areas are on the inside of the folds. Then roll or fold the linens together in one bundle.
• When carrying linens, be sure to carry them away from your body to avoid contaminating your clothes.
• If possible, bag linens in the patient's room. Avoid placing them on chairs, tables, or the floor. Don't sort or rinse linens in patient care areas. Place soiled linens in leak-proof bags.
• After you put the linens in the bag, close the bag securely. Then remove your gloves and wash your hands before carrying the bag to its appropriate destination.

Disposing of soiled dressings
• Dispose of all wound dressings in a way that confines and contains any blood or body fluids present. Avoid touching any soiled areas on the dressing.
• Usually, you'll need to wear nonsterile gloves to handle and remove soiled dressings. If the wound is large and draining, however, you'll also need to wear a gown and face shield (or mask and goggles).

Large dressings
• Immediately after removing a large dressing, fold it inward to enclose soiled areas within the dressing.

• Wrap the large dressing in the disposable linen-saver pad used during the dressing change.
• Drop the bundle into the bag inside the biohazard container. Continue wearing your gloves as you do so. Also use the bag in the biohazard container to hold other trash from the dressing change, including your gloves, gown (if disposable), and face shield (or mask). When you're finished, seal the bag and deposit it in the trash container in the patient's room.

Small dressings
• When removing a small dressing, enclose it in the disposable glove you used to remove the dressing. Holding the dressing in your gloved hand, pull the glove off with the inside out to contain the dressing inside it. Don't let your bare hand touch the dressing.
• Once you've sealed the dressing inside the disposable glove, discard both gloves and the dressing in the trash container in the patient's room.

Discarding disposable equipment
• When disposing of any object contaminated with potentially infectious materials, make sure to place it in an impervious bag. If the outside of the bag is visibly soiled, use double bagging. When the bag is about three-fourths full, secure it or seal it for disposal. Wear gloves when handling waste bags.
• When transporting a bag, hold it away from your body to prevent inadvertent injury from sharp objects that may protrude through the plastic.
• Tag or label all bags or other receptacles containing articles contaminated with potentially infectious material. This tag or label should read BIOHAZARD or bear the biohazard symbol.

• Whenever you lift a bag from a biohazard container, check for leaks. If you discover any, immediately place the leaking bag inside another biohazard bag.

Disposing of body fluids
• Consult institutional policy for handling infectious wastes. Large amounts of secretions, excretions, or bulk blood may be carefully poured into a sanitary sewer.

Category-specific procedures

Acid-fast bacillus isolation

This isolation procedure prevents the spread of pulmonary tuberculosis (TB). It should be used with patients who have pulmonary or laryngeal TB.

Implementation
• Keep the patient in a specially ventilated (negative air pressure) private room with the door shut. Usually, patients infected with the same organism may share a room.
• Wear a mask only if the patient is coughing and does not reliably cover his mouth. Wear a gown only if needed to prevent gross contamination of clothing. Gloves aren't necessary.
• Wash your hands after touching the patient or potentially contaminated articles and before caring for another patient.
• Objects are rarely involved in the transmission of TB. However, you

should thoroughly clean and disinfect contaminated items or discard them.

Blood and body fluid precautions

These precautions prevent the spread of infections transmitted by direct or indirect contact with blood or body fluids.

Implementation
• Provide a private room for patients whose hygiene is poor. Otherwise, a private room is optional.
• Wear gloves for all anticipated contact with blood, secretions, mucous membranes, or any body fluid.
• Wash your hands thoroughly after any patient contact in which you didn't wear gloves.
• Wear a gown, a plastic apron, a mask, or goggles if secretions, blood, or body fluids are likely to soil clothing or skin, or splash in the face.
• Make sure soiled, reusable articles are contained securely enough to prevent leaking. Double-bag only if the outside of the bag is visibly soiled.
• Place needles and other sharp instruments in puncture-resistant, rigid needle containers. Don't recap needles.

Contact isolation

This procedure prevents the spread of highly transmissible or epidemiologically important pathogens that do not warrant strict isolation. Contact isolation applies to diagnoses such as Group A *Streptococcus* endometritis; impetigo; *Staphylococcus aureus* or Group A *Streptococcus* pneumonia; rabies; rubella; scabies; scalded skin syndrome; major skin, wound, or burn infections; vaccinia; primary disseminated herpes simplex; and infection or colonization with resistant bacteria.

In infants and young children, this procedure applies to acute respiratory infections, influenza, infectious pharyngitis, and viral pneumonia.

In neonates, this procedure applies to gonococcal conjunctivitis, staphylococcal furunculosis, and neonatal disseminated herpes simplex.

Implementation
• Keep the patient in a private room. Usually, patients infected with the same organism may share a room. During outbreaks, infants and young children with the same respiratory condition may share a room.
• Wear a mask. If soiling is likely, wear a gown. Wear gloves if touching infective material.
• Wash your hands after touching the patient or potentially contaminated articles and before caring for another patient.

Drainage and secretion precautions

These precautions keep pathogens from spreading by direct or indirect contact with purulent material or drainage from an infected body site. Use them with patients who have conjunctivitis; minor or limited abscesses; or minor or limited burn, skin, wound, or pressure sore infections.

Implementation

• The patient doesn't need a private room.

• You don't need a mask when approaching the patient. Wear a gown if soiling is likely, and wear gloves for touching infective material.

• Wash your hands after touching the patient or potentially contaminated articles and before caring for another patient.

• Discard contaminated articles, or bag and label such articles and send them for decontamination and reprocessing.

Enteric precautions

These steps prevent the spread of pathogens by direct or indirect contact with feces. Use them in patients with amebic dysentery; cholera; coxsackievirus disease; acute diarrhea with suspected infection; echovirus disease; encephalitis caused by enteroviruses; *Clostridium difficile* or *Staphylococcus* enterocolitis; enteroviral infection; or gastroenteritis caused by *Campylobacter, Cryptosporidium, Dientamoeba fragilis, Escherichia coli, Giardia lamblia, Salmonella, Shigella, Vibrio parahaemolyticus;* or *Yersinia enterocolitica.*

Use them also in patients with hand, foot, and mouth disease; hepatitis A; herpangina; viral meningitis caused by enteroviruses; necrotizing enterocolitis; pleurodynia; poliomyelitis; typhoid fever; or viral pericarditis, viral myocarditis, or enteroviral meningitis.

Implementation

• Assess the patient's hygiene. Does he fail to wash his hands after touching infective material? Does he contaminate the environment with infec-

tive material or share contaminated articles with other patients? Usually, patients infected with the same organisms may share a room.

• A mask isn't needed when approaching the patient. Wear a gown if soiling is likely, and wear gloves if you'll be touching infective material.

• Wash your hands after touching the patient or potentially contaminated articles and before caring for another patient.

• Discard contaminated articles, or bag and label such articles and send them for decontamination and reprocessing.

Neutropenic isolation

Neutropenic isolation (also known as protective or reverse isolation) protects patients who are at increased risk for infection from contact with potential pathogens. Although deleted from CDC guidelines because of lack of evidence support its efficacy, it's still used in many institutions. This procedure is used primarily for patients with extensive noninfected burns, leukopenia, or a depressed immune system and for those who are receiving immunosuppressive treatments.

Implementation

• Provide a private room equipped with special ventilation, if possible. Place neutropenic isolation cards on the door to warn visitors.

• Keep supplies in a clean enclosed cart or an outide anteroom.

• Wash your hands with an antiseptic agent before putting on gloves to prevent bacterial growth on gloved skin. Wash your hands again after leaving the room.

• Put on a clean mask each time

you enter the patient's room. Use gowns and gloves according to universal precaution recommendations.
• Don't allow visits by anyone known to be infected or ill. Show all visitors how to put on masks before entering the patient's room, and tell them to remove them only after leaving the room.
• Don't perform invasive procedures, such as urethral catheterization, unless absolutely necessary, because these procedures risk serious infection in the patient with impaired resistance. Avoid transporting the patient out of the room; if he must be moved, gown and mask him first.
• Because the patient doesn't have a contagious disease, materials leaving the room need no special precautions, and the room requires no special cleaning after discharge.
• For patients with temporarily increased susceptibility, such as those who have undergone bone marrow transplantation, provide a patient-isolator unit and use sterile linens, gowns, gloves, and head and shoe coverings, if necessary. In such cases, all other items taken into the room should be sterilized as well.

Implementation period
• Acquired immunodeficiency syndrome: until white blood cell count reaches 1,000/mm³ or less, or according to hospital guidelines
• Agranulocytosis: until remission
• Burns, noninfected, extensive: until skin surface heals substantially
• Dermatitis, noninfected vesicular, bullous, or eczematous disease (when severe and extensive): until skin surface heals substantially
• Immunosuppressive therapy: until patient's immunity is adequate
• Lymphomas and leukemia, especially in late stages of Hodgkin's disease or acute leukemia: until clinical improvement is substantial.

Respiratory isolation

This procedure prevents the spread of infectious diseases transmitted by airborne pathogens that are breathed, sneezed, or coughed into the environment.

Implementation
• Provide a private room with private toilet facilities and an anteroom, if possible. If necessary, two patients with the same infection may share a room.
• For a patient with measles, provide a room with negative air pressure that is vented directly to the outside of the building.
• Keep the room door closed at all times to isolate the patient's airborne secretions. Put a respiratory isolation card on the door to notify anyone entering the room.
• Keep all respiratory isolation supplies outside the patient's room in an isolation cart or anteroom.
• Wash your hands before entering and after leaving the room and also during patient care if you've handled respiratory tract secretions.
• Ensure that all visitors wear masks and, if necessary, gowns. Ensure that everyone puts on and removes masks and gowns properly.
• If the patient has a highly contagious respiratory disease, you may discard your mask and gloves in a lined, covered receptacle outside the patient's room. Thus, you'll be outside the room (with the door shut behind you) before removing your protective garb.
• Remember to discard the mask and gloves right at the door. Carrying them away from the patient's immediate area promotes contamination.
• Instruct the patient to cover his mouth with a facial tissue while coughing or sneezing to control the

spread of airborne droplets. Tape an impervious bag to the bedside so he can discard tissues correctly.

• Place all sputum specimens from respiratory isolation patients in impervious, labeled containers and send them to the laboratory.

• Place all items that have come in direct contact with the patient — such as linens, trash, and nondisposable utensils or instruments — in a single impervious bag before removal from the room. Place this bag inside a second bag if it is punctured or visibly contaminated.

Implementation period

• Diphtheria (pharyngeal): until nose and throat cultures taken 24 hours after ending treatment are negative for causative organisms

• Epiglottitis, meningitis, and pneumonia caused by *Haemophilus influenzae*: until 4 hours after start of effective therapy

• Erythema infectiosum: until 7 days after onset

• Hemorrhagic fevers (such as Lassa fever, Marburg virus disease): for the duration of the illness

• Herpes zoster (shingles): for the duration of the illness

• Measles (rubeola): until 4 days after start of rash (for duration of illness in immunocompromised patients)

• Meningitis (*H. influenzae* or *Neisseria meningitidis* known or suspected): until 4 hours after start of effective therapy

• Meningococcemia: until 24 hours after start of effective therapy

• Mumps: until 9 days after onset of swelling

• Pertussis (whooping cough): until 7 days after start of effective therapy or 3 weeks after onset of paroxysms, if untreated

• Plague (pneumonic): until 3 days after start of effective therapy

• Pneumonia (*H. influenzae, N. meningitidis*): until 4 hours after start of effective therapy

• Rabies: for the duration of the illness

• Rubella (congenital syndrome): for first year after birth unless nasopharyngeal cultures are negative for causative organism after age 3 months

• Rubella (German measles): until 7 days after onset of rash

• Smallpox (variola): for the duration of the illness

Strict isolation

This procedure prevents the spread of highly contagious or virulent pathogens that are transmitted by both air and contact. This procedure should be used in cases of pharyngeal diphtheria, viral hemorrhagic fevers, pneumonic plague, smallpox, chicken pox (varicella), and herpes zoster (localized in an immunocompromised patient or disseminated).

Implementation

• Provide a private room (with negative air pressure ventilation) and keep the door closed. Usually, patients infected with the same organism may share a room. Patients with viral hemorrhagic fevers or smallpox need special room ventilation.

• Wear a mask, a gown, and gloves when entering the room.

• Wash your hands after touching the patient or potentially contaminated articles and before caring for another patient.

CHAPTER 9

Troubleshooting:
Spotting and correcting equipment problems

I.V. equipment

Peripheral I.V. lines

SIGNS AND SYMPTOMS	POSSIBLE CAUSES	INTERVENTIONS
Local complications		
Phlebitis • Tenderness at tip of and above venipuncture device • Redness at tip of catheter and along vein • Puffy area over vein • Vein hard on palpation • Possible fever	• Poor blood flow around venipuncture device • Friction from catheter movement in vein • Venipuncture device left in vein too long • Clotting at catheter tip (thrombophlebitis) • Drug or solution with high or low pH or high osmolarity	• Remove venipuncture device. • Apply warm soaks. • Notify doctor if patient has fever. Document patient's condition and your interventions. ***Prevention*** • Restart the infusion using a larger vein for an irritating solution, or restart with smaller-gauge device to ensure adequate blood flow. • Use a filter to lower the risk of phlebitis. • Tape device securely to prevent motion.
Extravasation • Swelling at and above I.V. site (may extend along entire limb) • Discomfort, burning, or pain at site (but may be painless) • Tight feeling at site • Decreased skin temperature around site • Blanching at site • Continuing fluid infusion even when vein is occluded (although rate may decrease) • Absent backflow of blood	• Venipuncture device dislodged from vein, or perforated vein	• Remove venipuncture device. Infiltrate site with antidote, if needed. • Apply ice (early) or warm soaks (later) to aid absorption. Elevate limb. • Monitor for pulse and capillary refill. • Restart infusion above infiltration site or in another limb. • Document patient's condition and your interventions. ***Prevention*** • Check site often. • Don't obscure area above site with tape. • Teach patient to observe I.V. site and report pain or swelling.

Peripheral I.V. lines *(continued)*

SIGNS AND SYMPTOMS	POSSIBLE CAUSES	INTERVENTIONS
Local complications *(continued)*		
Catheter dislodgment • Loose tape • Catheter partly backed out of vein • Solution infiltrating	• Loosened tape, or tubing snagged in bed linens, resulting in partial retraction of catheter • pulled out by confused patient	• If no infiltration occurs, retape without pushing catheter back into vein. If pulled out, apply pressure to I.V. site with sterile dressing. ***Prevention*** • Tape venipuncture securely on insertion.
Occlusion • No increase in flow rate when I.V. container is raised • Blood backflow in line • Discomfort at insertion site	• I.V. flow interrupted • Heparin lock not flushed • Blood backflow in line when patient walks • Line clamped too long	• Use mild flush injection. Don't force it. If unsuccessful, reinsert I.V. line. ***Prevention*** • Maintain I.V. flow rate. • Flush promptly after intermittent piggyback administration. • Have patient walk with his arm folded to his chest to reduce risk of blood backflow.
Vein irritation or pain at I.V. site • Pain during infusion • Possible blanching if vasospasm occurs • Red skin over vein during infusion • Rapidly developing signs of phlebitis	• Solution with high or low pH or high osmolarity, such as 40 mEq/liter of potassium chloride, phenytoin, and some antibiotics (vancomycin, erythromycin, and nafcillin)	• Decrease the flow rate. • Try using an electronic flow device to achieve a steady flow. ***Prevention*** • Dilute solutions before administration. For example, give antibiotics in 250-ml solution rather than in 100-ml. If drug has low pH, ask pharmacist if drug can be buffered with sodium bicarbonate. (Refer to hospital's policy.) • If long-term therapy of irritating drug is planned, ask doctor to use central I.V. line.

(continued)

Peripheral I.V. lines *(continued)*

SIGNS AND SYMPTOMS	POSSIBLE CAUSES	INTERVENTIONS
Local complications *(continued)*		
Severed catheter • Leakage from catheter shaft	• Catheter inadvertently cut by scissors • Reinsertion of needle into catheter	• If broken part is visible, attempt to retrieve it. If unsuccessful, notify the doctor. • If portion of catheter enters bloodstream, place tourniquet above I.V. site to prevent progression of broken part, and immediately notify doctor and radiology department. • Document patient's condition and your interventions. ***Prevention*** • Don't use scissors around I.V. site. • Never reinsert needle into catheter. • Remove unsuccessfully inserted catheter and needle together.
Hematoma • Tenderness at venipuncture site • Bruised area around site • Inability to advance or flush I.V. line	• Vein punctured through opposite wall at time of insertion • Leakage of blood from needle displacement	• Remove venipuncture device. • Apply pressure and warm soaks to affected area. • Recheck for bleeding. • Document patient's condition and your interventions. ***Prevention*** • Choose a vein that can accommodate size of venipuncture device. • Release tourniquet as soon as successful insertion is achieved.

Peripheral I.V. lines *(continued)*

SIGNS AND SYMPTOMS	POSSIBLE CAUSES	INTERVENTIONS
Local complications *(continued)*		
Venous spasm • Pain along vein • Flow rate sluggish when clamp completely open • Blanched skin over vein	• Severe vein irritation from irritating drugs or fluids • Administration of cold fluids or blood • Very rapid flow rate (with fluids at room temperature)	• Apply warm soaks over vein and surrounding area. • Decrease flow rate. ***Prevention*** • Use a blood warmer for blood or packed red blood cells.
Vasovagal reaction • Sudden collapse of vein during venipuncture • Sudden pallor, sweating, faintness, dizziness, and nausea • Decreased blood pressure	• Vasospasm from anxiety or pain	• Lower head of bed. • Have patient take deep breaths. • Check vital signs. ***Prevention*** • Prepare patient for therapy to relieve his anxiety. • Use local anesthetic to prevent pain.
Thrombosis • Painful, reddened, and swollen vein • Sluggish or stopped I.V. flow	• Injury to endothelial cells of vein wall, allowing platelets to adhere and thrombi to form	• Remove venipuncture device; restart infusion in opposite limb if possible. • Apply warm soaks. • Watch for I.V. therapy-related infection. ***Prevention*** • Use proper venipuncture techniques to reduce injury to vein.
Thrombophlebitis • Severe discomfort • Reddened, swollen, and hardened vein	• Thrombosis and inflammation	• Follow interventions for thrombosis. ***Prevention*** • Check site frequently. Remove venipuncture device at first sign of redness and tenderness.

(continued)

Peripheral I.V. lines *(continued)*

SIGNS AND SYMPTOMS	POSSIBLE CAUSES	INTERVENTIONS
Local complications *(continued)*		
Nerve, tendon, or ligament damage • Extreme pain (similar to electrical shock when nerve is punctured), numbness, and muscle contraction • Delayed effects, including paralysis, numbness, and deformity	• Improper venipuncture technique, resulting in injury to surrounding nerves, tendons, or ligaments • Tight taping or improper splinting with armboard	• Stop procedure. *Prevention* • Don't repeatedly penetrate tissues with venipuncture device. • Don't apply excessive pressure when taping; don't encircle limb with tape. • Pad armboards and tape securing armboards if possible.
Systemic complications		
Circulatory overload • Discomfort • Neck vein engorgement • Respiratory distress • Increased blood pressure • Crackles • Increased difference between fluid intake and output	• Roller clamp loosened to allow run-on infusion • Flow rate too rapid • Miscalculation of fluid requirements	• Raise the head of the bed. • Administer oxygen as needed. • Notify the doctor. • Give drugs as ordered. *Prevention* • Use pump, controller, or rate minder for elderly or compromised patients. • Recheck calculations of fluid requirements. • Monitor infusion frequently.
Systemic infection (septicemia or bacteremia) • Fever, chills, and malaise for no apparent reason • Contaminated I.V. site, usually with no visible signs of infection at site	• Failure to maintain aseptic technique during insertion or site care • Severe phlebitis, which can set up ideal conditions for organism growth • Poor taping that permits venipuncture device to	• Notify the doctor. • Administer medications as prescribed. • Culture the site and device. • Monitor vital signs. *Prevention* • Use scrupulous aseptic technique when handling solutions and tubing, inserting venipuncture device, and discontinuing infusion.

Peripheral I.V. lines *(continued)*

SIGNS AND SYMPTOMS	POSSIBLE CAUSES	INTERVENTIONS
Systemic complications *(continued)*		
Systemic infection *(continued)*	move, which can introduce organisms into bloodstream • Prolonged indwelling time • Compromised immune system	• Secure all connections. • Change I.V. solutions, tubing, and venipuncture device at recommended times. • Use I.V. filters.
Speed shock • Flushed face, headache • Tightness in chest • Irregular pulse • Syncope • Rapid hypertension • Shock • Cardiac arrest	• Too rapid injection of drug, causing plasma concentration to reach toxic levels • Improper administration of bolus infusion (especially additives)	• Discontinue infusion. • Begin infusion of dextrose 5% in water at keep-vein-open rate. • Notify doctor. ***Prevention*** • Check infusion guidelines before giving drugs. • Dilute drugs with compatible solutions.
Air embolism • Respiratory distress • Unequal breath sounds • Chest pain, dyspnea • Anxiety • Weak, rapid pulse • Increased central venous pressure • Decreased blood pressure • Loss of consciousness	• Solution container empty • Solution container empties, and added container pushes air down the line	• Discontinue infusion. • Place patient in left lateral Trendelenburg's position to allow air to enter right atrium and disperse via pulmonary artery. • Administer oxygen. • Notify doctor. • Document patient's condition and your interventions. ***Prevention*** • Purge tubing of air completely before starting infusion. • Use air-detection device on pump or air-eliminating filter proximal to I.V. site. • Secure connections.

(continued)

Peripheral I.V. lines *(continued)*

SIGNS AND SYMPTOMS	POSSIBLE CAUSES	INTERVENTIONS
Local complications *(continued)*		
Allergic reaction • Itching • Watery eyes and nose • Bronchospasm • Wheezing • Urticarial rash • Edema at I.V. site • Anaphylactic reaction, which may occur within minutes or up to 1 hour after exposure (flushing, chills, anxiety, agitation, itching, palpitations, paresthesia, throbbing in ears, wheezing, coughing, seizures, cardiac arrest)	• Allergens, such as medications	• If reaction occurs, stop infusion immediately. • Maintain patent airway. • Notify doctor. • Administer antihistaminic steroid and antipyretic drugs, as ordered. • Give 0.2 to 0.5 ml of 1:1,000 aqueous epinephrine subcutaneously, as ordered. Repeat at 3-minute intervals and as needed. ***Prevention*** • Obtain patient's allergy history. Be aware of cross-allergies. • Assist with test dosing. • Monitor patient carefully during first 15 minutes of administration of a new drug.

Central venous lines

SIGNS AND SYMPTOMS	POSSIBLE CAUSES	INTERVENTIONS
Pneumothorax, hemothorax, chylothorax, hydrothorax • Chest pain • Dyspnea • Cyanosis • Decreased breath sounds on affected side	• Lung puncture by catheter during insertion or exchange over a guide wire • Large blood vessel puncture with bleeding inside or outside lung	• Notify doctor. • Remove catheter or assist with removal. • Administer oxygen as ordered. • Set up and assist with chest tube insertion. • Document all interventions.

Central venous lines *(continued)*

SIGNS AND SYMPTOMS	POSSIBLE CAUSES	INTERVENTIONS
Pneumothorax, hemothorax, chylothorax, hydrothorax *(continued)* • With hemothorax, decreased hemoglobin because of blood pooling • Abnormal chest X-ray • Apprehension	• Lymph node puncture with leakage of lymph fluid • Infusion of solution into chest area through infiltrated catheter	**Prevention** • Position patient head down with a rolled towel between his scapulae to dilate and expose the internal jugular or subclavian vein as much as possible during catheter insertion. • Assess for early signs of fluid infiltration (swelling in the shoulder, neck, chest, and arm). • Ensure that the patient is immobilized and prepared for insertion; active patients may need to be sedated or taken to the operating room. • Minimize patient activity after insertion, especially with a peripheral catheter.
Air embolism • Respiratory distress • Chest pain • Unequal breath sounds • Weak, rapid pulse • Increased central venous pressure • Decreased blood pressure • Churning murmur over precordium • Alteration or loss of consciousness • Anxiety	• Intake of air into central venous system during catheter insertion or tubing changes, or inadvertent opening, cutting, or breaking of catheter	• Clamp catheter immediately. • Place patient in left lateral Trendelenburg's position so air can enter the right atrium and pulmonary artery. Maintain this position for 20 to 30 minutes. • Don't recommend Valsalva's maneuver because a large air intake worsens the condition. • Administer oxygen. • Notify the doctor. • Document interventions.

(continued)

Central venous lines *(continued)*

SIGNS AND SYMPTOMS	POSSIBLE CAUSES	INTERVENTIONS
Air embolism *(continued)*		***Prevention*** • Purge all air from tubing before hookup. • Teach patient to perform Valsalva's maneuver during catheter insertion and tubing changes. • Use air-eliminating filters or an infusion device with air-detection capability. • Use luer-lock tubing, tape the connections, or use locking devices for all connections.
Thrombosis • Edema at puncture site • Erythema • Ipsilateral swelling of arm, neck, and face • Pain along vein • Fever, malaise • Jugular vein distention	• Sluggish flow rate • Composition of catheter material (polyvinylchloride catheters are more thrombogenic) • Hematopoietic status of patient • Preexisting limb edema • Infusion of irritating solutions • Repeated or long-term use of same vein • Preexisting cardiovascular disease • Simultaneous administration of or inadequate flushing between incompatible medications	• Notify doctor. • Remove catheter, if necessary. • Infuse dose of heparin or thrombolytic agents, if ordered. • Apply warm, wet compresses locally. • Don't use limb on affected side for subsequent venipuncture. • Verify thrombosis with diagnostic studies. ***Prevention*** • Maintain steady flow rate with infusion pump, or flush catheter at regular intervals. • Use catheters made of less thrombogenic materials or catheters coated to prevent thrombosis. • Dilute irritating solutions. • Use 0.22-micron filter for infusions. • Ensure compatibility of medications, and flush adequately.

Central venous lines *(continued)*

SIGNS AND SYMPTOMS	POSSIBLE CAUSES	INTERVENTIONS
Infection • Redness, warmth, tenderness, swelling at insertion or exit site • Possible exudate of purulent material • Local rash or pustules • Fever, chills, malaise • Leukocytosis • Nausea and vomiting • Elevated urine glucose level	• Failure to maintain aseptic technique during catheter insertion or care • Failure to comply with dressing change protocol • Wet or soiled dressing remaining on site • Immunosuppression • Irritated suture line • Contaminated catheter or solution • Frequent opening of catheter or long-term use of single I.V. access site	• Monitor temperature frequently. • Monitor vital signs closely. • Culture the site. • Re-dress aseptically. • Use antibiotic ointment locally, as needed. • Treat systemically with antibiotics or antifungals, depending on culture results and doctor's order. • Draw central and peripheral blood cultures; if the same organism appears in both, then catheter is primary source and should be removed. • If cultures don't match but are positive, the catheter may be removed, or the infection may be treated through the catheter. • Treat patients with antibiotics, as ordered. • If the catheter is removed, culture its tip. • Document interventions. ***Prevention*** • Maintain sterile technique using sterile gloves, masks, and gowns when appropriate. • Observe dressing-change protocols. • Teach patient about restrictions on swimming, bathing, and other physical activities. (The doctor may allow these ac- *(continued)*

TROUBLESHOOTING

Central venous lines *(continued)*

SIGNS AND SYMPTOMS	POSSIBLE CAUSES	INTERVENTIONS
Infection *(continued)*		tivities with adequate white blood cell count.) • Change wet or soiled dressing immediately. • Change dressing more frequently if catheter is located in femoral area or near tracheostomy. Perform tracheostomy care after catheter care. • Examine solution for cloudiness and turbidity before infusing; check fluid container for leaks. • Monitor urine glucose level in patients receiving total parenteral nutrition (TPN); if greater than 2+, suspect early sepsis. • Use a 0.22-micron filter (or a 1.2-micron filter for 3-in-1 TPN solutions). • Change the catheter frequently. • Keep the system closed as much as possible.

Infusion control devices

When the alarm goes off, check for the following.

PROBLEMS	INTERVENTIONS
Air in the line	While setting up, make sure all air is out of the line, including air trapped in Y-injection sites. Also, check that the connections are secure and the container is filled properly. Withdraw any air from a piggyback port with a syringe or an air-eliminating filter. A wet-air detector may give a false reading.
Infusion completed	Reset the pump as ordered or discontinue the infusion. A slow keep-vein-open flow rate will usually keep the I.V. line patent as long as enough fluid remains.
Empty container	Check for adequate fluid levels in the I.V. container, and have another container available before the last one runs out.
Low battery	Battery life varies; keep the machine plugged in on AC power as much as possible, especially while the patient is in bed. If the alarm goes off, plug in the machine immediately, or power may be lost for a while (usually a half hour to several hours).
Occlusion	Check that all clamps are open, look for kinked tubing, and check the patency of the venipuncture device.
Rate change	Check that the infusion control device displays the ordered rate. The patient or a family member may have tampered with the controls.
Open door	The door should be closed; it may not shut if the device isn't set up properly (for example, if the cassette isn't inserted all the way).
Malfunction	A mechanical failure usually must be handled by the biomedical engineering department or the manufacturer. Disconnect the infusion control device. Label it clearly with a sign that says BROKEN and indicate the specific problem.

I.V. flow rates

PROBLEMS AND POSSIBLE CAUSES	INTERVENTIONS
Flow rate too fast	
Clamp manipulated by patient or visitor	Instruct the patient not to touch the clamp, and place tape over it. Restrain him or administer the I.V. solution with an infusion pump or a controller if necessary.
Tubing disconnected from catheter	Wipe the distal end of the tubing with luer-lock connections with alcohol, reinsert firmly into the catheter hub, and apply tape at the connection site.
Change in patient position	Use an infusion pump or a controller to ensure the correct flow rate.
Bevel against vein wall (positional cannulation)	Manipulate the venipuncture device, and place a 2″ × 2″ gauze pad under or over the catheter hub to change the angle. Reset the flow clamp at the desired rate. If necessary, remove and reinsert the venipuncture device.
Flow clamp drifting from patient movement	Place tape below the clamp.
Flow rate too slow	
Venous spasm after insertion	Apply warm soaks over site.
Venous obstruction from bending arm	Secure the I.V. line with an arm board if necessary.
Pressure change (from decreased fluid in bottle)	Readjust the flow rate.
Elevated blood pressure	Readjust flow rate. Use an infusion pump or a controller to ensure correct rate.
Cold solution	Allow the solution to warm to room temperature before hanging the bag.
Change in solution viscosity from drug added	Readjust the flow rate.
I.V. container too low or patient's arm or leg too high	Hang the container higher or remind the patient to keep his arm below heart level.
Bevel against vein wall (positional cannulation)	Withdraw the needle slightly, or place a folded 2″ × 2″ gauze pad over or under the catheter hub to change the angle.

I.V. flow rates *(continued)*

PROBLEMS AND POSSIBLE CAUSES	INTERVENTIONS
Flow rate too slow *(continued)*	
Excess tubing dangling below insertion site	Replace the tubing with a shorter piece, or tape the excess tubing to the I.V. pole below the flow clamp (making sure that the tubing is not kinked).
Venipuncture device too small	Remove the venipuncture device in use, and insert a larger-bore venipuncture device or use an infusion pump.
Infiltration or clotted venipuncture device	Remove the venipuncture device in use, and insert a new venipuncture device.
Kinked tubing	Check the tubing over its entire length and unkink it.
Clogged filter	Remove the filter and replace it with a new one.
Tubing compressed at clamped area	Massage or milk the tubing by pinching and wrapping it around a pencil four or five times. Then quickly pull the pencil out of the coiled tubing.

Infusion interruptions

When an infusion stops, systematically assess the I.V. system—from the patient to the fluid container—for potential trouble areas.

Check the I.V. site

Check for infiltration or phlebitis, which may slow or stop the flow rate.

Check for patency

Evaluate the I.V. device for patency, which may be affected by several factors.

• If the patient's limb is flexed or lying directly on the I.V. site, increased blood pressure may stop the flow. Reposition the limb as necessary.

• The tip of the needle may be against the vein wall or a venous valve. Lift up or pull back the venipuncture device to reestablish the I.V. flow.

• If the patient's arm is wrapped with tape, a tourniquet effect may reduce the flow rate. Taping the I.V. site too tightly can cause the same problem. Release or remove tape. Then reapply it.

• Smaller venipuncture devices may kink or fold, impeding I.V. flow. Pull the device back to reestablish flow.

• Local edema or poor tissue perfusion from disease can block venous flow. Move the I.V. line to an unaffected site.

• Infusion of incompatible fluids or medications may cause a precipitate to form. This can block the I.V. tubing and venipuncture device, and may even expose the patient to a life-threatening embolism. Always check the compatibility of medications and I.V. solutions before administration. Replace the venipuncture device if it's occluded.

Check the filter

Make sure that the in-line filter is the right size and type. I.V. fluids are usually run through a 0.22- or 0.45-micron filter that eliminates air and microorganisms from the system. Single-use filters shouldn't be used for in-line filtration — only for drawing up a medication or administering a bolus dose.

If you use the wrong size or type of filter, the solution may not pass through it. For example, drugs such as amphotericin B and lymphocyte immune globulin (Atgam) consist of molecules too large to pass through a 0.22-micron filter; they'd rapidly block the filter and stop the I.V. flow. If necessary, replace the filter.

A filter that's used longer than recommended may become blocked by minute particles and microorganisms. Not only will the I.V. flow stop, but the patient may become exposed to bacterial toxins and sepsis. The interval between filter changes usually ranges from 24 to 48 hours, depending on the manufacturer's instructions. Change the filter if necessary.

Check clamps

Be sure that the flow clamps are open. Check all clamps, including the roller clamp and any clamps on secondary sets, such as a slide clamp on a filter. (A roller clamp may also become jammed if the roller is pushed up too far.)

Check tubing

Determine if the tubing is kinked or if the patient is lying on it. Also check whether the tubing remains crimped where a clamp was tightened around it. If so, gently squeezing the area between your fingers will usually round out the tubing to its original shape.

Check air vents

If you're using an evacuated glass container, you need an air vent to make the solution flow. Insert one as necessary. With a volume-control set, an air vent is usually located at the top of the calibrated chamber. If the solution flow stops, check the patency of this vent and the position of the vent clamp. To check patency, follow the manufacturer's instructions.

Check fluid level

Observe the fluid level in the I.V. container. If it's empty, replace it as ordered. If the solution is cold, it may be causing venous spasm and thus decreasing the flow rate. Applying warm compresses may relieve venous spasm and help increase the flow rate. Make sure subsequent solutions are at room temperature. Finally, check to see if the spike at the end of the administration set has been pushed far enough into the container to allow the solution to flow.

If you can't identify the problem with this series of checks, the I.V. line should be removed and restarted at a different site. Be sure to document the episode in the patient's chart.

Vascular access ports

PROBLEMS AND POSSIBLE CAUSES	INTERVENTIONS
Inability to flush vascular access port (VAP) or withdraw blood	
• Kinked tubing or closed clamp	• Check tubing or clamp.
• Catheter lodged against vessel wall	• Reposition the patient. • Teach the patient to change his position to free the catheter from the vessel wall. • Raise the arm that's on the same side as the catheter. • Roll the patient to the opposite side. • Have the patient cough, sit up, or take a deep breath. • Infuse 10 ml of 0.9% sodium chloride solution into the catheter. • Regain access to the catheter or VAP using a new sterile needle.
• Incorrect needle placement • Needle not advanced through septum	• Regain access to the device. • Teach the home care patient to push down firmly on the noncoring needle in the septum and to verify needle position by aspirating for a blood return.
• Clot formation	• Assess patency by trying to flush the VAP while the patient changes position. • Notify the doctor; obtain an order for urokinase instillation. • Teach the patient to recognize clot formation, to notify the doctor if it occurs, and to avoid forcibly flushing the VAP.
• Kinked catheter, catheter migration, port rotation	• Notify the doctor immediately. • Tell the patient to notify the doctor if he has difficulty using the VAP.
Inability to palpate the VAP	
• Deeply implanted port	• Note the portal chamber scar to locate the correct spot for palpation. • Use deep palpation technique. • Ask another nurse to locate the VAP. • Use a 1½" or 2" noncoring needle to gain access to the VAP.

Cardiovascular monitors and devices

Blood pressure readings

PROBLEMS AND POSSIBLE CAUSES	INTERVENTIONS
False-high reading	
Cuff too small	Make sure the cuff bladder is 20% wider than the circumference of the arm or leg being used for measurement.
Cuff wrapped too loosely, reducing its effective width	Tighten the cuff.
Slow cuff deflation, causing venous congestion in the arm or leg	Never deflate the cuff more slowly than 2 mm Hg per heartbeat.
Tilted mercury column	Read pressures with the mercury column vertical.
Poorly timed measurement – after patient has eaten, ambulated, appeared anxious, or flexed arm muscles	Postpone blood pressure measurement or help the patient relax before taking pressures.
False-low reading	
Incorrect position of arm or leg	Make sure the arm or leg is level with the patient's heart.
Mercury column below eye level	Read the mercury column at eye level.
Failure to notice auscultatory gap (sound fades out for 10 to 15 mm Hg, then returns)	Estimate systolic pressure by palpation before actually measuring it. Then check this pressure against the measured pressure.
Inaudible low-volume sounds	Before reinflating the cuff, instruct the patient to raise the arm or leg to decrease venous pressure and amplify low-volume sounds. After inflating the cuff, tell the patient to lower the arm or leg. Then deflate the cuff and listen. If you still fail to detect low-volume sounds, chart the palpated systolic pressure.

▶

Cardiac monitors

PROBLEMS AND POSSIBLE CAUSES	INTERVENTIONS
False-high-rate alarm	
Monitor interpreting large T waves as QRS complexes, which doubles the rate	Reposition electrodes to lead where QRS complexes are taller than the T waves.
Skeletal muscle activity	Place electrodes away from major muscle masses.
False-low-rate alarm	
Shift in electrical axis caused by patient movement, making QRS complexes too small to register	Reapply electrodes. Set gain so that height of complex exceeds 1 millivolt.
Low amplitude of QRS complex	Increase gain dial.
Poor electrode-skin contact	Reapply electrodes.
Low amplitude	
Gain dial set too low	Increase gain.
Poor contact between skin and electrodes; dried gel; broken or loose leadwires; poor connection between patient and monitor; malfunctioning monitor; physiologic loss of amplitude of QRS complex	Check connections on all leadwires and monitoring cable. Replace or reapply electrodes as necessary.
Wandering baseline	
Poor electrode placement or contact with skin	Reposition or replace electrodes.
Thoracic movement with respirations	Reposition electrodes.
Artifact (waveform interference)	
Patient having seizures, chills, or anxiety	Notify doctor and treat patient as ordered. Keep patient warm and reassure him.
Patient movement	Help patient relax.
Electrodes applied improperly	Check electrodes and reapply, if necessary.
Static electricity	Make sure cables don't have exposed connectors. Change static-causing bedclothes.

(continued)

Cardiac monitors *(continued)*

PROBLEMS AND POSSIBLE CAUSES	INTERVENTIONS
Artifact (waveform interference) *(continued)* Electrical short circuit in lead-wires or cable	Replace broken equipment. Use stress loops to apply leadwires.
Interference from decreased room humidity	Regulate humidity to 40%.
Broken leadwires or cable Tension on leadwires due to repeated pulling	Replace and retape leadwires, taping part of wire into a loop. This absorbs tension that would otherwise tug at the ends of the wire.
Cables and leadwires cleaned with alcohol or acetone, causing brittleness	Clean cable and leadwires with soapy water. *Do not let cable ends get wet.* Replace cable as necessary.
60-cycle interference (fuzzy baseline) Electrical interference from other equipment in room	Attach electrical equipment to common ground, checking plugs for loose prongs
Patient's bed improperly grounded	Attach bed ground to the room's common ground.
Skin excoriation under electrode Patient allergic to electrode adhesive	Remove electrodes and apply nonallergenic electrodes and tape.
Electrode remaining on skin too long	Remove electrode, clean site, and reapply electrode at new site.

▶

Intra-aortic balloon pumps

When your patient undergoes intra-aortic balloon counterpulsation (IABC), you must respond immediately to any equipment problems. This chart describes the problems most often encountered in the Model 700 IABP Control System, a popular device.

PROBLEMS AND POSSIBLE CAUSES	INTERVENTIONS
High gas leakage (automatic mode only)	
Balloon leakage or abrasion	Check for blood in tubing. Stop pumping. Contact the doctor to remove the balloon.
Condensation in extension tubing, volume limiter disk, or both	Remove condensate from tubing and volume limiter disk. Refill, autopurge, and resume pumping.
Kink in balloon catheter or tubing	Check catheter and tubing for kinks and loose connections. Refill and resume pumping.
Tachycardia (rapid flow of helium causing insufficient fill pressure)	Change wean control to 1:2 or operate in ON (manual) mode. *Note:* Gas alarms are off in manual mode. Autopurge balloon every 1 to 2 hours, and monitor balloon pressure waveform closely.
Malfunctioning or loose volume limiter disk	Replace or tighten volume limiter disk. Refill, autopurge, and resume pumping.
System leak	Perform leak test.
Balloon line block (automatic mode only)	
Kink in balloon catheter or tubing	Check catheter and tubing for kinks. Refill and resume pumping.
Balloon catheter not unfurled; sheath or balloon positioned too high	Contact doctor to verify placement; balloon may have to be repositioned or inflated manually.
Condensation in tubing, volume limiter disk, or both	Remove condensate from tubing and volume limiter disk. Refill, autopurge, and resume pumping.
Balloon too large for aorta	Decrease volume control percentage by one notch.
Malfunctioning volume limiter disk or incorrect volume limiter disk size	Replace volume limiter disk, refill, autopurge, and resume pumping.

(continued)

TROUBLESHOOTING

Intra-aortic balloon pumps *(continued)*

PROBLEMS AND POSSIBLE CAUSES	INTERVENTIONS
No electrocardiogram (ECG) trigger	
Inadequate signal	Adjust ECG gain, and change lead or trigger mode.
Lead disconnected	Replace lead.
Improper ECG input mode (skin or monitor) selected	Adjust ECG input to appropriate mode (skin or monitor).
No arterial pressure trigger	
Arterial line damped	Flush line.
Arterial line open to atmosphere	Check connections on arterial pressure line.
Trigger mode change	
Trigger mode changed while pumping	Resume pumping.
Irregular heart rhythm	
Patient in irregular rhythm (such as atrial fibrillation or ectopic beats)	Change to R or QRS sense (if necessary) to accommodate irregular rhythm.
Erratic atrioventricular (AV) pacing	
Demand for paced rhythm occurs while in atrioventricular sequential trigger mode	Change to pacer reject trigger or QRS sense.
Noisy ECG signal	
Malfunctioning leads	Replace leads; check ECG cable.
Electrocautery in use	Switch to arterial pressure trigger.
Internal trigger	
Trigger mode set on internal 80 beats/minute	Select alternative trigger if patient has a heartbeat or rhythm. *Caution:* Use internal trigger only during cardiopulmonary bypass surgery or cardiac arrest.

Intra-aortic balloon pumps *(continued)*

PROBLEMS AND POSSIBLE CAUSES	INTERVENTIONS
Purge incomplete	
OFF button pressed during autopurge, interrupting purge cycle	Initiate autopurge again or initiate pumping.
High fill pressure	
Malfunctioning volume limiter disk	Replace volume limiter disk, refill, autopurge, and resume pumping.
Occluded vent line or valve	Attempt to resume pumping. If this fails to correct problem, contact manufacturer.
No balloon drive	
No volume limiter disk	Insert volume limiter disk, and lock it securely in place.
Tubing disconnected	Reconnect tubing, refill, autopurge, and pump.
Incorrect timing	
INFLATE and DEFLATE controls improperly set	Place INFLATE and DEFLATE controls at set midpoints. Reassess timing and readjust.
Low volume percentage	
Volume control percentage not on 100%	Assess cause of decreased volume and reset if necessary.

►

Pacemakers

Life-threatening arrhythmias can result when the patient's pacemaker sends an impulse too weak to stimulate the heart (failure to capture). In addition, the pacemaker may fail to detect ventricular depolarization (failure to sense), or to send an impulse at all (failure to fire). Below are rhythm strips that compare these problems with a normal strip as well as lists of possible causes and interventions.

Normal
The location of the spike is your first clue that the pacemaker is functioning normally.

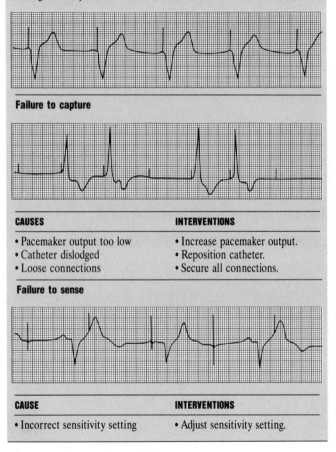

Failure to capture

CAUSES	INTERVENTIONS
• Pacemaker output too low	• Increase pacemaker output.
• Catheter dislodged	• Reposition catheter.
• Loose connections	• Secure all connections.

Failure to sense

CAUSE	INTERVENTIONS
• Incorrect sensitivity setting	• Adjust sensitivity setting.

TROUBLESHOOTING

Pacemakers *(continued)*

Failure to fire

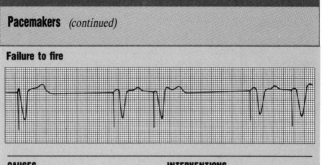

CAUSES	INTERVENTIONS
• Loose lead hookups	• Secure lead hookups.
• Dead battery	• Replace battery.
• Malfunctioning pulse generator	• Replace pulse generator.

Arterial lines

PROBLEMS	POSSIBLE CAUSES	INTERVENTIONS
Damped waveform Appearing as a small waveform with a slow rise in the anacrotic limb and a reduced or nonexistent dicrotic notch, a damped waveform may result from interference with transmission of the physiologic signal to the transducer.	Air in the system	Check the system for air, paying particular attention to the tubing and the transducer's diaphragm. If you find air, aspirate it or force it from the system through a stopcock port. Never flush any fluid containing air bubbles into the patient.
	Loose connection	Check and tighten all connections.
	Clotted catheter tip	Attempt to aspirate the clot. If you're successful, flush the line. If you're not successful, avoid flushing the line; you could dislodge the clot.

(continued)

Arterial lines *(continued)*

PROBLEMS	POSSIBLE CAUSES	INTERVENTIONS
Damped waveform *(continued)*	Catheter tip resting against the arterial wall	Reposition the catheter by carefully rotating it or pulling it back slightly. Anticipate possible change in catheter placement site and assist as appropriate.
	Kinked tubing	Unkink the tubing.
	Inadequately inflated pressure infuser bag	Inflate the pressure infuser bag to 300 mm Hg.
Drifting waveform Waveform floats above and below the baseline.	Temperature change in the flush solution	Allow the temperature of the flush solution to stabilize before the infusion.
	Kinked or compressed monitor cable	Check the cable and relieve the kink or compression.
Inability to flush the arterial line or to withdraw blood Activating the continuous flush device fails to move the flush solution, and blood can't be withdrawn from the stopcock.	Incorrectly positioned stopcocks	Properly reposition the stopcocks.
	Kinked tubing	Unkink the tubing.
	Inadequately inflated pressure infuser bag	Inflate the pressure infuser bag to 300 mm Hg.
	Clotted catheter tip	Attempt to aspirate the clot. If you're successful, flush the line. If you're not successful, avoid flushing the line; you could dislodge the clot.
	Catheter tip resting against the arterial wall	Reposition the catheter insertion area, and flush the catheter. Or reposition the catheter by carefully rotating it or pulling it back slightly.

Arterial lines *(continued)*

PROBLEMS	POSSIBLE CAUSES	INTERVENTIONS
Inability to flush the arterial line or to withdraw blood *(continued)*	Position of the insertion area	Check the position of the insertion area, and change it as indicated. For radial and brachial arterial lines, use an armboard to immobilize the area. With a femoral arterial line, keep the head of the bed at a 45-degree angle or less to prevent catheter kinking.
Artifact Waveform tracings follow an erratic pattern or fail to appear as a recognizable diagnostic pattern.	Electrical interference	Check electrical equipment in the room.
	Patient movement	Ask the patient to lie quietly while you try to read the monitor.
	Catheter whip or fling (excessive catheter tip movement)	Shorten the tubing, if possible.
False-high pressure reading Arterial pressure exceeds the patient's normal pressure without a significant change in baseline clinical findings. Before responding to this high pressure, recheck the system to make sure that the reading is accurate.	Improper calibration	Recalibrate the system.
	Transducer positioned below the phlebostatic axis	Relevel the transducer with the phlebostatic axis.
	Catheter kinked	Unkink the catheter.
	Clotted catheter tip	Attempt to aspirate the clot. If you're successful, flush the line. If you're not successful, avoid flushing the line; you could dislodge the clot.
	Catheter tip resting against the arterial line	Flush the catheter, or reposition it by carefully rotating it or pulling it back slightly.

(continued)

Arterial lines *(continued)*

PROBLEMS	POSSIBLE CAUSES	INTERVENTIONS
False-high pressure reading *(continued)*	I.V. tubing too long	Shorten the tubing by removing extension tubing (if used), or replace the administration set with a set that has shorter tubing.
	Small air bubbles in tubing close to patient	Remove air bubbles.
False-low pressure reading Arterial pressure drops below the patient's normal pressure without a significant change in baseline clinical findings. Before responding to this low pressure, recheck the system to ensure that the reading is accurate.	Improper calibration	Recalibrate the system.
	Transducer positioned above the level of the phlebostatic axis	Relevel the transducer with the phlebostatic axis.
	Loose connections	Check and tighten all connections.
	Catheter kinked	Unkink the catheter.
	Clotted catheter tip	Attempt to aspirate the clot. If you're successful, flush the line. If you're not successful, avoid flushing the line; you could dislodge the clot.
	Catheter tip resting against the arterial line	Reposition the catheter insertion area, and flush the catheter. Or reposition the catheter by carefully rotating it or pulling it back slightly.
	I.V. tubing too long	Shorten the tubing by removing the extension tubing (if used), or replace the administration set with a set having shorter tubing.
	Large air bubble close to the transducer	Reprime the transducer.

Arterial lines *(continued)*

PROBLEMS	POSSIBLE CAUSES	INTERVENTIONS
No waveform No waveform appears on the monitor.	No power supply	Turn on the power.
	Loose connections	Check and tighten all connections.
	Stopcocks turned off to the patient	Position the stopcocks properly. Make sure that the transducer is open to the catheter.
	Transducer disconnected from the monitor module	Reconnect the transducer to the monitor module.
	Occluded catheter tip	Attempt to aspirate the clot. If you're successful, flush the line. If you're not successful, avoid flushing the line; you could dislodge the clot.
	Catheter tip resting against the arterial wall	Flush the catheter, or reposition it by carefully rotating it or pulling it back slightly.

TROUBLESHOOTING

Arterial line accidental removal

If the patient removes his arterial line, he's in danger of hypovolemic shock from blood loss. Here's what to do.

Stanching blood flow
• Apply direct pressure to the insertion site immediately, and send someone to call the doctor. Maintain firm, direct pressure on the insertion site for 5 to 10 minutes to encourage clot formation because arterial blood flows under extremely high intravascular pressure.
• Check the patient's I.V. line and, if ordered, increase the flow rate temporarily to compensate for blood loss.

When the bleeding stops
• Apply a sterile pressure dressing.
• Reassess the patient's level of consciousness (LOC), and comfort and reassure him; losing large quantities of blood may have a significant psychological as well as physiologic impact.
• Estimate the amount of blood loss

from what you see and from changes in the patient's blood pressure and heart rate.
• Help the doctor reinsert the catheter, ensuring that the patient's arm is immobilized and the tubing and catheter secured.
• Withdraw blood for a complete blood count and arterial blood gas analysis, as ordered.

Ongoing care
• Closely monitor the patient's vital signs, LOC, skin color, temperature, and circulation to the extremity.
• Watch for further bleeding or hematoma.
• Decrease the I.V. flow rate to the previous level after the patient has stabilized.

Respiratory monitors and devices

Pulse oximeters

To maintain a continuous display of SaO$_2$ levels, you'll need to keep the monitoring site clean and dry. Make sure the skin doesn't become irritated from adhesives used to keep disposable probes in place. You may need to change the site if this happens. Disposable probes that irritate the skin also can be replaced by nondisposable models that don't need tape.

Another common problem with pulse oximeters is the failure of the devices to obtain a signal. Your first reaction if this happens should be to check the patient's vital signs. If they're sufficient to produce a signal, then check for the following problems.

Poor connection
See if the sensors are properly aligned. Make sure that wires are intact and securely fastened and that the pulse oximeter is plugged into a power source.

Inadequate or intermittent blood flow to the site
Check the patient's pulse rate and capillary refill time, and take corrective action if blood flow to the site is decreased. This may mean loosening restraints, removing tight-fitting clothes, taking off a blood pressure cuff, or checking arterial and I.V. lines. If none of these interventions works, you may need to find an alternate site. Finding a site with proper circulation may also prove challenging when a patient is receiving vasoconstrictive drugs.

Equipment malfunctions
Remove the pulse oximeter from the patient, set the alarm limits at 85% and 100%, and try the instrument on yourself or another healthy person. This will tell you if the equipment is working correctly.

SV̄O₂ monitors

During continuous mixed venous oxygen saturation (SV̄O₂) monitoring, you'll need to be alert for signals of equipment malfunction so that you can distinguish them from changes in your patient's condition and respond appropriately. This chart identifies the common problems, their causes, and nursing interventions.

PROBLEMS AND POSSIBLE CAUSES	INTERVENTIONS
Low-intensity alarm sounds	
Inadequate blood flow past the catheter tip	• Look for and straighten any obvious kinks in the catheter.
	• Follow hospital procedure to ensure patency of the distal lumen.
	• Check for proper connection between the optical module and the computer.
Damaged fiber-optic filaments	• Replace the catheter.
Damped intensity	
Blood clot over the catheter tip	• Follow hospital procedure to ensure patency of the distal lumen.
Wedging of the catheter tip	• Reposition the catheter.
Erratic intensity	
Blood clot over the catheter tip	• Follow hospital procedure to ensure patency of the distal lumen.
Wedging of the catheter tip	• Reposition the catheter.
High-intensity alarm sounds	
Catheter tip pressing against the vessel wall	• Reposition catheter, examine the pressure waveform to confirm proper position.
Catheter floating distally into a wedge position	• Check balloon status and confirm proper position by examining the pressure waveform.
	• Reposition catheter as needed.

(continued)

S$\bar{v}o_2$ monitors *(continued)*

PROBLEMS AND POSSIBLE CAUSES	INTERVENTIONS
LOW-LIGHT message Poor connection between the catheter and optical module	• Disconnect the catheter from the optical module, close the lid, and place the optical module out of direct light. If the LOW-LIGHT message disappears, the problem lies with the catheter. Check the connection and reattach as needed.
Defective optical module	• Replace the optical module.
Poor connection between the optical module and the computer	• Check the connections, and reconnect as needed. Turn off the computer for a few seconds and turn it back on. You'll hear two beeps if the computer is functional and connections are secure.
Damaged fiber-optic filaments	• Gently manipulate the catheter, particularly around the insertion site. If this doesn't solve the problem, replace the catheter.
CAL FAIL message Unsuccessful preinsertion calibration	• Verify a correct attachment between the catheter and the optical module; then repeat calibration. • If the CAL FAIL message still appears, replace the optical module.
Dashes in oxygen saturation display Improper preinsertion calibration	• Verify a correct attachment between the catheter and the optical module; then repeat calibration.
Optical module malfunction	• If dashes continue to appear, replace the optical module and repeat calibration.
Catheter damage	• Gently manipulate the catheter. If the monitor does not compute a range, replace the catheter and repeat calibration.
Catheter tip improperly positioned	• Reposition the catheter.
Loss of electronic memory	• Determine the cause of the power loss. Repeat calibration.

▶

Ventilators

Most ventilators have alarms to warn you of hazardous situations—for instance, when inspiratory pressure rises too high or drops too low. Use the chart below to help you respond quickly and effectively to a ventilator alarm.

PROBLEMS AND POSSIBLE CAUSES	INTERVENTIONS
Low pressure	
Tube disconnected from ventilator	Reconnect the tube to the ventilator.
Endotracheal (ET) tube displaced above vocal cords or tracheostomy tube extubated	If extubation or displacement has occurred, open the patient's airway, manually ventilate the patient, and call the doctor.
Leaking tidal volume from low cuff pressure (from an underinflated or ruptured ET cuff or a leak in the cuff or one-way valve)	Listen for a whooshing sound (an air leak) around the tube; check cuff pressure. If you can't maintain pressure, the doctor may insert a new tube.
Ventilator malfunction	Disconnect the patient from the ventilator, and manually ventilate him if necessary. Get another ventilator.
Leak in ventilator circuitry (from loose connection or hole in tubing, loss of temperature-sensing device, or cracked humidification container)	Make sure all connections are intact. Check the humidification container and the tubing for holes or leaks, and replace if necessary.
High pressure	
Increased airway pressure or decreased lung compliance caused by worsening disease	Auscultate the lungs for evidence of increasing lung consolidation, barotrauma, or wheezing. Call the doctor if indicated.
Patient biting on ET tube	If needed, insert a bite-block.
Secretions in airway	Suction or have the patient cough.
Condensate in large-bore tubing	Remove any condensate.

(continued)

Ventilators *(continued)*

PROBLEMS AND POSSIBLE CAUSES	INTERVENTIONS
High pressure *(continued)*	
Intubation of right mainstem bronchus	Check tube position. If it has slipped, call the doctor, who may need to reposition it.
Patient coughing, gagging, or trying to talk	If the patient is fighting the ventilator in any way, he may need sedation or a neuromuscular blocker, as ordered.
Chest wall resistance	Reposition the patient if his position limits chest expansion. If ineffective, give prescribed analgesic.
Malfunctioning high-pressure relief valve	Have the faulty equipment replaced.
Bronchospasm, pneumothorax, or barotrauma	Assess the patient for the cause. Report disorder to the doctor, and treat as ordered.
Spirometer or low exhaled tidal volume, or low exhaled minute volume	
Power interruption	Check all electrical connections.
Loose connection or leak in delivery system	Make sure all connections in the delivery system are secure; check for leaks.
Leaking cuff or inadequate cuff seal	Listen for leak with stethoscope. Reinflate cuff according to hospital policy. Replace cuff if necessary.
Leaking chest tube	Check all chest tube connections. Be sure that the water seal is intact; then notify the doctor.
Increased airway resistance in a patient on a pressure-cycled ventilator	Auscultate lungs for signs of airway obstruction, barotrauma, or lung consolidation.
Disconnected spirometer	Make sure the spirometer is connected.
Any change that sets off the high- or low-pressure alarms and prevents delivery of full air volume	See interventions for high- and low-pressure alarms.
Malfunctioning volume measuring device	Alert respiratory therapist to replace device.

Ventilators *(continued)*

PROBLEMS AND POSSIBLE CAUSES	INTERVENTIONS
High respiratory rate	
Anxious patient	Assess the patient for the cause. Dispel patient's fears if possible; sedate, if necessary.
Patient in pain	Position patient comfortably. Administer medication for pain as ordered.
Secretions in airway	Suction patient.
Low positive end-expiratory pressure (PEEP)-continuous positive airway pressure	
Leak in system	Check that all connections are secure. Check for holes in tubing and replace if necessary.
Mechanical failure of PEEP mechanism	Discontinue PEEP and call respiratory therapist.

◄

► LIFE-THREATENING EFFECTS

Accidental extubation

If an endotracheal or tracheostomy tube is removed accidentally (or deliberately by a patient), take these steps immediately.

Endotracheal tube

• Remove any remaining part of the tube.
• Ventilate the patient using common resuscitation techniques or a hand-held resuscitation bag.
• Notify the doctor.
• Restrain the patient if he's extubated himself.
• After the tube is reinstated, periodically check its position and the condition of the tape holding it. For a secure fit, anchor the tape from the nape of the patient's neck to and around the tube.

Tracheostomy tube

• Remove any remaining part of the tube.
• Keep the stoma open with a Kelly clamp and try to insert a new tube. If you can't get the tube in, insert a suction catheter instead, and thread the tube over the catheter.
• If you still can't establish an effective airway and you no longer detect a pulse, call a code. Then either ventilate with a face mask and resuscitation bag, or remove the Kelly clamp to close the stoma and perform mouth-to-mouth resuscitation until the doctor arrives. If air leaks from the stoma, cover it with an occlusive dressing.

Note: Don't leave the patient alone until you've established that he has an effective airway and can breathe comfortably.

• After the patient has a new tracheostomy tube in place and can breathe more easily, provide him with supplemental humidified oxygen until he receives a full evaluation.

• Monitor the patient's vital signs, skin color, and level of consciousness, and, unless contraindicated, elevate the head of his bed.

Chest drains

PROBLEMS	INTERVENTIONS
Patient rolls over on drainage tubing, causing obstruction	• Reposition patient and remove any kinks in tubing. • Auscultate for decreased breath sounds and percuss for dullness, indicating fluid accumulation, or for hyperresonance, indicating air accumulation.
Dependent loops in tubing trap fluids and prevent effective drainage	• Make sure chest drainage unit sits below patient's chest level. If necessary, raise the bed slightly to increase gravity flow. Remove kinks in tubing. • Monitor for decreased breath sounds and percuss for dullness.
No drainage appears in the collection chamber	• If draining blood or other fluid, suspect a clot or obstruction in the tubing. Gently milk the tubing to expel the obstruction, if hospital policy permits. • Monitor the patient for lung-tissue compression caused by accumulated pleural fluid.
Substantial increase in bloody drainage, indicating possible active bleeding or drainage of old blood	• Monitor patient's vital signs. Look for increased pulse rate, decreased blood pressure, and orthostatic changes that may indicate acute blood loss. • Measure drainage every 15 to 30 minutes to determine if it's occurring continuously or in one gush caused by position changes.
No bubbling in the suction-control chamber	• Check for obstructions in the tubing. Make sure connections are tight. • Check that suction apparatus is turned on. Increase suction slowly until you see gentle bubbling.

Chest drains *(continued)*

PROBLEMS	INTERVENTIONS
Loud, vigorous bubbling in the suction-control chamber	• Turn down the suction source until bubbling is just visible.
Constant bubbling in the water-seal chamber	• Assess the chest drainage unit and tubing for air leak. • If air leak isn't noted in the external system, notify physician immediately. Leaking and trapping of air in the pleural space can result in a tension pneumothorax.
Evaporation causes the water level in the suction-control chamber to drop below desired −20 cm H_2O	• Using a syringe and needle, add water or 0.9% sodium chloride solution through resealable diaphragm on back of suction-control chamber.
Patient has trouble breathing immediately after a special procedure. Chest drainage unit is improperly placed on his bed, interfering with drainage	• Raise the head of the bed and reposition the unit so that gravity promotes drainage. • Perform a quick respiratory assessment, and take his vital signs. Check to ensure that there's enough water in the water-seal and suction-control chambers.
As bed lowers, the chest drainage unit gets caught under the bed; the tubing comes apart and becomes contaminated	• Clamp the chest tube proximal to the latex connection tubing. • Irrigate the tubing, using the sealed jar of sterile water or 0.9% sodium chloride solution kept at the patient's bedside. • Insert the distal end of the chest tube into the jar of fluid until the end is 2 to 4 cm below the top of the water. Unclamp the chest tube. • Have another nurse obtain a new closed chest drainage system and set it up. • Attach the chest tube to the new unit.

Gastrointestinal tubes

Nasoenteric-decompression tubes

If your patient's nasoenteric-decompression tube appears to be obstructed, notify the doctor right away. He may order measures, such as the following, to restore patency quickly and efficiently.

• First, disconnect the tube from the suction source and irrigate with 0.9% sodium chloride solution. Use gravity flow to help clear the obstruction, unless ordered otherwise.

• If irrigation doesn't reestablish patency, the tube may be obstructed by its position against the gastric mucosa. Gentle tugging may help. For a double-lumen tube, such as a Salem pump, irrigate the pigtail port (blue) with 10 to 30 ml of air to help move the tube away from the mucosa.

If these measures don't work, the tube may be kinked and may need additional manipulation. Before proceeding:

• Never reposition or irrigate a nasoenteric-decompression tube (without a doctor's order) in a patient who has had GI surgery.

• Avoid manipulating a tube in a patient who had the tube inserted during surgery. To do so may disturb new sutures.

• Don't try to reposition the tube in a patient who was difficult to intubate (because of an esophageal stricture, for example).

T tubes

T tubes, typically inserted in the common bile duct after cholecystectomy, may become blocked by viscous bile or clots. Notify the doctor and take these steps while you wait for him to arrive.

• Unclamp the T tube (if it was clamped before and after a meal), and connect the tube to a closed gravity-drainage system.

• Inspect the tube carefully to detect any kinks or obstructions.

• Irrigate the tube with normal saline solution, if ordered, and prepare the patient for direct X-ray of the common bile duct (cholangiography). Briefly describe these measures to reduce the patient's apprehension and promote cooperation.

Total parenteral nutrition setups

PROBLEMS AND SIGNS AND SYMPTOMS	INTERVENTIONS
Clotted catheter Interrupted flow rate, hypoglycemia, no blood return	• Reposition patient on his side. Attempt to aspirate clot. If clot remains, use urokinase according to institution's policy.
Dislodged catheter Catheter out of the vein, anterior chest pain, neck pain	• Place a sterile gauze pad on the site and apply pressure if catheter is completely out. For partial displacement, call doctor. • Prepare for X-ray and repositioning with guide wire or removal and replacement.
Air embolism Chest pain, tachycardia, hypotension, fear, seizures, loss of consciousness, cardiac arrest	• Clamp the catheter. • Place patient in Trendelenburg's position on left side. Give oxygen, as ordered. • If cardiac arrest occurs, begin cardiopulmonary resuscitation.
Thrombosis Erythema, edema, or pain at insertion site or along vein; ipsilateral swelling of arm, neck, and face; tachycardia	• Anticipate prompt catheter removal. • Administer heparin, as ordered. • Prepare for venous flow study, as ordered.
Too-rapid infusion Nausea, headache, lethargy, hyperglycemia	• Check the infusion rate. • Check the infusion pump.
Extravasation Swelling or pain around the insertion site	• Stop the infusion and assess for cardiopulmonary abnormalities. • Take a chest X-ray, as needed.
Hypoglycemia Headache, sweating, dizziness, palpitations	• Give I.V. dextrose (10% as infusion, 50% as I.V. bolus), as ordered. • Avoid abrupt increases or decreases in total parenteral nutrition (TPN) flow rate; wean slowly from TPN.
Cracked or broken tubing Fluid leakage	• Apply a padded hemostat above the break to prevent air from entering the line.
Sepsis Fever, chills, leukocytosis, positive blood cultures, glucose intolerance	• Remove catheter and culture the tip. • Give appropriate antibiotics.

TROUBLESHOOTING

Tube feedings

PROBLEMS	INTERVENTIONS
Tube obstruction or clogging	• Flush the tube with warm water or cranberry juice. If necessary, replace the tube. • Flush the tube with 50 ml of water after each feeding to remove excess sticky formula, which could occlude the tube.
Aspiration of gastric secretions	• Discontinue feeding immediately. • Perform tracheal suction of aspirated contents if possible. • Notify the doctor. Prophylactic antibiotics and chest physiotherapy may be ordered. • Check tube placement before feeding to prevent complications.
Nasal or pharyngeal irritation or necrosis	• Change the tube's position. If necessary, replace the tube. • Provide frequent oral hygiene using mouthwash or lemon-glycerin swabs. Use petroleum jelly on cracked lips.
Vomiting, bloating, diarrhea, or cramps	• Reduce the flow rate. • As ordered, administer metoclopramide to increase GI motility. • Warm the formula. • For 30 minutes after feeding, position the patient on his right side with his head elevated to facilitate gastric emptying. • Notify the doctor. He may reduce the amount of formula being given during each feeding.

Neurologic monitors

▶ Damped ICP waveforms

An intracranial pressure (ICP) waveform that looks like the one shown below signals a problem with the transducer or monitor. Check for line obstruction, and determine if the transducer needs rebalancing.

PROBLEMS	INTERVENTIONS
Transducer or monitor needs re-calibration	• Turn stopcock off to patient. • Open transducer's stopcock to air, and balance transducer. • Recalibrate transducer and monitor.
Air in line	• Turn stopcock off to patient. • Using a syringe, flush air out through an open stopcock port with sterile 0.9% sodium chloride solution. *Note:* Never use heparin to flush the intracranial pressure (ICP) line. You could accidentally inject some of the drug into the patient and cause bleeding. • Rebalance and recalibrate transducer and monitor.
Loose connection in line	• Check tubing and stopcocks for possible moisture, which may indicate a loose connection. • Turn stopcock off to patient; then tighten all connections. • Make sure the tubing is long enough to allow patient to turn his head without straining tubing. This may prevent further problems.
Disconnection in line	• Turn stopcock off to patient immediately. (Rapid cerebrospinal fluid loss through a ventricular catheter may allow ICP to drop precipitously, causing brain herniation.) • Replace equipment to reduce risk of infection.

(continued)

Damped waveforms *(continued)*

PROBLEMS	INTERVENTIONS
Change in patient's position	• Reposition transducer's balancing port level with Monro's foramen. • Rebalance and recalibrate transducer and monitor. *Remember:* Always balance and recalibrate at least once every 4 hours and whenever the patient is repositioned.
Tubing, catheter, or screw occluded with blood or brain tissue	• Notify doctor. He may want to irrigate the screw or catheter with a small amount (0.1 ml) of sterile 0.9% sodium chloride solution. *Important:* Never irrigate the screw or catheter yourself.

CHAPTER 10

Drug administration:
Reviewing the methods

Administration guidelines

▶

Precautions for drug administration

Whenever you administer any medication, observe the following precautions to ensure that you're giving the right drug in the right dose to the right patient.

Check the order
Check the order on the patient's medication record against the doctor's order.

Check the label
Check the label on the medication three times before administering it to be sure you're administering the prescribed medication in the prescribed dose. Check it when you take the container from the shelf or drawer, right before pouring the medication into the medication cup or drawing it into the syringe, and before returning the container to the shelf or drawer. If you're administering a unit-dose medication, check the label for the third time immediately after pouring the medication and again before discarding the wrapper. (Remember, don't open a unit-dose medication until you're at the patient's bedside.)

Confirm the patient's identity
Before giving the medication, confirm the patient's identity by checking his name, room number, and bed number on his wristband. Then check again that you have the correct medication.

Always explain the procedure to the patient, and provide privacy.

Have a written order
Make sure you have a written order for every medication given. Verbal orders should be signed by the doctor within the specified time period.

Give labeled medications
Don't give medication from a poorly labeled or unlabeled container. Don't attempt to label or reinforce drug labels yourself. This must be done by a pharmacist.

Monitor medications
Never give a medication poured or prepared by someone else. Never allow your medication cart or tray out of your sight. Never return unwrapped or prepared medications to stock containers. Instead, dispose of them, and notify the pharmacy.

Respond to patients' questions
If the patient questions you about his medication or the dosage, check his medication record again. If the medication is correct, reassure him. Make sure you tell him about any changes in his medication or dosage. Instruct him, as appropriate, about possible adverse reactions. Ask him to report anything that he feels may be an adverse reaction.

◀

Topical administration

▶

Topical medications

Topical drugs, such as lotions and ointments, are applied directly to the skin. They're commonly used for local, rather than systemic, effects. Typically, they must be applied two or three times a day for full therapeutic effect.

Equipment

Patient's medication record and chart • prescribed medication • sterile tongue blades • gloves • sterile 4″ × 4″ gauze pads • transparent semipermeable dressing • adhesive tape • solvent (such as cottonseed oil) • cotton-tipped applicators, cotton gloves, or terry cloth scuffs, if necessary.

Implementation

• Explain the procedure to the patient because, after discharge, he may have to apply the medication by himself.
• Wash your hands to prevent cross-contamination, and glove your dominant hand.
• Help the patient to a comfortable position, and expose the area to be treated. Make sure the skin or mucous membrane is intact (unless the medication has been ordered to treat a skin lesion). Application of medication to broken or abraded skin may cause unwanted systemic absorption and result in further irritation.
• If necessary, clean the skin of debris. You may have to change the glove if it becomes soiled.

To apply a paste, a cream, or an ointment

• Open the container. Place the cap upside down to avoid contaminating its inner surface.
• Remove a tongue blade from its sterile wrapper, and cover one end of it with medication from the tube or jar. Then transfer the medication from the tongue blade to your gloved hand.
• Apply the medication to the affected area with long, smooth strokes that follow the direction of hair growth, at top right.

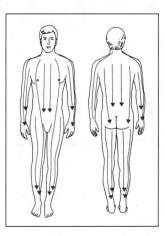

This technique avoids forcing medication into hair follicles, which can cause irritation and lead to folliculitis. Avoid excessive pressure when applying the medication because it could abrade the skin or cause the patient discomfort.
• When applying medication to the patient's face, use cotton-tipped applicators for small areas, such as under the eyes. For larger areas, use a sterile gauze pad, and follow the directions shown below.

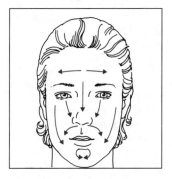

• To prevent contamination of the medication, use a new sterile tongue blade each time you remove medication from the container.

To remove an ointment

• Gently swab ointment from the patient's skin using a sterile 4″ × 4″ gauze pad saturated with a solvent, such as cottonseed oil. Remove any remaining oil by wiping the area with a clean sterile gauze pad. Don't wipe too hard because you could irritate the skin.

To apply other topical medications

• To apply shampoos, follow package directions. Apply medication using your fingertips, or instruct the patient to do so, as shown below. Massage it into the scalp if appropriate.

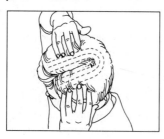

• To apply aerosol sprays, shake the container, if indicated, to mix the medication. Hold the container 6″ to 12″ (15 to 30 cm) from the skin, or follow the manufacturer's recommendation. Spray the medication evenly over the treatment area to apply a thin film.
• To apply powders, dry the skin surface and apply a thin layer of powder over the treatment area.
• To protect applied medications and prevent them from soiling the patient's clothes, tape a sterile gauze pad or a transparent semipermeable dressing over the treated area. If you're applying topical medication to his hands or feet, cover the site with cotton gloves for the hands or terry cloth scuffs for the feet.

• Assess the patient's skin for signs of irritation, allergic reaction, or breakdown.

Special considerations

• To prevent skin irritation from an accumulation of medication, never apply medication without first removing previous applications.
• Always wear gloves to prevent absorption by your skin.
• Never apply ointment to the eyelids or ear canal unless ordered. The ointment may congeal and occlude the tear duct or ear canal.
• Inspect the treated area frequently for any adverse (for instance, allergic) reaction.

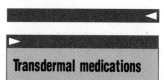

Transdermal medications

Given through an adhesive disk or measured dose of ointment applied to the skin, transdermal drugs deliver constant, controlled medication directly into the bloodstream for a prolonged systemic effect.

Medications currently available in transdermal form include nitroglycerin, used to control angina; scopolamine, used to treat motion sickness; estradiol, for postmenopausal hormone replacement; clonidine, used to treat hypertension; and fentanyl, a narcotic analgesic used to control chronic pain.

Nitroglycerin ointment dilates coronary vessels for 2 to 12 hours; a nitroglycerin disk can produce the same effect for as long as 24 hours.

The scopolamine disk can relieve motion sickness for as long as 72 hours; transdermal estradiol lasts for 72 hours to 1 week; clonidine lasts for 7 days; and fentanyl lasts up to 72 hours.

Equipment

Patient's medication record and chart • prescribed medication (disk or ointment) • application strip or measuring paper (for nitroglycerin ointment) • adhesive tape • plastic wrap (optional for nitroglycerin ointment) or semipermeable dressing. Optional: gloves.

Implementation

• Wash your hands and, if necessary, put on gloves.
• Make sure that any previously applied medication has been removed from the skin.

To apply transdermal ointment

• Place the prescribed amount of ointment on the application strip or measuring paper, taking care not to get any on your skin.
• Apply the strip to any dry, hairless area of the body. Don't rub the ointment into the skin.
• Tape the application strip and ointment to the skin. If desired, cover the application strip with the plastic wrap, and tape the wrap in place.

To apply a transdermal disk

• Open the package and remove the disk.
• Without touching the adhesive surface, remove the clear plastic backing.
• Apply the disk to a dry, hairless area—behind the ear, for example, as with scopolamine. Avoid any area that may cause uneven absorption, such as skin folds or scars, or any irritated or damaged skin. Don't apply the disk below the elbow or knee.

After applying transdermal medications

• Store the medication as ordered.
• Instruct the patient to keep the area around the disk or ointment as dry as possible.

• If you didn't wear gloves, wash your hands immediately after applying the disk or ointment to avoid absorbing the drug yourself.

Special considerations

• Reapply daily transdermal medications at the same time every day to ensure a continuous effect, but alternate the application sites to avoid skin irritation.
• Before applying nitroglycerin ointment, obtain the patient's baseline blood pressure. Obtain another blood pressure reading 5 minutes after applying the ointment. If blood pressure has dropped significantly and the patient has a headache, notify the doctor immediately. If blood pressure has dropped, but the patient has no symptoms, instruct him to lie still until blood pressure returns to normal.
• Before reapplying nitroglycerin ointment, remove the plastic wrap, the application strip, and any ointment remaining on the skin at the previous site.
• When applying a scopolamine disk, instruct the patient not to drive or operate machinery until his response to the drug has been determined.
• Warn a patient using clonidine disks to check with his doctor before using any over-the-counter cough preparations because they may counteract the effects of the drug.

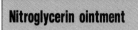

Nitroglycerin ointment

Unlike most topical medications, nitroglycerin ointment is used for its transdermal systemic effect. It's used to dilate the arteries and veins, thus improving cardiac perfusion in a patient with cardiac ischemia or angina pectoris.

Nitroglycerin ointment is prescribed by the inch, and comes with a rectangular piece of ruled paper to be used in applying the medication.

Equipment

Patient's medication record and chart • ointment • ruled paper • plastic wrap or a transparent semipermeable dressing • adhesive tape • sphygmomanometer. Optional: gloves.

Implementation

• Start by taking the patient's baseline blood pressure to compare it with later readings.
• Put on gloves if you wish to avoid contact with the medication.
• Squeeze the prescribed amount of ointment onto the ruled paper, as shown below.

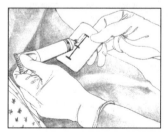

• After measuring the correct amount of ointment, tape the paper, drug side down, directly to the skin. Some health care facilities require you to use the paper to apply the medication to the patient's skin, usually on the chest or arm. Spread a thin layer of ointment over a 3″ (8-cm) area.
• For increased absorption, the doctor may request that you cover the site with plastic wrap or a transparent semipermeable dressing, as shown below.

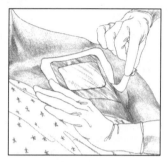

• After 5 minutes, record the patient's blood pressure. If it has dropped significantly and he has a headache (from vasodilation of blood vessels in his head), notify the doctor immediately. He may reduce the dose.
• If the patient's blood pressure has dropped but he has no adverse reactions, instruct him to lie still until it returns to normal.

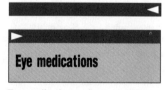

Eye medications

Eye medications – drops or ointments – serve diagnostic and therapeutic purposes. During an eye examination, eye medications can be used to anesthetize the eye, dilate the pupil, and stain the cornea to identify anomalies. Therapeutic uses include eye lubrication and treatment of such conditions as glaucoma and infections.

Equipment and preparation

Patient's medication record and · chart • prescribed eye medication • sterile cotton balls • gloves • warm water or 0.9% sodium chloride solution • sterile gauze pads • facial tissue. Optional: ocular dressing.

Make sure the medication is labeled for ophthalmic use. Then check the expiration date. Remember to date the container after first use.

Inspect ocular solutions for cloudiness, discoloration, and precipitation, but remember that some eye medications are suspensions and normally appear cloudy. Don't use any solution that appears abnormal.

Implementation

• Make sure you know which eye to treat because different medications or doses may be ordered for each eye.
• Put on gloves.
• If the patient has an eye dressing, remove it by pulling it down and away from his forehead. Avoid contaminating your hands.
• To remove exudates or meibomian gland secretions, clean around the eye with sterile cotton balls or sterile gauze pads moistened with warm water or 0.9% sodium chloride solution. Have the patient close his eye; then gently wipe the eyelids from the inner to outer canthus. Use a fresh cotton ball or gauze pad for each stroke.
• Have the patient sit or lie in the supine position. Instruct him to tilt his head back and toward his affected eye so that excess medication can flow away from the tear duct, minimizing systemic absorption through nasal mucosa.
• Remove the dropper cap from the medication container, and draw the medication into it.
• Before instilling eyedrops, instruct the patient to look up and away.

This moves the cornea away from the lower lid and minimizes the risk of touching it with the dropper.

To instill eyedrops

• Steady the hand that's holding the dropper by resting it against the patient's forehead. With your other hand, pull down the lower lid of the affected eye, and instill the drops in the conjunctival sac. Never instill eyedrops directly onto the eyeball.

 When teaching elderly patients how to instill eyedrops, keep in mind that they may have difficulty sensing drops in the eye. Suggest chilling the medication slightly; the cold drops should enhance placement sensation.

To apply eye ointment

• Squeeze a small ribbon of medication on the edge of the conjunctival sac from the inner to the outer canthus, as shown below. Cut off the ribbon by turning the tube.

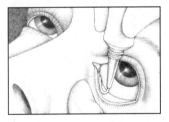

After instilling eyedrops or applying ointment

• Instruct the patient to close his eyes gently, without squeezing the lids shut. If you instilled drops, tell him to blink. If you've applied ointment, tell him to roll his eyes behind closed lids to help distribute the medication over the eyeball.
• Use a clean tissue to remove any excess medication leaking from the eye. Use a fresh tissue for each eye to prevent cross-contamination.

• Apply a new eye dressing, if necessary.
• Remove and discard gloves. Then wash your hands.

Special considerations

• When administering an eye medication that may be absorbed systemically, press your thumb on the inner canthus for 1 to 2 minutes after instillation while the patient closes his eyes.
• To maintain the drug container's sterility, never touch the tip of the dropper or bottle to the eye area. Discard any solution remaining in the dropper before returning it to the bottle. If the dropper or bottle tip has become contaminated, discard it, and use another sterile dropper.

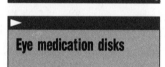

Eye medication disks

Small and flexible, the oval disk can release medication (such as pilocarpine) in the eye for up to 1 week. Floating between the eyelids and the sclera, the disk stays in the eye while the patient sleeps and even during swimming and other athletic activities. The disk frees the patient from having to remember to instill his eye medication. Eye moisture or contact lenses don't adversely affect the disk.

Equipment

Patient's medication record and chart • prescribed eye medication • sterile gloves.

Implementation

• Make sure you know which eye to treat because different medications

or doses may be ordered for each eye.

To insert an eye medication disk

• Insert the disk at bedtime to minimize initial blurring.
• Wash your hands, and put on sterile gloves.
• Press your fingertip against the disk so that it sticks lengthwise across your fingertip.
• Gently pull the patient's lower eyelid away from the eye, and place the disk in the conjunctival sac. It should lie horizontally, as shown below, not vertically. The disk will adhere to the eye naturally.

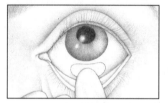

• Pull the lower eyelid out, up, and over the disk. Tell the patient to blink several times. If the disk is still visible, pull the lower lid out and over the disk again. Tell him that once the disk is in place, he can adjust its position by pressing his finger against his closed lid. Warn him not to rub his eye or move the disk across the cornea.
• If the disk falls out, rinse the disk in cool water, and reinsert it. If the disk appears bent, replace it.
• If both eyes are being treated with medication disks, replace both disks at the same time.
• If the disk repeatedly slips out of position, reinsert it under the upper eyelid. To do this, gently lift and evert the upper eyelid, and insert the disk in the conjunctival sac. Then gently pull the lid back into position, and tell the patient to

blink several times. The more he uses the disk, the easier it should be for him to retain it. If not, notify the doctor.

To remove an eye medication disk
• To remove the disk with one finger, put on sterile gloves and evert the lower eyelid to expose the disk. Then use the forefinger of your other hand to slide the disk onto the lid and out of the patient's eye. To use two fingers, evert the lower lid with one hand to expose the disk. Then pinch it with the thumb and forefinger of your other hand, and remove it.
• If the disk is located in the upper eyelid, apply long circular strokes to the closed eyelid with your finger until you can see the disk in the corner of the eye. Then, place your finger directly on the disk, move it to the lower sclera, and remove it as you would a disk located in the lower lid.

Special considerations
• If the patient will continue therapy with an eye medication disk after discharge, teach him to insert and remove it himself. Have him demonstrate the techniques for you.
• Explain that mild reactions are common but should subside within the first 6 weeks of use. Foreign-body sensation in the eye, mild tearing or redness, increased mucous discharge, eyelid redness, and itchiness can occur. Blurred vision, stinging, swelling, and headaches can occur with pilocarpine, specifically. Tell him to report persistent or severe symptoms.

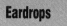

Eardrops

Eardrops may be instilled to treat infection and inflammation, to soften cerumen for later removal, to produce local anesthesia, or to facilitate removal of an insect trapped in the ear.

Equipment and preparation
Patient's medication record and chart • prescribed eardrops • light source • facial tissue or cotton-tipped applicator. Optional: cotton ball, bowl of warm water.

First, warm the medication to body temperature in the bowl of warm water, or carry it in your pocket for 30 minutes before administration. If necessary, test the temperature of the medication by placing a drop on your wrist. (If the medication is too hot, it may burn the patient's eardrum.) To avoid injuring the ear canal, check the dropper before use to make sure it's not chipped or cracked.

Implementation
• Wash your hands.
• Confirm the patient's identity by asking his name and checking the name, room number, and bed number on his wristband.
• Have the patient lie on the side opposite the affected ear.
• Straighten the patient's ear canal. For an adult, pull the auricle up and back.

AGE ALERT For an infant or child under age 3, gently pull the auricle down and back—the ear canal is straighter at this age.
• Using a light source, examine the ear canal for drainage. If you find any, clean the canal with the tissue or cotton-tipped applicator because drainage can reduce the medication's effectiveness.

any, clean the canal with the tissue or cotton-tipped applicator because drainage can reduce the medication's effectiveness.

• Compare the label on the eardrops to the order on the patient's medication record. Check the label again while drawing the medication into the dropper. Check the label for the final time before returning the eardrops to the shelf or drawer.

• To avoid damaging the ear canal with the dropper, gently rest the hand holding the dropper against the patient's head. Straighten the patient's ear canal once again, and instill the ordered number of drops. To avoid patient discomfort, aim the dropper so that the drops fall against the sides of the ear canal, not on the eardrum. Hold the ear canal in position until you see the medication disappear down the canal. Then release the ear.

• Instruct the patient to remain on his side for 5 to 10 minutes to allow the medication to run down into the ear canal.

• Tuck the cotton ball (if ordered) loosely into the opening of the ear canal to prevent the medication from leaking out. Be careful not to insert it too deeply into the canal because this would prevent drainage of secretions and increase pressure on the eardrum.

• Clean and dry the outer ear.

• If ordered, repeat the procedure in the other ear after 5 to 10 minutes.

• Assist the patient into a comfortable position.

• Wash your hands.

Special considerations

• Remember that some conditions make the normally tender ear canal even more sensitive, so be especially gentle when performing this procedure.

• To prevent injury to the eardrum, never insert a cotton-tipped applicator into the ear canal past the point where you can see the tip. After applying eardrops to soften cerumen, irrigate the ear as ordered to facilitate its removal.

• If the patient has vertigo, keep the side rails of his bed up, and assist him as necessary during the procedure. Also, move slowly and unhurriedly to avoid exacerbating his vertigo.

• If necessary, teach the patient to instill the eardrops correctly so that he can continue treatment at home. Review the procedure, and let the patient try it himself while you observe.

Nasal medications

Nasal medications may be instilled by means of drops, a spray (using an atomizer), or an aerosol (using a nebulizer). Most drugs instilled by these methods produce local rather than systemic effects. Drops can be directed at a specific area; sprays and aerosols diffuse medication throughout the nasal passages. Nasal medications include vasoconstrictors, antiseptics, anesthetics, and corticosteroids.

Equipment

Patient's medication record and chart • prescribed medication • emesis basin (for nose drops) • facial tissue. Optional: pillow, piece of soft rubber or plastic tubing, gloves.

Implementation

• Wash your hands. Put on gloves, if necessary.

To instill nose drops

• Draw up some medication into the dropper.

• To reach the ethmoidal and sphenoidal sinuses, have the patient lie on his back with his neck hyperextended and his head tilted back over the edge of the bed. Support his head with one hand to prevent neck strain.

• To reach the maxillary and frontal sinuses, have the patient lie on his back with his head toward the affected side and hanging slightly over the edge of the bed. Ask him to rotate his head laterally after hyperextension, and support his head with one hand to prevent neck strain.

• To relieve ordinary nasal congestion, help the patient to a reclining or supine position with his head tilted slightly toward the affected side. Aim the dropper upward, toward the patient's eye, rather than downward toward his ear.

• Insert the dropper about ⅓" (0.8 cm) into the nostril. Make sure it doesn't touch the sides of the nostril to avoid contaminating the dropper or making the patient sneeze.

• Instill the prescribed number of drops, observing the patient for any signs of discomfort.

• Keep the patient's head tilted back for at least 5 minutes, and have him breathe through his mouth to prevent drops from leaking and to allow time for the medication to work.

• Keep an emesis basin handy so that the patient can expectorate any medication that flows into the oropharynx and mouth. Wipe excess medication from the patient's face with facial tissues.

• Return the dropper to the bottle and close it tightly.

To use a nasal spray

• Have the patient sit upright with his head upright.

• Remove the protective cap from the atomizer.

• Occlude one of the patient's nostrils, and insert the atomizer tip about ½" (1.2 cm) into the open nostril. Position the tip straight up toward the inner canthus of the eye.

• Depending on the drug, have the patient hold his breath or inhale. Then squeeze the atomizer once quickly and firmly—just enough to coat the inside of the nose. Excessive force may propel the medication into the patient's sinuses and cause a headache. Repeat the procedure in the other nostril, as ordered.

• So that the medication has time to work, tell the patient to keep his head tilted back for several minutes, to breathe slowly through his nose, and not to blow his nose.

To use a nasal aerosol

• Insert the medication cartridge according to the manufacturer's directions. Shake it well before each use, and remove the protective cap.

• Hold the aerosol between your thumb and index finger (index finger on top of the cartridge).

• Tilt the patient's head back slightly, and carefully insert the adapter tip in one nostril. Depending on the medication, tell the patient to hold his breath or inhale.

• Press your fingers together firmly to release one measured dose of medication.

• Shake the aerosol and repeat the procedure to instill medication into the other nostril.

• Remove the cartridge, and wash the nasal adapter in lukewarm water daily. Allow the adapter to dry before reinserting the cartridge.

DRUG
ADMINISTRATION

Special considerations

 For a child or an uncooperative patient, place a short piece of tubing on the dropper end to avoid damaging mucous membranes.

• Tell patient not to blow his nose for at least 2 minutes afterward.

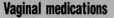

Vaginal medications

Vaginal medications include suppositories, creams, gels, and ointments. These medications can be inserted as topical treatment for infection (particularly *Trichomonas vaginalis* and monilial vaginitis) or inflammation, or as a contraceptive. Suppositories melt when they contact the vaginal mucosa, and their medication diffuses topically—as effectively as creams, gels, and ointments.

Vaginal medications usually come with a disposable applicator that enables placement of medication in the anterior and posterior fornices. Vaginal administration is most effective when the patient can remain lying down afterward to retain the medication.

Equipment

Patient's medication record and chart • prescribed medication and applicator, if needed • gloves • water-soluble lubricant • small sanitary pad.

Implementation

• If possible, plan to give vaginal medications at bedtime when the patient is recumbent.
• Wash your hands, explain the procedure to the patient, and provide privacy.

• Ask the patient to void.
• Ask the patient if she would rather insert the medication herself. If so, provide appropriate instructions. If not, proceed with the following steps.
• Help her into the lithotomy position.
• Expose only the perineum.

To insert a suppository

• Remove the suppository from the wrapper, and lubricate it with water-soluble lubricant.
• Put on gloves, and expose the vagina by spreading the labia.
• If you see any discharge, wash the area with several cotton balls soaked in warm, soapy water. Clean each side of the perineum and then the center, using a fresh cotton ball for each stroke. While the labia are still separated, insert the suppository about 3″ to 4″ (7.6 to 10 cm) into the vagina.

To insert ointments, creams, or gels

• Fit the applicator to the tube of medication and gently squeeze the tube to fill the applicator with the prescribed amount of medication. Lubricate the applicator tip.
• Put on gloves, and expose the vagina.
• Insert the applicator about 2″ (5 cm) in the patient's vagina and administer the medication by depressing the plunger on the applicator.
• Instruct the patient to remain supine with her knees flexed for 5 to 10 minutes to allow medication to flow into the posterior fornix.

After vaginal insertion

• Remove and discard your gloves.
• Wash the applicator with soap and warm water and store or discard it, as appropriate. Label it so it will be used only for the same patient.

• To prevent the medication from soiling the patient's clothing and bedding, provide a sanitary pad.

• Help the patient return to a comfortable position, and advise her to remain in bed as much as possible for the next several hours.

• Wash your hands thoroughly.

Special considerations

• Refrigerate vaginal suppositories that melt at room temperature.

• If possible, teach the patient how to insert vaginal medication. She may have to administer it herself after discharge. Give her a patient-teaching sheet if one is available.

• Instruct the patient not to wear a tampon after inserting vaginal medication because it would absorb the medication and decrease its effectiveness.

Respiratory administration

Hand-held oropharyngeal inhalers

Hand-held inhalers include the metered-dose inhaler or nebulizer, the turbo-inhaler, and the nasal inhaler. These devices deliver topical medications to the respiratory tract, producing local and systemic effects. The mucosal lining of the respiratory tract absorbs the inhalant almost immediately. Examples of inhalants are bronchodilators, used to improve airway patency and facilitate mucous drainage, and mucolytics, which liquefy tenacious bronchial secretions.

Equipment

Patient's medication record and chart • metered-dose inhaler, turbo-inhaler, or nasal inhaler • prescribed medication • 0.9% sodium chloride solution.

Implementation
To use a metered-dose inhaler

• Shake the inhaler bottle. Remove the cap, and insert the stem into the small hole on the flattened portion of the mouthpiece, as shown below.

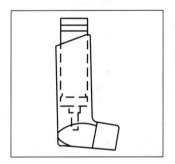

• Have the patient exhale. Place the inhaler about 1″ (2.5 cm) in front of his open mouth.

• As you push the bottle down against the mouthpiece, instruct the patient to inhale slowly through his mouth and to continue inhaling until his lungs feel full. Compress the bottle against the mouthpiece only once.

• Remove the inhaler and tell the patient to hold his breath for several seconds. Then instruct him to exhale slowly through pursed lips to keep distal bronchioles open, allowing increased absorption and diffusion of the drug.

• Have the patient gargle with 0.9% sodium chloride solution, if desired, to remove medication from the mouth and back of the throat.

To use a turbo-inhaler
• Hold the mouthpiece in one hand, and with the other hand, slide the sleeve away from the mouthpiece as far as possible, as shown below.

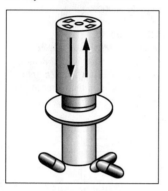

• Unscrew the tip of the mouthpiece by turning it counterclockwise.
• Press the colored portion of the medication capsule into the propeller stem of the mouthpiece. Screw the inhaler together again.
• Holding the inhaler with the mouthpiece at the bottom, slide the sleeve all the way down and then up again to puncture the capsule and release the medication. Do this only once.
• Have the patient exhale completely and tilt his head back. Instruct him to place the mouthpiece in his mouth, close his lips around it, and inhale once. Tell him to hold his breath for several seconds.
• Remove the inhaler from the patient's mouth, and tell him to exhale as much air as possible.
• Repeat the procedure until all the medication in the device is inhaled.
• Have the patient gargle with 0.9% sodium chloride solution, if desired.

To use a holding chamber (InspirEase)
• Insert the inhaler into the mouthpiece of the holding chamber and shake the inhaler. Then place the mouthpiece into the opening of the holding device and twist the mouthpiece to lock it in place.
• Extend the holding device, have the patient exhale, and place the mouthpiece in his mouth.
• Press down on the inhaler once. Then have the patient inhale slowly and deeply, collapsing the bag completely. If he breathes incorrectly, the bag will make a whistling sound. Tell the patient to hold his breath for 5 to 10 seconds and then exhale slowly into the bag. Then repeat the inhaling and exhaling steps.
• Have the patient wait 1 to 2 minutes and then repeat the procedure, if ordered.
• Disconnect the holding chamber from the mouthpiece, rinse both in lukewarm water, and allow them to air-dry.

Special considerations
Teach the patient how to use the inhaler so that he can continue treatments after discharge, if necessary. Explain that overdosage can cause the medication to lose its effectiveness. Tell him to record the date and time of each inhalation and his response.

Be aware that some oral respiratory drugs may cause restlessness, palpitations, nervousness, and other systemic effects. They can also cause hypersensitivity reactions, such as rash, urticaria, or bronchospasm.

Administer oral respiratory drugs cautiously to patients with heart disease because these drugs may potentiate coronary insufficiency, cardiac arrhythmias, or hypertension. If paradoxical bronchospasm occurs, discontinue the drug and call the doctor. He'll prescribe another drug.

Enteral administration

Oral medications

Because oral drug administration is usually the safest, most convenient, and least expensive, most drugs are administered by this route. Drugs for oral administration are available in many forms: tablets, enteric-coated tablets, capsules, syrups, elixirs, oils, liquids, suspensions, powders, and granules. Some require special preparation before administration, such as mixing with juice to make them more palatable.

Oral drugs are sometimes prescribed in higher dosages than their parenteral equivalents, because after absorption through the GI system, they are broken down by the liver before they reach the systemic circulation.

Equipment
Patient's medication record and chart • prescribed medication • medication cup. Optional: appropriate vehicle (such as jelly or applesauce) for crushed pills commonly used with children or elderly patients, or juice, water, or milk for liquid medications; and mortar and pestle for crushing pills.

Implementation
• Wash your hands.
• Assess the patient's condition, including level of consciousness and vital signs, as needed. Changes in

the patient's condition may warrant withholding medication.
• Give the patient his medication and, as needed, an appropriate vehicle or liquid to aid swallowing, minimize adverse effects, or promote absorption. If appropriate, crush the medication to facilitate swallowing.
• Stay with the patient until he has swallowed the drug. If he seems confused or disoriented, check his mouth to make sure he has swallowed it. Return and reassess the patient's response within 1 hour after giving the medication.

Special considerations
• To avoid damaging or staining the patient's teeth, give acid or iron preparations through a straw. An unpleasant-tasting liquid can usually be made more palatable if taken through a straw because the liquid contacts fewer taste buds.
• If the patient can't swallow a whole tablet or capsule, ask the pharmacist if the drug is available in liquid form or if it can be administered by another route. If not, ask him if you can crush the tablet or open the capsule and mix it with food.

Drug delivery through a nasogastric tube or gastrostomy button

Besides providing an alternate means of nourishment, the nasogastric (NG) tube allows direct instillation of medication into the GI system of patients who can't ingest it orally. The gastrostomy button, inserted into an established stoma, lies flush with the skin and receives a feeding tube.

Equipment and preparation

Patient's medication record and chart • prescribed medication • towel or linen-saver pad • 50- or 60-ml piston-type catheter-tip syringe • feeding tubing • two 4″ × 4″ gauze pads • stethoscope • gloves • diluent (juice, water, or a nutritional supplement) • cup for mixing medication and fluid • spoon • 50-ml cup of water • rubber band • gastrostomy tube and funnel, if needed. Optional: pill-crushing equipment, clamp (if not already attached to tube).

Gather equipment for use at bedside. Liquids should be at room temperature to avoid abdominal cramping. Make sure the cup, syringe, spoon, and gauze are clean.

Implementation
To give a drug through an NG tube

• Wash your hands, and put on gloves.
• Unpin the tube from the patient's gown. To avoid soiling the sheets during the procedure, fold back the bed linens, and drape the patient's chest with a towel or linen-saver pad.
• Help the patient into Fowler's position, if her condition allows.
• After unclamping the tube, auscultate the patient's abdomen about 3″ (8 cm) below the sternum, while you gently insert 10 cc of air into the tube with the 50- or 60-ml syringe. You should hear the air bubble entering the stomach. Gently draw back on the piston of the syringe. The appearance of gastric contents implies that the tube is patent and in the stomach.
• If no gastric contents appear or if you meet resistance, the tube may be lying against the gastric mucosa. Withdraw the tube slightly, or turn the patient to free it.

• Clamp the tube, detach the syringe, and lay the end of the tube on the 4″ × 4″ gauze pad.
• If the medication is in tablet form, crush it before mixing with the diluent. (Make sure the particles are small enough to pass through the eyes at the distal end of the tube.) Open capsules and pour them into the diluent. Pour liquid medications into the diluent and stir well.
• Reattach the syringe, without the piston, to the end of the tube. Holding the tube upright at a level slightly above the patient's nose, open the clamp, and pour in the medication slowly and steadily, as shown below.

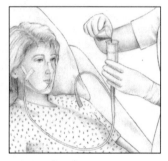

• To prevent air from entering the patient's stomach, hold the tube at a slight angle, and add more medication before the syringe empties.
• If the medication flows smoothly, slowly give the entire dose. If it doesn't flow, it may be too thick. If so, dilute it with water. If you suspect tube placement is inhibiting flow, stop the procedure, and reevaluate the placement.
• Watch the patient's reaction, and stop immediately if she shows signs of discomfort.
• As the last of the medication flows out of the syringe, start to irrigate the tube by adding 30 to 50 ml of water (15 to 30 ml for a child). Irrigation clears medication from the

tube and reduces the risk of clogging.
• When the water stops flowing, clamp the tube. Detach the syringe, and discard it properly.
• Fasten the tube to the patient's gown, and make the patient comfortable.
• Leave the patient in Fowler's position, or on her right side with her head partially elevated, for at least 30 minutes to facilitate flow and prevent esophageal reflux.

To give a drug through a gastrostomy button
• Assist the patient into an upright position.
• Put on gloves, and open the safety plug on top of the device.
• Attach the feeding tube set to the button.
• Remove the piston from the catheter-tipped syringe and insert the tip into the distal end of the feeding tube.
• Pour the prescribed medication into the syringe and allow it to flow into the stomach.
• After instilling all of the medication, pour 30 to 50 ml of water into the syringe and allow it to flow through the tube.
• When all the water has been delivered, remove the feeding tube and replace the safety plug. Keep the patient in semi-Fowler's position for 30 minutes after giving the medication.

Special considerations
• If you must give a tube feeding as well as instill medication, give the medication first to ensure that the patient receives it all.
• If residual stomach contents exceed 100 ml, withhold the medication and feeding, and notify the doctor. Excessive contents may indicate intestinal obstruction or paralytic ileus.

• If the NG tube is on suction, turn it off for 20 to 30 minutes after giving medication.

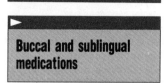

Buccal and sublingual medications

Certain drugs are given buccally (between the patient's cheek and teeth) or sublingually (under the patient's tongue) to bypass the digestive tract and facilitate their absorption into the bloodstream.

Drugs given buccally include erythrityl tetranitrate. Drugs given sublingually include ergotamine tartrate, erythrityl tetranitrate, isoproterenol hydrochloride, isosorbide dinitrate, and nitroglycerin. When using either administration method, you must observe the patient carefully to ensure that he doesn't swallow the drug or suffer mucosal irritation.

Equipment
Patient's medication record and chart • prescribed medication • medication cup.

Implementation
• Wash your hands.
• For buccal administration, place the tablet in the patient's buccal pouch, between the cheek and teeth.
• For sublingual administration, place the tablet under the patient's tongue.
• Instruct the patient to keep the medication in place until it dissolves completely to ensure absorption.
• Caution him against chewing the tablet or touching it with his tongue to prevent accidental swallowing.

• Tell him not to smoke before the drug has dissolved because nicotine's vasoconstrictive effects slow absorption.

Special considerations
• Don't give liquids because some buccal tablets may take up to 1 hour to be absorbed.
• Tell the patient with angina to wet the nitroglycerin tablet with saliva and to keep it under his tongue until it's fully absorbed.

Rectal suppositories or ointment

A rectal suppository is a small, solid, medicated mass, usually cone-shaped, with a cocoa-butter or glycerin base. It may be inserted to stimulate peristalsis and defecation or to relieve pain, vomiting, and local irritation. An ointment is a semisolid medication used to produce local effects. It may be applied externally to the anus or internally to the rectum.

Equipment and preparation
Patient's medication record and chart • rectal suppository or tube of ointment and ointment applicator • 4″ × 4″ gauze pads • gloves • water-soluble lubricant. Optional: bedpan.

Store rectal suppositories in the refrigerator until needed to prevent softening and possible decreased effectiveness of the medication. A softened suppository is also difficult to handle and insert. To harden it again, hold the suppository (in its wrapper) under cold running water.

Implementation
Wash your hands.

To insert a rectal suppository
• Place the patient on his left side in Sims' position. Drape him with the bedcovers, exposing only the buttocks. Put on gloves. Unwrap the suppository, and lubricate it with water-soluble lubricant.
• Lift the patient's upper buttock with your nondominant hand to expose the anus.
• Instruct the patient to take several deep breaths through his mouth to relax the anal sphincter and reduce anxiety during drug insertion.
• Using the index finger of your dominant hand, insert the suppository—tapered end first—about 3″ (8 cm) until you feel it pass the internal anal sphincter, as shown below.

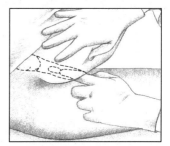

• Direct the suppository's tapered end toward the side of the rectum so it contacts the membranes.
• Encourage the patient to lie quietly and, if applicable, to retain the suppository for the correct length of time. Press on the anus with a gauze pad, if necessary, until the urge to defecate passes.
• Discard the used equipment.

To apply an ointment
• For external application, wear gloves or use a gauze pad to spread medication over the anal area.
• To apply internally, attach the applicator to the tube of ointment, and coat the applicator with water-soluble lubricant.

• Expect to use about 1″ (2 cm) of ointment. To gauge how much pressure to use during application, try squeezing a small amount from the tube before you attach the applicator.

• Lift the patient's upper buttock with your nondominant hand to expose the anus.

• Tell the patient to take several deep breaths through his mouth to relax the anal sphincter and reduce discomfort during insertion. Then gently insert the applicator, directing it toward the umbilicus, as shown below.

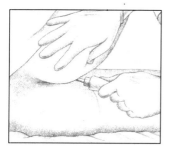

• Squeeze the tube to eject medication.

• Remove the applicator, and place a folded 4″ × 4″ gauze pad between the patient's buttocks to absorb excess ointment. Disassemble the tube and applicator. Recap the tube. Clean the applicator with soap and warm water. Remove and discard gloves. Then wash your hands thoroughly.

Special considerations

• Because the intake of food and fluid stimulates peristalsis, a suppository for relieving constipation should be inserted about 30 minutes before mealtime to help soften the stool and faciliate defecation. A medicated retention suppository should be inserted between meals.

• Tell the patient not to expel the suppository. If retaining it is difficult, put him on a bedpan.

• Make sure the patient's call button is handy, and watch for his signal because he may be unable to suppress the urge to defecate.

• Be sure to inform the patient that the suppository may discolor his next bowel movement.

Parenteral administration

Subcutaneous injection

Subcutaneous injection allows slower, more sustained drug administration than intramuscular injection. Drugs and solutions for subcutaneous injections are injected through a relatively short needle, using meticulous sterile technique.

Equipment and preparation

Patient's medication record and chart • prescribed medication • needle of appropriate gauge and length • gloves • 1- to 3-ml syringe • alcohol sponges. Optional: antiseptic cleaning agent, filter needle, insulin syringe, insulin pump.

Inspect the medication to make sure it's not cloudy and doesn't contain precipitates.

Wash your hands. Select a needle of the proper gauge and length.

 An average adult patient requires a 25G ⅝″ needle; an infant, a child, or an elderly or thin patient usually requires a 25G to 27G ½″ needle.

DRUG ADMINISTRATION

For single-dose ampules
Wrap the neck of the ampule in an alcohol sponge, and snap off the top. If desired, attach a filter needle to the needle, and withdraw the medication. Tap the syringe to clear air from it. Cover the needle with the needle sheath. Before discarding the ampule, check the label against the patient's medication record. Discard the filter needle and the ampule. Attach the appropriate needle to the syringe.

For single-dose or multidose vials
Reconstitute powdered drugs according to the label's instructions. Clean the vial's rubber stopper with an alcohol sponge. Pull the syringe plunger back until the volume of air in the syringe equals the volume of drug to be withdrawn from the vial. Insert the needle into the vial. Inject the air, invert the vial, and keep the needle's bevel tip below the level of the solution as you withdraw the prescribed amount of medication. Cover the needle with the needle sheath. Tap the syringe to clear any air from it. Check the drug label against the patient's medication record before returning the multidose vial to the shelf or drawer or before discarding the single-dose vial.

Implementation
• Select the injection site from those shown at top right, and tell the patient where you'll be giving the injection.

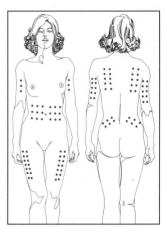

• Put on gloves. Position and drape the patient if necessary.
• Clean the injection site with an alcohol sponge. Loosen the protective needle sheath.
• With your nondominant hand, pinch the skin around the injection site firmly to elevate the subcutaneous tissue, forming a 1″ (2-cm) fat fold, as shown below.

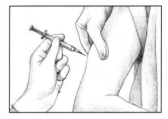

• Holding the syringe in your dominant hand (while pinching the skin around the injection site with the index finger and thumb of your nondominant hand), grip the needle sheath between the fourth and fifth fingers of your nondominant hand, and pull back to uncover the needle. Don't touch the needle.
• Position the needle with its bevel up.

• Tell the patient she'll feel a prick as the needle is inserted. Insert the needle quickly in one motion at a 45-degree or 90-degree angle, as shown below, depending on needle length and the amount of subcutaneous tissue at the site. Some drugs, such as heparin, should always be injected at a 90-degree angle.

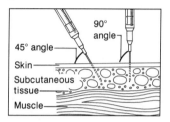

• Release the skin to avoid injecting the drug into compressed tissue and irritating the nerves.
• Pull the plunger back slightly to check for blood return. If none appears, slowly inject the drug. If blood appears upon aspiration, withdraw the needle, prepare another syringe, and repeat the procedure.
• After injection, remove the needle at the same angle used for insertion. Cover the site with an alcohol sponge, and massage the site gently.
• Remove the alcohol sponge, and check the injection site for bleeding or bruising.
• Dispose of injection equipment according to hospital policy.

Special considerations
Don't aspirate for blood return when giving insulin or heparin. It's not necessary with insulin and may cause a hematoma with heparin.

Repeated injections in the same site can cause lipodystrophy. A natural immune response, this complication can be minimized by rotating injection sites.

Intradermal injection

Used primarily for diagnostic purposes, as in allergy or tuberculin testing, intradermal injections are administered in small amounts, usually 0.5 ml or less, into the outer layers of the skin. Because little systemic absorption takes place, this type of injection is used primarily to produce a local effect.

The ventral forearm is the most commonly used site because of its easy access and lack of hair. In extensive allergy testing, the outer aspect of the upper arms may be used, as well as the area of the back between the scapulae.

Equipment
Patient's medication record and chart • prescribed medication • tuberculin syringe with a 26G or 27G ½" to ⅝" needle • gloves • alcohol sponges.

Implementation
• Locate an injection site from those shown below, and tell the patient where you will be giving the injection.

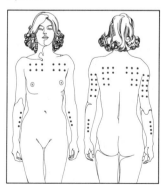

• Instruct the patient to sit up and to extend her arm and support it on a flat surface with the ventral forearm exposed.
• Put on gloves.
• With an alcohol sponge, clean the surface of the ventral forearm about two or three fingerbreadths distal to the antecubital space. Be sure the test site you have chosen is free of hair and blemishes. Allow the skin to dry completely before administering the injection.
• While holding the patient's forearm in your hand, stretch the skin taut with your thumb.
• With your free hand, hold the needle at a 15-degree angle to the patient's arm, with its bevel up.
• Insert the needle about ⅛" below the epidermis. Stop when the needle's bevel tip is under the skin, and inject the antigen slowly. You should feel some resistance as you do this, and a wheal should form as you inject the antigen, as shown below.

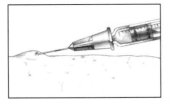

If no wheal forms, you have injected the antigen too deeply; withdraw the needle, and administer another test dose at least 2" (5 cm) from the first site.
• Withdraw the needle at the same angle at which it was inserted. Do not rub the site. This could irriate the underlying tissue, which may affect test results.
• Circle each test site with a marking pen, and label each site according to the recall antigen given. Instruct the patient to refrain from washing off the circles until the test is completed.

• Dispose of needles and syringes according to hospital policy.
• Remove and discard your gloves.
• Assess the patient's response to the skin testing in 24 to 48 hours.

Special considerations
In patients hypersensitive to the test antigens, a severe anaphylactic response can result. This requires immediate epinephrine injection and other emergency resuscitation procedures. Be especially alert after giving a test dose of penicillin or tetanus antitoxin.

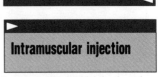

Intramuscular injection

Intramuscular (I.M.) injections deposit medication deep into well-vascularized muscle for rapid systemic action and absorption of up to 5 ml.

Equipment and preparation
Patient's medication record and chart • prescribed medication • diluent or filter needle, if needed • 3- to 5-ml syringe • 20G to 25G 1" to 3" needle • gloves • alcohol sponges.
   The prescribed medication must be sterile. The needle may be packaged separately or already attached to the syringe. Needles used for I.M. injections are longer than subcutaneous needles because they reach deep into the muscle. Needle length also depends on the injection site, the patient's size, and the amount of subcutaneous fat covering the muscle. A larger needle gauge accommodates viscous solutions and suspensions.
   Check the drug for abnormal changes in color and clarity. If in doubt, ask the pharmacist.

Wipe the stopper of the vial with alcohol, and draw up the prescribed amount of medication.

Provide privacy and explain the procedure to the patient. Position and drape him appropriately, making sure that the site is well-lit and exposed.

Implementation

• Wash your hands, and select an appropriate injection site. Avoid a site that is inflamed, edematous, or irritated, or that contains moles, birthmarks, scar tissue, or other lesions. Dorsogluteal or ventrogluteal muscles are used most commonly, as shown below.

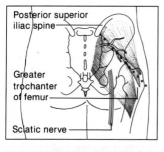

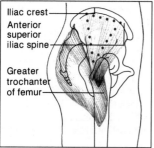

• The deltoid muscle may be used for injections of 2 ml or less, as shown at top right.

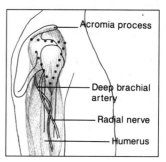

• The vastus lateralis is used most often in children; the rectus femoris may be used in infants, as shown below.

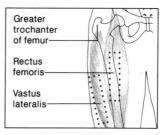

• Remember to rotate sites for patients who require repeated injections.
• Position and drape the patient appropriately.
• Loosen, but don't remove, the needle sheath.
• Gently tap the site to stimulate nerve endings and minimize pain. Clean it by moving an alcohol sponge in circles increasing in diameter to about 2″ (5 cm). Allow the skin to dry; alcohol stings in the puncture.
• Put on gloves. With the thumb and index finger of your nondominant hand, gently stretch the skin.
• With the syringe in your dominant hand, remove the needle sheath with the free fingers of the other hand.

• Position the syringe perpendicular to the skin surface and a couple of inches from the skin. Tell the patient that he will feel a prick. Then quickly and firmly thrust the needle into the muscle.

• Pull back slightly on the plunger to aspirate for blood. If none appears, inject the medication slowly and steadily to let the muscle distend gradually. You should feel little or no resistance. Gently but quickly remove the needle at a 90-degree angle.

• If blood appears, the needle is in a blood vessel. Withdraw it, prepare a fresh syringe, and inject another site.

• Using a gloved hand, apply gentle pressure to the site with the used alcohol sponge. Massage the relaxed muscle, unless contraindicated, to distribute the drug and promote absorption.

• Inspect the site for bleeding or bruising. Apply pressure or ice as necessary.

• Discard all equipment properly. Don't recap needles; put them in an appropriate biohazard container to avoid needle-stick injuries.

Special considerations

• To slow absorption, some drugs are dissolved in oil. Mix them well before use.

• Never inject into the gluteal muscles of a child who has been walking for less than a year.

• If the patient must have repeated injections, consider numbing the area with ice before cleaning it. If you must inject more than 5 ml, divide the solution, and inject it at two sites.

• Urge the patient to relax the muscle to reduce pain and bleeding.

• I.M. injections can damage local muscle cells and elevate serum enzyme levels (creatine kinase), which can be confused with elevated lev-

els caused by myocardial infarction. Diagnostic tests can differentiate the two.

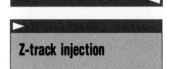

Z-track injection

This method of intramuscular injection prevents leakage, or tracking, into the subcutaneous tissue. Typically, it's used to administer drugs that irritate and discolor subcutaneous tissue – primarily iron preparations, such as iron dextran. It may also be used in elderly patients who have decreased muscle mass. Lateral displacement of the skin during the injection helps to seal the drug in the muscle.

This procedure requires careful attention to technique because leakage into subcutaneous tissue can cause patient discomfort and may permanently stain some tissues.

Equipment and preparation

Patient's medication record and chart • two 20G 1" to 3" needles • prescribed medication • gloves • 3- to 5-ml syringe • two alcohol sponges.

Wash your hands. Make sure the needle you're using is long enough to reach the muscle. As a rule of thumb, a 200-pound patient requires a 2" needle; a 100-pound patient, a 1¼" to 1½" needle.

Attach one needle to the syringe, and draw up the prescribed medication. Then draw 0.2 to 0.5 cc of air (depending on hospital policy) into the syringe. Remove the first needle, and attach the second to prevent tracking the medication through the subcutaneous tissue as the needle is inserted.

Implementation

• Place the patient in the lateral position, exposing the gluteal muscle to be used as the injection site. The patient may also be placed in the prone position. Put on gloves.

• Clean an area on the upper outer quadrant of the patient's buttock with an alcohol sponge.

• Displace the skin laterally by pulling it away from the injection site. To do so, place your finger on the skin surface, and pull the skin and subcutaneous layers out of alignment with the underlying muscle. In doing so, you should move the skin about 1″ (2.5 cm).

• Insert the needle at a 90-degree angle in the site where you initially placed your finger, as shown below.

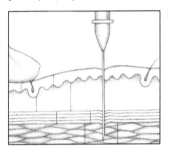

• Aspirate for blood return; if none appears, inject the drug slowly, followed by the air. Injecting air after the drug helps clear the needle and prevents tracking the medication through subcutaneous tissues as the needle is withdrawn.

• Wait 10 seconds before withdrawing the needle to ensure dispersion of the medication.

• Withdraw the needle slowly. Then release the displaced skin and subcutaneous tissue to seal the needle track, as shown at top right.

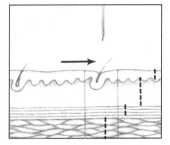

• Don't massage the injection site or allow the patient to wear a tight-fitting garment over the site because it could force the medication into subcutaneous tissue.

• Encourage the patient to walk or move about in bed to facilitate absorption of the drug from the injection site.

• Discard the needles and syringe in an appropriate biohazard container. Do not recap needles to avoid needle-stick injuries.

• Remove and discard your gloves.

Special considerations

• Never inject more than 5 ml of solution into a single site using the Z-track method. Alternate gluteal sites for repeat injections.

• If the patient is on bed rest, encourage active range-of-motion (ROM) exercises, or perform passive ROM exercises to facilitate absorption from the injection site.

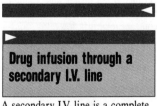

Drug infusion through a secondary I.V. line

A secondary I.V. line is a complete I.V. set connected to the lower Y-port (secondary port) of a primary line instead of to the I.V. catheter or needle. It features an

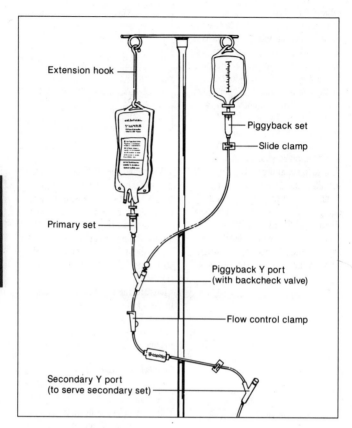

I.V. container, long tubing, and either a microdrip or a macrodrip system, and it can be used for continuous or intermittent drug infusion. When used continuously, it permits drug infusion and titration while the primary line maintains a constant total infusion rate.

A secondary I.V. line used only for intermittent drug administration is called a piggyback set. In this case, the primary line maintains venous access between drug doses. A piggyback set includes a small I.V. container, short tubing, and usually a macrodrip system, and it connects to the primary line's upper Y-port (piggyback port), as shown above.

Equipment and preparation

Patient's medication record and chart • prescribed I.V. medication • diluent, if necessary • prescribed I.V. solution • administration set with secondary injection port • 22G 1" needle • alcohol sponges • 1" adhesive tape • time tape • labels • infusion pump • extension hook and solution for intermittent piggyback infusion.

Wash your hands. Inspect the I.V. container for cracks, leaks, or contamination, and check compatibility with the primary solution. See if the primary line has a secondary injection port.

If necessary, add the drug to the secondary I.V. solution. To do so, remove any seals from the secondary container, and wipe the main port with an alcohol sponge. Inject the prescribed medication and agitate the solution to mix the medication. Label the I.V. mixture. Insert the administration set spike, and attach the needle. Open the flow clamp, and prime the line. Then close the flow clamp.

Some medications come in vials for hanging directly on an I.V. pole. In this case, inject diluent directly into the medication vial. Then spike the vial, prime the tubing, and hang the set.

Implementation

• If the drug is incompatible with the primary I.V. solution, replace the primary solution with a fluid that's compatible with both solutions, and flush the line before starting the drug infusion.
• Hang the container of the secondary set and wipe the injection port of the primary line with an alcohol sponge.
• Insert the needle from the secondary line into the injection port, and tape it securely to the primary line.
• To run the container of the secondary set by itself, lower the primary set's container with an extension hook. To run both containers simultaneously, place them at the same height.
• Open the clamp, and adjust the drip rate. For continuous infusion, set the secondary solution to the desired drip rate; then adjust the primary solution to the desired total infusion rate.
• For intermittent infusion, wait until the secondary solution is completely infused; then adjust the primary drip rate, as required. If the secondary solution tubing is being reused, close the clamp on the tub-

ing, and follow the hospital's policy: Either remove the needle and replace it with a new one, or leave it taped in the injection port, and label it with the time it was first used. Leave the empty container in place until you replace it with a new dose of medication at the prescribed time. If the tubing won't be reused, discard it appropriately with the I.V. container.

Special considerations

• If hospital policy allows, use a pump for drug infusion. Put a time tape on the secondary container to help prevent an inaccurate administration rate.
• When reusing secondary tubing, change it according to hospital policy, usually every 48 to 72 hours. Inspect the injection port for leakage with each use; change it more often if needed.
• Except for lipids, don't piggyback a secondary I.V. line to a total parenteral nutrition line because it risks contamination.

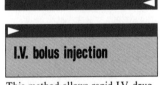

I.V. bolus injection

This method allows rapid I.V. drug administration to quickly achieve peak levels in the bloodstream. It may also be used for drugs that can't be given I.M. because they're toxic or the patient has reduced ability to absorb them. And it may be used to deliver drugs that can't be diluted.

Bolus doses may be injected directly into a vein or through an existing I.V. line or implanted vascular access port (VAP).

Equipment and preparation

Patient's medication record and chart • prescribed drug • 20G needle and syringe • diluent, if necessary • tourniquet • povidone-iodine sponge • alcohol sponge • sterile 2″ × 2″ gauze pad • gloves • adhesive bandage • tape. Optional: winged-tip needle with catheter and second syringe (and needle) filled with 0.9% sodium chloride solution, noncoring needle for VAP, heparin flush solution.

Draw the drug into the syringe, and dilute it if necessary.

Implementation

Wash your hands, and put on gloves.

To give direct injections

• Select the largest vein suitable to dilute the drug and minimize irritation.
• Apply a tourniquet above the site to distend the vein, and clean the site with an alcohol or povidone-iodine sponge, working outward in a circle.
• If you're using the needle of the drug syringe, insert it at a 30-degree angle with the bevel up. The bevel should reach ¼″ (0.6 cm) into the vein. Insert a winged-tip needle bevel up, tape the wings in place when you see blood return, and attach the syringe containing the drug.
• Check for blood backflow.
• Remove the tourniquet, and inject the drug at the ordered rate.
• Check for blood backflow to ensure that the needle remained in place and all of the injected medication entered the vein.
• For a winged-tip needle, flush the line with 0.9% sodium chloride solution from the second syringe to ensure complete delivery.
• Withdraw the needle, and apply pressure to the site with the sterile

gauze pad for at least 3 minutes to prevent hematoma.
• Use an adhesive bandage when the bleeding stops.

To inject through an existing I.V. line

• Check the compatibility of the medication.
• Close the flow clamp, wipe the injection port with an alcohol sponge, and inject the drug as you would a direct injection.
• Open the flow clamp, and readjust the flow rate.
• If the drug isn't compatible with the I.V. solution, flush the line with 0.9% sodium chloride solution before and after the injection.

To use a vascular access port

• Wash your hands, put on gloves, and clean the site three times with an alcohol sponge or a povidone-iodine sponge.
• Palpate for the septum, anchor the port between your thumb and first two fingers of your nondominant hand, and give the injection.

Special considerations

• If the existing I.V. line is capped, making it an intermittent infusion device, verify patency and placement of the device before injecting the medication. Then flush the device with normal saline solution, administer the medication, and follow with the appropriate flush.
• Immediately report any signs of acute allergic reaction or anaphylaxis. If extravasation occurs, stop the injection, estimate the amount of infiltration, and notify the doctor.
• When giving diazepam or chlordiazepoxide hydrochloride through a winged-tip needle or I.V. line, flush with bacteriostatic water to prevent precipitation.

Special administration

Epidural analgesics

In this procedure, the doctor injects or infuses medication into the epidural space, thus into cerebrospinal fluid, so it can bypass the blood-brain barrier.

Epidural analgesia helps manage pain, including postoperative pain, and is especially useful in patients with cancer or degenerative joint disease.

Equipment and preparation

Patient's medication record and chart • prescribed epidural solutions • volume infusion device and epidural infusion tubing (depending on hospital policy) • transparent dressing or sterile gauze pads • epidural tray • labels for epidural infusion line • silk tape.

Make sure that the pharmacy has been notified ahead of time regarding the medication order because epidural solutions require special preparation.

Implementation

• Tell the patient he'll feel some pain as the catheter is inserted.
• Put the patient on his side in the knee-chest position, or have him sit on the edge of the bed and lean over a bedside table.
• After the catheter is in place, as shown below, prime the infusion device, confirm medication and infusion rate, and adjust the device.
• After the infusion tubing is connected to the epidural catheter, connect the tubing to the infusion pump. Tape all connection sites, and apply a label that says EPIDURAL INFUSION.
• Tell the patient to report any feeling of pain, which may require an increased infusion rate.
• Change the dressing over the exit site every 24 to 48 hours or as specified.

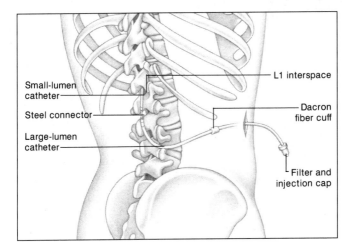

Small-lumen catheter

Steel connector

Large-lumen catheter

L1 interspace

Dacron fiber cuff

Filter and injection cap

Special considerations

• After starting the infusion, assess the patient's respiratory rate and blood pressure every 2 hours for 8 hours, then every 4 hours for 8 hours, then once per shift unless ordered otherwise. Notify the doctor if respiratory rate is below 10 breaths/minute or systolic blood pressure is less than 90 mm Hg.

• Assess the patient's sedation level, mental status, and pain relief every hour initially, then every 2 to 4 hours, until adequate pain control is achieved.

• If the patient is receiving a local anesthetic, assess lower extremity motor strength every 2 to 4 hours. If sensory and motor loss occurs, large motor nerve fibers have been affected, and dosage may need to be decreased.

• The patient should always have a peripheral I.V. line open to allow administration of emergency drugs.

• Don't give analgesics by other routes because such administration increases the risk of respiratory depression.

CHAPTER 11

Drug dosages and indications:
Ensuring effective therapy

Dosage calculations

Dosage finder

Dosage calculations

Tips for simplifying dosage calculations

Incorporate units of measure in the calculation

This incorporation helps protect you from one of the most common dosage calculation errors – the incorrect unit of measure. When you include units of measure in the calculation, those in the numerator and the denominator cancel each other out and leave the correct unit of measure in the answer. The following example uses units of measure in calculating a drug with a usual dose of 4 mg/kg for a 55-kg patient:

• State the problem in a proportion:

$$4 \text{ mg} : 1 \text{ kg} :: X \text{ mg} : 55 \text{ kg}$$

• Solve for X by applying the principle that the product of the means equals the product of the extremes:

$$1 \text{ kg} \times X \text{ mg} = 4 \text{ mg} \times 55 \text{ kg}$$

• Divide and cancel out the units of measure that appear in the numerator and denominator:

$$X = \frac{4 \text{ mg} \times 55 \text{ kg}}{1 \text{ kg}}$$

$$X = 220 \text{ mg}$$

Check zeros and decimal places

Suppose you receive an order to administer 0.1 mg of epinephrine S.C., but the only epinephrine on hand is a 1-ml ampule that contains 1 mg of epinephrine. To calculate the volume for injection, use the ratio and proportion method:

• State the problem in a proportion:

$$1 \text{ mg} : 1 \text{ ml} :: 0.1 \text{ mg} : X \text{ ml}$$

• Solve for X by applying the principle that the product of the means equals the product of the extremes:

$$1 \text{ ml} \times 0.1 \text{ mg} = 1 \text{ mg} \times X \text{ ml}$$

• Divide and cancel out the units of measure that appear in the numerator and denominator, carefully checking the decimal placement:

$$\frac{1 \text{ ml} \times 0.1 \text{ mg}}{1 \text{ mg}} = X$$

$$0.1 \text{ ml} = X$$

Recheck calculations that seem unusual

If, for instance, a calculation yields an answer that suggests you administer 25 tablets, you've probably made an error and should recheck your figures carefully. If you still have doubts, review your calculations with another health care professional.

Reviewing ratios and proportions

A ratio is a mathematical expression of the relationship between two things. A proportion is a set of two equal ratios. A ratio may be expressed with a fraction, such as ⅓, or with a colon, such as 1:3.

When ratios are expressed as fractions in a proportion, their cross products are equal, as indicated below:

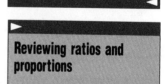

Proportion
$$\frac{2}{4} \diagdown\!\!\!\!\diagup \frac{5}{10}$$

Cross products
$$2 \times 10 = 4 \times 5$$

When ratios are expressed using colons in a proportion, the product of the means equals the product of the extremes:

Proportion
means
↓   ↓
3 : 30 :: 4 : 40
↑ extremes ↑

Product of means
and extremes
$$30 \times 4 = 3 \times 40$$

Whether fractions or ratios are used in a proportion, they must appear in the same order on both sides of the equal sign. When the ratios are expressed as fractions, the units in the numerators must be the same, and the units in the denominators must be the same (although they do not have to be the same as the units in the numerators). The example below demonstrates this principle:

$$\frac{mg}{kg} = \frac{mg}{kg}$$

If the ratios in a proportion are expressed with colons, the units of the first term on the left side of the equal sign must be the same as the units of the first term on the right side. In other words, the units of the mean on one side of the equal sign must match the units of the extreme on the other side, and vice versa. The example below demonstrates this principle:

mg : kg :: mg : kg

Determining the number of tablets to administer

Calculating the number of tablets to administer lends itself to the use of ratios and proportions. Follow this four-step process.
1. Set up the first ratio with the known tablet strength.
2. Set up the second ratio with the unknown quantity.
3. Use these ratios in a proportion.
4. Solve for X, applying the principle that the product of the means equals the product of the extremes.

For example, suppose a drug order calls for propranolol 100 mg P.O. q.i.d., but the only available form of propranolol is 40-mg tablets.

1. Set up the first ratio with the known tablet strength:

40 mg : 1 tab

2. Set up the second ratio with the desired dose and the unknown number of tablets:

100 mg : X tab

3. Use these ratios in a proportion:

40 mg : 1 tab :: 100 mg: X tab

4. Solve for X, applying the principle that the product of the means equals the product of the extremes:

$$1 \text{ tab} \times 100 \text{ mg} = 40 \text{ mg} \times X \text{ tab}$$
$$\frac{1 \text{ tab} \times 100 \text{ mg}}{40 \text{ mg} \times X \text{ tab}}$$
$$2\frac{1}{2} \text{ tab} = X$$

DRUG DOSAGES & INDICATIONS

> ### Determining the amount of liquid medication to administer

To calculate this amount, you can also use ratios and proportions. Follow the same four-step process used in determining the number of tablets to administer.

For example, a patient is to receive 750 mg of amoxicillin oral suspension. The label reads *Amoxicillin (Amoxicillin Trihydrate) 250 mg/5 ml*. The bottle contains 100 ml. How many milliliters of amoxicillin solution should the patient receive?

To solve this problem:

1. Set up the first ratio with the known liquid medication's strength:

$$250 \text{ mg} : 5 \text{ ml}$$

2. Set up the second ratio with the desired dose and the unknown quantity:

$$750 \text{ mg} : X \text{ ml}$$

3. Use these ratios in a proportion:

$$250 \text{ mg} : 5 \text{ ml} :: 750 \text{ mg} : X \text{ ml}$$

4. Solve for X by applying the principle that the product of the means equals the product of the extremes:

$$5 \text{ ml} \times 750 \text{ mg} = 250 \text{ mg} \times X \text{ ml}$$

$$\frac{5 \text{ ml} \times 750 \text{ mg}}{250 \text{ mg}} = X$$

$$15 \text{ ml} = X$$

> ### Administering drugs available in varied concentrations

Drugs such as epinephrine, heparin, and allergy serums are available in varied concentrations. So you must consider the drug's concentration when calculating dosages. Otherwise, you could make a serious – even lethal – medication error. To avoid a dosage error, make sure that drug concentrations are part of the calculation.

For example, a drug order calls for 0.2 mg epinephrine S.C. stat. The ampule is labeled 1 ml of 1:1,000 epinephrine. You need to calculate the correct volume of drug to inject:

1. Determine the strength of the solution based on its unlabeled ratio:

$$1{:}1{,}000 \text{ epinephrine} = 1 \text{ g}/1{,}000 \text{ ml}$$

2. Set up a proportion with this information and the desired dose:

$$1 \text{ g} : 1{,}000 \text{ ml} :: 0.2 \text{ mg} : X \text{ ml}$$

Before you can perform this calculation, however, you must convert grams to milligrams by using the conversion 1 g = 1,000 mg.

3. Restate the proportion with the converted units and solve for X:

$$1{,}000 \text{ mg} : 1{,}000 \text{ ml} :: 0.2 \text{ mg} : X \text{ ml}$$

$$1{,}000 \text{ ml} \times 0.2 \text{ mg} = 1{,}000 \text{ mg} \times X \text{ ml}$$

$$\frac{1{,}000 \text{ ml} \times 0.2 \text{ mg}}{1{,}000 \text{ mg}} = X$$

$$0.2 \text{ ml} = X$$

Calculating I.V. drip and flow rates

To compute drip and flow rates, set up a fraction showing the solution volume to be delivered over the prescribed duration. For example, if a patient is to receive 100 ml of solution within 1 hour, the fraction is:

$$\frac{100 \text{ ml}}{60 \text{ min}}$$

Next, multiply the fraction by the drip factor (the number of drops contained in 1 ml) to determine the drip rate (the number of drops per minute to be infused).

The drip factor varies among I.V. sets and appears on the package containing the I.V. tubing administration set. Following the manufacturer's directions for drip factor is a crucial step. Standard sets have drip factors of 10, 15, or 20 drops/ml. A microdrip (minidrip) set has a drip factor of 60 drops/ml.

Use the following equation to determine the drip rate:

$$\frac{\text{total no. of ml}}{\text{total no. of min}} \times \frac{\text{drip}}{\text{factor}} = \text{drops/min}$$

The equation applies to solutions that infuse over many hours or to such small-volume infusions as those used for antibiotics, which are given less than 1 hour.

You can modify the equation by first determining the number of milliliters to be infused over 1 hour (the flow rate). Next, divide the flow rate by 60 minutes. Multiply the result by the drip factor to determine the number of drops per minute. You'll also use the flow rate when working with infusion pumps to set the number of milliliters to be delivered in 1 hour.

Quick calculation of drip rates

Besides the equation and its modified version, quicker computation methods exist. To administer solutions via a microdrip, adjust the flow rate (number of milliliters per hour) to equal the drip rate (number of drops per minute). Using the equation, divide the flow rate by 60 minutes and multiply by the drip factor, which also equals 60. Because the flow rate and drip factor are equal, the two arithmetic operations cancel each other. For example, if flow rate is 125 ml/hr, the equation would be:

$$\frac{125 \text{ ml}}{60 \text{ min}} \times 60 = \text{drip rate (125)}$$

Rather than spend the time solving the equation, you can simply use the number assigned to the flow rate as the drip rate.

For sets that deliver 15 drops/ml, the flow rate divided by 4 equals the drip rate. For sets with a drip factor of 10, the flow rate divided by 6 equals the drip rate.

To determine how many micrograms (mcg) of a drug are in a milliliter of solution, use this equation:

$$\text{mcg/ml} = \text{mg/ml} \times 1,000$$

To express drip rates in mcg per kilogram (kg) per minute, you must know the solution's concentration (mcg/ml), the patient's weight (kg), and the infusion rate (ml/hr):

$$\text{mcg/kg/min} = \frac{\text{mcg/ml} \times \text{ml/min}}{\text{body wt (kg)}}$$

To find ml/min, divide ml/hr by 60.

You can also convert ml/hour from a dosage given in mcg/kg/min:

$$\text{ml/hr} = \frac{\text{wt (kg)} \times \text{mcg/kg/min}}{\text{mcg/ml}} \times 60$$

Estimating body surface area in adults

Place a straightedge from the patient's height in the left-hand column to his weight in the right-hand column. The intersection of this line with the center scale reveals the body surface area. The adult nomogram is especially useful in calculating dosages for chemotherapy.

HEIGHT	BODY SURFACE AREA	WEIGHT
cm 200 — 79 inch 78 195 — 77 76 190 — 75 74 185 — 73 72 180 — 71 70 175 — 69 68 170 — 67 66 165 — 65 64 160 — 63 62 155 — 61 60 150 — 59 58 145 — 57 56 140 — 55 54 135 — 53 52 130 — 51 50 125 — 49 48 120 — 47 46 115 — 45 44 110 — 43 42 105 — 41 40 cm 100 — 39 in	2.80 m^2 2.70 2.60 2.50 2.40 2.30 2.20 2.10 2.00 1.95 1.90 1.85 1.80 1.75 1.70 1.65 1.60 1.55 1.50 1.45 1.40 1.35 1.30 1.25 1.20 1.15 1.10 1.05 1.00 0.95 0.90 0.86 m^2	kg 150 — 330 lb 145 — 320 140 — 310 135 — 300 130 — 290 125 — 280 120 — 270 115 — 260 110 — 250 105 — 240 100 — 230 — 220 95 — 210 90 — 200 85 — 190 80 — 180 75 — 170 70 — 160 65 — 150 60 — 140 55 — 130 50 — 120 45 — 110 — 105 — 100 40 — 95 — 90 — 85 35 — 80 — 75 — 70 kg 30 — 66 lb

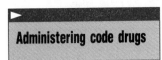

Administering code drugs

Adenosine

Indicated for paroxysmal supraventricular tachycardia with atrioventricular node conduction.

Dosage

6 mg I.V. initially as a rapid bolus over 1 to 3 seconds. If no response in 1 to 2 minutes, give 12 mg I.V.

Nursing considerations

• Adverse effects, such as flushing, disappear quickly because the drug has a short half-life.
• Follow each dose with a 20-ml flush of 0.9% sodium chloride solution to ensure drug delivery.

Atropine sulfate

Indicated for sinus bradycardia with hemodynamic compromise or with frequent ventricular ectopic beats, and for ventricular asystole.

Dosage

0.5 mg for bradycardia or 1 mg for asystole, I.V. push over 1 to 2 minutes; may be repeated every 3 to 5 minutes to a maximum of 2 mg.

Nursing considerations

• Monitor for paradoxical initial bradycardia, especially in patients who are receiving small doses (0.4 to 0.6 mg).
• Monitor fluid intake and urine output.
• May induce tachycardia.

Bretylium tosylate

Indicated for resistant ventricular fibrillation or tachycardia.

Dosage

For resistant ventricular fibrillation, 5 mg/kg I.V. push followed by defibrillation; if ventricular fibrillation persists, increase to 10 mg/kg and repeat every 5 minutes (maximum dose: 30 to 35 mg/kg). *For resistant ventricular tachycardia,* 5 to 10 mg/kg diluted to 50 ml with dextrose 5% in water (D_5W) and infused I.V. over 8 to 10 minutes. Dose can be repeated in 1 to 2 hours, then every 6 to 8 hours if ventricular tachycardia persists. Or give as a continuous infusion at 2 mg/min.

Nursing considerations

• Not a first-line drug; use only if ventricular fibrillation isn't converted by lidocaine and defibrillation, if ventricular fibrillation recurs despite lidocaine therapy, or if lidocaine and procainamide fail to control ventricular tachycardia associated with palpable pulse.

Dobutamine hydrochloride

Indicated for patients with low cardiac output, hypotension, and pulmonary congestion.

Dosage

Infuse 2.5 to 10 mcg/kg/min; use the smallest effective dose, as indicated by hemodynamic parameters.

Nursing considerations

• May induce reflex peripheral vasodilation
• Monitor heart rate closely; an increase of 10% or more may worsen myocardial ischemia.

Dopamine hydrochloride

Indicated for hypotension with bradycardia.

Dosage

1 to 5 mcg/kg/min initially, titrated until the desired response is achieved.

DRUG DOSAGES & INDICATIONS

Nursing considerations
• Drug effects vary with dosage: At 0.5 to 2 mcg/kg/min, drug dilates renal and mesenteric vessels without increasing heart rate or blood pressure; at 2 to 10 mcg/kg/min, it increases cardiac output without peripheral vasoconstriction; at over 10 mcg/kg/min, it causes peripheral vasoconstriction.

Epinephrine hydrochloride
Indicated for cardiac arrest.

Dosage
1 mg I.V. (10 ml of 1:10,000 solution); repeat every 3 to 5 minutes if necessary.

Nursing considerations
• May be given endotracheally at 2 to 2½ times the I.V. dose if I.V. line can't be established quickly.
• Intracardiac injection indicated only if venous and endotracheal routes are unavailable.

Lidocaine hydrochloride
Indicated for ventricular tachycardia (VT), ventricular ectopy, and ventricular fibrillation (VF). Prophylactic administration in uncomplicated MI is no longer recommended unless VT and VF persist after defibrillation and administration of epinephrine.

Dosage
1 to 1.5 mg/kg I.V. bolus as a loading dose at 25 to 50 mg/min. Repeat bolus dose every 3 to 5 minutes until arrhythmias subside or adverse reactions develop, to a maximum of 3 mg/kg (300 mg over 1 hour). Simultaneously, set up a continuous I.V. infusion at 1 to 4 mg/min. (Dilute 1 g of lidocaine in 250 ml of D_5W for a 0.4% solution, or 4 mg/ml.)

Nursing considerations
• Administer half the bolus dose to elderly patients, patients weighing less than 50 kg, and those with congestive heart failure or hepatic disease.
• Improves response to defibrillation when patient is in ventricular fibrillation.
• May be given endotracheally at 2 to 2½ times the I.V. dose if an I.V. line can't be established quickly.

Magnesium sulfate
Indicated for treatment of VF, VT, or torsades de pointes and for prevention of post-MI arrhythmias.

Dosage
2 to 6 g I.V. over several minutes, followed by continuous I.V. infusion of 3 to 20 mg/min administered over 5 to 48 hours.

Nursing considerations
• Monitor serum magnesium levels.

Nitroglycerin
Indicated for congestive heart failure associated with MI and for unstable angina.

Dosage
5 mcg/min I.V. infusion initially, increasing by 5 mcg/min every 3 to 5 minutes until response occurs.

Nursing considerations
• Monitor for hypotension, which could worsen myocardial ischemia.
• Mean dosage range is 50 to 500 mcg/min; most patients will respond to 200 mcg/min or less.
• Use special I.V. tubing supplied by the manufacturer; up to 80% of drug binds to plastic in normal I.V. administration sets.

Nitroprusside sodium
Indicated for heart failure and hypertensive crisis.

Dosage

Dissolve 50 mg in 2 to 3 ml of D_5W; then mix with 250 to 1,000 ml of D_5W, depending on desired concentration. Infuse at 0.3 to 10 mcg/kg/min, titrating until the desired effect is achieved. The therapeutic dosage ranges from 0.5 to 8 mcg/kg/min.

Nursing considerations

• Wrap container in opaque material to prevent drug deterioration.
• Monitor blood pressure with an intra-arterial line.
• Large doses given at fast infusion rates increase the risk of cyanide toxicity. Measure cyanide levels, and monitor for acidosis; if toxicity is suspected, start treatment without test results.

Norepinephrine hydrochloride

Indicated for severe hypotension with low total peripheral resistance.

Dosage

Mix 4 mg of norepinephrine bitartrate per 1,000 ml of D_5W or 0.9% sodium chloride solution to yield a 4 mcg/ml solution. Initially, give 2 to 3 ml (8 to 12 μg base) per minute I.V. Adjust flow to establish and maintain a low-normal blood pressure; average rate of maintenance infusion is 2 to 4 μg/min.

Nursing considerations

• Contraindicated in hypovolemia.
• Monitor blood pressure with intra-arterial line; blood pressure measurements with a standard cuff may be falsely low.
• Cardiac output may increase or decrease, depending on vascular resistance, left ventricular function, and reflex response.
• Avoid prolonged use; drug may cause ischemia of vital organs.

Procainamide hydrochloride

Indicated for ventricular arrhythmias, such as premature ventricular contractions or tachycardia, when lidocaine is contraindicated or ineffective.

Dosage

100 mg by slow I.V. push every 5 minutes, no faster than 25 to 50 mg/min, until arrhythmias disappear, adverse reactions develop, or 1 g has been given. When arrhythmias disappear, give continuous I.V. infusion of 2 to 6 mg/min.

Nursing considerations

• Lower the dosage for patients with renal failure.
• Too-rapid infusion will cause acute hypotension.
• Monitor electrocardiogram carefully; if QRS complex widens more than 50% or if QT interval is prolonged, notify doctor and discontinue infusion, as ordered.

Verapamil hydrochloride

Indicated for atrial fibrillation, atrial flutter, or multifocal atrial tachycardia. Also used to help treat narrow QRS complex paroxysmal supraventricular tachycardia.

Dosage

5 to 10 mg I.V. push over 2 minutes with electrocardiogram and blood pressure monitoring. Repeat dose in 30 minutes if no response.

Nursing considerations

• Use cautiously and in lower doses for patients receiving beta blockers.
• Monitor for hypotension, severe bradycardia, and congestive heart failure (CHF).
• Because verapamil may decrease myocardial contractility, it can aggravate CHF in patients with severe left ventricular dysfunction.

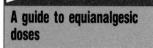

A guide to equianalgesic doses

Narcotic agonists

The standard narcotic agonist dose, 10 mg of morphine sulfate I.M., is used to calculate equally effective (equianalgesic) doses of other narcotic agonists. This method is useful when a patient must be switched from one narcotic agonist to another with no change in dose effectiveness. This chart lists equianalgesic doses of selected narcotic agonists.

DRUG	DOSE
codeine	120 mg P.O.
morphine	10 mg I.M.
hydromorphone	1.5 mg I.M.
levorphanol	2 mg I.M.
(Levo-Dromoran)	
meperidine	75 to 100 mg I.M.
methadone	8 to 10 mg I.M.
(Dolophine)	
fentanyl	0.1 to 0.2 mg I.M.
oxymorphone	1 to 1.5 mg I.M.
(Numorphan)	

Mixed narcotic agonist-antagonists

This chart lists equianalgesic doses (based on the standard dose of 10 mg of morphine sulfate I.M.) for mixed narcotic agonist-antagonists.

DRUG	DOSE
morphine	10 mg I.M.
buprenorphine	0.3 mg I.M.
butorphanol	2 mg I.M.
dezocine	10 mg I.M.
nalbuphine	10 mg I.M.
pentazocine	30 mg I.M.

Critical elements of medication teaching

As patients become more responsible for their own care, it's important that you supply them with all the information they need to enable them to fully comply with their treatment plan. Accurate written information is crucial for any patient, but it's especially so for the young, the elderly, and those with any cognitive impairments. When preparing your written medication teaching plan, be sure to include the following points:
• name, dosage, and action of the drug
• frequency and times of administration
• special storage and preparation instructions
• drugs (including over-the-counter products) and foods (including additives) to avoid
• special comfort or safety measures and precautions
• adverse effects and possible signs and symptoms of toxicity
• warnings about discontinuing the medication.

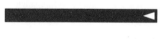

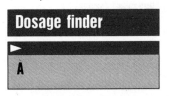

Dosage finder

A

acebutolol (Monitan, Sectral)
• Hypertension. *Adults:* 400 mg P.O. either as a single daily dose or divided b.i.d. Patients may receive up to 1,200 mg daily.
• Ventricular arrhythmias. *Adults:* 400 mg P.O. daily divided b.i.d. Dosage is then increased to provide an adequate response. Usual dosage is 600 to 1,200 mg daily.

acetazolamide (Diamox, Diamox Sequels)
acetazolamide sodium (Diamox Parenteral, Diamox Sodium)
• Open-angle glaucoma. *Adults:* 250 mg to 1 g daily P.O. divided q.i.d., not to exceed 1 g/day.
• Secondary glaucoma. *Adults:* 250 mg q 4 hours; 250 mg P.O. b.i.d.; or 500 mg followed by 125 to 150 mg q 4 hours.

acetic acid (Domeboro Solution, VSol HC Otic)
• External ear canal infection. *Adults and children:* 4 to 6 drops into ear canal t.i.d. or q.i.d., or insert saturated wick for first 24 hours, then continue with instillations.
• Prophylaxis of swimmer's ear. *Adults and children:* 2 drops in each ear b.i.d.

acetohexamide (Dimelor, Dymelor)
• Adjunct to diet to lower the blood glucose level in patients with Type II diabetes (non-insulin-dependent diabetes mellitus). *Adults:* initially, 250 mg P.O. daily before breakfast; may increase dosage q 5 to 7 days (by 250 to 500 mg) as needed to maximum of 1.5 g daily, divided

b.i.d. or t.i.d. before meals.
• To replace insulin therapy in Type II diabetes. *Adults:* if insulin dosage is less than 20 units daily, insulin may be stopped and oral therapy started with 250 mg P.O. daily, before breakfast, increased as above if needed. If insulin dosage is 20 to 40 units daily, start oral therapy with 250 mg P.O. daily, before breakfast, while reducing insulin dosage 25% to 30% daily or every other day, depending on response to oral therapy.

acetylcysteine (Airbron, Mucomyst, Mucosol, Parvolex)
• Pneumonia, bronchitis, tuberculosis, cystic fibrosis, emphysema, atelectasis (adjunct), complications of thoracic surgery and cardiovascular surgery. *Adults and children:* 1 to 2 ml of 10% to 20% solution by direct instillation into trachea as often as every hour; or 3 to 5 ml of 20% solution, or 6 to 10 ml of 10% solution, by nebulization q 2 to 6 hours p.r.n.

acyclovir (Zovirax)
• Initial genital herpes; limited, non-life-threatening mucocutaneous herpes simplex virus infections in immunocompromised patients. *Adults and children:* apply sufficient quantity to adequately cover all lesions q 3 hours six times daily for 7 days.

acyclovir sodium (Zovirax)
• Treatment of initial and recurrent episodes of mucocutaneous HSV-1 and HSV-2 infections in immunocompromised patients; severe initial episodes of genital herpes in patients who are not immunocompromised. *Adults and children over age 11:* 5 mg/kg given at a constant rate over a period of 1 hour by I.V. infusion q 8 hours for 7 days (5 days for genital herpes). *Children under age 12:* 250 mg/m^2 given at a

constant rate over a period of 1 hour by I.V. infusion q 8 hours for 7 days (5 days for genital herpes).
• Treatment of initial genital herpes. *Adults:* 200 mg P.O. q 4 hours while awake (a total of five capsules daily). Treatment should continue for 10 days.
• Intermittent therapy for recurrent genital herpes. *Adults:* 200 mg P.O. q 4 hours while awake (a total of five capsules daily). Treatment should continue for 5 days. Initiate therapy at the first sign of recurrence.
• Chronic suppressive therapy for recurrent genital herpes. *Adults:* 200 mg P.O. t.i.d. for up to 6 months.
• Treatment for chicken pox. *Adults and children:* 20 mg/kg P.O. q.i.d. for 5 days. Start therapy as soon as symptoms appear.

albuterol (Proventil Inhaler, Ventolin Inhaler)
albuterol sulfate (Proventil, Proventil Repetabs, Ventolin)
• Prevention and treatment of bronchospasm in patients with reversible obstructive airway disease. *Adults and children over age 13:* 1 to 2 inhalations q 4 to 6 hours. More frequent administration or greater number of inhalations isn't recommended. Oral tablets: 2 to 4 mg t.i.d. or q.i.d.; maximum dosage is 8 mg q.i.d. Extended-release tablets: 4 to 8 mg q 12 hours; maximum dosage is 16 mg b.i.d.
    Children ages 6 to 13: 2 mg (1 teaspoon) P.O. t.i.d. or q.i.d. *Children ages 2 to 5:* 0.1 mg/kg P.O. t.i.d., not to exceed 2 mg (1 teaspoon) t.i.d. *Adults over age 65:* 2 mg P.O. t.i.d. or q.i.d.
• Prevention of exercise-induced asthma. *Adults:* 2 inhalations 15 minutes before exercise.

alprazolam (Xanax)
Controlled Substance Schedule IV
• Anxiety and tension. *Adults:* Usual starting dosage is 0.25 to 0.5 mg t.i.d. Maximum total daily dosage is 4 mg in divided doses. In elderly or debilitated patients, usual starting dosage is 0.25 mg b.i.d. or t.i.d.

aluminum acetate (Burow's solution) (Acid Mantle Creme, Buro-sol)
aluminum sulfate and calcium acetate (modified Burow's solution) (Bluboro Powder, Domeboro Powder and Tablets)
• Mild skin irritation from exposure to soaps, detergents, chemicals, diaper rash, acne, scaly skin, eczema. *Adults and children:* apply p.r.n.
• Skin inflammation, insect bites, poison ivy or other contact dermatoses, swelling, athlete's foot. *Adults and children:* mix powder or tablet with 1 pint of lukewarm tap water, and apply for 15 to 30 minutes every 4 to 8 hours; bandage loosely.

aluminum hydroxide (AlternaGEL, Amphojel)
• Antacid. *Adults:* 600 mg P.O. (5 to 10 ml of most products) 1 hour after meals and h.s.; 300- or 600-mg tablet, chewed before swallowing, taken with milk or water five to six times daily after meals and h.s.
• Hyperphosphatemia in renal failure. *Adults:* 500 mg to 2 g P.O. b.i.d. to q.i.d.

ambenonium chloride (Mytelase)
• Symptomatic treatment of myasthenia gravis in patients who can't take neostigmine bromide or pyridostigmine bromide. *Adults:* dosage must be individualized for each patient, but usually ranges from 5 to 25 mg P.O. t.i.d. to q.i.d. Starting dosage usually is 5 mg P.O. t.i.d. to q.i.d. Increase gradually and adjust

at 1- to 2-day intervals to avoid drug accumulation and overdose.

amikacin sulfate (Amikin)
• Serious infections caused by sensitive strains of *Pseudomonas aeruginosa, Escherichia coli, Proteus, Klebsiella, Serratia, Enterobacter, Acinetobacter, Providencia, Citrobacter,* and *Staphylococcus;* meningitis. *Adults and children with normal renal function:* 15 mg/kg/day divided q 8 to 12 hours I.M. or I.V. (in 100 to 200 ml D$_5$W or 0.9% sodium chloride solution administered over 30 to 60 minutes). *Neonates with normal renal function:* Initially, 10 mg/kg I.V. followed by 7.5 mg/kg q 12 hours.
• Uncomplicated urinary tract infections. *Adults:* 250 mg I.M. or I.V. b.i.d.
• Dosage adjustments are necessary in renal failure.

amiloride hydrochloride (Midamor)
• Hypertension; edema associated with congestive heart failure (CHF), usually in patients who are also taking thiazide or other potassium-wasting diuretics. *Adults:* Usual dosage is 5 mg P.O. daily. Dosage may be increased to 10 mg daily, if necessary. Maximum dosage is 20 mg/day.

aminophylline (Aminophyllin)
• Symptomatic relief of bronchospasm. *Patients not currently receiving theophylline who require rapid relief of symptoms:* Loading dose is 6 mg/kg (equivalent to 4.7 mg/kg anhydrous theophylline) I.V. slowly (less than or equal to 25 mg/kg/min); then maintenance infusion. *Adults (nonsmokers):* 0.7 mg/kg/hour I.V. for 12 hours; then 0.5 mg/kg/hour. *Otherwise healthy adult smokers:* 1 mg/kg/hour I.V. for 12 hours; then 0.8 mg/kg/hour. *Older patients and adults with cor pulmo-*

nale: 0.6 mg/kg/hour I.V. for 12 hours; then 0.3 mg/kg/hour. *Adults with CHF or liver disease:* 0.5 mg/kg/hour I.V. for 12 hours; then 0.1 to 0.2 mg/kg/hour. *Children ages 9 to 16:* 1 mg/kg/hour I.V. for 12 hours; then 0.8 mg/kg/hour. *Children ages 6 months to 9 years:* 1.2 mg/kg/hour I.V. for 12 hours; then 1 mg/kg/hour.

Patients currently receiving theophylline: Aminophylline infusions of 0.63 mg/kg (0.5 mg/kg anhydrous theophylline) will increase plasma levels of theophylline by 1 mcg/ml. Some clinicians recommend a dose of 3.1 mg/kg (2.5 mg/kg anhydrous theophylline) if no obvious signs of theophylline toxicity are present.
• Chronic bronchial asthma. *Adults:* 600 to 1,600 mg P.O. daily divided t.i.d. or q.i.d. *Children:* 12 mg/kg P.O. daily divided t.i.d. or q.i.d. *Note:* Rectal dosage is the same as that recommended for oral dosage.

amiodarone hydrochloride (Cordarone)
• Recurrent ventricular fibrillation and recurrent hemodynamically unstable ventricular tachycardia refractory to other antiarrhythmics. *Adults:* Loading dose is 5 to 10 mg/kg by I.V. infusion over 20 minutes to 2 hours via central line. Alternatively (and where available), a loading dose of 5 mg/kg I.V. over 20 minutes to 2 hours using a central line. Then repeated 2 to 3 times in 24 hours to a maximum of 1.2 g. Or, give loading dosage of 800 to 1,600 mg P.O. daily for 1 to 3 weeks until initial therapeutic response occurs, then 650 to 800 mg P.O. daily for 1 month. Maintenance dosage is 200 to 600 mg P.O. daily.

amitriptyline hydrochloride (Elavil, Emitrip, Endep, Enovil, Levate)
• Treatment of depression. *Adults:* 50 to 100 mg P.O. h.s., increasing to

150 mg daily; maximum dosage is
300 mg daily if needed. Or 20 to 30
mg I.M. q.i.d. *Elderly patients and
adolescents:* 10 mg P.O. usually t.i.d.
and 20 mg h.s. daily.

amlodipine besylate (Norvasc)

• Hypertension. *Adults:* Initially,
5 mg P.O. daily; maximum dosage is
10 mg once daily. Dosage is then
adjusted according to patient response and tolerance. Small, fragile,
or elderly patients or those with hepatic insufficiency should receive
2.5 mg daily.
• Chronic, stable or vasospastic
(Prinzmetal's [variant]) angina.
Adults: Initially, 10 mg P.O. daily.
Small, fragile, or elderly patients or
those with hepatic insufficiency
should receive 5 mg daily.

ammonium chloride

• Metabolic alkalosis, chloride replacement. *Adults and children:* I.V.
dose (in milliequivalent [mEq])
equals the serum chloride deficit
(in mEq/ml) multiplied by the extracellular fluid volume (estimated
as 20% of the body weight in kilo-
grams). Patient should be given
one-half the calculated volume, then
be reassessed.
• As an acidifying agent. *Adults:*
4 to 12 g P.O. daily in divided
doses. *Children:* 75 mg/kg P.O. daily
in four divided doses.

amoxapine (Asendin)

• Treatment of depression. *Adults:*
initial dosage is 50 mg P.O. b.i.d. or
t.i.d. May increase to 100 mg b.i.d.
or t.i.d. on third day of treatment.
Increases above 300 mg daily
should be made only if 300 mg
daily has been ineffective during a
trial period of at least 2 weeks.
When effective dosage is established, entire dose (not exceeding
300 mg) may be given at bedtime.

amoxicillin (Amoxil)

• Systemic infections, acute and
chronic urinary or respiratory tract
infections caused by susceptible
strains of gram-positive and gram-
negative organisms. *Adults and children 20 kg and over:* 250 to 500 mg
P.O. q 8 hours. *Children under 20
kg:* 20 mg/kg P.O. daily, divided into
doses given q 8 hours. In severe infections, 40 mg/kg P.O. daily in divided doses q 8 hours or 500 mg/m²
to 1 g/m² P.O. in divided doses q 8
hours.
• Uncomplicated gonorrhea. *Adults
and children over 45 kg:* 3 g P.O.
with 1 g probenecid given as a single dose.
• Endocarditis prophylaxis for dental procedure. *Adults:* Initially, 3 g
P.O. 1 hour before procedure, then
1.5 g 6 hours later. *Children:* Initially, 50 mg/kg P.O. 1 hour before
procedure, then one-half of initial
dose 6 hours later.
• Dosage adjustments are necessary
in renal failure.

amoxicillin and clavulanate potassium (Augmentin)

• Lower respiratory infections, otitis media, sinusitis, skin and skin
structure infections, and urinary
tract infections (UTIs) caused by
susceptible strains of gram-positive
and gram-negative organisms.
Adults: 250 mg (based on the
amoxicillin component) P.O. q 8
hours. For more severe infections,
500 mg q 8 hours. *Children:* 20 to
40 mg/kg/day (based on the amoxicillin component) given in divided
doses q 8 hours.

ampicillin, ampicillin sodium, ampicillin trihydrate (Omnipen, Principen)

• Systemic infections, acute and
chronic UTIs caused by susceptible
strains of gram-positive and gram-
negative organisms. *Adults and children 20 kg or over:* 250 to 500 mg

P.O. daily, divided into doses given q 6 hours; or 2 to 12 g I.M. or I.V. daily, divided into doses given q 4 to 6 hours. *Children 20 kg or under:* 50 to 100 mg/kg P.O. daily, divided into doses given q 6 hours; or 100 to 200 mg/kg I.M. or I.V. daily, divided into doses given q 6 hours.
• Meningitis. *Adults:* 8 to 14 g I.V. daily in divided doses q 3 to 4 hours. *Children:* Up to 300 mg/kg I.V. daily in divided doses q 3 to 4 hours.
• Uncomplicated gonorrhea. *Adults and children over 45 kg:* 3.5 g P.O. with 1 g probenecid given as a single dose.
• Endocarditis prophylaxis for dental procedure. *Adults:* 1 to 2 g I.M. or I.V. with gentamicin 30 minutes before procedure, then repeated 6 hours after initial dose. *Children:* 50 mg/kg I.M. or I.V. with gentamicin 2 mg/kg 30 minutes before procedure, then one-half of initial dose given 6 hours later.

amrinone lactate (Inocor)
• Short-term management of CHF. *Adults:* Initially, 0.75 mg/kg I.V. bolus over 2 to 3 minutes. Then begin maintenance infusion of 5 to 10 mcg/kg/minute. Additional bolus of 0.75 mg/kg may be given 30 minutes after start of therapy. Total daily dosage should not exceed 10 mg/kg.

amyl nitrite
• Relief of angina pectoris. *Adults and children:* 0.18 to 0.3 ml by inhalation (one glass ampule) p.r.n.
• Antidote for cyanide poisoning. *Adults and children:* 0.3 ml by inhalation for 30 to 60 seconds q 5 minutes until conscious.

anthralin (Anthra-Derm)
• Psoriasis, chronic dermatitis. *Adults and children:* apply thin layer daily. Concentrations range

from 0.1% to 1%; start with lowest and increase if necessary.

antihemophilic factor (AHF)
• Treatment of bleeding in patients with hemophilia A. *Adults and children:* For minor hemorrhaging into muscles and joints, 8 to 10 IU/kg I.V. q 8 to 12 hours for 1 or more days. For overt bleeding, initial dosage of 15 to 25 IU/kg I.V., followed by 8 to 15 IU/kg every 8 to 12 hours for 3 or 4 days. To treat massive bleeding or hemorrhaging involving major organs, initial dose of 40 to 50 IU/kg I.V., followed by 20 to 25 IU/kg q 8 to 12 hours.

apraclonidine hydrochloride (Iopidine)
• Prevention or control of intraocular pressure elevations after laser surgery. *Adults:* Instill 1 drop of 1% solution in the eye 1 hour before initiation of surgery on the anterior segment, followed by 1 drop immediately after completion of surgery.

artificial tears (Isopto Tears, Liquifilm Tears)
• Insufficient tear production. *Adults and children:* Instill 1 to 2 drops in eye t.i.d., q.i.d., or p.r.n.
• Moderate-to-severe dry eye syndromes, including keratoconjunctivitis sicca. *Adults:* Insert 1 rod daily into inferior cul-de-sac. Some patients may require twice-daily use.

astemizole (Hismanal)
• Symptomatic relief in chronic idiopathic urticaria and seasonal allergic rhinitis. *Adults and children over age 12:* 10 mg P.O. daily.

atenolol (Tenormin)
• Hypertension. *Adults:* Initially, 50 mg P.O. daily as a single dose. Dosage may be increased to 100 mg once daily after 7 to 14 days. Daily dosages greater than 100 mg are unlikely to produce further benefit.

Dosage adjustment is necessary in patients with creatinine clearance below 35 ml/minute.

• Angina pectoris. *Adults:* 50 mg P.O. once daily. May increase to 100 mg daily after 7 days for optimal effect. May give as much as 200 mg daily.

• Reduction of mortality and reinfarction in acute myocardial infarction (MI). *Adults:* 5 mg I.V. over 5 minutes, followed by another 5 mg I.V. 10 minutes later; after an additional 10 minutes, administer 50 mg P.O., followed by 50 mg P.O. in 12 hours. Thereafter, give 100 mg P.O. daily as single dose or 50 mg b.i.d. for at least 7 days.

• Dosage adjustments may be necessary in patients with renal insufficiency.

atropine sulfate (Atropisol, Isopto Atropine)

• Acute iritis and uveitis. *Adults:* Instill 1 to 2 drops of solution in eye up to 4 times daily, or apply small amount of ointment to conjunctival sac up to 3 times daily. *Children:* Instill 1 to 2 drops of 0.5% solution into eye up to 3 times daily or apply a small strip of ointment to conjunctival sac up to 3 times daily.

• Cycloplegic refraction. *Adults:* Instill 1 to 2 drops of 1% solution 1 hour before refracting. *Children:* Instill 1 to 2 drops of 0.5% solution in each eye b.i.d. for 1 to 3 days before eye examination and 1 hour before refraction.

auranofin (Ridaura)

• Rheumatoid arthritis (RA). *Adults:* 6 mg P.O. daily, administered either as 3 mg b.i.d. or 6 mg once daily. After 6 months, may be increased to 9 mg daily.

aurothioglucose (Solganal) gold sodium thiomalate

• RA. *Adults:* For aurothioglucose, initially 10 mg I.M., followed by

25 mg for second and third doses at weekly intervals. Then, 50 mg weekly until 1 g has been given. If improvement occurs without toxicity, continue 25 to 50 mg at 3- to 4-week intervals indefinitely as maintenance therapy. *Adults:* For gold sodium thiomalate, initially 10 mg I.M., followed by 25 mg in 1 week. Then 50 mg weekly until 14 to 20 doses have been given. If improvement occurs without toxicity, continue 25 to 50 mg q 2 weeks for four doses; then 25 to 50 mg q 3 weeks for four doses; then 25 to 50 mg q month indefinitely as maintenance therapy. If relapse occurs during maintenance therapy, resume injections at weekly intervals. *Children ages 6 to 12:* For aurothioglucose, one-quarter usual adult dosage. Alternatively, 1 mg/kg I.M. once weekly for 20 weeks. *Children:* For gold sodium thiomalate, 1 mg/kg I.M. weekly for 20 weeks. If response is good, may be given q 3 to 4 weeks indefinitely.

azathioprine (Imuran)

• Immunosuppression in kidney transplantation. *Adults and children:* Initially, 3 to 5 mg/kg P.O. or I.V. daily, usually beginning on day of transplantation. Maintained at 1 to 3 mg/kg daily (dosage varies considerably according to patient response).

• Treatment of severe, refractory RA. *Adults:* Initially, 1 mg/kg taken as a single dose or as two doses. If patient response is not satisfactory after 6 to 8 weeks, dosage may be increased by 0.5 mg/kg daily (up to a maximum of 2.5 mg/kg daily) at 4-week intervals.

azithromycin (Zithromax)

• Acute bacterial exacerbations of chronic obstructive pulmonary disease (COPD) caused by *Haemophilus influenzae, Moraxella (Branhamella) catarrhalis,* or *Streptococcus pneumoniae;* mild community-acquired pneumonia caused by *H. influenzae* or *S. pneumoniae;* uncomplicated skin and skin structure infections caused by *Staphylococcus aureus, Streptococcus pyogenes,* or *Streptococcus agalactiae;* and second-line therapy of pharyngitis or tonsillitis caused by *S. pyogenes. Adults and adolescents age 16 and older:* Initially, 500 mg P.O. as a single dose on day 1, followed by 250 mg daily on days 2 through 5. Total cumulative dose is 1.5 g.

• Nongonococcal urethritis or cervicitis caused by *Chlamydia trachomatis. Adults and adolescents age 16 and older:* 1 g P.O. as a single dose.

aztreonam (Azactam)
• Urinary tract, respiratory tract, intra-abdominal, gynecologic, or skin infections; or septicemia caused by aerobic organisms. *Adults:* 500 mg to 2 g I.V. or I.M. q 8 to 12 hours. For severe systemic or life-threatening infections, 2 g q 6 to 8 hours may be given. Maximum dosage is 8 g daily.

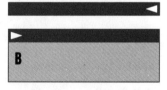

B

bacampicillin hydrochloride (Spectrobid)
• Upper and lower respiratory tract, urinary tract, and skin infections caused by susceptible organisms. *Adults and children weighing more than 25 kg:* 400 to 800 mg P.O. q 12 hours. *Children weighing less than 25 kg:* 25 to 50 mg/kg P.O. q 12 hours.
• Gonorrhea. *Adults and children weighing more than 25 kg:* Usual dosage is 1.6 g plus 1 g probenecid given as a single dose.

bacitracin
• Ocular infections. *Adults and children:* Instill small amount in conjunctival sac several times daily or p.r.n. until favorable response is observed.

baclofen (Lioresal)
• Spasticity in multiple sclerosis (MS), spinal cord injury. *Adults:* initially, 5 mg t.i.d. for 3 days, then 10 mg t.i.d. for 3 days, 15 mg t.i.d. for 3 days, 20 mg t.i.d. for 3 days. Increase according to response up to maximum of 80 mg daily.

beclomethasone dipropionate (Beclovent, Vanceril)
• Steroid-dependent asthma. *Adults:* 2 to 4 inhalations t.i.d. or q.i.d. Maximum dosage is 20 inhalations daily. *Children ages 6 to 12:* 1 to 2 inhalations t.i.d. or q.i.d. Maximum dosage is 10 inhalations daily.

beclomethasone dipropionate (Beconase AQ, Beconase Nasal Inhaler, Vancenase AQ, Vancenase Nasal Inhaler)
• Relief of symptoms of seasonal or perennial rhinitis; prevention of recurrence of nasal polyps after surgical removal. *Adults and children over age 12:* usual dosage is 1 spray (42 mcg) in each nostril two to four times daily (total dosage is 168 to 336 mcg daily). Most patients require 1 spray in each nostril t.i.d. (252 mcg daily). Not recommended for children under age 12.

benazepril hydrochloride (Lotensin)
• Hypertension. *Adults:* Initially, 10 mg daily. Usual dosage is 20 to 40 mg daily in 1 or 2 doses.

benzonatate (Tessalon)
• Nonproductive cough. *Adults and children over age 10:* 100 mg P.O. t.i.d.; up to 600 mg/day.

benzoyl peroxide (Oxy 5, Oxy 10, Oxy Cover, PanOxyl)
• Acne. *Adults and children:* Apply once daily to q.i.d., depending on tolerance and effect.

benzquinamide hydrochloride (Emete-Con)
• Nausea and vomiting associated with anesthesia and surgery. *Adults:* 50 mg I.M. (0.5 to 1 mg/kg); may repeat in 1 hour and thereafter q 3 to 4 hours, p.r.n. Or 25 mg (0.2 to 0.4 mg/kg) I.V. as single dose, administered slowly.

benztropine mesylate (Cogentin)
• Drug-induced extrapyramidal disorders (except tardive dyskinesia). *Adults:* 1 to 4 mg P.O. or I.M. once or twice daily.
• Acute dystonic reaction. *Adults:* 2 mg I.V. or I.M., followed by 1 to 2 mg P.O. b.i.d. to prevent recurrence.
• Parkinsonism. *Adults:* 0.5 to 6 mg P.O. daily. Initial dose is 0.5 to 1 mg. Increase by 0.5 mg q 5 to 6 days. Adjust dosage to meet individual requirements.

betamethasone acetate betamethasone sodium phosphate (Celestone Soluspan)
• Severe inflammation and immunosuppression. *Adults:* 0.6 to 7.2 mg P.O. daily or 0.5 to 9 mg into joint or soft tissue daily.

betaxolol hydrochloride (Betoptic)
• Chronic open-angle glaucoma and ocular hypertension. *Adults:* Instill 1 drop 0.5% solution in eyes b.i.d. or 1 to 2 drops 0.25% solution in eyes b.i.d.

betaxolol hydrochloride (Kerlone)
• Hypertension. *Adults:* Initially, 10 mg P.O. once daily. Full antihypertensive effect should occur in 7 to 14 days. May increase dosage to 20 mg P.O. once daily.

biperiden hydrochloride (Akineton) biperiden lactate (Akineton Lactate)
• Extrapyramidal disorders. *Adults:* 2 mg P.O. daily, b.i.d., or t.i.d., depending on severity. Usual dosage is 2 mg daily. Or 2 mg I.M. or I.V. q ½ hour, not to exceed four doses or 8 mg total daily.
• Parkinsonism. *Adults:* 2 mg P.O. t.i.d. or q.i.d.

bisacodyl (Bisacolax, Dulcolax, Fleet Bisacodyl)
• Chronic constipation; preparation for delivery, surgery, or rectal or bowel examination. *Adults and children age 12 and over:* 10 to 15 mg P.O. in evening or before breakfast, or 10 mg P.R. for evacuation before examination or surgery. Up to 30 mg may be used for thorough evacuation needed for examinations or surgery. *Children ages 6 to 12:* 5 mg P.O. or P.R. h.s. or before breakfast.

bismuth subgallate (Devrom) bismuth subsalicylate (Pepto-Bismol)
• Mild, nonspecific diarrhea. *Adults:* 1 to 2 tablets P.O. chewed or swallowed whole t.i.d. (subgallate). *Adults:* 30 ml or 2 tablets P.O. q ½ to 1 hour up to a maximum of eight doses and for no longer than 2 days (subsalicylate). *Children ages 9 to 12:* 15 ml or 1 tablet P.O. *Children ages 6 to 9:* 10 ml or two-thirds of a tablet P.O. *Children ages 3 to 6:* 5 ml or one-third of a tablet P.O.

bitolterol mesylate (Tornalate)
• Prevention and treatment of bronchial asthma and bronchospasm. *Adults and children over age 12:* To prevent: 2 inhalations q 8 hours. To treat: 2 inhalations at an interval of at least 1 to 3 minutes followed by a third inhalation if needed. In either case, dosage should not exceed 3 inhalations q 6 hours or 2 inhalations q 4 hours.

brompheniramine maleate (Dimetane, Histaject Modified)
• Rhinitis, allergy symptoms. *Adults:* 4 to 8 mg P.O. t.i.d. or q.i.d.; (timed-release) 8 to 12 mg P.O. b.i.d. or t.i.d.; or 5 to 20 mg q 6 to 12 hours I.M., I.V., or S.C. Maximum dosage is 40 mg daily. *Children over age 6:* 2 to 4 mg P.O. t.i.d. or q.i.d.; or (timed-release) 8 to 12 mg q 12 hours; or 0.5 mg/kg I.M., I.V., or S.C. daily divided t.i.d. or q.i.d. *Children under age 6:* 0.5 mg/kg P.O., I.M., I.V., or S.C. daily divided t.i.d. or q.i.d. (*Note:* Children under age 12 should use only as directed by a doctor.)

bumetanide (Bumex)
• Edema (CHF, hepatic and renal disease). *Adults:* 0.5 to 2 mg P.O. once daily. If diuretic response is not adequate, a second or third dose may be given at 4- to 5-hour intervals. Maximum dosage is 10 mg/day. May be administered parenterally when P.O. is not feasible. Usual initial dose is 0.5 to 1 mg I.V. or I.M. If response is not adequate, a second or third dose may be given at 2- to 3-hour intervals. Maximum dosage is 10 mg/day.

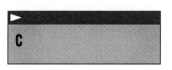

C

calamine (liniment, 15% calamine; lotion, 8% calamine; ointment, 17% calamine)
• Topical astringent and protectant for itching, poison ivy and poison oak, nonpoisonous insect bites, mild sunburn, minor skin irritations. *Adults and children age 2 or older:* apply p.r.n.

calcitonin (Calcimar, Cibacalcin, Miacalcin)
• Paget's disease of bone (osteitis deformans). *Adults:* initially, 100 international units (IU) of calcitonin (salmon) daily, S.C. or I.M. Maintenance dosage is 50 to 100 IU daily or every other day. Alternatively, give calcitonin (human) 0.5 mg S.C. daily. If patient obtains sufficient improvement, dosage may be reduced to 0.25 mg daily two or three times per week. Some patients may need as much as 1 mg daily.
• Hypercalcemia. *Adults:* 4 IU/kg I.M. q 12 hours (calcitonin salmon).
• Postmenopausal osteoporosis. *Adults:* 100 IU I.M. or S.C. daily (calcitonin salmon).

calcitriol (Calcijex, Rocaltrol)
• Management of hypocalcemia in patients undergoing chronic renal dialysis. *Adults:* initially, 0.25 mcg P.O. daily. Dosage may be increased by 0.25 mcg daily at 2- to 4-week intervals. Maintenance dosage is 0.25 mcg every other day up to 0.5 to 1.25 mcg daily.
• Management of hypoparathyroidism and pseudohypoparathyroidism. *Adults and children over age 1:* initially, 0.25 mcg P.O. daily. Dosage may be increased at 2- to 4-week

intervals. Maintenance dosage is 0.25 to 2 mcg daily.

calcium acetate, calcium chloride, calcium gluceptate, calcium gluconate, calcium lactate

• Hypocalcemic emergency. *Adults:* 7 to 14 mEq calcium I.V. May be given as a 10% calcium gluconate solution, 2% to 10% calcium chloride solution, or 22% calcium gluceptate solution. *Children:* 1 to 7 mEq calcium I.V. *Infants:* up to 1 mEq calcium I.V.

• Hypocalcemic tetany. *Adults:* 4.5 to 16 mEq calcium I.V., repeated until tetany is controlled. *Children:* 0.5 to 0.7 mEq calcium I.V. 3 to 4 times a day until tetany is controlled. *Neonates:* 2.4 mEq I.V. daily in divided doses.

• Adjunctive treatment of cardiac arrest. *Adults:* 0.027 to 0.054 mEq calcium chloride I.V., or 4.5 to 6.3 mEq calcium gluceptate I.V., or 2.3 to 3.7 mEq calcium gluconate I.V. *Children:* 0.27 mEq/kg calcium chloride I.V., repeated in 10 minutes if necessary; determine serum calcium levels before continuing.

• Adjunctive treatment of magnesium intoxication. *Adults:* initially, 7 mEq I.V. Subsequent doses must be based upon the patient's response.

• During exchange transfusions. *Adults:* 1.35 mEq concurrently with each 100 ml of citrated blood. *Neonates:* 0.45 mEq after each 100 ml of citrated blood.

• Hyperphosphatemia. *Adults:* 1,334 to 2,000 mg P.O. calcium acetate t.i.d. with meals. Most dialysis patients will require 3 to 4 tablets with each meal.

• Dietary supplement. *Adults:* 500 mg to 2 g P.O. daily.

calcium carbonate (Calcilac, Chooz, Genalac, Titralac, Tums, Tums Liquid Extra Strength)

• Antacid, calcium supplement. *Adults:* 350 mg to 1.5 g P.O. or 2 pieces of chewing gum 1 hour after meals and h.s., p.r.n.

captopril (Capoten)

• Hypertension. *Adults:* 25 mg P.O. b.i.d. or t.i.d. initially. If blood pressure not controlled in 1 to 2 weeks, dosage may be increased to 50 mg t.i.d. If not controlled after another 1 to 2 weeks, add a diuretic to regimen. If further blood pressure reduction is necessary, can raise dosage up to 150 mg t.i.d. while continuing diuretic. Maximum dosage is 450 mg daily. Daily dose may also be administered b.i.d.

• CHF; to reduce risk of death and slow development of heart failure after MI. *Adults:* 6.25 to 12.5 mg P.O. t.i.d. initially. May be gradually increased to 50 mg t.i.d. Maximum dosage is 450 mg daily.

carbamazepine (Tegretol)

• Generalized tonic-clonic and complex-partial (psychomotor) seizures, mixed seizure patterns. *Adults and children over age 12:* initially, 200 mg P.O. b.i.d. May increase by 200 mg P.O. daily, in divided doses at 6- to 8-hour intervals. Adjust to minimum effective level when control is achieved. *Children under age 12:* 100 mg P.O. b.i.d. Increased at weekly intervals by 100 mg P.O. daily.

• Trigeminal neuralgia. *Adults:* initially, 100 mg P.O. b.i.d. with meals. Increase by 100 mg q 12 hours until pain is relieved. Don't exceed 1.2 g daily. Maintenance dosage is 200 to 400 mg P.O. b.i.d.

carbenicillin indanyl sodium (Geocillin)

• Urinary tract infection (UTI) and prostatitis caused by susceptible organisms. *Adults:* 382 to 764 mg P.O. q.i.d. *Note:* Use drug only in patients whose creatinine clearance equals or exceeds 10 ml/min to ensure adequate bladder concentrations.

carisoprodol (Rela, Soma)
• As an adjunct in acute, painful musculoskeletal conditions. *Adults and children over age 12:* 350 mg P.O. t.i.d. and h.s. Not recommended for children under age 12.

carteolol (Cartrol)
• Hypertension. *Adults:* Initially, 2.5 mg P.O. as single daily dose. May gradually increase to 5 or 10 mg as a single daily dose.

castor oil (Alphamul, Emulsoil)
• Preparation for rectal or bowel examination or surgery; acute constipation (rarely). *Adults:* 15 to 60 ml P.O. *Children over age 2:* 5 to 15 ml P.O. *Children under age 2:* 1 to 5 ml P.O. *Infants:* up to 4 ml P.O. Increased dose produces no greater effect.

cefaclor (Ceclor)
• Otitis media and infections of respiratory or urinary tracts, skin, and soft tissue caused by susceptible organisms. *Adults:* 250 to 500 mg P.O. q 8 hours. Total daily dosage should not exceed 4 g. *Children:* 20 mg/kg P.O. daily in divided doses q 8 hours, not to exceed 1 g/day.

cefadroxil (Duricef, Ultracef)
• Urinary tract, skin, and soft-tissue infections caused by susceptible organisms. *Adults:* 500 mg to 2 g P.O. daily, depending on the infection treated. Usually given in once-daily or b.i.d. doses. *Children:* 30 mg/kg daily in two divided doses.
• Dosage adjustments are necessary in renal failure.

cefamandole nafate (Mandol)
• Serious respiratory, genitourinary, skin and soft-tissue, and bone and joint infections; septicemia; peritonitis from susceptible organisms. *Adults:* 500 mg to 1 g q 4 to 8 hours. In life-threatening infections, up to 2 g q 4 hours may be needed. *Infants and children:* 50 to 100 mg/kg daily in equally divided doses q 4 to 8 hours. May be increased to total daily dosage of 150 mg/kg (not to exceed maximum adult dose) for severe infections.

Total daily dosage is same for I.M. or I.V. administration and depends on susceptibility of organism and severity of infection. Cefamandole should be injected deep I.M. into a large muscle mass, such as the gluteus or the lateral aspect of the thigh.

cefazolin sodium (Ancef, Kefzol, Zolicef)
• Serious respiratory, genitourinary, skin and soft-tissue, and bone and joint infections; septicemia; and endocarditis caused by susceptible organisms. *Adults:* 250 mg I.M. or I.V. q 8 hours to 1.5 g q 6 hours. Maximum dosage is 12 g/day in life-threatening situations. *Children over age 1 month:* 25 to 50 mg/kg/day or 1.25 g/m²/day I.M. or I.V. in 3 or 4 divided doses.

Total daily dosage is same for I.M. or I.V. administration and depends on susceptibility of organism and severity of infection. Cefazolin should be injected deep I.M. into a large muscle mass, such as the gluteus or the lateral aspect of the thigh.

cefixime (Suprax)
• Uncomplicated UTI; otitis media; acute bronchitis; acute exacerbations of chronic bronchitis, pharyngitis, or tonsillitis. *Adults and children over age 12 or over 50 kg:* 400 mg P.O. daily in one or two doses.

Children under age 12 or under 50 kg: 8 mg/kg P.O. daily in one or two doses.
• Dosage adjustments are necessary in renal failure.

cefmetazole sodium (Zefazone)
• Lower respiratory tract infections. *Adults:* 2 g I.V. q 6 to 12 hours for 5 to 14 days.
• UTIs caused by *E. coli. Adults:* 2 g I.V. q 12 hours.
• Prophylaxis in patients undergoing vaginal hysterectomy. *Adults:* 2 g I.V. 30 to 90 minutes before surgery as a single dose; or 1 g I.V. 30 to 90 minutes before surgery, repeated in 8 and 16 hours.
• Prophylaxis in patients undergoing abdominal hysterectomy. *Adults:* 1 g I.V. 30 to 90 minutes before surgery, repeated in 8 and 16 hours.
• Prophylaxis in patients undergoing cesarean section. *Adults:* 2 g I.V. as a single dose after clamping cord; or 1 g I.V. after clamping cord, repeated in 8 and 16 hours.
• Prophylaxis in patients undergoing colorectal surgery. *Adults:* 2 g I.V. as a single dose 30 to 90 minutes before surgery. Some clinicians follow with additional 2-g doses in 8 and 16 hours.
• Prophylaxis in high-risk patients undergoing cholecystectomy. *Adults:* 1 g I.V. 30 to 90 minutes before surgery, repeated in 8 and 16 hours.

cefonicid sodium (Monocid)
• Serious lower respiratory, urinary tract, skin, and skin-structure infections; septicemia; and bone and joint infections caused by susceptible organisms. *Adults:* Usual dosage is 1 g I.V. or I.M. q 24 hours. In life-threatening infections, 2 g q 24 hours.
Total daily dosage is same for I.M. or I.V. administration and depends on susceptibility of organism and severity of infection. Cefonicid

should be injected deep I.M. into a large muscle mass, such as the gluteus or the lateral aspect of the thigh.
• Dosage adjustments are necessary in renal failure.

cefoperazone sodium (Cefobid)
• Serious respiratory tract, intra-abdominal, gynecologic, and skin infections; bacteremia; and septicemia caused by susceptible organisms. *Adults:* Usual dosage is 1 to 2 g q 12 hours I.M. or I.V. In severe infections or infections caused by less sensitive organisms, the total daily dosage or frequency may be increased up to 16 g/day in certain situations.
• Dosage adjustments are necessary in renal failure.

cefotaxime sodium (Claforan)
• Serious lower respiratory, urinary, central nervous system (CNS), gynecologic, and skin infections; bacteremia; and septicemia caused by susceptible organisms. *Adults and children weighing more than 50 kg:* Usual dosage is 1 g I.V. or I.M. q 6 to 8 hours. Up to 12 g daily can be administered in life-threatening infections. *Children ages 1 month to 12 years weighing less than 50 kg:* 50 to 180 mg/kg/day in four or six equally divided doses. Higher doses are reserved for serious infections (such as meningitis). *Neonates ages 1 to 4 weeks:* 50 mg/kg I.V. q 8 hours. *Neonates ages 0 to 1 week:* 50 mg/kg I.V. q 12 hours.
Total daily dosage is same for I.M. or I.V. administration and depends on susceptibility of organism and severity of infection. Cefotaxime should be injected deep I.M. into a large muscle mass, such as the gluteus or the lateral aspect of the thigh.
• Dosage adjustments are necessary in renal failure.

cefotetan disodium (Cefotan)

• Serious urinary, lower respiratory, gynecologic, skin, intra-abdominal, and bone and joint infections caused by susceptible organisms. *Adults:* 1 to 2 g I.V. or I.M. q 12 hours for 5 to 10 days. Up to 6 g daily in life-threatening infections.

Total daily dosage is same for I.M. or I.V. administration and depends on the susceptibility of the organism and severity of infection. Cefotetan should be injected deep I.M. into a large muscle mass, such as the gluteus or the lateral aspect of the thigh.

• Dosage adjustments are necessary in renal failure.

cefoxitin sodium (Mefoxin)

• Serious respiratory, genitourinary, skin, soft-tissue, bone and joint, blood, and intra-abdominal infections caused by susceptible organisms. *Adults:* 1 to 2 g q 6 to 8 hours for uncomplicated infections. Up to 12 g daily in life-threatening infections. *Children:* 80 to 160 mg/kg daily given in four to six equally divided doses.

Total daily dosage is same for I.M. or I.V. administration and depends on susceptibility of organism and severity of infection. Cefoxitin should be injected deep I.M. into a large muscle mass, such as the gluteus or lateral aspect of the thigh.

• Dosage adjustments are necessary in renal failure.

cefpodoxime proxetil (Vantin)

• Acute, community-acquired pneumonia caused by strains of *Haemophilus influenzae* or *Streptococcus pneumoniae* that don't produce beta-lactamase. *Adults:* 200 mg P.O. q 12 hours for 14 days.

• Uncomplicated gonorrhea in men and women; rectal gonococcal infections in women. *Adults:* 200 mg P.O. as a single dose. Follow with doxycycline, 100 mg P.O. b.i.d. for 7 days.

• Uncomplicated skin and skin structure infections caused by *Staphylococcus aureus* or *Streptococcus pyogenes. Adults:* 400 mg P.O. q 12 hours for 7 to 14 days.

• Acute otitis media caused by *S. pneumoniae, H. influenzae,* or *Moraxella (Branhamella) catarrhalis. Children age 6 months and older:* 5 mg/kg (not to exceed 200 mg) P.O. q 12 hours for 10 days.

• Pharyngitis or tonsillitis caused by *S. pyogenes. Adults:* 100 mg P.O. q 12 hours for 10 days. *Children age 6 months and older:* 5 mg/kg (not to exceed 100 mg) P.O. q 12 hours for 10 days.

• Uncomplicated UTIs caused by *Escherichia coli, Klebsiella pneumoniae, Proteus mirabilis,* or *Staphylococcus saprophyticus. Adults:* 100 mg P.O. q 12 hours for 7 days.

cefprozil (Cefzil)

• Pharyngitis or tonsillitis caused by *Streptococcus pyogenes. Adults:* 500 mg P.O. daily for at least 10 days.

• Otitis media caused by *Streptococcus pneumoniae, Haemophilus influenzae,* or *Moraxella (Branhamella) catarrhalis. Infants and children ages 6 months to 12 years:* 15 mg/kg P.O. q 12 hours for 10 days.

• Secondary bacterial infections of acute bronchitis and acute bacterial exacerbation of chronic bronchitis caused by *S. pneumoniae, H. influenzae,* or *M. catarrhalis. Adults:* 500 mg P.O. q 12 hours for 10 days.

• Uncomplicated skin and skin structure infections caused by *S. pyogenes* or *Staphylococcus aureus. Adults:* 250 mg P.O. b.i.d. or 500 mg daily to b.i.d.

• Dosage adjustments are necessary in renal failure.

ceftazidime (Ceptaz, Fortaz, Tazicef, Tazidime)

• Bacteremia, septicemia, and serious respiratory, urinary, gynecologic, intra-abdominal, CNS, and skin infections caused by susceptible organisms. *Adults and children age 12 and over:* 1 g I.V. or I.M. q 8 to 12 hours; up to 6 g daily in life-threatening infections. *Children ages 1 month to 12 years:* 30 to 50 mg/kg I.V. q 8 hours. *Neonates ages 0 to 4 weeks:* 30 mg/kg I.V. q 12 hours.

Total daily dosage is same for I.M. or I.V. administration and depends on susceptibility of organism and severity of infection. Ceftazidime should be injected deep I.M. into a large muscle mass, such as the gluteus or lateral aspect of the thigh.

• Dosage adjustments are necessary in renal failure.

ceftizoxime sodium (Cefizox)

• Bacteremia, septicemia, meningitis, and serious respiratory, urinary, gynecologic, intra-abdominal, bone and joint, and skin infections caused by susceptible organisms. *Adults:* Usual dosage is 1 to 2 g I.V. or I.M. q 8 to 12 hours. In life-threatening infections, up to 2 g q 4 hours.

Total daily dosage is same for I.M. or I.V. administration and depends on susceptibility of organism and severity of infection. Ceftizoxime should be injected deep I.M. into a large muscle mass, such as the gluteus or lateral aspect of the thigh.

• Dosage adjustments are necessary in renal failure.

ceftriaxone sodium (Rocephin)

• Bacteremia, septicemia, and serious respiratory, urinary, gynecologic, intra-abdominal, and skin infections caused by susceptible organisms. *Adults:* 1 to 2 g I.M. or

I.V. once daily or in equally divided doses twice daily. Total daily dosage should not exceed 4 g. *Children:* 50 to 75 mg/kg, given in divided doses every 12 hours.

• Meningitis. *Adults and children:* 100 mg/kg given in divided doses every 12 hours. May give loading dose of 75 mg/kg.

Total daily dosage is same for I.M. or I.V. administration and depends on susceptibility of organism and severity of infection. Ceftriaxone should be injected deep I.M. into a large muscle mass, such as the gluteus or lateral aspect of the thigh.

cefuroxime sodium (Kefurox, Zinacef)

• Serious lower respiratory, urinary tract, skin and skin-structure infections; bone and joint infections; septicemia; meningitis; gonorrhea; perioperative prophylaxis. *Adults and children age 12 and over:* Usual dosage is 750 mg to 1.5 g I.M. or I.V. q 8 hours, usually for 5 to 10 days. For life-threatening infections and infections caused by less susceptible organisms, 1.5 g I.M. or I.V. q 6 hours; for bacterial meningitis, up to 3 g I.V. q 8 hours. *Children and infants over age 3 months:* 50 to 100 mg/kg I.M. or I.V. daily. Some clinicians give 100 to 150 mg/kg/day in equally divided doses q 6 to 8 hours. Higher doses are administered for meningitis. However, some clinicians prefer other agents for meningitis.

Total daily dosage is same for I.M. or I.V. administration and depends on susceptibility of organism and severity of infection. Cefuroxime should be injected deep I.M. into a large muscle mass, such as the gluteus or lateral aspect of the thigh.

• Pharyngitis, tonsillitis, lower respiratory infection, UTI. *Adults and children age 12 and over:* 250

mg P.O. q 12 hours. *Children and infants over age 3 months:* 125 mg P.O. q 12 hours.
• Otitis media. *Children age 2 and older:* 250 mg P.O. q 12 hours. *Infants and children under age 2:* 125 mg P.O. q 12 hours. *Note:* Compliance may be a problem when treating otitis media in children. The tablets are not chewable and may be difficult for a child to swallow. The drug has an unpleasant taste, so tablets should not be crushed. An alternative drug may be considered.
• Dosage adjustments are necessary in renal failure.

cephalexin hydrochloride (Keftab)
• Otitis media and respiratory, genitourinary, skin and soft-tissue, or bone and joint infections caused by susceptible organisms. *Adults:* 250 mg to 1 g P.O. q 6 hours. *Children:* 6 to 12 mg/kg P.O. q 6 hours. Maximum dosage is 25 mg/kg q 6 hours.
• Dosage adjustments are necessary in renal failure.

cephalothin sodium (Ceporacin, Keflin)
• Serious respiratory, genitourinary, GI, skin and soft-tissue, bone and joint infections; septicemia; endocarditis; meningitis. *Adults:* 500 mg to 1 g I.M. or I.V. (or intraperitoneally) q 4 to 6 hours; in life-threatening infections, up to 2 g q 4 hours. *Children:* 80 to 160 mg/kg/ day I.V. in divided doses q 4 to 6 hours; dosage should be proportionately less depending on age, weight, and severity of infection.

Cephalothin should be injected deep I.M. into a large muscle mass, such as the gluteus or lateral aspect of the thigh. I.V. route is preferable in severe or life-threatening infections.
• Dosage adjustments are necessary in renal failure.

cephapirin sodium (Cefadyl)
• Serious respiratory, genitourinary, GI, skin and soft-tissue, bone and joint infections (including osteomyelitis); septicemia; endocarditis. *Adults:* 500 mg to 1 g I.V. or I.M. q 4 to 6 hours up to 12 g daily. *Children over age 3 months:* 10 to 20 mg/kg I.V. or I.M. q 6 hours; dosage depends on age, weight, and severity of infection.

Cephapirin should be injected deep I.M. into a large muscle mass, such as the gluteus or lateral aspect of the thigh.
• Dosage adjustments are necessary in renal failure.

cephradine (Anspor, Velosef)
• Serious respiratory, genitourinary, GI, skin and soft-tissue, bone and joint infections; septicemia; endocarditis. *Adults:* 250 to 500 mg P.O. q 6 hours. Severe or chronic infections may require larger or more frequent dosages (up to 1 g P.O. q 6 hours). *Children over age 9 months:* 25 to 50 mg/kg P.O. daily in divided doses.
• Otitis media. *Adults and children:* 75 to 100 mg/kg P.O. daily, not to exceed 4 g daily.

Larger dosages (up to 1 g q.i.d.) may be given for severe or chronic infections in all patients regardless of age and weight.
• Dosage adjustments are necessary in renal failure.

chenodiol (Chenix)
• Dissolution of radiolucent cholesterol stones (gallstones) when systemic disease or age precludes surgery. *Adults:* 250 mg P.O. b.i.d. for the first 2 weeks, followed, as tolerated, by weekly increases of 250 mg/day, up to 13 to 16 mg/kg/ day for up to 24 months.

chloramphenicol, chloramphenicol palmitate, chloramphenicol sodium succinate (Chloromycetin)

• *Haemophilus influenzae* meningitis, brain abscesses, bacteremia, acute *Salmonella typhi* infection and meningitis, or other serious infections. *Adults and children:* 50 to 100 mg/kg P.O. or I.V. daily, divided q 6 hours. Maximum dosage is 100 mg/kg daily. *Premature infants, neonates age 2 weeks or under, and children and infants with immature metabolic processes:* 25 mg/kg I.V. or P.O. daily. I.V. route must be used to treat meningitis.
• Superficial infections of the skin caused by susceptible bacteria. *Adults and children:* Rub into affected area b.i.d. or t.i.d.
• External ear canal infection. *Adults and children:* 2 to 3 drops into ear canal t.i.d or q.i.d.
• Surface bacterial infection involving conjunctiva or cornea. *Adults and children:* Instill 2 drops of solution in eye every hour until condition improves, or instill q.i.d., depending on severity of infection. Apply small amount of ointment to lower conjunctival sac at bedtime as supplement to drops. To use ointment alone, apply small amount to lower conjunctival sac q 3 to 6 hours or more frequently if necessary. Continue until condition improves.

chlordiazepoxide (Libritabs) chlordiazepoxide hydrochloride (Librium, Lipoxide)

Controlled Substance Schedule IV
• Mild-to-moderate anxiety and tension. *Adults:* 5 to 10 mg t.i.d. or q.i.d. *Children over age 6:* 5 mg P.O. b.i.d. to q.i.d. Maximum dosage is 10 mg P.O. b.i.d. or t.i.d.
• Severe anxiety and tension. *Adults:* 20 to 25 mg t.i.d. or q.i.d.
• Withdrawal symptoms of acute alcoholism. *Adults:* 50 to 100 mg P.O.,

I.M., or I.V. Maximum dosage is 300 mg daily.
• Preoperative apprehension and anxiety. *Adults:* 5 to 10 mg P.O. t.i.d. or q.i.d. on day preceding surgery; or 50 to 100 mg I.M. 1 hour before surgery.

(*Note:* Parenteral form not recommended for children under age 12.)

chlorothiazide (Diuril)

• Edema, hypertension. *Adults:* 500 mg to 2 g P.O. or I.V. daily or in two divided doses.
• Diuresis, hypertension. *Children ages 2 to 12:* 1 g P.O. once daily or in divided doses. *Children ages 6 months to 2 years:* 20 mg/kg P.O. or I.V. daily in divided doses. *Children under age 6 months:* may require 10 to 30 mg/kg P.O. or I.V. daily in two divided doses.

chlorphenesin carbamate (Maolate)

• As an adjunct in short-term, acute, painful musculoskeletal conditions. *Adults:* Initial dosage is 800 mg P.O. t.i.d. Maintenance dosage is 400 mg P.O. q.i.d. for maximum of 8 weeks.

chlorpromazine hydrochloride (Chlorpromanyl, Largactil, Thorazine, Thor-Prom)

• Psychosis. *Adults:* 50 to 75 mg P.O. daily in two to four divided doses, increased by 25 to 50 mg twice weekly until symptoms are controlled. Or 25 to 50 mg I.M. q 1 to 4 hours, p.r.n. *Children age 6 months and over:* 0.55 mg/kg P.O. or I.M. q 4 to 6 hours; or 1.1 mg/kg P.R. q 6 to 8 hours. Maximum I.M. dose is 40 mg in children under age 5 or weighing less than 22.7 kg, and 75 mg in children ages 5 to 12 or weighing 22.7 to 45.5 kg.
• Intractable hiccups. *Adults:* 25 to 50 mg P.O. or I.M. t.i.d. or q.i.d.
• Acute intermittent porphyria and

tetanus. *Adults:* 25 to 50 mg I.M. t.i.d. or q.i.d.

chlorpropamide (Diabinese, Glucamide)

• Adjunct to diet to lower blood glucose level in patients with non-insulin-dependent (Type II) diabetes mellitus. *Adults:* 250 mg P.O. daily with breakfast or in divided doses if GI disturbances occur. Dosage may first be increased after 5 to 7 days because of extended duration of action, then may be increased q 3 to 5 days by 125 mg, if needed, to maximum of 500 mg daily. *Adults over age 65:* initial dosage should be in the range of 100 to 125 mg daily.

• To change from insulin to oral therapy. *Adults:* If insulin dosage is less than 40 units daily, insulin may be stopped and oral therapy started as above. If it's 40 units or more daily, start oral therapy as above with insulin reduced 50%. Further reductions should reflect patient response.

chlorzoxazone (Paraflex, Parafon Forte DSC)

• As an adjunct in acute, painful musculoskeletal conditions. *Adults:* 250 to 750 mg t.i.d. or q.i.d. *Children:* 20 mg/kg daily in divided doses t.i.d. or q.i.d.

cholestyramine (Cholybar, Questran)

• Primary hyperlipidemia, pruritus, and diarrhea from excess bile acid; as adjunctive therapy to reduce elevated serum cholesterol levels in patients with primary hypercholesterolemia; to reduce the risks of atherosclerotic coronary artery disease and MI. *Adults:* 4 g P.O. once or twice daily. Maintenance dosage is 8 to 16 mg daily. Maximum daily dosage is 24 g. Questran contains 4 g of cholestyramine.

choline magnesium trisalicylate (Trilisate)

• Rheumatoid arthritis (RA), osteoarthritis, or other polyarthritic or inflammatory conditions. *Adults:* Initially, 1.5 to 2.5 g P.O. daily either as a single dose h.s. or in divided doses. Dosage is adjusted according to patient response. Dosage range is 1 to 4.5 g daily.

• Juvenile rheumatoid arthritis. *Children:* 60 to 100 mg/kg/day in divided doses q 6 to 8 hours.

• Mild to moderate pain and fever. *Adults:* 2 to 3 g P.O. daily in divided doses q 4 to 6 hours. *Children:* 10 to 15 mg/kg/day q 4 hours, up to 60 to 80 mg/kg/day.

choline salicylate (Arthropan)

• RA, osteoarthritis, minor pain or fever. *Adults and children over age 12:* 1 teaspoon (870 mg) P.O. every 3 to 4 hours p.r.n. If tolerated and needed, dose may be increased to 2 teaspoons. Do not exceed 6 teaspoons daily.

• Relief of pain from inflamed gums. *Adults and children over age 2:* apply 1 cm of gel to affected area q 3 to 4 hours and h.s., p.r.n.

cimetidine (Tagamet)

• Duodenal ulcer (short-term treatment). *Adults and children over age 16:* 300 mg P.O. q.i.d. with meals and h.s. Alternatively, may give 400 mg P.O. b.i.d. or 800 mg once daily h.s. Continue treatment for 4 to 6 weeks unless endoscopy shows healing. Maintenance dosage is 400 mg h.s. *Parenteral:* 300 mg diluted to 20 ml with 0.9% sodium chloride solution or other compatible I.V. solution by I.V. push over no less than 2 minutes q 6 hours. Or 300 mg diluted in 50 ml of D_5W or other compatible I.V. solution by I.V. infusion over 15 to 20 minutes q 6 hours. Or 300 mg I.M. q 6 hours (no dilution necessary). To increase dosage, give 300-mg doses more frequently to maximum daily dosage of 2,400 mg.

• Active benign gastric ulcer. *Adults:* 300 mg q.i.d. with meals and h.s. for up to 8 weeks.

• Pathologic hypersecretory conditions (such as Zollinger-Ellison syndrome, systemic mastocytosis, and multiple endocrine adenomas). *Adults and children over age 16:* 300 mg P.O. q.i.d. with meals and h.s., adjusted as needed. Maximum daily dosage is 2,400 mg. *Parenteral:* 300 mg diluted to 20 ml with 0.9% sodium chloride solution or other compatible I.V. solution by I.V. push over at least 2 minutes q 6 hours. Or 300 mg diluted in 50 ml of D_5W or other compatible I.V. solution infused over 15 to 20 minutes q 6 hours. To increase dosage, give 300-mg doses more frequently to maximum daily dosage of 2,400 mg.

• Gastroesophageal reflux disease. *Adults:* 800 mg b.i.d. or 400 mg q.i.d. before meals and h.s.

cinoxacin (Cinobac)

• Initial or recurrent UTIs caused by susceptible organisms. *Adults and children over age 12:* 1 g P.O. daily in two to four divided doses for 7 to 14 days. Not recommended for children under age 12.

ciprofloxacin (Cipro)

• Mild-to-moderate UTIs caused by susceptible bacteria. *Adults:* 250 mg P.O. or I.V. q 12 hours.

• Infectious diarrhea, mild-to-moderate respiratory tract infections, bone and joint infections, and severe or complicated UTIs. *Adults:* 500 mg P.O. q 12 hours or 400 mg I.V. q 12 hours.

• Severe or complicated infections of the respiratory tract, bones, joints, skin, or skin structures. *Adults:* 750 mg P.O. q 12 hours.

• Dosage adjustments are necessary for patients in renal failure.

clarithromycin (Biaxin)

• Pharyngitis or tonsillitis caused by *Streptococcus pyogenes. Adults:* 250 mg P.O. q 12 hours for 10 days.

• Acute maxillary sinusitis caused by *Streptococcus pneumoniae. Adults:* 500 mg P.O. q 12 hours for 14 days.

• Acute exacerbations of chronic bronchitis caused by *Moraxella (Branhamella) catarrhalis* or *S. pneumoniae;* pneumonia caused by *S. pneumoniae* or *Mycoplasma pneumoniae. Adults:* 250 mg P.O. q 12 hours for 7 to 14 days.

• Acute exacerbations of chronic bronchitis caused by *Haemophilus influenzae. Adults:* 500 mg P.O. q 12 hours for 7 to 14 days.

• Uncomplicated skin and skin structure infections caused by *Staphylococcus aureus* or *Streptococcus pyogenes. Adults:* 250 mg P.O. q 12 hours for 7 to 14 days.

clemastine fumarate (Tavist, Tavist-1)

• Rhinitis, allergy symptoms. *Adults and children over age 12:* 1.34 mg P.O. q 12 hours.

clindamycin hydrochloride
clindamycin palmitate hydrochloride
clindamycin phosphate (Cleocin)

• Infections caused by sensitive organisms. *Adults:* 150 to 450 mg P.O. q 6 hours; or 300 mg I.M. or I.V. q 6, 8, or 12 hours. Up to 2,700 mg I.M. or I.V. daily, divided q 6, 8, or 12 hours. May be used for severe infections. *Children over age 1 month:* 8 to 20 mg/kg/day P.O. in divided doses q 6 hours; or 15 to 40 mg/kg/day I.M. or I.V. in divided doses q 6 hours.

• Acne vulgaris. *Adults:* Apply thin film of topical solution to affected areas b.i.d.

clofibrate (Atromid-S, Claripex)

• Hyperlipidemia. *Adults:* 2 g P.O. daily in four divided doses. Some patients may respond to lower doses as assessed by serum lipid monitoring. Should not be used in children.

clomiphene citrate (Clomid)

• To induce ovulation. *Women:* 50 to 100 mg P.O. daily for 5 days, starting any time; or 50 to 100 mg P.O. daily starting on day 5 of menstrual cycle (first day of menstrual flow is day 1). Repeat until conception occurs or until three courses of therapy are completed.

clonazepam (Klonopin, Rivotril)

Controlled Substance Schedule IV
• Absence and atypical absence seizures; akinetic and myoclonic seizures. *Adults:* initial dosage should not exceed 1.5 mg P.O. daily in three divided doses. May be increased by 0.5 to 1 mg q 3 days until seizures are controlled. Maximum recommended daily dosage is 20 mg. *Children up to age 10 or weighing less than 30 kg:* 0.01 to 0.03 mg/kg P.O. daily (not to exceed 0.05 mg/kg daily), divided q 8 hours. Increase dosage by 0.25 to 0.5 mg every third day to a maximum maintenance dosage of 0.1 to 0.2 mg/kg daily.

clonidine hydrochloride (Catapres, Catapres-TTS, Dixarit)

• Essential, renal, or malignant hypertension. *Adults:* Initially, 0.1 mg P.O. b.i.d., increased by 0.1 to 0.2 mg/day on a weekly basis. Usual dosage range is 0.2 to 0.8 mg daily in divided doses; infrequently, dosage may rise as high as 2.4 mg daily. No dosing recommendations for children.

Or apply transdermal patch to a hairless area of intact skin on the upper arm or torso once every 7 days.

clorazepate dipotassium (Gen-XENE, Tranxene)

Controlled Substance Schedule IV
• Acute alcohol withdrawal. *Adults:* Day 1 — 30 mg P.O. initially, followed by 30 to 60 mg P.O. in divided doses; day 2 — 45 to 90 mg P.O. in divided doses; day 3 — 22.5 to 45 mg P.O. in divided doses; day 4 — 15 to 30 mg P.O. in divided doses; taper daily dosage to 7.5 to 15 mg.
• Anxiety. *Adults:* 15 to 60 mg P.O. daily.

clotrimazole (Canesten, Lotrimin 1%, Mycelex, Mycelex-G)

• Superficial fungal infections. *Adults and children:* apply a thin layer and massage into affected and surrounding area, morning and evening, for 1 to 8 weeks.
• Vulvovaginal candidiasis. *Adults:* Two 100-mg vaginal tablets daily h.s. for 3 consecutive days; or one 500-mg vaginal tablet daily h.s. for 3 days; or 1 applicatorful vaginal cream daily h.s. for 7 to 14 days.

cloxacillin sodium (Cloxapen, Tegopen)

• Systemic infections caused by susceptible organisms. *Adults and children over 20 kg:* 250 to 500 mg P.O. q 6 hours. *Children 20 kg or less:* 50 to 100 mg/kg P.O. daily, divided into doses given q 6 hours.

codeine phosphate codeine sulfate

Controlled Substance Schedule II
• Mild-to-moderate pain. *Adults:* 15 to 60 mg P.O. or 15 to 60 mg (phosphate) S.C. or I.M. q 4 hours, p.r.n. or around the clock. *Children over age 1:* 0.5 mg/kg P.O., S.C., or I.M. q 4 hours, p.r.n. or around the clock.
• Nonproductive cough. *Adults:* 10 to 20 mg P.O. q 4 to 6 hours. Maximum dosage is 120 mg/day. *Chil-*

dren ages 6 to 12: 5 to 10 mg P.O. q 4 to 6 hours. Maximum dosage is 60 mg/day.

colestipol hydrochloride (Colestid)
• Primary hypercholesterolemia. *Adults:* 5 to 30 g P.O. daily or in two four divided doses.

cortisone acetate (Cortone Acetate)
• Adrenal insufficiency, allergy, inflammation. *Adults:* 25 to 300 mg P.O. or I.M. daily or on alternate days.

cosyntropin (Cortrosyn)
• Diagnostic test of adrenocortical function. *Adults and children age 2 years and over:* 0.25 mg I.M. or I.V. (unless label prohibits I.V. administration). *Children under age 2:* 0.125 mg I.M. or I.V.

co-trimoxazole (trimethoprim-sulfamethoxazole) (Bactrim, Septra)
• UTIs and shigellosis. *Adults:* 160 mg trimethoprim and 800 mg sulfamethoxazole (double-strength tablet) q 12 hours for 10 to 14 days in UTIs and for 5 days in shigellosis. For simple cystitis or acute urethral syndrome, may give one to three double-strength tablets as a single dose. *Children age 2 months and over:* 8 mg/kg trimethoprim and 40 mg/kg sulfamethoxazole daily in two divided doses q 12 hours (10 days for UTIs; 5 days for shigellosis).
• Otitis media. *Children age 2 months and over:* 8 mg/kg trimethoprim and 40 mg/kg sulfamethoxazole daily, in two divided doses q 12 hours for 10 days.
• *Pneumocystis carinii* pneumonia. *Adults and children age 2 months and over:* 20 mg/kg trimethoprim and 100 mg/kg sulfamethoxazole daily, in equally divided doses q 6 hours for 14 days.

• Chronic bronchitis. *Adults:* 160 mg trimethoprim and 800 mg sulfamethoxazole q 12 hours for 10 to 14 days.
  Note: Not recommended for infants younger than age 2 months.

cromolyn sodium (Intal)
• Adjunct in treatment of severe perennial bronchial asthma. *Adults and children over age 5:* 2 metered sprays using inhaler q.i.d. at regular intervals. Also available as aqueous solution given by nebulizer.

cyclobenzaprine hydrochloride (Flexeril)
• Short-term treatment of muscle spasm. *Adults:* 10 mg P.O. t.i.d. for 7 days. Maximum dosage is 60 mg daily for 2 to 3 weeks.

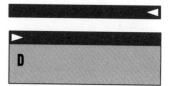

dantrolene sodium (Dantrium, Dantrium I.V.)
• Spasticity and sequelae secondary to severe chronic disorders (multiple sclerosis, cerebral palsy, spinal cord injury, stroke). *Adults:* 25 mg P.O. daily. Increase gradually in increments of 25 mg at 4- to 7-day intervals to maximum of 400 mg daily. *Children:* 0.5 mg/kg daily P.O. b.i.d. Increase gradually, as needed, by 0.5 mg/kg daily to a maximum of 100 mg q.i.d.

demeclocycline hydrochloride (Declomycin)
• Infections caused by susceptible organisms. *Adults:* 150 mg P.O. q 6 hours, or 300 mg P.O. q 12 hours. *Children over age 8:* 6 to 12 mg/kg P.O. daily, divided q 6 to 12 hours.
• Gonorrhea. *Adults:* 600 mg P.O.

initially, then 300 mg P.O. q
12 hours for 4 days (total 3 g).

desipramine hydrochloride (Norpramin, Pertofrane)
• Depression. *Adults:* 100 to 200 mg
P.O. daily in divided doses, increasing to maximum of 300 mg daily.
Alternatively, the entire dose may
be given at bedtime. *Elderly patients and adolescents:* 25 to 100 mg
P.O. daily, increasing gradually to a
maximum of 150 mg daily.

desmopressin acetate (DDAVP, Stimate)
• Pituitary diabetes insipidus, temporary polyuria and polydipsia associated with pituitary trauma.
Adults: 0.1 to 0.4 ml intranasally
daily in one to three doses. May
administer injectable form in dosage of 0.5 to 1 ml I.V. or S.C. daily,
usually in two divided doses. *Children ages 3 months to 12 years:*
0.05 to 0.3 ml intranasally daily in
one or two doses.
• Hemophilia A and von Willebrand's disease. *Adults and children:*
0.3 mcg/kg diluted in 0.9% sodium
chloride solution I.V. infused over
15 to 30 minutes. Dose may be repeated if necessary.

dexamethasone (Decadron, Hexadrol)
dexamethasone acetate (Decadron-LA)
dexamethasone sodium phosphate (Decadron Phosphate, Hexadrol Phosphate)
• Inflammatory conditions, allergic
reactions, neoplasias. *Adults:*
0.75 to 9 mg/day P.O.; or 0.5 to 9
mg/day (phosphate) I.M.; or 4 to 16
mg (acetate) I.M. into joint or soft
tissue q 1 to 3 weeks; or 0.8 to 1.6
mg (acetate) into lesions q 1 to 3
weeks.

• Cerebral edema. *Adults:* initially,
10 mg (phosphate) I.V., then 4 to
6 mg I.M. q 6 hours for 2 to 4 days,
then tapered over 5 to 7 days.

dexamethasone, ophthalmic (Maxidex Ophthalmic Suspension)
dexamethasone sodium phosphate (Decadron Phosphate Ophthalmic, Maxidex Ophthalmic)
• Uveitis; iridocyclitis; inflammatory
conditions of eyelids, conjunctiva,
cornea, anterior segment of globe;
corneal injury from chemical or
thermal burns, or penetration of
foreign bodies; allergic conjunctivitis. *Adults and children:* Instill 1 to
2 drops into conjunctival sac. In severe disease, drops may be used
hourly, tapering off as condition improves. In mild conditions, drops
may be used four to six times daily.
Treatment may extend from a few
days to several weeks.

dexamethasone sodium phosphate, nasal (Decadron Phosphate)
• Allergic or inflammatory conditions, nasal polyps. *Adults:* 2 sprays
in each nostril b.i.d. or t.i.d. Maximum dosage is 12 sprays daily.
Children ages 6 to 12: 1 or 2 sprays
in each nostril b.i.d. Maximum dosage is 8 sprays daily.
  Each spray delivers 0.1 mg dexamethasone sodium phosphate equal
to 0.084 mg dexamethasone.

dextromethorphan hydrobromide (Benylin DM, Hold, St. Joseph Cough Suppressant for Children, Sucrets Cough Control Formula)
• Nonproductive cough. *Adults:*
10 to 20 mg P.O. q 4 hours, or 30
mg q 6 to 8 hours. Or 60 mg b.i.d.
(controlled-release liquid) twice
daily. Maximum dosage is 120 mg/
day. *Children ages 6 to 12:* 5 to
10 mg P.O. q 4 hours, or 15 mg q 6

to 8 hours. Or 30 mg b.i.d. (controlled-release liquid) twice daily. Maximum dosage is 60 mg/day. *Children ages 2 to 6:* 2.5 to 5 mg P.O. q 4 hours, or 7.5 mg q 6 to 8 hours. Maximum dosage is 30 mg/day.

diazepam (Novodipam, Valium)
Controlled Substance Schedule IV
• Tension, anxiety, as adjunct in seizure disorders or skeletal muscle spasm. *Adults:* 2 to 10 mg P.O. t.i.d. or q.i.d. Or 15 to 30 mg of extended-release capsule once daily. Or 5 to 10 mg I.V. initially, up to 30 mg in 1 hour or possibly more for cardioversion or status epilepticus, depending on response. *Children over age 6 months:* 1 to 2.5 mg P.O. t.i.d. or q.i.d. *Children age 5 and older:* 1 mg I.V. slowly q 2 to 5 minutes to maximum of 10 mg. Repeat q 2 to 4 hours. *Children ages 30 days to 5 years:* 0.2 to 0.5 mg I.V. slowly q 2 to 5 minutes to maximum of 5 mg. Repeat q 2 to 4 hours.

diclofenac sodium (Voltaren)
• Ankylosing spondylitis. *Adults:* 25 mg P.O. q.i.d. and h.s.
• Osteoarthritis. *Adults:* 50 mg P.O. b.i.d. or t.i.d., or 75 mg P.O. b.i.d.

dicloxacillin sodium (Dynapen)
• Systemic infections caused by susceptible organisms. *Adults and children over 40 kg:* 125 to 250 mg P.O. given q 6 hours. *Children:* 25 to 50 mg/kg P.O. daily, divided into doses given q 6 hours.

dicyclomine hydrochloride (Antispas, Bentyl)
• Adjunctive therapy for peptic ulcers and other functional GI disorders. *Adults:* Initially, 20 mg P.O. q.i.d. increased to 40 mg q.i.d., or 20 mg I.M. q 4 to 6 hours. Always adjust dosage according to patient's needs and response. *Children age 2*

and over: 10 mg P.O. t.i.d. or q.i.d. *Children ages 6 months to 2 years:* 5 to 10 mg P.O. t.i.d. or q.i.d.

dienestrol (DV, Ortho Dienestrol)
• Atrophic vaginitis and kraurosis vulvae. *Postmenopausal women:* One to two intravaginal applications of cream daily for 1 to 2 weeks (as directed); then half that dose for the same period. A maintenance dosage of 1 application one to three times a week may be ordered.

diethylstilbestrol (DES) diethylstilbestrol diphosphate (Honvol, Stilphostrol)
• Prostate cancer. *Men:* Initially, 1 to 3 mg P.O. daily, possibly reduced to 1 mg daily. Or 50 mg (diphosphate) P.O. t.i.d., increased up to 200 mg or more as needed t.i.d. Or 0.5 g I.V., followed by 1 g daily for 5 or more days as needed. Maintenance dosage is 0.25 to 0.5 g I.V. once or twice a week.
• Advanced metastatic breast cancer. *Men and postmenopausal women:* 15 mg P.O. daily.

diflunisal (Dolobid)
• Mild-to-moderate pain and osteoarthritis. *Adults:* 500 to 1,000 mg P.O. daily in two divided doses, usually q 12 hours. Maximum dosage is 1,500 mg daily. *Adults over age 65:* Start with one-half the usual adult dosage.

digitoxin (Crystodigin)
• CHF, paroxysmal supraventricular tachycardia, atrial fibrillation and flutter. *Adults:* Loading dose is 1.2 to 1.6 mg P.O. in divided doses over 24 hours; average maintenance dosage is 0.15 mg daily (range: 0.05 to 0.3 mg daily). *Children ages 2 to 12:* Loading dose is 0.03 mg/kg or 0.75 mg/m^2 P.O. in divided doses over 24 hours; maintenance dosage is one-tenth of loading dose or 0.003 mg/kg or 0.075 mg/m^2 daily. Monitor

closely for toxicity. *Children ages 1 to 2:* Loading dose is 0.04 mg/kg P.O. in divided doses over 24 hours; maintenance dosage is 0.004 mg/kg daily. Monitor closely for toxicity. *Children ages 2 weeks to 1 year:* Loading dose is 0.045 mg/kg P.O. in divided doses over 24 hours; maintenance dosage is 0.0045 mg/kg daily. Monitor closely for toxicity. *Premature infants, neonates, severely ill older infants:* Loading dose is 0.022 mg/kg or 0.3 to 0.35 mg/m² P.O. in divided doses over 24 hours; maintenance dosage is 0.0022 mg/kg daily. Monitor closely for toxicity.

digoxin (Lanoxicaps, Lanoxin)

• CHF, paroxysmal supraventricular tachycardia, atrial fibrillation and flutter. *Adults:* Loading dose is 0.5 to 1 mg I.V. or P.O. in divided doses over 24 hours; maintenance dosage is 0.125 to 0.5 mg I.V. or P.O. daily (average 0.25 mg). Larger doses are often needed for treatment of arrhythmias, depending on patient response. Smaller loading and maintenance dosages should be given to patients with impaired renal function. *Adults over age 65:* 0.125 mg P.O. daily as maintenance dosage. Frail or underweight elderly patients may require only 0.0625 mg daily or 0.125 mg every other day. *Children over age 2:* Loading dose is 0.02 to 0.04 mg/kg P.O. divided q 8 hours over 24 hours; I.V. loading dose is 0.015 to 0.035 mg/kg; maintenance dosage is 0.012 mg/kg P.O. daily divided q 12 hours. *Children ages 1 month to 2 years:* Loading dose is 0.035 to 0.060 mg/kg P.O. in three divided doses over 24 hours; I.V. loading dose is 0.03 to 0.05 mg/kg; maintenance dosage is 0.01 to 0.02 mg/kg P.O. daily divided q 12 hours. *Neonates under age 1 month:* Loading dose is 0.035 mg/kg P.O. divided q 8 hours over 24 hours; I.V.

loading dose is 0.02 to 0.03 mg/kg; maintenance dosage is 0.01 mg/kg P.O. daily divided q 12 hours. *Premature infants:* Loading dose is 0.025 mg/kg I.V. in three divided doses over 24 hours; maintenance dosage is 0.01 mg/kg I.V. daily divided q 12 hours.

dihydroergotamine mesylate (D.H.E. 45)

• Short-term treatment of vascular or migraine headache. *Adults:* 1 mg I.M. or I.V. May repeat q 1 to 2 hours, p.r.n., up to total of 3 mg. Maximum weekly dosage is 6 mg.

dihydrotachysterol (Hytakerol)

• Hypocalcemia associated with hypoparathyroidism and pseudohypoparathyroidism. *Adults:* Initially, 0.75 to 2.5 mg P.O. daily for several days. Maintenance dosage is 0.2 to 1.5 mg daily, as required for normal serum calcium. Average dosage is 0.6 mg daily. *Children:* Initially, 1 to 5 mg for several days. Maintenance dosage is 0.5 to 1.5 mg daily, as required for normal serum calcium.
• Prophylaxis of hypocalcemic tetany following thyroid surgery. *Adults:* 0.25 mg P.O. daily (with calcium supplements).

diltiazem hydrochloride (Cardizem, Cardizem CD, Cardizem SR)

• Management of vasospastic (also called Prinzmetal's or variant) angina and classic chronic stable angina pectoris. *Adults:* 30 mg P.O. t.i.d. or q.i.d. before meals and h.s. Dosage may be gradually increased to a maximum of 360 mg/day. Alternatively, 120 or 180 mg P.O. (dual-release capsule), titrated as needed and tolerated to maximum dosage of 480 mg daily.
• Hypertension. *Adults:* 180 to 240 mg daily P.O. (extended-release capsule) initially. Alternatively, 60 to 120 mg P.O. (sustained-release cap-

sule). Increase dosage as needed and tolerated to maximum of 360 mg/day.

dimenhydrinate (Dramamine)

• Nausea, vomiting, dizziness of motion sickness (treatment and prevention). *Adults:* 50 mg P.O. q 4 hours, or 100 mg q 4 hours if drowsiness is not objectionable; or 50 mg I.M., p.r.n.; or 50 mg I.V. diluted in 10 ml of 0.9% sodium chloride solution, injected over 2 minutes. *Children ages 6 to 12:* 25 to 50 mg P.O. q 6 to 8 hours, not to exceed 150 mg in 24 hours. *Children ages 2 to 6:* 12.5 to 25 mg P.O. q 6 to 8 hours, not to exceed 75 mg in 24 hours.

diphenhydramine hydrochloride (Benadryl, Benylin Cough)

• Rhinitis, allergy symptoms. *Adults:* 25 to 50 mg P.O. t.i.d. or q.i.d.; or 10 to 50 mg deep I.M. or I.V. Maximum dosage is 400 mg/day. *Children under age 12:* 5 mg/kg daily P.O., deep I.M., or I.V. divided q.i.d. Maximum dosage is 300 mg/day.
• Nonproductive cough. *Adults:* 25 mg P.O. q 4 hours (not to exceed 150 mg/day). *Children ages 6 to 12:* 12.5 mg P.O. q 4 hours (not to exceed 75 mg/day). *Children ages 2 to 6:* 6.25 mg P.O. q 4 hours (not to exceed 25 mg/day). Children under age 12 should use only as directed by a doctor.

diphenoxylate hydrochloride with atropine sulfate (Lomotil)

• Acute, nonspecific diarrhea. *Adults:* Initially, 5 mg P.O. q.i.d.; then adjust dosage. *Children ages 2 to 12:* 0.3 to 0.4 mg/kg P.O. daily in four divided doses, using liquid form only. For maintenance, initial dose may be reduced by as much as 75%. Not for use in children under age 2.

dipivefrin 0.1% (Propine)

• To reduce intraocular pressure in chronic open-angle glaucoma. *Adults:* For initial glaucoma therapy, instill 1 drop in eye q 12 hours.

dipyridamole (Persantine)

• Inhibition of platelet adhesion in prosthetic heart valves, in combination with warfarin or aspirin. *Adults:* 75 to 100 mg P.O. q.i.d.
• As an alternative to exercise in thallium myocardial perfusion imaging. *Adults:* 0.142 mg/kg/min I.V. infused over 4 minutes. Inject thallium within 5 minutes of infusion.

disopyramide (Rythmodan) disopyramide phosphate (Norpace, Norpace CR, Rythmodan-LA)

• Premature ventricular contractions (unifocal, multifocal, or coupled); ventricular tachycardia not severe enough to require electrocardioversion. *Adults over 50 kg:* Usual maintenance dosage is 150 mg P.O. q 6 hours; for patients who weigh less than 50 kg or those with renal, hepatic, or cardiac impairment, dosage is highly individualized. May give sustained-release capsule q 12 hours. *Recommended dosage in advanced renal insufficiency:* creatinine clearance 30 to 40 ml/min, 100 mg P.O. q 8 hours; creatinine clearance 15 to 30 ml/min, 100 mg q 12 hours; creatinine clearance less than 15 ml/min, 100 mg q 24 hours. *Children ages 12 to 18:* 6 to 15 mg/kg daily. *Children ages 4 to 12:* 10 to 15 mg/kg daily. *Children ages 1 to 4:* 10 to 20 mg/kg daily. *Children under age 1:* 10 to 30 mg/kg daily.

All children's dosages should be divided into equal amounts and given q 6 hours.

docusate calcium (Surfak)
docusate potassium (Dialose)
docusate sodium (Colace)

• Stool softener. *Adults:* 50 to
300 mg P.O. daily until bowel movements return to normal. *Children
ages 6 to 12:* 40 to 120 mg (docusate sodium) P.O. daily. *Children
ages 3 to 6:* 20 to 60 mg (docusate
sodium) P.O. daily. *Children under
age 3:* 10 to 40 mg (docusate sodium) P.O. daily. Higher doses are
for initial therapy. Dosage is adjusted according to individual response. Usual dosage in children
and adults with minimal need is
50 to 150 mg (docusate calcium)
P.O. daily.

doxazosin mesylate (Cardura)

• Essential hypertension. *Adults:*
Initially, 1 mg P.O. daily. Based on
response, daily dosage may be increased to 2 mg and thereafter to
4 mg, 8 mg, and 16 mg, if necessary.

doxepin hydrochloride
(Sinequan, Triadapin)

• Treatment of depression. *Adults:*
initially, 50 to 75 mg P.O. daily in
divided doses, increased as needed
to maximum of 300 mg daily. Alternatively, entire dosage may be given
at bedtime.

doxycycline hyclate
(Vibramycin)

• Infections caused by sensitive organisms, including *Rickettsiae,
Chlamydia,* and *Mycoplasma.
Adults:* 100 mg P.O. q 12 hours on
first day, then 100 mg P.O. daily; or
200 mg I.V. on first day in one or
two infusions, then 100 to 200 mg
I.V. daily. *Children over age 8 and
weighing less than 45 kg:* 4.4 mg/kg
P.O. or I.V. daily, divided q 12 hours
first day, then 2.2 to 4.4 mg/kg
daily. For children weighing more
than 45 kg, dosage is same as
adults.

Give I.V. infusion slowly (minimum 1 hour). Infusion must be
completed within 12 hours (within
6 hours if using lactated Ringer's
solution or D$_5$W in lactated Ringer's solution).
• Gonorrhea in patients allergic to
penicillin. *Adults:* 200 mg P.O. initially, followed by 100 mg P.O. at
bedtime, then 100 mg P.O. b.i.d. for
3 days; or 300 mg P.O. initially and
repeat dose in 1 hour.
• Primary or secondary syphilis in
pregnant patients allergic to penicillin. *Adults:* 300 mg P.O. daily in
divided doses for at least 10 days.
• *Chlamydia trachomatis* infection,
nongonococcal urethritis, and uncomplicated urethral, endocervical,
or rectal infections; prophylaxis for
rape victims. *Adults:* 100 mg P.O.
b.i.d. for at least 7 days.
• Chemoprophylaxis for malaria in
travelers to areas where chloro-
quine-resistant *Plasmodium falci-
parum* is endemic and mefloquine is
contraindicated. *Adults:* 100 mg P.O.
once daily. Begin prophylaxis 1 to
2 days before travel to malarious
area, continue daily while in affected area, and continue for 4
weeks after return from the malarious area. *Children over age 8:* 2 mg/
kg P.O. daily as a single dose, not
to exceed 100 mg daily. Employ the
same dosage schedule as for adults.

**DRUG DOSAGES &
INDICATIONS**

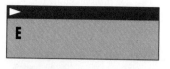

E

enalapril maleate
(Enalaprilat Vasotec I.V., Vasotec)
• Hypertension. *Adults:* Initially,
5 mg P.O. once daily, then adjust
according to response. Usual dosage range is 10 to 40 mg daily as a
single dose or two divided doses.
By I.V. infusion, give 1.25 mg q
6 hours over 5 minutes.
• Adjunct in heart failure. *Adults:*
Initially, 2.5 mg P.O. b.i.d. Usual
dosage range is 5 to 20 mg daily in
2 divided doses; maximum dose is
40 mg.

enoxacin (Penetrex)
• Uncomplicated UTIs. *Adults:*
200 mg P.O. q 12 hours for 7 days.
• Severe or complicated UTIs.
Adults: 400 mg P.O. q 12 hours for
14 days.
• Uncomplicated urethral or endocervical gonorrhea. *Adults:* 400 mg
P.O. as a single dose. Follow with
doxycycline therapy to treat possible coexisting chlamydial infection.

ephedrine sulfate
(Vatronol Nose Drops)
• Nasal congestion. *Adults and children:* apply 3 to 4 drops 0.5% solution or a small amount of jelly to
nasal mucosa. Use no more frequently than q 4 hours.

ergotamine tartrate
**(Ergomar, Ergostat, Gynergen,
Medihaler Ergotamine)**
• Vascular or migraine headache.
Adults: initially, 2 mg P.O. sublingually; may repeat at 30-minute intervals as needed. Do not exceed
6 mg/24 hours or 10 mg/week. Inhaled forms: Begin with 1 inhalation; repeat in 5 minutes if attack
persists. Do not exceed 4 inhala-

tions/24 hours or 15 inhalations/
week.
  Patients may also use rectal suppositories. Initially, 2 mg rectally at
onset of attack, repeated in 1 hour
p.r.n. Maximum dose is 2 suppositories per attack or 5 suppositories
per week.

erythromycin base (E-Mycin, Eryc)
erythromycin estolate (Ilosone)
erythromycin ethylsuccinate (E.E.S., Pediamycin)
erythromycin glucceptate (Ilotycin)
erythromycin lactobionate (Erythrocin)
erythromycin stearate (Erythrocin)
• Acute pelvic inflammatory disease
(PID) caused by *Neisseria gonorrhoeae. Women:* 500 mg I.V. (gluceptate, lactobionate) q 6 hours for
3 days; then 250 mg (base, estolate,
stearate) or 400 mg (ethylsuccinate)
P.O. q 6 hours for 7 days.
• Endocarditis prophylaxis for dental procedures in patients allergic
to penicillin. *Adults:* 1 g (base, estolate, stearate) or 800 to 1,600 mg
(ethylsuccinate) P.O. 1 hour before
procedure, then 500 mg (base, estolate, stearate) or 400 to 800 mg
(ethylsuccinate) P.O. 6 hours later.
• Mild-to-moderately severe respiratory tract, skin, and soft-tissue infections caused by sensitive group
A beta-hemolytic streptococci, *Dip-
lococcus pneumoniae, Mycoplasma
pneumoniae, Corynebacterium diph-
theriae, Bordetella pertussis,* and
Listeria monocytogenes. Adults:
250 to 500 mg (base, estolate, stearate) P.O. q 6 hours; or 400 to 800
mg (ethylsuccinate) P.O. q 6 hours;
or 15 to 20 mg/kg I.V. daily, as continuous infusion or divided q 6
hours. *Children:* 30 to 50 mg/kg
(oral erythromycin salts) P.O. daily,
divided q 6 hours; or 15 to 20 mg/
kg I.V. daily, divided q 4 to 6 hours.
• Syphilis. *Adults:* 500 mg (base, es-

tolate, stearate) P.O. q.i.d. for 15 days.
• Legionnaire's disease. *Adults:* 500 mg to 1 g I.V. or P.O. (base, estolate, stearate) or 800 to 1,600 mg (ethylsuccinate) q 6 hours for 21 days.
• Uncomplicated urethral, endocervical, or rectal infections where tetracyclines are contraindicated. *Adults:* 500 mg (base, estolate, stearate) or 800 mg (ethylsuccinate) P.O. q.i.d. for at least 7 days.
• Urogenital *Chlamydia trachomatis* infections during pregnancy. *Women:* 500 mg (base, estolate, stearate) P.O. q.i.d. for at least 7 days or 250 mg (base, estolate, stearate) or 400 mg (ethylsuccinate) P.O. q.i.d. for at least 14 days.

estrogens, conjugated (Premarin)
• Abnormal uterine bleeding (hormonal imbalance). *Women:* 25 mg I.V. or I.M. Repeat in 6 to 12 hours.
• Primary ovarian failure, osteoporosis. *Women:* 1.25 mg P.O. daily in cycles of 3 weeks on and 1 week off.
• Hypogonadism. *Women:* 2.5 mg P.O. b.i.d. or t.i.d. for 20 consecutive days each month.
• Vasomotor menopausal symptoms. *Women:* 0.3 to 1.25 mg P.O. daily in cycles of 3 weeks on and 1 week off.
• Osteoporosis. *Postmenopausal women:* 0.625 mg P.O. daily in cycles of 3 weeks on, 1 week off.
• Palliative treatment of inoperable prostate cancer. *Men:* 1.25 to 2.5 mg P.O. t.i.d.
• Palliative treatment of breast cancer. *Men and postmenopausal women:* 10 mg P.O. t.i.d. for 3 or more months.
• Atrophic vaginitis, kraurosis vulvae. *Women:* 2 to 4 g intravaginally once daily on a cyclical basis (3 weeks on, 1 week off).

estrone (Estrone-A, Estronol, Theelin Aqueous)
• Atrophic vaginitis and menopausal symptoms. *Women:* 0.1 to 0.5 mg I.M. two or three times weekly.
• Female hypogonadism and primary ovarian failure. *Women:* 0.1 to 1 mg I.M. weekly in single or divided doses.
• Palliative treatment of inoperable prostate cancer. *Men:* 2 to 4 mg I.M. 2 to 3 times weekly.

ethacrynate sodium (Edecrin) ethacrynic acid (Edecrin)
• Acute pulmonary edema. *Adults:* 50 to 100 mg of ethacrynate sodium I.V. slowly over several minutes.
• Edema. *Adults:* 50 to 200 mg ethacrynic acid P.O. daily. Refractory cases may require up to 200 mg b.i.d. *Children:* Initial dose is 25 mg P.O., cautiously increased in 25-mg increments daily until desired effect is achieved.

ethinyl estradiol (Estinyl, Feminone)
• Hypogonadism. *Women:* 0.05 mg P.O. daily to t.i.d. for 2 weeks a month, followed by 2 weeks of progesterone therapy; continue for 3 to 6 monthly dosing cycles, followed by 2 months off.
• Menopausal symptoms. *Women:* 0.02 to 0.05 mg P.O. daily for cycles of 3 weeks on and 1 week off.
• Palliative treatment of metastatic breast cancer. *Women:* 1 mg P.O. t.i.d. for at least 3 months.
• Palliative treatment of inoperable metastatic prostate cancer. *Men:* 0.15 to 2 mg P.O. daily.

ethosuximide (Zarontin)
• Absence seizures. *Adults and children over age 6:* initially, 250 mg P.O. b.i.d. May increase by 250 mg q 4 to 7 days up to 1.5 g daily. *Children ages 3 to 6:* 250 mg P.O. daily or 125 mg P.O. b.i.d. May in-

crease by 250 mg q 4 to 7 days up to 1.5 g daily.

ethotoin (Peganone)
• Generalized tonic-clonic or complex-partial (psychomotor) seizures. *Adults:* initially, 250 mg P.O. q.i.d. after meals. May increase slowly over several days to 3 g daily divided q.i.d. *Children:* initially, 250 mg P.O. b.i.d. May increase up to 250 mg P.O. q.i.d.

etodolac (Lodine)
• Acute and chronic management of osteoarthritis and pain. *Adults:* 200 to 400 mg P.O. q 6 to 8 hours p.r.n. Maximum dosage is 1,200 mg/day.

etretinate (Tegison)
• Recalcitrant psoriasis, including the erythrodermic and generalized pustular types. *Adults:* initially, 0.75 to 1 mg/kg daily in divided doses. Don't exceed maximum initial dosage of 1.5 mg/kg daily. After initial response, begin maintenance dosage of 0.5 to 0.75 mg/kg daily.

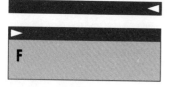

F

famotidine (Pepcid)
• Duodenal ulcer. *Adults:* for acute therapy, 40 mg P.O. once daily h.s.; for maintenance therapy, 20 mg P.O. once daily h.s.
• Pathologic hypersecretory conditions (such as Zollinger-Ellison syndrome). *Adults:* 20 mg P.O. q 6 hours. As much as 160 mg q 6 hours may be administered.
• Hospitalized patients with intractable ulcers or hypersecretory conditions, or patients who cannot take oral medication. *Adults:* 20 mg I.V. q 12 hours.

felodipine (Plendil)
• Hypertension. *Adults:* Initially, 5 mg P.O. daily. Usual dosage is 5 to 10 mg P.O. daily; maximum dosage, 20 mg daily. Allow 2 weeks between dosage adjustments. *Elderly adults and patients with impaired hepatic function:* 5 mg P.O. daily; maximum, 10 mg daily. Adjust dosage as for adults.

fenoprofen calcium (Nalfon)
• RA and osteoarthritis. *Adults:* 300 to 600 mg P.O. q.i.d. Maximum dosage is 3.2 g daily.
• Mild-to-moderate pain. *Adults:* 200 mg P.O. q 4 to 6 hours, p.r.n.

fludrocortisone acetate (Florinef)
• Adrenal insufficiency (partial replacement), adrenogenital syndrome. *Adults:* 0.1 to 0.2 mg P.O. daily.

flunisolide (AeroBid)
• Steroid-dependent asthma. *Adults and children over age 6:* 2 inhalations (500 mcg) b.i.d., do not exceed 4 inhalations b.i.d.

flunisolide (Nasalide)
• Relief of symptoms of seasonal or perennial rhinitis. *Adults:* starting dosage is 2 sprays (50 mcg) in each nostril b.i.d. Total daily dosage is 200 mcg. If necessary, dosage may be increased to 2 sprays in each nostril t.i.d. Maximum total daily dosage is 8 sprays in each nostril (400 mcg daily). *Children ages 6 to 14:* starting dosage is 1 spray (25 mcg) in each nostril t.i.d. or 2 sprays (50 mcg) in each nostril b.i.d. Total daily dosage is 150 to 200 mcg. Maximum total daily dosage is 4 sprays in each nostril (200 mcg daily).

Not recommended for children under age 6.

fluoxetine hydrochloride (Prozac)
• Depression, obsessive-compulsive disorder. *Adults:* Initially, 20 mg P.O. in the morning; dosage increased according to patient response. May be given b.i.d. in the morning and at noon. Maximum dosage is 80 mg/day.

fluphenazine decanoate (Prolixin Decanoate)
fluphenazine enanthate (Prolixin Enanthate)
fluphenazine hydrochloride (Permitil, Permitil Concentrate, Prolixin, Prolixin Concentrate)
• Psychotic disorders. *Adults:* 12.5 to 25 mg of long-acting esters (fluphenazine decanoate and enanthate) I.M. or S.C. q 1 to 6 weeks. Maintenance dosage is 25 to 100 mg, p.r.n. *Adults:* Initially, 1.25 to 10 mg fluphenazine hydrochloride P.O. daily in divided doses q 6 to 8 hours; may increase cautiously to 20 mg daily. Higher doses (50 to 100 mg) have been given. Maintenance dosage is 1 to 5 mg P.O. daily. I.M. doses are one-third to one-half of oral doses. Lower dosages for geriatric patients (1 to 2.5 mg daily).
   Note: Prolixin Concentrate and Permitil Concentrate are 10 times more concentrated than Prolixin elixir (5 mg/ml vs. 0.5 mg/ml). Check dosage carefully.

flurbiprofen sodium (Ocufen Liquifilm)
• Inhibition of intraoperative miosis. *Adults:* Instill 1 drop approximately every ½ hour, beginning 2 hours before surgery. Give a total of 4 drops.

furosemide (Furoside, Lasix, Myrosemide, Uritol)
• Acute pulmonary edema. *Adults:* 40 mg I.V. injected slowly; then 80 mg I.V. in 1 to 1½ hours if needed.

• Edema. *Adults:* 20 to 80 mg P.O. daily in morning; second dose can be given in 6 to 8 hours; carefully titrated up to 600 mg daily if needed. Or 20 to 40 mg I.M. or I.V., increased by 20 mg q 2 hours until desired response is achieved. I.V. dose should be given slowly over 1 to 2 minutes. *Infants and children:* 2 mg/kg P.O. daily, increased by 1 to 2 mg/kg in 6 to 8 hours if needed; carefully titrated up to 6 mg/kg daily if needed.
• Hypertension. *Adults:* 40 mg P.O. b.i.d. Adjust dosage according to response.

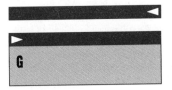

gemfibrozil (Lopid)
• Type IV hyperlipidemia (hypertriglyceridemia), Type V hyperlipidemia, and severe hypercholesterolemia unresponsive to diet and other drugs. *Adults:* 1,200 mg P.O. administered in two divided doses. Usual dosage range is 900 to 1,500 mg daily. If no beneficial effect is seen after 3 months of therapy, drug should be discontinued.

gentamicin sulfate (Garamycin)
• Serious infections caused by susceptible organisms. *Adults with normal renal function:* 3 mg/kg I.M. or I.V. infusion (in 50 to 200 ml of 0.9% sodium chloride solution or D₅W infused over 30 minutes to 2 hours) daily in divided doses q 8 hours. May be given by direct I.V. push if necessary. For life-threatening infections, patient may receive up to 5 mg/kg/day in three or four divided doses. *Children with normal renal function:* 2 to 2.5 mg/kg I.M. or I.V. infusion q 8 hours. *Infants and neonates over age 1 week with*

normal renal function: 2.5 mg/kg I.M. or I.V. infusion q 8 hours. *Neonates under age 1 week:* 2.5 mg/kg I.V. q 12 hours. For I.V. infusion, dilute in 0.9% sodium chloride solution or D₅W and infuse over 30 minutes to 2 hours.

• Meningitis. *Adults:* Systemic therapy as above; may also use 4 to 8 mg intrathecally daily. *Children:* Systemic therapy as above; may also use 1 to 2 mg intrathecally daily.

• Endocarditis prophylaxis for GI or genitourinary procedure or surgery. *Adults:* 1.5 mg/kg I.M. or I.V. 30 to 60 minutes before procedure or surgery and q 8 hours after, for two doses. Given medication separately with aqueous penicillin G or ampicillin. *Children:* 2.5 mg/kg I.M. or I.V. 30 to 60 minutes before procedure or surgery and q 8 hours after, for two doses. Give medication separately with aqueous penicillin G or ampicillin.

• External ocular infections caused by susceptible organisms. *Adults and children:* Instill 1 to 2 drops in eye q 4 hours. In severe infections, may use up to 2 drops q 1 hour. Apply ointment to lower conjunctival sac b.i.d. or t.i.d.

• Primary and secondary bacterial infections; superficial burns; skin ulcers; and infected lacerations, abrasions, insect bites, or minor surgical wounds. *Adults and children over age 1:* Rub in small amount gently t.i.d. or q.i.d., with or without gauze dressing.

• Dosage adjustments are necessary in renal failure.

• Posthemodialysis to maintain therapeutic blood levels. *Adults:* 1 to 1.7 mg/kg I.M. or I.V. infusion after each dialysis. *Children:* 2 mg/kg I.M. or I.V. infusion after each dialysis.

glipizide (Glucotrol)

• Adjunct to diet to lower blood glucose level in patients with non-insulin-dependent diabetes mellitus (Type II). *Adults:* initially, 5 mg P.O. daily given before breakfast. Elderly patients or those with liver disease may be started on 2.5 mg. Usual maintenance dosage is 10 to 15 mg. Maximum recommended daily dosage is 40 mg.

• Replacement for insulin therapy. *Adults:* if insulin dosage is less than 20 units daily, insulin may be discontinued.

glucagon

• Hypoglycemia. *Adults and children over 20 kg:* 1 mg S.C., I.M., or I.V. *Children 20 kg or under:* 0.5 mg S.C., I.M., or I.V. May repeat within 15 minutes if necessary. I.V. glucose must be given if patient fails to respond. When patient responds, give additional carbohydrate immediately.

• Diagnostic aid for radiologic examination. *Adults:* 0.25 to 2 mg I.V. or I.M. before initiation of radiologic procedure.

glyburide (DiaBeta, Micronase)

• Adjunct to diet to lower blood glucose level in patients with non-insulin-dependent (type II) diabetes mellitus. *Adults:* Initially, 2.5 to 5 mg P.O. daily administered with breakfast. Patients who are more sensitive to antidiabetic drugs should be started at 1.25 mg daily. Usual maintenance dosage is 1.25 to 20 mg daily, administered either as a single dose or in divided doses. Alternatively, micronized formula may be used. Initial dosage is 1.5 to 3 mg daily. Patients who are more sensitive to antidiabetic agents should be started at 0.75 mg daily.

• To replace insulin therapy. *Adults:*

if insulin dosage is less than 20 units daily, insulin may be discontinued.

glycerin
(Fleet Babylax, Sani-Supp)
• Constipation. *Adults and children over age 6:* 3 g as a rectal suppository; or 5 to 15 ml as an enema. *Children under age 6:* 1 to 1.5 g as a rectal suppository; or 2 to 5 ml as an enema.

gold sodium thiomalate
(Myochrysine)
(See aurothioglucose).

gonadotropin, human chorionic
(Antuitrin, A.P.L., Chorex 5, Follutein, Pregnyl, Profasi HP)
• Anovulation and infertility. *Women:* 10,000 units I.M. 1 day after last dose of menotropins.
• Hypogonadism. *Men:* 500 to 1,000 units I.M. three times weekly for 3 weeks, then twice weekly for 3 weeks; or 4,000 units I.M. three times weekly for 6 to 9 months, then 2,000 units I.M. three times weekly for 3 more months.
• Nonobstructive cryptorchidism. *Boys ages 4 to 9:* 5,000 units I.M. every other day for four doses.

guaifenesin (Baytussin, GG-CEN, Naldecon Senior EX, Robitussin)
• Expectorant. *Adults:* 200 to 400 mg P.O. q 4 hours. Maximum dosage is 2,400 mg/day. *Children ages 6 to 12:* 100 to 200 mg P.O. q 4 hours. Maximum dosage is 1,200 mg/day. *Children ages 2 to 5:* 50 to 100 mg P.O. q 4 hours. Maximum dosage is 600 mg/day.

guanadrel sulfate (Hylorel)
• Hypertension. *Adults:* Initially, 5 mg P.O. b.i.d. Dosage can be adjusted until blood pressure is controlled. Most patients require dosages of 20 to 75 mg/day, usually given b.i.d.

guanethidine monosulfate
(Ismelin)
• Moderate-to-severe hypertension (usually given with other antihypertensives). *Adults:* Initially, 10 mg P.O. daily. Increase by 10 mg at weekly to monthly intervals, p.r.n. Usual dosage is 25 to 50 mg daily. Some patients may require up to 300 mg.

guanfacine hydrochloride (Tenex)
• Hypertension. *Adults:* Initially, 1 mg P.O. daily h.s. Dosage may be increased to 2 mg P.O. h.s. after 3 to 4 weeks, as needed. Dosage may be further increased to 3 mg P.O. h.s. after an additional 3 to 4 weeks, as needed. Average dosage is 1 to 3 mg daily.

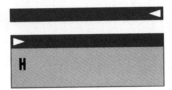

H

DRUG DOSAGES & INDICATIONS

haloperidol (Haldol, Peridol)
haloperidol decanoate (Haldol Decanoate, Haldol LA)
• Psychotic disorders. *Adults and children over age 12:* Dosage varies for each patient. Initial range is 0.5 to 5 mg P.O. b.i.d. or t.i.d.; or 2 to 5 mg I.M. q 4 to 8 hours, increasing rapidly if necessary for prompt control. Maximum dosage is 100 mg P.O. daily. *Children ages 3 to 12:* 0.05 to 0.15 mg/kg P.O. daily. Severely disturbed children may require higher dosages.
• Chronic psychotic patients who require prolonged therapy. *Adults:* 50 to 100 mg I.M. (decanoate) q 4 weeks.
• Control of tics, vocal utterances in Tourette syndrome. *Adults:* 0.5 to 5 mg P.O. b.i.d. or t.i.d., increasing p.r.n. *Children ages 3 to 12:* 0.075 mg/kg P.O. daily.

hydralazine hydrochloride (Apresoline)

• Essential hypertension (oral, alone, or in combination with other antihypertensives); reduction of afterload in severe CHF (with nitrates); and severe essential hypertension (parenteral to lower blood pressure quickly). *Adults:* Initially, 10 mg P.O. q.i.d.; gradually increased to 50 mg q.i.d. Maximum recommended dosage is 200 mg daily, but some patients may require 300 to 400 mg daily. Can be given b.i.d. for CHF. Give I.V. 10 to 20 mg slowly and repeat as necessary, generally q 4 to 6 hours. Switch to oral antihypertensives as soon as possible. Inject I.M. – 20 to 40 mg; repeat as necessary, generally q 4 to 6 hours. Switch to oral antihypertensives as soon as possible. *Children:* Initially, 0.75 mg/kg P.O. daily in four divided doses (25 mg/m² daily). May increase gradually to ten times this dosage if necessary. Give I.V. slowly 1.7 to 3.5 mg/kg daily or 50 to 100 mg/m² daily in four to six divided doses. Inject I.M. 1.7 to 3.5 mg/kg daily or 50 to 100 mg/m² daily in four to six divided doses.

hydrochlorothiazide (Diuchlor H, Esidrix, HydroDIURIL)

• Edema. *Adults:* Initially, 25 to 100 mg P.O. daily or intermittently for maintenance dosage. *Children ages 2 to 12:* 37.5 to 100 mg P.O. daily in two divided doses. *Children ages 6 months to 2 years:* 12.5 to 37.5 mg/kg P.O. daily in two divided doses. *Children under age 6 months:* Up to 3.3 mg/kg P.O. daily divided b.i.d.
• Hypertension. *Adults:* 25 to 50 mg P.O. daily or in divided doses. Daily dosage increased or decreased according to blood pressure.

hydrocortisone (Acticort 100, Cort-Dome, Dermacort)
hydrocortisone acetate (Cortaid, Cortamed, Cortef, Corticreme)
hydrocortisone valerate (Westcort Cream)

• Inflammation of corticosteroid-responsive dermatoses; adjunctive typical management of seborrheic dermatitis of scalp; may be safely used on face, groin, armpits, and under breasts. *Adults and children:* clean area; apply cream, lotion, ointment, foam, or aerosol sparingly daily to q.i.d. For aerosol application, shake can well. Direct spray onto affected area from a distance of 6″ (15 cm). Apply for only 3 seconds (to avoid freezing tissues). Apply to dry scalp after shampooing; no need to massage or rub medication into scalp after spraying. Apply daily until acute phase is controlled, then reduce dosage to one to three times a week as needed.

hydrocortisone (Cortef, Cortenema, Hydrocortone)
hydrocortisone acetate (Cortifoam, Hydrocortone Acetate)
hydrocortisone cypionate (Cortef)
hydrocortisone sodium phosphate (Hydrocortone Phosphate)
hydrocortisone sodium succinate (A-hydroCort, Solu-Cortef)

• Severe inflammation, adrenal insufficiency. *Adults:* 5 to 30 mg P.O. b.i.d., t.i.d., or q.i.d. (as much as 80 mg P.O. q.i.d. may be given in acute situations); or initially, 100 to 250 mg (succinate) I.M. or I.V., then 50 to 100 mg I.M., as indicated; or 15 to 240 mg (phosphate) I.M. or I.V. q 12 hours; or 5 to 75 mg (acetate) into joints and soft tissue. Dosage varies with size of joint. Local anesthetics are commonly injected with dose.

• Shock. *Adults:* Initially, 50 mg/kg (succinate) I.V., repeated in 4 hours. Repeat dosage q 24 hours as needed. Alternatively, 100 to 500 mg to 2 g q 2 to 6 hours. *Children:* 186 to 280 mg/kg (phosphate or succinate) I.M. or I.V. t.i.d.

hydroxyprogesterone caproate (Delalutin, Gesterol L.A.)

• Abnormal uterine bleeding. *Women:* 375 mg I.M. q 4 weeks. Stop after four cycles.

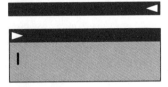

ibuprofen (Advil, Motrin, Nuprin, Rufen)

• Mild-to-moderate pain. *Adults:* 400 mg P.O. q 4 to 6 hours.
• Rheumatoid arthritis or osteoarthritis. *Adults:* 300 to 800 mg P.O. t.i.d. or q.i.d., not to exceed 3.2 g daily.

idoxuridine (Herplex, Stoxil)

• Herpes simplex keratitis. *Adults and children:* Instill 1 drop of solution into conjunctival sac q 1 hour during day and q 2 hours at night, or apply ointment to conjunctival sac q 4 hours or five times daily, with last dose at bedtime. Therapy should not be continued longer than 21 days.

imipenem-cilastatin (Primaxin)

• Severe lower respiratory and urinary tract, skin and skin-structure, bone, joint, intra-abdominal and gynecologic infections; bacterial septicemia; endocarditis. *Adults:* 500 to 750 mg I.M. q 12 hours, or 250 mg to 1 g by I.V. infusion over 20 to 30 minutes q 6 to 8 hours. Maximum dosage is 50 mg/kg/day or 4 g daily, whichever is less.

• Don't administer by direct I.V. bolus injection.
• Dosage adjustments are necessary in renal failure.

imipramine hydrochloride (Tofranil) imipramine pamoate (Tofranil-PM)

• Depression. *Adults:* 75 to 100 mg P.O. or I.M. daily in divided doses, increased in 25- to 50-mg increments up to maximum dosage of 300 mg daily. Alternatively, the entire dosage may be given at bedtime. (I.M. route rarely used.)
• Childhood enuresis. *Children over age 12:* 25 mg P.O. 1 hour before bedtime. If no response occurs within 1 week, increase dosage to 75 mg. Don't exceed 2.5 mg/kg/day. *Children ages 6 to 12:* 25 mg P.O. 1 hour before bedtime. If no response occurs within 1 week, increase dosage to 50 mg.

indomethacin (Indocin)

• Moderate-to-severe arthritis, ankylosing spondylitis. *Adults:* 25 mg P.O. or rectally b.i.d. or t.i.d. with food or antacids; may increase dosage by 25 mg daily q 7 days up to a maximum of 200 mg daily. Alternatively, sustained-release capsules (75 mg) may be given: 75 mg initially in the morning or at bedtime, followed, if necessary, by 75 mg b.i.d.
• Acute gouty arthritis. *Adults:* 50 mg P.O. t.i.d. Reduce dosage as soon as possible, then discontinue drug. Sustained-release capsules shouldn't be used for this condition.

insulin, regular insulin (beef or pork — Iletin II; Regular Iletin I and II; Velosulin)
prompt insulin zinc suspension (Semilente MC)
isophane insulin suspension (NPH) (Beef or Pork — NPH Iletin II, Insulatard Human, NPH Iletin II)
isophane insulin, human, suspension (Humulin N, Insulatard, Novolin N)
isophane insulin suspension with insulin injection (Actraphane HM, Humulin 50/50, Humulin 70/30, Novolin 70/30)
insulin zinc suspension (Lente, Lente Iletin II)
insulin zinc, human, suspension (Humulin L, Novolin L)
protamine zinc insulin (PZI) suspension (Protamine Zinc & Iletin I and II)
insulin zinc suspension, extended (Humulin U, Ultralente Insulin)
• Diabetic ketoacidosis (use regular insulin only). *Adults:* 25 to 150 units I.V. immediately, then additional doses q 1 hour based on blood glucose level until patient is out of acidosis, then q 6 hours S.C. thereafter. *Alternative dosage schedule:* 50 to 100 units I.V. and 50 to 100 units S.C. stat; additional doses may be given q 2 to 6 hours based on blood glucose levels; or 0.33 units/kg I.V. bolus, followed by 0.1 units/kg/hour I.V. by continuous infusion. Continue infusion until blood glucose level drops to 250 mg/dl; then start S.C. insulin q 6 hours. *Children:* 1 to 2 units/kg in two divided doses, one given I.V. and the other S.C., followed by 0.5 to 1 unit/kg I.V. q 1 to 2 hours. Or 0.1 unit/g I.V. bolus, then 0.1 unit/ kg hourly by continuous I.V. infusion until blood glucose level drops to 250 mg/dl; then start S.C. insulin. Preparation of infusion: Add 100 units regular insulin and 1 g al-

bumin to 100 ml of 0.9% sodium chloride solution. Insulin concentration will be 1 unit/ml. (Albumin adsorbs to plastic, preventing loss of the insulin to plastic.)
• Types I and II diabetes mellitus, diabetes mellitus inadequately controlled by diet and oral antidiabetic medications. *Adults and children:* prescribed regimen adjusted according to patient's blood and urine glucose concentrations.

ipecac syrup
• To induce vomiting in poisoning. *Adults and children age 12 and over:* 30 ml P.O., followed by 200 to 300 ml of water. *Children ages 1 to 12:* 15 ml P.O., followed by about 200 ml of water or milk. *Children ages 6 months to 1 year:* 5 ml P.O., followed by 100 to 200 ml of water or milk; may repeat dose once after 20 minutes if needed.

ipratropium bromide (Atrovent)
• Maintenance treatment of bronchospasm associated with chronic obstructive pulmonary disease. *Adults:* 1 to 2 inhalations (26 mcg) q.i.d.; additional inhalations may be needed. Alternatively, 250 to 500 mg dissolved in 0.9% sodium chloride and administered by nebulizer q 4 to 6 hours. Total inhalations should not exceed 12 in 24 hours.

isocarboxazid (Marplan)
• Depression. *Adults:* 30 mg P.O. daily in divided doses, reduced to 10 to 20 mg daily when condition improves. Not recommended for children under age 16.

isoproterenol hydrochloride (Isuprel, Isuprel Mistometer)
isoproterenol sulfate (Medihaler-Iso)
• Bronchial asthma and reversible bronchospasm. *Adults:* 10 to 15 mg (hydrochloride) sublingually q 6 to

8 hours. *Children:* 5 to 10 mg (hydrochloride) sublingually q 6 to 8 hours. Not recommended for children younger than age 6.
• Bronchospasm. *Adults and children:* acute dyspneic episodes: 1 inhalation (sulfate) initially. May repeat, if needed, after 2 to 5 minutes. Maintenance dosage is 1 to 2 inhalations 4 to 6 times daily. May repeat once more 10 minutes after second dose. No more than three doses should be administered for each attack.

isosorbide (Ismotic)
• Short-term reduction of intraocular pressure from glaucoma. *Adults:* Initially, 1.5 g/kg P.O. Usual dosage range is 1 to 3 g/kg.

isosorbide dinitrate (Isordil)
• Acute anginal attacks (sublingual and chewable tablets only); prophylaxis of anginal attacks; treatment of chronic ischemic heart disease (by preload reduction). *Adults:* Sublingual form—2.5 to 5 mg under the tongue for prompt relief of anginal pain, repeated q 5 to 10 minutes (maximum of three doses for each 30-minute period). Or 2.5 to 10 mg q 2 to 3 hours for prophylaxis. Chewable form—5 to 10 mg p.r.n. for acute attack or q 2 to 3 hours for prophylaxis, but only after initial test dose of 5 mg to determine risk of severe hypotension. Oral form—5 to 30 mg P.O. t.i.d. or q.i.d. for prophylaxis only (use smallest effective dose). Sustained-release form—40 mg P.O. q 6 to 12 hours.

isotretinoin (Accutane)
• Severe cystic acne unresponsive to conventional therapy. *Adults and adolescents:* 0.5 to 2 mg/kg P.O. daily given in two divided doses and continued for 15 to 20 weeks.

isoxsuprine hydrochloride (Vasodilan)
• Adjunct for relief of symptoms associated with cerebrovascular insufficiency or peripheral vascular disorders. *Adults:* 10 to 20 mg P.O. t.i.d. or q.i.d.

isradipine (DynaCirc)
• Essential hypertension. *Adults:* Initially, 2.5 mg P.O. b.i.d. alone or with thiazide diuretic. Adjust dosage based on tolerance and response to a maximum of 20 mg b.i.d.

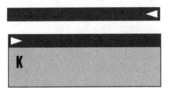

kanamycin sulfate (Kantrex)
• Serious infections caused by sensitive *Escherichia coli, Proteus, Enterobacter aerogenes, Klebsiella pneumoniae, Serratia marcescens, Mycobacterium* and *Acinetobacter. Adults and children with normal renal function:* 15 mg/kg deep I.M. injection into upper outer quadrant of buttocks or I.V. infusion (diluted 500 mg/200 ml of 0.9% sodium chloride solution or D_5W infused over 30 to 60 minutes) daily divided q 8 to 12 hours. Maximum daily dosage is 1.5 g. *Patients with impaired renal function:* Doses or frequency of administration should be altered. In all patients, keep peak serum concentrations between 15 and 30 mcg/ml, and trough serum concentrations between 5 and 10 mcg/ml. *Neonates:* 15 mg/kg I.M. or I.V. daily divided q 12 hours.
• Adjunctive treatment in hepatic coma. *Adults:* 8 to 12 g P.O. daily in divided doses.
• Preoperative bowel sterilization. *Adults:* 1 g P.O. q 1 hour for 4 doses, then q 4 hours for 4 doses;

or 1 g P.O. q 1 hour for 4 doses, then q 6 hours for 36 to 72 hours.
• Intraperitoneal irrigation. *Adults:* Instill 500 mg in 20 ml of sterile distilled water via catheter into wound after patient fully recovers from anesthesia and neuromuscular blocking agent effects.
• Wound irrigation. *Adults:* Up to 2.5 mg/ml in 0.9% sodium chloride irrigation solution.
• Dosage adjustments are necessary in renal failure.

kaolin, pectin, activated attapulgite mixtures (Donnagel-MB, Kao-Con, Kaopectate, Kaopectate Concentrate, Kao-tin, Kapectolin, K-C, K-P, K-Pek)
• Mild, nonspecific diarrhea. *Adults:* 60 to 120 ml P.O. after each bowel movement. *Children over age 12:* 60 ml P.O. after each bowel movement. *Children ages 6 to 12:* 30 to 60 ml P.O. after each bowel movement. *Children ages 3 to 6:* 15 to 30 ml P.O. after each bowel movement.

ketorolac tromethamine (Toradol)
• Short-term management of pain. *Adults:* 30 to 60 mg I.M. as a loading dose, followed by one-half of the loading dose (15 or 30 mg) q 6 hours on a regular schedule or p.r.n. Subsequent doses should be based on patient response. If pain returns before 6 hours, dose may be increased by as much as 50% (up to 60 mg); if pain relief continues for 8 to 12 hours, increase interval between doses or reduce dose. The recommended maximum dosage is 150 mg on the first day and 120 mg/day thereafter. Alternatively, the drug may be used orally on a short-term basis (up to 15 days); dosage is 10 mg P.O. q 4 to 6 hours, p.r.n., up to a maximum of 40 mg/day.

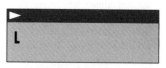

labetalol hydrochloride (Normodyne, Trandate)
• Hypertension. *Adults:* 100 mg P.O. b.i.d. with or without a diuretic. Dosage may be increased to 200 mg b.i.d. after 2 days. Further dosage increases may be made q 1 to 3 days until optimal response is reached. Usual maintenance dosage is 200 to 400 mg b.i.d.
• Severe hypertension and hypertensive emergencies. *Adults:* Make an infusion containing 1 mg/ml by adding 200 mg of labetalol to 160 mg D_5W. Infuse at 2 mg/minute until a satisfactory response is obtained. Then stop the infusion. May repeat q 6 to 12 hours.
  Alternatively, administer by repeated I.V. injection: Initially, give 20 mg I.V. slowly over 2 minutes. May repeat injections of 40 to 80 mg q 10 minutes until maximum daily dosage of 300 mg is reached.

lactulose (Cephulac, Cholac, Chronulac, Constilac, Lactulax)
• Constipation. *Adults:* 15 to 30 ml P.O. daily.
• Prevention and treatment of portal-systemic encephalopathy, including hepatic precoma and coma in patients with severe hepatic disease. *Adults:* Initially, 20 to 30 g (30 to 45 ml) P.O. t.i.d. or q.i.d. until two or three soft stools are produced daily. Usual dosage is 60 to 100 g daily in divided doses. Can also be given by retention enema: 200 g (300 ml) diluted with 700 ml of water or saline solution and administered q 4 to 6 hours p.r.n.

levodopa (Dopar, Larodopa)
• Idiopathic parkinsonism, postencephalitic parkinsonism, and symp-

tomatic parkinsonism after carbon monoxide or manganese intoxication or in association with cerebral arteriosclerosis. *Adults and children over age 12:* Initially, 0.5 to 1 g P.O. daily divided into two or more doses with food; increase by no more than 0.75 g daily q 3 to 7 days, until usual daily maximum dosage of 8 g is reached. Higher dosage requires close supervision.

Levodopa is administered orally with food in dosages carefully adjusted to individual requirements.

levodopa-carbidopa (Sinemet, Sinemet CR)

• Idiopathic parkinsonism, postencephalitic parkinsonism, and symptomatic parkinsonism resulting from carbon monoxide or manganese intoxication. *Adults:* 1 tablet of 25 mg carbidopa/100 mg levodopa P.O. t.i.d., followed by an increase of 1 tablet every day or every other day as necessary, up to a maximum daily dosage of 8 tablets. Tablets containing 25 mg carbidopa/250 mg levodopa or 10 mg carbidopa/100 mg levodopa are substituted as required to obtain maximum response. Titrate optimal daily dosage for each patient.

levothyroxine sodium (Eltroxin, Levoid, Levothroid, Levoxine, Synthroid)

• Cretinism. *Children under age 1:* Initially, 0.025 to 0.05 mg P.O. daily, increased by 0.05 mg q 4 to 6 weeks, as needed.

• Myxedema coma. *Adults:* 0.2 to 0.5 mg I.V. If no response occurs in 24 hours, additional 0.1 to 0.3 mg I.V., followed by parenteral maintenance dosage of 0.05 to 0.2 mg I.V. daily. After condition stabilizes, switch to oral maintenance.

• Thyroid hormone replacement. *Adults:* Initially, 0.025 to 0.05 mg P.O. daily, increased by 0.025 mg q 2 to 4 weeks until desired response

occurs. Maintenance dosage is 0.1 to 0.4 mg P.O. daily. May be administered I.V. or I.M. when P.O. ingestion is precluded for long periods. *Adults over age 65:* 0.0125 to 0.025 mg P.O. daily. May be increased by 0.025 mg at 3- to 4-week intervals, depending on response. *Children:* Initially, 0.025 to 0.05 mg P.O. daily in children under age 1, or 3 to 5 mcg/kg P.O. daily in children age 1 or older; dosage is gradually increased by 0.025 to 0.05 mg P.O. q 1 to 4 weeks until desired response occurs.

lidocaine hydrochloride (LidoPen Auto-Injector, Xylocaine)

• Ventricular arrhythmias from MI, cardiac manipulation, or digitalis glycosides; ventricular tachycardia. *Adults:* 50 to 100 mg (1 to 1.5 mg/kg) by I.V. bolus at 25 to 50 mg/min. Give half this amount to elderly patients, patients weighing less than 50 kg, and those with CHF or hepatic disease. Repeat bolus q 3 to 5 minutes until arrhythmias subside or adverse reactions develop. Don't exceed 300-mg total bolus during a 1-hour period. At same time, begin constant infusion of 1 to 4 mg/min. If single bolus has been given, repeat smaller bolus 15 to 20 minutes after start of infusion to maintain serum level. After 24 hours of continuous infusion, decrease rate by half. Or give I.M. dose of 200 to 300 mg in deltoid muscle only, followed by second I.M. dose 60 to 90 minutes later, if needed. *Children:* 1 mg/kg by I.V. bolus, followed by infusion of 30 mcg/kg/min.

lindane (GBH, Kwell, Kwellada, Scabene)

• Parasitic infestation (scabies, pediculosis). *Adults and children:* cream or lotion — apply thin layer over entire skin surface (with special attention to folds, creases, interdigital spaces, and genital area) for scabies, or to hairy areas for pediculosis. After 12 hours, wash off drug. If second application is needed, wait 1 week before repeating; never apply more than twice in a week. Shampoo—apply 30 ml undiluted to affected area and work into lather for 4 to 5 minutes. Rinse thoroughly and rub with dry towel.

liothyronine sodium (Cytomel)
• Congenital hypothyroidism. *Infants and children:* 5 mcg P.O. daily. Increase dosage as needed in increments of 5 mcg daily every 3 to 4 days until optimal response is achieved.
• Myxedema. *Adults:* Initially, 5 mcg daily, increased by 5 to 10 mcg q 1 or 2 weeks, then increased by 12.5 to 25 mcg daily q 1 to 2 weeks. Maintenance dosage is 50 to 100 mcg daily.
• Nontoxic goiter. *Adults:* Initially, 5 mcg P.O. daily; may be increased by 5 to 10 mcg daily q 1 to 2 weeks. Usual maintenance dosage is 75 mcg daily.
• Thyroid hormone replacement. *Adults:* Initially, 25 mcg P.O. daily, increased by 12.5 to 25 mcg q 1 to 2 weeks until satisfactory response occurs. Usual maintenance dosage is 25 to 75 mcg daily.
• T_3 suppression test to differentiate hyperthyroidism from euthyroidism. *Adults:* 75 to 100 mcg P.O. daily for 7 days.

liotrix (T_3/T_4) (Euthroid, Thyrolar)
• Hypothyroidism—dosages are expressed in thyroid equivalents and must be tailored to the patient's deficit. *Adults and children:* Initially, 15 to 30 mg P.O. daily, increased by 15 to 30 mg q 1 to 2 weeks until desired response is achieved; with children, increase dosage q 2 weeks. *Adults over age 65:* Initially, 15 to 30 mg. Usual adult dosage

doubled q 6 to 8 weeks until desired response occurs.

lisinopril (Prinivil, Zestril)
• Hypertension. *Adults:* Initially, 10 mg P.O. daily (5 mg P.O. daily for patient receiving diuretic). Most patients are well controlled on 20 to 40 mg daily as a single dose.

lithium carbonate (Carbolith, Duralith, Eskalith, Eskalith CR, Lithane, Lithizine, Lithobid, Lithonate, Lithotabs)
lithium citrate (Cibalith-S)
• Prevention or control of mania. *Adults:* 300 to 600 mg P.O. up to q.i.d., increasing on the basis of blood levels to achieve optimal dosage. Recommended therapeutic lithium blood levels: 1 to 1.5 mEq/liter for acute mania; 0.6 to 1.2 mEq/liter for maintenance therapy; and 2 mEq/liter as maximum.
   (Note: 5 ml of lithium citrate—liquid—contains 8 mEq of lithium equal to 300 mg of lithium carbonate.)

lomefloxacin (Maxaquin)
• Acute bacterial exacerbations of chronic bronchitis caused by *Haemophilus influenzae* or *Moraxella (Branhamella) catarrhalis. Adults:* 400 mg P.O. daily for 10 days.
• Uncomplicated UTIs (cystitis) caused by *Escherichia coli, Klebsiella pneumoniae, Proteus mirabilis,* or *Staphylococcus saprophyticus. Adults:* 400 mg P.O. daily for 10 days.
• Complicated UTIs caused by *E. coli, K. pneumoniae, P. mirabilis,* and *Pseudomonas aeruginosa;* possibly effective against infections caused by *Citrobacter diversus* or *Enterobacter cloacae. Adults:* 400 mg P.O. daily for 14 days.
• Prophylaxis of infections after transurethral surgical procedures. *Adults:* 400 mg P.O. 2 to 6 hours before surgery as a single dose.

• Dosage adjustments are necessary in renal failure.

loperamide
(Imodium, Imodium A-D)
• Acute, nonspecific diarrhea. *Adults:* initially, 4 mg P.O., then 2 mg after each unformed stool. Maximum dosage is 16 mg/day. *Children ages 8 to 12:* 10 ml P.O. t.i.d. on first day. (Subsequent doses of 5 ml/10 kg of body weight may be administered after each unformed stool.) *Children ages 5 to 8:* 10 ml P.O. b.i.d. on first day. *Children ages 2 to 5:* 5 ml P.O. t.i.d. on first day.
• Chronic diarrhea. *Adults:* initially, 4 mg P.O., then 2 mg after each unformed stool until diarrhea subsides. Adjust dosage to individual response.

loracarbef (Lorabid)
• Secondary bacterial infections of acute bronchitis. *Adults:* 200 to 400 mg P.O. q 12 hours for 7 days.
• Acute bacterial exacerbations of chronic bronchitis. *Adults:* 400 mg P.O. q 12 hours for 7 days.
• Pneumonia. *Adults:* 400 mg P.O. q 12 hours for 14 days.
• Pharyngitis or tonsillitis. *Adults:* 400 mg P.O. q 12 hours for 10 days. *Children:* 15 mg/kg P.O. daily in divided doses q 12 hours for 10 days.
• Acute otitis media. *Children:* 30 mg/kg P.O. daily (oral suspension) in divided doses q 12 hours for 10 days.
• Uncomplicated skin and skin structure infections. *Adults:* 200 mg P.O. q 12 hours for 7 days.
• Impetigo. *Children:* 15 mg/kg P.O. daily in divided doses q 12 hours for 7 days.
• Uncomplicated cystitis. *Adults:* 200 mg P.O. daily for 7 days.
• Uncomplicated pyelonephritis. *Adults:* 400 mg P.O. q 12 hours for 7 days.
• Dosage adjustments are necessary in patients with renal failure. If creatinine clearance is 10 to 49 ml/min/1.73 m², give 50% of the usual dose at the same interval. Alternatively, give the usual dose at twice the interval. If creatine clearance is <10 ml/min/1.73 m², give the usual dose every 3 to 5 days. Patients receiving hemodialysis should be given another dose following the dialysis session.

lovastatin (Mevacor)
• Reduction of low-density lipoprotein and total cholesterol levels in patients with primary hypercholesterolemia (Types IIa and IIb). *Adults:* Initially, 20 mg P.O. once daily with the evening meal. For patients with severely elevated cholesterol levels (for example, over 300 mg/dl), the initial dosage should be 40 mg daily. The recommended daily dosage range is 20 to 80 mg in single or divided doses.

lypressin (Diapid)
• Pituitary diabetes insipidus. *Adults and children:* 1 or 2 sprays (approximately 2 USP posterior pituitary pressor units/spray) in either or both nostrils q.i.d. and an additional dose at bedtime, if needed, to prevent nocturia.

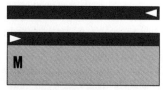

magnesium oxide
(Mag-Ox 400, Maox, Uro-Mag)
• Antacid. *Adults:* 140 mg P.O. with water or milk after meals and h.s.
• Laxative. *Adults:* 4 g P.O. with water or milk, usually h.s.
• Oral replacement therapy in mild hypomagnesemia. *Adults:* 400 to 840 mg P.O. daily. Monitor serum magnesium response.

magnesium salicylate (Doan's Pills, Magan, Mobidin)
• Arthritis. *Adults:* 545 mg to 1.2 g P.O. t.i.d. or q.i.d., not to exceed 9.6 g daily.

magnesium salts (magnesium citrate, magnesium hydroxide, magnesium sulfate)
• Constipation; bowel evacuation before surgery. *Adults and children over age 12:* 11 to 25 g magnesium citrate P.O. daily as a single or divided dose; 2.4 to 4.8 g (30 to 60 ml) magnesium hydroxide P.O. daily as a single or divided dose; or 10 to 30 g magnesium sulfate P.O. daily as a single or divided dose. *Children ages 6 to 12:* 5.5 to 12.5 g magnesium citrate P.O. daily; 1.2 to 2.4 g (15 to 30 ml) magnesium hydroxide P.O. daily; or 5 to 10 g magnesium sulfate P.O. daily. *Children ages 2 to 6:* 2.7 to 6.25 g magnesium citrate P.O. daily; 0.4 to 1.2 g (5 to 15 ml) magnesium hydroxide P.O. daily; or 2.5 to 5 g magnesium sulfate P.O. daily.

magnesium sulfate
• Hypomagnesemia. *Adults:* 1 g or 8.12 mEq of 50% solution (2 ml) I.M. q 6 hours for four doses, depending on serum magnesium level.
• Severe hypomagnesemia (serum magnesium 0.8 mEq/liter or less, with symptoms). *Adults:* 5 g or 50 mEq of 50% solution I.V. in 1 liter of solution over 3 hours. Subsequent dosage based on magnesium level.
• Hypomagnesemic seizures. *Adults:* 1 to 2 g (as 10% solution) I.V. over 15 minutes, then 1 g I.M. q 4 to 6 hours, based on magnesium level.
• Seizures secondary to hypomagnesemia in acute nephritis. *Children:* 0.2 ml/kg of 50% solution I.M. q 4 to 6 hours, p.r.n.; or 100 mg/kg of 1% to 3% solution I.V. very slowly, based on response and magnesium level.

mannitol (Osmitrol)
• To reduce intracranial pressure. *Adults and children over age 12:* 1.5 to 2 g/kg as a 15% to 25% solution I.V. over 30 to 60 minutes.

meclizine hydrochloride (Antivert, Bonine)
• Dizziness. *Adults:* 25 to 100 mg P.O. daily in divided doses. Dosage varies with patient response.
• Motion sickness. *Adults:* 25 to 50 mg P.O. 1 hour before travel, repeated daily for duration of journey.

meclofenamate sodium (Meclomen)
• RA and osteoarthritis. *Adults:* 200 to 400 mg/day P.O. in three or four equally divided doses.

medroxyprogesterone acetate (Amen, Curretab, Cycrin, Depo-Provera, Provera)
• Abnormal uterine bleeding caused by hormonal imbalance. *Women:* 5 to 10 mg P.O. daily for 5 to 10 days beginning on the 16th day of menstrual cycle. If patient has received estrogen, 10 mg P.O. daily for 10 days beginning on 16th day of cycle.
• Secondary amenorrhea. *Women:* 5 to 10 mg P.O. daily for 5 to 10 days.
• Prevention of pregnancy. *Women:* Inject 150 mg deep I.M. within 5 days of onset of menses; within 5 days of birth (if not nursing); or at 6 weeks postpartum, if nursing. Repeat dose q 3 months.

menotropins (Pergonal)
• Anovulation. *Women:* 1 ampule (75 IU follicle-stimulating hormone [FSH] and 75 IU luteinizing hormone [LH]) I.M. daily for 7 to 12 days, then 5,000 to 10,000 units of human chorionic gonadotropin (HCG) I.M. 1 day after last dose of menotropins. Repeat for one to

three menstrual cycles until ovulation occurs.
• Infertility with ovulation. *Women:* 1 ampule I.M. daily for 9 to 12 days, followed by 10,000 units of HCG I.M. 1 day after last dose of menotropins. Repeat for two menstrual cycles and then double the dose (2 ampules) daily for 9 to 12 days, followed by 10,000 units HCG I.M. 1 day after last dose of menotropins. Repeat for two menstrual cycles.
• Infertility. *Men:* 1 ampule I.M. three times weekly (given concomitantly with 2,000 units HCG twice weekly) for at least 4 months.

meperidine hydrochloride (Demerol)
Controlled Substance Schedule II
• Moderate-to-severe pain. *Adults:* 50 to 150 mg P.O., I.M., or S.C. q 3 to 4 hours, p.r.n. or around the clock. *Children:* 1 to 1.8 mg/kg P.O., I.M., or S.C. q 4 to 6 hours. Maximum dosage is 100 mg q 4 hours, p.r.n. or around the clock.

mephenytoin (Mesantoin)
• Generalized tonic-clonic or complex-partial (psychomotor) seizures. *Adults:* 50 to 100 mg P.O. daily. May increase by 50 to 100 mg at weekly intervals up to 200 mg P.O. t.i.d. *Children:* initially, 50 to 100 mg P.O. daily or 100 to 450 mg/ m^2 P.O. daily in three divided doses. May increase slowly by 50 to 100 mg at weekly intervals up to 200 mg P.O. t.i.d., divided q 8 hours. Dosage must be adjusted individually.

mephobarbital (Mebaral)
Controlled substance schedule IV
• Generalized tonic-clonic or absence seizures. *Adults:* 400 to 600 mg P.O. daily or in divided doses. *Children:* 6 to 12 mg/kg P.O. daily, divided q 6 to 8 hours (smaller doses are given initially and increased over 4 to 5 days as needed).

mesoridazine besylate (Serentil)
• Alcoholism. *Adults and children over age 12:* 25 mg P.O. b.i.d. up to maximum of 200 mg daily.
• Behavioral problems associated with chronic brain syndrome. *Adults and children over age 12:* 25 mg P.O. t.i.d. up to maximum of 300 mg daily.
• Psychoneurotic manifestations (anxiety). *Adults and children over age 12:* 10 mg P.O. t.i.d. up to maximum of 150 mg daily.
• Schizophrenia. *Adults and children over age 12:* initially, 50 mg P.O. t.i.d. or 25 mg I.M. repeated in 30 to 60 minutes, p.r.n.

metaproterenol sulfate (Alupent, Metaprel)
• Acute episodes of bronchial asthma. *Adults and children:* 2 to 3 inhalations no more often than q 3 to 4 hours. Maximum of 12 inhalations daily.
• Bronchial asthma and reversible bronchospasm. *Adults:* 20 mg P.O. q 6 to 8 hours. *Children over age 9 or weighing over 27 kg:* 20 mg P.O. q 6 to 8 hours. *Children ages 6 to 9 or weighing less than 27 kg:* 10 mg P.O. q 6 to 8 hours. Not recommended for children under age 6.

methicillin sodium (Staphcillin)
• Systemic infections caused by susceptible organisms. *Adults:* 4 to 12 g I.M. or I.V. daily, divided into doses given q 4 to 6 hours. *Children:* 150 to 200 mg/kg I.M. or I.V. daily, divided into doses given q 4 to 6 hours.

methimazole (Tapazole)
• Hyperthyroidism. *Adults:* 5 mg P.O. t.i.d. if mild; 10 to 15 mg P.O. t.i.d. if moderately severe; and 20 mg P.O. t.i.d. if severe. Continue until patient is euthyroid, then start

maintenance dosage of 5 mg daily to t.i.d. Maximum dosage is 150 mg daily. *Children:* 0.4 mg/kg daily divided q 8 hours. Continue until patient is euthyroid, then start maintenance dosage of 0.2 mg/kg daily divided q 8 hours.

methocarbamol (Robaxin)

• As an adjunct in acute, painful musculoskeletal conditions. *Adults:* 1.5 g P.O. q.i.d. for 2 to 3 days, then 1 g P.O. q.i.d., or no more than 500 mg (5 ml) I.M. into each gluteal region. May repeat q 8 hours. Or 1 to 3 g (10 to 30 ml) I.V. daily directly into vein at 3 ml/minute, or 10 ml added to no more than 250 ml of D_5W or 0.9% sodium chloride solution. Maximum dosage is 3 g daily.

• Supportive therapy in tetanus management: *Adults:* 1 to 2 g by direct I.V. or 1 to 3 g as I.V. infusion q 6 hours. *Children:* 15 mg/kg I.V. q 6 hours.

methotrexate
methotrexate sodium (Rheumatrex)

• Trophoblastic tumors. *Adults:* 15 to 30 mg P.O. or I.M. daily for 5 days. Repeated after 1 or more weeks based on response.

• RA. *Adults:* Initially, 7.5 mg P.O. weekly, either in a single dose or divided as 2.5 mg P.O. every 12 hours for three doses once a week. Dosage may be gradually increased to a maximum of 20 mg weekly.

methyldopa (Aldomet)

• Hypertension, hypertensive crisis. *Adults:* Initially, 250 mg P.O. b.i.d. to t.i.d. in first 48 hours, increased as needed q 2 days. May give entire daily dosage in the evening or h.s. Dosage may need adjustment if other antihypertensive drugs are added to or deleted from therapy. Maintenance dosage is 500 mg to 2 g daily in two to four divided doses. Maximum recommended

daily dosage is 3 g. Or 250 to 500 mg I.V. q 6 hours, diluted in D_5W and administered over 30 to 60 minutes. Switch to oral antihypertensives as soon as possible. *Children:* Initially, 10 mg/kg P.O. daily in two to four divided doses; or 20 to 40 mg/kg I.V. daily in four divided doses. Increase dosage daily until desired response occurs. Maximum daily dosage is 65 mg/kg or 3 g, whichever is less.

metoclopramide hydrochloride (Maxeran, Reglan)

• To prevent or reduce nausea and vomiting induced by cisplatin and other chemotherapeutic drugs. *Adults:* 1 to 2 mg/kg I.V. q 30 minutes before therapy, then repeated q 2 hours for two doses, then q 3 hours for three doses.

• To facilitate small-bowel intubation and to aid in radiologic examinations. *Adults:* 10 mg (2 ml) I.V. as a single dose over 1 to 2 minutes. *Children ages 6 to 14:* 2.5 to 5 mg (0.5 to 1 ml) I.V. *Children under age 6:* 0.1 mg/kg I.V.

• Delayed gastric emptying secondary to diabetic gastroparesis. *Adults:* 10 mg P.O. 30 minutes before meals and h.s. for 2 to 8 weeks, depending on response.

• Gastroesophageal reflux. *Adults:* 10 to 15 mg P.O. q.i.d., p.r.n. Take 30 minutes before meals.

metoprolol tartrate (Lopressor)

• Hypertension (may be used alone or in combination with other antihypertensives). *Adults:* 50 mg b.i.d. or 100 mg P.O. once daily initially, up to 100 to 450 mg daily in two or three divided doses.

• Early intervention in acute MI. *Adults:* Three injections of 5-mg I.V. boluses q 2 minutes. Then, starting 15 minutes after last dose, administer 50 mg P.O. q 6 hours for 48 hours. Maintenance dosage is 100 mg P.O. b.i.d.

mexiletine hydrochloride (Mexitil)
• Refractory ventricular arrhythmias, including ventricular tachycardia and PVCs. *Adults:* 200 to 400 mg P.O. followed by 200 mg q 8 hours. May increase dose to 400 mg q 8 hours if satisfactory control is not obtained. Some patients may respond well to an every-12-hour schedule. May give up to 450 mg q 12 hours.

mezlocillin sodium (Mezlin)
• Infections caused by susceptible organisms. *Adults:* 100 to 300 mg/kg I.V. or I.M. daily given in four to six divided doses. Usual dosage is 3 g q 4 hours or 4 g q 6 hours. For serious infections, up to 24 g daily may be administered. *Children under age 12:* 200 to 300 mg/kg per day I.M. or I.V. in divided doses q 4 to 6 hours.
• Dosage adjustments are necessary in renal failure.

mineral oil (Agoral Plain, Kondremul, Petrogalar Plain)
• Constipation; preparation for bowel studies or surgery. *Adults:* 15 to 30 ml P.O. h.s.; or 120 ml as an enema. *Children:* 5 to 15 ml P.O. h.s.; or 30 to 60 ml as an enema.

minocycline hydrochloride (Minocin)
• Infections caused by sensitive organisms. *Adults:* Initially, 200 mg P.O., I.V.; then 100 mg q 12 hours or 50 mg P.O. q 6 hours. *Children over age 8:* Initially, 4 mg/kg P.O., I.V.; then 4 mg/kg P.O. daily, divided q 12 hours. Give I.V. in 500 to 1,000 ml of a compatible solution such as D$_5$W or 0.9% sodium chloride injection, over 6 hours.
• Gonorrhea in patients sensitive to penicillin. *Adults:* Initially, 200 mg; then 100 mg q 12 hours for 4 days.
• Syphilis in patients sensitive to penicillin. *Adults:* Initially, 200 mg;

then 100 mg q 12 hours for 10 to 15 days.
• Meningococcal carrier state. *Adults:* 100 mg P.O. q 12 hours for 5 days.
• Uncomplicated urethral, endocervical, or rectal infection. *Adults:* 100 mg b.i.d. for at least 7 days.
• Uncomplicated gonoccocal urethritis in men. *Adults:* 100 mg b.i.d. for 5 days.

minoxidil (Loniten)
• Severe hypertension. *Adults:* 5 mg P.O. initially as a single dose. Effective dosage range is usually 10 to 40 mg daily. Maximum dosage is 100 mg daily. *Children under age 12:* 0.2 mg/kg as a single daily dose. Effective dosage range usually is 0.25 to 1 mg/kg daily. Maximum dosage is 50 mg.

minoxidil, topical (Rogaine)
• Baldness (alopecia androgenetica) in men and women. *Adults:* apply 1 ml of 2% solution to affected area twice daily. Total daily dosage should not exceed 2 ml.

misoprostol (Cytotec)
• Prevention of gastric ulcers induced by anti-inflammatory drugs (NSAIDs) in elderly or debilitated patients at high risk for complications from gastric ulcer and in patients with a history of NSAID-induced ulcers. *Adults:* 200 mcg P.O. q.i.d. with food. May be decreased to 100 mcg P.O. q.i.d. if not tolerated.

morphine hydrochloride (Morphitec, M.O.S., M.O.S.-S.R.) morphine sulfate (Astramorph, Duramorph, MS Contin, Roxanol)
Controlled Substance Schedule II
• Severe pain. *Adults:* 5 to 20 mg S.C. or I.M.; 10 to 30 mg P.O. or 10 to 20 mg rectally q 4 hours p.r.n. or around the clock; or 2.5 to 15 mg I.V. injected slowly (over 4 to 5 minutes) diluted in 4 to 5 ml water for

injection. May also administer controlled-release tablets q 8 to 12 hours. As an epidural injection, 5 mg via an epidural catheter q 24 hours. *Children:* 0.1 to 0.2 mg/kg dose S.C. Maximum daily dosage is 15 mg.

In some situations, morphine may be administered by continuous I.V. infusion or by intraspinal and intrathecal injection.

mupirocin (Bactroban)
• Treatment of common bacterial skin infections caused by susceptible bacteria. *Adults and children:* apply to affected areas b.i.d. to t.i.d.

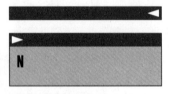

nabumetone (Relafen)
• Acute and chronic treatment of RA or osteoarthritis. *Adults:* Initially, 1,000 mg P.O. daily as a single dose or in divided doses b.i.d. Maximum daily dosage is 2,000 mg.

nadolol (Corgard)
• Angina pectoris. *Adults:* 40 mg P.O. once daily, initially. Dosage may be increased in 40- to 80-mg increments until optimal response occurs. Usual maintenance dosage range is 80 to 240 mg once daily.
• Hypertension. *Adults:* 40 mg P.O. once daily, initially. Dosage may be increased in 40- to 80-mg increments until optimal response occurs. Usual maintenance dosage is 80 to 320 mg once daily. Doses of 640 mg may be necessary in rare cases.

nafcillin sodium (Unipen)
• Systemic infections caused by susceptible organisms (methicillin-sensitive *Staphylococcus aureus*).

Adults: 2 to 4 g P.O. daily, divided into doses given q 6 hours; 2 to 12 g I.M. or I.V. daily, divided into doses given q 4 to 6 hours. *Children:* 50 to 100 mg/kg P.O. daily, divided into doses given q 4 to 6 hours; 100 to 200 mg/kg I.M. or I.V. daily, divided into doses given q 4 to 6 hours.

nalidixic acid (NegGram)
• Acute and chronic UTIs caused by susceptible gram-negative organisms (*Proteus, Klebsiella, Enterobacter,* and *Escherichia coli*). *Adults:* 1 g P.O. q.i.d. for 7 to 14 days; 2 g daily for long-term use. *Children over age 3 months:* 55 mg/kg P.O. daily divided q.i.d. for 7 to 14 days; 33 mg/kg daily for long-term use.

naphazoline hydrochloride (Privine)
• Nasal congestion. *Adults:* apply 2 drops or sprays of 0.05% solution to nasal mucosa q 3 to 4 hours. *Children ages 6 to 12:* 1 to 2 drops or sprays of 0.05% solution. Repeat q 3 to 6 hours, p.r.n. Use no longer than 3 to 5 days.

naproxen (Naprosyn)
naproxen sodium (Anaprox)
• Arthritis. *Adults:* 250 to 500 mg P.O. b.i.d. Maximum dosage is 1,000 mg daily.
• Mild-to-moderate pain. *Adults:* 500 mg P.O. to start, followed by 250 mg q 6 to 8 hours as needed. Maximum daily dosage should not exceed 1,375 mg.

neomycin sulfate (Mycifradin)
• Infectious diarrhea caused by enteropathogenic *Escherichia coli.* *Adults:* 50 mg/kg P.O. daily in four divided doses for 2 to 3 days. *Children:* 50 to 100 mg/kg P.O. daily divided q 4 to 6 hours for 2 to 3 days.
• Suppression of intestinal bacteria preoperatively. *Adults:* 1 g P.O. q 1 hour for four doses, then 1 g q 4

hours for the balance of the 24 hours. A saline cathartic should precede therapy. *Children:* 40 to 100 mg/kg P.O. daily divided q 4 to 6 hours. First dose should be preceded by saline cathartic.

• Adjunctive treatment in hepatic coma. *Adults:* 1 to 3 g P.O. q.i.d. for 5 to 6 days.

• Topical bacterial infections, burns, wounds, skin grafts, lesions, pruritus, trophic ulcerations, edema, and following surgical procedure. *Adults and children:* Rub in small amount gently b.i.d., t.i.d., or as directed.

• Dosage adjustments are necessary in renal failure.

neostigmine bromide (Prostigmin Bromide)
neostigmine methylsulfate (Prostigmin)

• Myasthenia gravis. *Adults:* 15 to 30 mg P.O. t.i.d. (range is 15 to 375 mg daily); or 0.5 to 2 mg I.M. or I.V. q 1 to 3 hours. Dosage must be individualized, depending on response and tolerance of adverse reactions. Therapy may be required day and night. *Children:* 7.5 to 15 mg P.O. t.i.d. to q.i.d.

A 1:1,000 injectable solution contains 1 mg/ml; a 1:2,000 solution contains 0.5 mg/ml.

netilmicin sulfate (Netromycin)

• Serious infections caused by aerobic gram-negative bacilli *(Pseudomonas aeruginosa* and some *Enterobacteriaceae)* resistant to gentamicin or tobramycin. *Adults and children over age 12:* 3 to 6.5 mg/kg/day by I.M. injection or I.V. infusion. May be given q 12 hours to treat serious UTIs and q 8 to 12 hours to treat serious systemic infections. *Children age 6 weeks to 12 years:* 5.5 to 8 mg/kg/day by I.M. injection or I.V. infusion given in doses of either 1.8 to 2.7 mg/kg q 8 hours or 2.7 to 4 mg/kg q 12 hours. *Neonates under age 6 weeks:* 4 to 6.5 mg/kg/day by

I.M. injection or I.V. infusion given as 2 to 3.25 mg/kg q 12 hours.

• Dosage adjustments are necessary in renal failure.

nicardipine (Cardene)

• Chronic stable angina (used alone or in combination with beta blockers). *Adults:* Initially, 20 mg P.O. t.i.d. Titrate dosage according to patient response. Usual dosage range is 20 to 40 mg P.O. t.i.d.

• Hypertension. *Adults:* Initially, 20 to 40 mg P.O. t.i.d. Increase dosage according to patient response.

nifedipine (Adalat, Adalat P.A., Procardia, Procardia XL)

• Vasospastic (Prinzmetal's or variant) angina and classic chronic stable angina pectoris, hypertension, and Raynaud's disease. *Adults:* Starting dose is 10 mg P.O. t.i.d. Usual effective dosage range is 10 to 20 mg t.i.d. Some patients may require up to 30 mg q.i.d. Maximum daily dosage is 180 mg.

• Hypertension. *Adults:* 30 to 60 mg P.O. (sustained-release form only) once daily. Titrate over 7- to 14-day period.

nimodipine (Nimotop)

• Improvement of neurologic deficits in patients after subarachnoid hemorrhage from ruptured congenital aneurysms. *Adults:* 60 mg P.O. every 4 hours for 21 days. Therapy should begin within 96 hours after subarachnoid hemorrhage.

nitrofurantoin (Furadantin, Furalan, Furan, Furanite, Macrodantin, Nitrofan)
nitrofurantoin macrocrystals (Macrodantin)

• Pyelonephritis, pyelitis, and cystitis due to susceptible *Escherichia coli, Staphylococcus aureus,* enterococci; certain strains of *Klebsiella, Proteus,* and *Enterobacter. Adults and children over age 12:* 50 to

100 mg P.O. q.i.d. with milk or meals. *Children ages 1 month to 12 years:* 5 to 7 mg/kg P.O. daily, divided q.i.d.
• Long-term suppression therapy. *Adults:* 50 to 100 mg P.O. daily at bedtime. *Children:* 1 to 2 mg/kg P.O. daily at bedtime.

nitroglycerin (Nitro-Bid, Nitro-Dur, Transderm-Nitro)

• Prophylaxis for chronic anginal attacks. *Adults:* One sustained-release capsule q 8 to 12 hours; or if using 2% ointment, start with ½" ointment, increasing by ½" increments until headache occurs, then decrease to previous dose. Range of dosage with ointment is ½" to 5". Usual dose is 1" to 2". Alternatively, transdermal disc or pad (Nitro-Dur or Transderm-Nitro) may be applied to hairless site once daily.
• Relief of acute angina pectoris, prophylaxis for anginal attacks when taken immediately before stressful events. *Adults:* One sublingual tablet (gr ¼₄₀₀, ⅟₂₀₀, ⅟₁₅₀, ⅟₁₀₀) dissolved under the tongue or in the buccal pouch immediately upon indication of anginal attack. May repeat q 5 minutes for 15 minutes. May repeat q 3 to 5 minutes to a maximum of three doses within a 15-minute period. Or, transmucosally, 1 to 3 mg q 3 to 5 hours during waking hours.
• Control of hypertension associated with surgery; treatment of CHF associated with MI; relief of acute angina pectoris; induction of controlled hypotension during surgery (by I.V. infusion). *Adults:* Initial infusion rate is 5 mcg/min. May be increased by 5 mcg/min q 3 to 5 minutes until a response is noted. If a 20 mcg/min rate doesn't produce a response, dosage may be increased by as much as 20 mcg/min q 3 to 5 minutes.

nitroprusside sodium (Nipride, Nitropress)

• Rapid reduction of blood pressure in hypertensive emergencies; hypotension control during anesthesia; reduction of preload and afterload in cardiac pump failure or cardiogenic shock (may be used with or without dopamine). *Adults:* 50-mg vial diluted with 2 to 3 ml of D_5W I.V. and then added to 250, 500, or 1,000 ml of D_5W. Infuse at 0.3 to 10 mcg/kg/min. Average dosage is 3 mcg/kg/min. Maximum infusion rate is 10 mcg/kg/min.
• Patients taking other antihypertensive drugs along with nitroprusside are very sensitive to this drug. Adjust dosage accordingly.

norepinephrine injection (Levophed)

• Restoration of blood pressure in acute hypotension. *Adults:* Initially, 8 to 12 mcg/min by I.V. infusion, then adjust to maintain normal blood pressure. Average maintenance dosage is 2 to 4 mcg/min. *Children:* Initially, 2 mcg/min or 2 mcg/m²/min by I.V. infusion, titrated to maintain desired blood pressure. For advanced cardiac life support, infuse initially at 0.1 mcg/kg/min.

norethindrone acetate (Aygestin, Norlutate)

• Amenorrhea, abnormal uterine bleeding. *Women:* 2.5 to 10 mg P.O. daily on days 5 to 25 of menstrual cycle.
• Endometriosis. *Women:* 5 mg P.O. daily for 14 days; then increase by 2.5 mg daily q 2 weeks up to 15 mg daily.

norfloxacin (Noroxin)

• Complicated and uncomplicated UTIs caused by various gram-negative and gram-positive bacteria, bacterial prostatitis. *Adults:* Complicated infection — 400 mg P.O. b.i.d.

for 10 to 21 days; uncomplicated infection—400 mg P.O. b.i.d. for 7 to 10 days. Do not exceed 800 mg/day. Patients with creatinine clearance below 30 ml/min should receive 400 mg/day for appropriate duration of therapy.

nortriptyline hydrochloride (Aventyl, Pamelor)
• Treatment of depression. *Adults:* 25 mg P.O. t.i.d. or q.i.d., gradually increasing to maximum of 150 mg daily. Alternatively, entire dose may be given at bedtime.

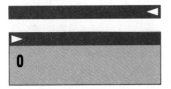

oatmeal (Aveeno)
• Emollient and demulcent for local irritation. *Adults and children:* Use as a lotion; 1 level tablespoon to a cup of warm water.
• Skin irritation, pruritus, common dermatoses, sunburn, dry skin. *Adults:* 1 packet in tub of warm water. *Children:* 1 to 2 rounded tablespoons in 3″ to 4″ (8 to 10 cm) of bath water. *Infants:* 2 or 3 level teaspoons, depending on size of bath.

ofloxacin (Floxin)
• Acute bacterial exacerbations of chronic bronchitis and pneumonia caused by susceptible organisms. *Adults:* 400 mg P.O. or I.V. q 12 hours for 10 days.
• Sexually transmitted diseases (STDs), such as acute uncomplicated urethral and cervical gonorrhea, nongonococcal urethritis and cervicitis, and mixed infections of urethra and cervix. *Adults:* Acute uncomplicated gonorrhea—400 mg P.O. or I.V. once as a single dose; cervicitis and urethritis—300 mg

P.O. or I.V. q 12 hours for 7 days.
• Mild-to-moderate skin and skin-structure infections. *Adults:* 400 mg P.O. or I.V. q 12 hours for 10 days.
• UTIs. *Adults:* Cystitis caused by *Escherichia coli* or *Klebsiella pneumoniae*—200 mg P.O. or I.V. q 12 hours for 3 days; cystitis caused by other organisms—200 mg P.O. or I.V. q 12 hours for 7 days.
• Complicated UTIs. *Adults:* 20 mg P.O. or I.V. q 12 hours for 10 days.
• Prostatitis. *Adults:* 300 mg P.O. or I.V. q 12 hours for 6 weeks.

omeprazole (Prilosec)
• Severe erosive esophagitis or poorly responsive gastroesophageal reflux disease (GERD). *Adults:* 20 mg P.O. daily for 4 to 8 weeks. (Patients with GERD should have failed initial therapy with an histamine$_2$ antagonist.)
• Pathologic hypersecretory conditions (such as Zollinger-Ellison syndrome). *Adults:* Initially, usual dosage is 60 mg P.O. daily with dosage titrated according to patient response. Daily dosages exceeding 80 mg should be given in divided doses. Dosages as high as 120 mg t.i.d. have been administered. Continue therapy as long as clinically indicated.
• Treatment of duodenal ulcer. *Adults:* 20 mg P.O. daily for 4 to 8 weeks.

ondansetron hydrochloride (Zofran)
• Prevention of nausea and vomiting associated with chemotherapy (including high-dose cisplatin). *Adults and children over age 4:* Administer three doses of 0.15 mg/kg I.V.; dilute drug in 50 ml of D_5W or 0.9% sodium chloride solution. Give first dose 30 minutes before chemotherapy; subsequent doses at 4 and 8 hours after first dose.

opium tincture (laudanum)
Controlled Substance Schedule II
opium tincture, camphorated (Paregoric)
Controlled Substance Schedule III
• Acute, nonspecific diarrhea.
Adults: 0.6 ml opium tincture
(range: 0.3 to 1 ml) P.O. q.i.d.; maximum dosage is 6 ml/day. Or 5 to
10 ml camphorated opium tincture
daily, b.i.d., t.i.d., or q.i.d. until diarrhea subsides. *Children:* 0.25 to
0.5 ml/kg camphorated opium tincture daily, b.i.d., t.i.d., or q.i.d. until
diarrhea subsides.

oxacillin sodium (Bactocill, Prostaphlin)
• Systemic infections caused by
Staphylococcus aureus. Adults: 2 to
4 g P.O. daily, divided into doses
given q 6 hours; 2 to 12 g I.M. or
I.V. daily, divided into doses given q
4 to 6 hours. *Children:* 50 to
100 mg/kg P.O. daily, divided into
doses given q 6 hours; 150 to
200 mg/kg I.M. or I.V. daily, divided
into doses given q 4 to 6 hours.

oxazepam (Serax)
Controlled Substance Schedule IV
• Alcohol withdrawal. *Adults:* 15 to
30 mg P.O. t.i.d. or q.i.d.
• Severe anxiety. *Adults:* 15 to
30 mg P.O. t.i.d. or q.i.d.
• Tension, mild-to-moderate anxiety.
Adults: 10 to 15 mg P.O. t.i.d. or
q.i.d.

oxymetazoline hydrochloride (Afrin, Duration, OcuClear)
• Nasal congestion. *Adults and chil-
dren over age 6:* apply 2 to 4 drops
or spray of 0.05% solution to nasal
mucosa b.i.d. *Children ages 2 to 6:*
apply 2 to 3 drops of 0.025% solution to nasal mucosa b.i.d. Use no
longer than 5 days. Dosage for
younger children has not been established.

• Relief of eye redness due to minor
eye irritations. *Adults and children
over age 6:* 1 to 2 drops in the conjunctival sac two to four times daily
(spaced at least 6 hours apart).

oxytetracycline hydrochloride
• Infections caused by sensitive
gram-negative or gram-positive organisms or *Rickettsia;* trachoma.
Adults: 250 mg P.O. q 6 hours; 100
mg I.M. q 8 to 12 hours; or 250 mg
I.M. as a single dose. *Children over
age 8:* 25 to 50 mg/kg P.O. daily, divided q 6 hours; or 15 to 25 mg/kg
I.M. daily, divided q 8 to 12 hours.
• Brucellosis. *Adults:* 500 mg P.O.
q.i.d. for 3 weeks with streptomycin
1 g I.M. q 12 hours first week, once
daily second week.
• Syphilis in patients sensitive to
penicillin. *Adults:* 30 to 40 g total
dosage P.O. divided equally over 10
to 15 days.
• Dosage adjustments are necessary
in renal failure.

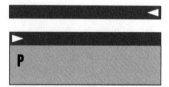

P

pancrelipase (Cotazym capsules)
• Exocrine pancreatic secretion insufficiency, cystic fibrosis in adults
and children, steatorrhea and other
disorders of fat metabolism secondary to insufficient pancreatic enzymes. *Adults and children:* Dose
must be titrated to patient's response. Dosage ranges from 1 to 3
capsules or tablets P.O. before or
with meals and 1 capsule or tablet
with snack; or 1 to 2 powder packets before meals or snacks.

paramethadione (Paradione)
• Refractory absence seizures.
Adults: initially, 300 mg P.O. t.i.d.
May increase by 300 mg weekly, up

to 600 mg q.i.d., if needed. *Children over age 6:* 0.9 g P.O. daily in divided doses t.i.d. or q.i.d. *Children ages 2 to 6:* 0.6 g P.O. daily in divided doses t.i.d. or q.i.d. *Children under age 2:* 0.3 g P.O. daily in divided doses b.i.d.

penbutolol sulfate (Levatol)
• Mild-to-moderate hypertension. *Adults:* 20 mg P.O. once daily. Usually given with other antihypertensive agents, such as thiazide diuretics.

penicillin G benzathine
• Congenital syphilis. *Children under age 2:* 50,000 units/kg I.M. as a single dose.
• Group A streptococcal upper respiratory infections. *Adults:* 1.2 million units I.M. in a single injection. *Children who weigh 27 kg or more:* 900,000 units I.M. in a single injection. *Children weighing less than 27 kg:* 300,000 to 600,000 units I.M. in a single injection.
• Prophylaxis of poststreptococcal rheumatic fever. *Adults and children:* 1.2 million units I.M. once a month or 600,000 units twice a month.
• Syphilis of less than 1 year's duration. *Adults:* 2.4 million units I.M. in a single dose.
• Syphilis of more than 1 year's duration. *Adults:* 2.4 million units I.M. weekly for 3 successive weeks.

penicillin G potassium
Moderate-to-severe systemic infections. *Adults:* 1.6 to 3.2 million units P.O. daily, divided into doses given q 6 hours (1 mg = 1,600 units); or 1.2 to 2.4 million units I.M. or I.V. daily, divided into doses given q 4 hours. *Children:* 25,000 to 100,000 units/kg P.O. daily, divided into doses given q 6 hours; or 25,000 to 300,000 units/kg I.M. or I.V. daily, divided into doses given q 4 hours.

penicillin G procaine
• Moderate-to-severe systemic infections. *Adults:* 600,000 to 1.2 million units I.M. daily as a single dose. *Children:* 300,000 units I.M. daily as a single dose.
• Uncomplicated gonorrhea. *Adults and children over age 12:* 1 g probenecid; then 30 minutes later, 4.8 million units of penicillin G procaine I.M., divided into two injection sites.
• Pneumococcal pneumonia. *Adults and children over age 12:* 300,000 to 600,000 units I.M. daily for 7 to 10 days.

penicillin G sodium
• Moderate-to-severe systemic infections. *Adults:* 1.2 to 24 million units I.M. or I.V. daily, divided into doses given q 4 hours. *Children:* 25,000 to 300,000 units/kg I.M. or I.V. daily, divided into doses given q 4 hours.
• Endocarditis prophylaxis for dental surgery. *Adults:* 2 million units I.V. or I.M. 30 to 60 minutes before procedure, then 1 million units 6 hours later.
• Dosage adjustments are necessary in renal failure.

penicillin V potassium
• Mild-to-moderate susceptible infections. *Adults:* 250 to 500 mg (400,000 to 800,000 units) P.O. q 6 hours. *Children:* 15 to 50 mg/kg (25,000 to 90,000 units/kg) P.O. daily, divided into doses given q 6 to 8 hours.
• Endocarditis prophylaxis for dental surgery. *Adults:* 2 g P.O. 30 to 60 minutes before procedure, then 1 g P.O. 6 hours afterwards. *Children weighing less than 30 kg:* Half the adult dose.

phenelzine sulfate (Nardil)
• Depression. *Adults:* 45 mg P.O. daily in divided doses, increasing rapidly to 60 mg daily. Then dosage can usually be reduced to 15 mg

daily. Maximum dosage is 90 mg daily.

phenobarbital (Barbita) phenobarbital sodium (Luminal Sodium)

Controlled Substance Schedule IV

• All forms of epilepsy, febrile seizures in children. *Adults:* 60 to 200 mg P.O. daily, divided t.i.d. or given as single dose at bedtime. *Children:* 3 to 6 mg/kg P.O. daily, usually divided q 12 hours but can be administered once daily.

• Status epilepticus. *Adults:* 200 to 600 mg as I.V. infusion no faster than 50 mg/minute. May give up to 20 mg/kg total. Administer in acute care or emergency area only. *Children:* 10 to 400 mg I.V. injection at a rate not exceeding 50 mg/minute.

• Sedation. *Adults:* 30 to 120 mg P.O. daily in two or three divided doses. *Children:* 3 to 5 mg/kg P.O. divided t.i.d.

• Insomnia. *Adults:* 100 to 200 mg P.O. or I.M.

phenylephrine hydrochloride (Neo-Synephrine)

• Hypotensive emergencies during spinal anesthesia. *Adults:* Initially, 0.10 to 0.2 mg I.V., then subsequent doses of 0.1 to 0.2 mg I.V. p.r.n.

• Maintenance of blood pressure during spinal or inhalation anesthesia. *Adults:* 2 to 3 mg S.C. or I.M. 3 to 4 minutes before anesthesia. *Children:* 0.044 to 0.088 mg/kg S.C. or I.M.

• Vasoconstrictor for regional anesthesia. *Adults:* 1 mg phenylephrine added to 20 ml local anesthetic.

• Mild-to-moderate hypotension. *Adults:* Initially, 2 to 5 mg S.C. or I.M. Alternatively, give 0.1 to 0.5 mg by slow I.V., repeated q 10 to 15 minutes.

• Paroxysmal supraventricular tachycardia. *Adults:* Initially, 0.5 mg by rapid I.V.; subsequent doses shouldn't exceed the preceding dose

by more than 0.1 to 0.2 mg and shouldn't exceed 1 mg.

• Severe hypotension and shock (including drug-induced). *Adults:* 10 mg in 500 ml of D_5W. Start at 100 to 180 drops per minute by I.V. infusion; then decrease to 40 to 60 drops per minute. Adjust to patient response.

• Mydriasis without cycloplegia. *Adults and children:* 1 or 2 drops of solution instilled before examination. May repeat in 10 to 60 minutes if needed.

• Nasal congestion. *Adults:* 2 or 3 drops or 1 to 2 sprays of 0.25% to 1% solution; or jelly or spray applied to nasal mucosa. *Children ages 6 to 12:* 2 to 3 drops or 1 to 2 sprays of 0.25% solution. *Children under age 6:* 2 to 3 drops or 1 to 2 sprays of 0.125% solution. Give drops, spray, or jelly q 4 hours p.r.n.

phenytoin (Dilantin)

• Control of tonic-clonic (grand mal) and complex partial (temporal lobe) seizures. *Adults:* Highly individualized. Initially, 100 mg P.O. t.i.d., increased in increments of 100 mg P.O. every 2 to 4 weeks until desired response is obtained. Usual range is 300 to 600 mg daily. If patient stabilizes with extended-release capsules, once-daily dosing with 300-mg extended-release capsules may be used as an alternative. *Children:* 5 mg/kg or 250 mg/m^2 P.O. daily b.i.d. or t.i.d. Maximum daily dosage is 300 mg.

• For patient requiring a loading dose. *Adults:* Initially, 1 g P.O. daily divided into three doses and administered at 2-hour intervals. Alternatively, 10 to 15 mg/kg I.V. at a rate not exceeding 50 mg/minute. Normal maintenance dosage instituted 24 hours later. *Children:* 5 mg/kg/day P.O. in two or three equally divided doses; subsequent dosage individualized to a maximum of 300 mg daily.

• Prevention and treatment of seizures occurring during neurosurgery. *Adults:* 100 to 200 mg I.M. q 4 hours during surgery and continued during the postoperative period.

• Status epilepticus. *Adults:* loading dose of 10 to 15 mg/kg I.V. (1 to 1.5 g may be needed) at a rate not exceeding 50 mg/minute, followed by maintenance doses of 100 mg P.O. or I.V. q 6 to 8 hours. *Children:* loading dose of 15 to 20 mg/kg I.V. at a rate not exceeding 1 to 3 mg/kg/minute, followed by highly individualized maintenance dosages.

pindolol (Visken)

• Hypertension. *Adults:* Initially, 5 mg P.O. b.i.d.; may be increased by 10 mg/day q 2 to 3 weeks up to a maximum of 60 mg/day.

piperacillin sodium (Pipracil)

• Infections caused by susceptible organisms. *Adults and children over age 12:* 100 to 300 mg/kg/day I.V. or I.M. divided q 4 to 6 hours. Usual dosage is 3 g q 4 hours (18 g/day). Maximum daily dosage is usually 24 g. Usually administered with an aminoglycoside. Dosage for children under age 12 has not been established.

• Prophylaxis of surgical infections. *Adults:* 2 g I.V. given 30 to 60 minutes before surgery. Depending on type of surgery, dose may be repeated during surgery, and once or twice more after surgery, according to the manufacturer. However, clinicians strongly discourage this practice.

• Dosage adjustments are necessary in renal failure.

piroxicam (Feldene)

• Osteoarthritis and rheumatoid arthritis. *Adults:* 20 mg P.O. once daily. If desired, the dosage may be divided.

potassium chloride (Kaon-Cl, Kay Ciel, Slow-K)

• Hypokalemia. *Adults:* 40 to 100 mEq P.O. daily in three or four divided doses for treatment; 20 mEq daily for prevention. Further dosage based on serum potassium levels. Use I.V. route when oral replacement isn't feasible or when hypokalemia is life-threatening. Usual dose is 20 mEq/hour in concentration of 40 mEq/liter or less. Total daily dosage not to exceed 150 mEq (3 mEq/kg in children).

pravastatin sodium (Pravachol)

• Reduction of low-density lipoprotein and total cholesterol levels in primary hypercholesterolemia (Types IIA and IIB). *Adults:* Initially, 10 or 20 mg h.s. daily; adjust dose q 4 weeks based on patient tolerance and response. Maximum daily dosage is 40 mg. Most elderly patients respond to daily dosage of 20 mg or less.

prazosin hydrochloride (Minipress)

• Mild-to-moderate hypertension (used alone or in combination with a diuretic or other antihypertensive drug); also used to decrease afterload in severe chronic CHF. *Adults:* P.O. test dose is 1 mg given before bedtime to prevent "first-dose syncope." Initial dosage is 1 mg t.i.d. Increase dosage slowly. Maximum daily dosage is 20 mg. Maintenance dosage is 6 to 15 mg daily in three divided doses, but a few patients have required larger dosages (up to 40 mg daily). If other antihypertensive drugs or diuretics are added to this drug, decrease prazosin dosage to 1 to 2 mg t.i.d. and retitrate.

prednisolone (Delta-Cortef, Prelone)
prednisolone acetate (Key-Pred, Predaject)
prednisolone sodium phosphate (Hydeltrasol, Key-Pred-SP, Pediapred)

• Severe inflammation or immuno-suppression. *Adults:* 2.5 to 15 mg P.O. b.i.d., t.i.d., or q.i.d.; 2 to 30 mg I.M. (acetate, phosphate) or I.V. (phosphate) q 12 hours; or 2 to 30 mg I.M. or I.V. (phosphate).

prednisone (Deltasone)

• Severe inflammation or immuno-suppression. *Adults:* 2.5 to 15 mg P.O. b.i.d., t.i.d., or q.i.d. Maintenance dosage is given once daily or every other day. Dosage must be individualized.

primidone (Myidone, Mysoline)

• Generalized tonic-clonic seizures, complex-partial (psychomotor) seizures. *Adults and children over age 8:* Initially, 100 to 125 mg P.O. h.s. on days 1 to 3, then 100 to 125 mg P.O. b.i.d. on days 4 to 6, then 100 to 125 mg P.O. on days 7 to 9, followed by maintenance dosage of 250 mg P.O. t.i.d. *Children under age 8:* Initially, 50 mg P.O. h.s., then 50 mg P.O. b.i.d., then 100 mg P.O. b.i.d., followed by maintenance dosage of 125 to 250 mg P.O. t.i.d.

probucol (Lorelco)

• Primary hypercholesterolemia. *Adults:* Two tablets (500 mg total) P.O. b.i.d. with morning and evening meals. Not recommended for children.

procainamide hydrochloride (Procan SR, Promine, Pronestyl, Pronestyl-SR)

• Life-threatening ventricular arrhythmias. *Adults:* 100 mg q 5 minutes by slow I.V. push, no faster than 25 to 50 mg/min until arrhythmias disappear, adverse reactions develop, or 1 g has been given. When arrhythmias disappear, give continuous infusion of 2 to 6 mg/min. Usual effective dose is 500 to 600 mg. If arrhythmias recur, repeat bolus as above and increase infusion rate. Alternatively, 0.5 to 1 g I.M. q 4 to 8 hours until oral therapy begins. For oral therapy, 50 mg/kg P.O. q 3 hours daily; average is 250 to 500 mg q 3 hours.

Sustained-release tablet may be used for maintenance dosing when treating ventricular tachycardia, atrial fibrillation, and paroxysmal atrial tachycardia. Dosage is 500 mg to 1 g q 6 hours.)

prochlorperazine (Compazine, Stemetil)

• Preoperative nausea control. *Adults:* 5 to 10 mg I.M. 1 to 2 hours before induction of anesthesia, repeated once in 30 minutes if necessary; or 5 to 10 mg I.V. 15 to 30 minutes before induction of anesthesia, repeated once if necessary; or 20 mg/liter of D_5W and 0.9% sodium chloride solution by I.V. infusion, added to infusion 15 to 30 minutes before induction. Maximum parenteral dosage is 40 mg/day.
• Severe nausea, vomiting. *Adults:* 5 to 10 mg P.O. t.i.d. or q.i.d.; or 15 mg sustained-release form P.O. on arising; or 10 mg sustained-release form P.O. q 12 hours; or 25 mg rectally b.i.d.; or 5 to 10 mg I.M. injected deep into upper outer quadrant of gluteal region. Repeat q 3 to 4 hours, p.r.n. Maximum I.M. dosage is 40 mg/day.

procyclidine hydrochloride (Kemadrin, PMS Procyclidine, Procyclid)

• Parkinsonism, muscle rigidity. *Adults:* Initially, 2 to 2.5 mg P.O. t.i.d. after meals. Increase as needed to 5 mg P.O. t.i.d. after meals and occasionally 5 mg P.O. h.s. daily.

progesterone (Gesterol, Progestaject, Progestasert)

• Amenorrhea. *Women:* 5 to 10 mg I.M. daily for 6 to 8 days, usually beginning 8 to 10 days before anticipated start of menses.
• Dysfunctional uterine bleeding. *Women:* 5 to 10 mg I.M. daily for six doses. Give oil solution via deep I.M. injection and check sites frequently for irritation. Rotate sites.
• Contraception (as an intrauterine device). *Women:* Progestasert system inserted into uterine cavity. Replace after 1 year.

propantheline bromide (Pro-Banthine)

• Adjunctive treatment of peptic ulcer, irritable bowel syndrome, and other GI disorders; to reduce duodenal motility during diagnostic radiologic procedures. *Adults:* 15 mg P.O. t.i.d. before meals and 30 mg h.s., up to 60 mg q.i.d. For elderly patients, 7.5 mg P.O. t.i.d. before meals.

propranolol hydrochloride (Inderal, Inderal LA)

• Management of angina pectoris. *Adults:* 10 to 20 mg t.i.d. or q.i.d. Or one 80-mg sustained-release capsule daily. Dosage may be increased at 7- to 10-day intervals. Usual optimal dosage is 160 to 240 mg daily.
• Reduction of mortality after MI. *Adults:* 180 to 240 mg P.O. daily in divided doses, beginning 5 to 21 days after MI has occurred. Usually administered t.i.d. to q.i.d.

• Supraventricular, ventricular, and atrial arrhythmias; tachyarrhythmias caused by excessive catecholamine action during anesthesia, hyperthyroidism, and pheochromocytoma. *Adults:* 0.5 to 3 mg I.V. diluted in 50 ml of D_5W or 0.9% sodium chloride solution infused slowly, not to exceed 1 mg/minute. After 3 mg have been infused, another dose may be given in 2 minutes and subsequent doses no sooner than q 4 hours. May be diluted and infused slowly. Usual maintenance dosage is 10 to 30 mg P.O. t.i.d. or q.i.d.
• Hypertension. *Adults:* Initially, 80 mg P.O. daily in two to four divided doses or the sustained-release form once daily. Increase at 3- to 7-day intervals to maximum daily dosage of 640 mg. Usual maintenance dosage is 160 to 480 mg daily.
• Prevention of frequent, severe, or disabling migraine or vascular headache. *Adults:* Initially, 80 mg P.O. daily in divided doses or 1 sustained-release capsule. Usual maintenance dosage is 160 to 240 mg daily divided t.i.d. or q.i.d.

propylthiouracil (PTU) (Propyl-Thyracil)

• Hyperthyroidism. *Adults:* 100 to 150 mg P.O. t.i.d., up to 300 mg q 8 hours in severe cases. Continue until patient is euthyroid; then start maintenance dosage of 100 to 150 mg daily to t.i.d. *Children over age 10:* 150 to 300 mg P.O. t.i.d. Continue until patient is euthyroid; then start maintenance dosage of 25 mg t.i.d. to 100 mg b.i.d. *Children ages 6 to 10:* 50 to 150 mg P.O. in divided doses q 8 hours.
• Preparation for thyroidectomy. *Adults and children:* 200 mg q 4 to 6 hours on first day; once full control of symptoms is achieved, dosage gradually reduced to maintenance levels.

DRUG DOSAGES & INDICATIONS

• Thyrotoxic crisis. *Adults and children:* same doses as for hyperthyroidism, with concomitant iodine therapy and propranolol.

protriptyline hydrochloride (Triptil, Vivactil)
• Treatment of depression. *Adults:* 15 to 40 mg P.O. daily in divided doses, increasing gradually to maximum of 60 mg daily.

pseudoephedrine hydrochloride (Sudafed)
• Nasal and eustachian tube decongestant. *Adults:* 60 mg P.O. q 4 hours. Maximum dosage is 240 mg/day. *Children ages 6 to 12:* 30 mg P.O. q 4 hours. Maximum dosage is 120 mg daily. *Children ages 2 to 6:* 15 mg P.O. q 4 hours. Maximum dosage is 60 mg/day.
• Relief of nasal congestion. *Adults:* 120 mg q 12 hours.

pyridostigmine bromide (Mestinon, Mestinon Supraspan, Mestinon Timespan, Regonol)
• Myasthenia gravis. *Adults:* 60 to 120 mg P.O. q 3 or 4 hours. Usual dosage is 600 mg daily but higher dosage may be needed (up to 1,500 mg daily). Give $1/30$ of oral dose I.M. or I.V. Dosage must be adjusted for each patient, depending on response and tolerance of adverse reactions. Alternatively, may give 180 to 540 mg timed-release tablets (1 to 3 tablets) b.i.d., with at least 6 hours between doses.

Q

quinapril hydrochloride (Accupril)
• Hypertension. *Adults:* Initially, 10 mg daily. Adjust dosage based on patient response at 2 week intervals. Most patients are controlled at 20, 40, or 80 mg daily, as a single dose or in 2 divided doses.

quinidine gluconate (62% quinidine base) (Quinaglute Dura-Tabs)
quinidine polygalacturonate (60.5% quinidine base) (Cardioquin)
quinidine sulfate (83% quinidine base) (Cin-Quin, Quine, Quinidex Extentabs, Quinora)
• Atrial flutter or fibrillation. *Adults:* 200 mg quinidine sulfate or equivalent base P.O. q 2 to 3 hours for 5 to 8 doses with subsequent daily increases until sinus rhythm is restored or toxic effects develop. Administer quinidine only after digitalization to avoid increasing atrioventricular conduction. Maximum dosage is 3 to 4 g daily.
• Paroxysmal supraventricular tachycardia. *Adults:* 400 to 600 mg I.M. quinidine gluconate q 2 to 3 hours until toxic effects develop or arrhythmia subsides.
• Premature atrial contractions; PVCs; paroxysmal atrioventricular junctional rhythm; paroxysmal atrial tachycardia; paroxysmal ventricular tachycardia; maintenance after cardioversion of atrial fibrillation or flutter. *Adults:* Test dose is 200 mg P.O. or I.M., then monitor vital signs before beginning therapy. Quinidine sulfate or equivalent base 200 to 400 mg P.O. q 4 to 6 hours; or initially, quinidine gluconate 600 mg I.M., then up to 400 mg q 2 hours, p.r.n.; or quinidine gluconate 800 mg (10 ml of the commercially available solution) added to 40 ml of D_5W, given by I.V. infusion at 16 mg (1 ml)/minute. *Children:* Test dose is 2 mg/kg; then give 3 to 6 mg/kg q 2 to 3 hours for 5 doses P.O. daily.

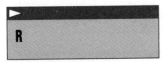

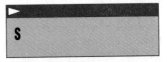

ramipril (Altace)

• Essential hypertension. *Adults:* Initially, 2.5 mg P.O. once daily. Increase dosage based on patient response. Maintenance dosage is 2.5 to 20 mg daily, as a single dose or in divided doses.

ranitidine (Zantac)

• Duodenal and gastric ulcer (short-term treatment); pathologic hypersecretory conditions, such as Zollinger-Ellison syndrome. *Adults:* 150 mg P.O. b.i.d. or 300 mg once daily h.s. Dosages up to 6 g/day may be prescribed for patients with Zollinger-Ellison syndrome. May also be administered parenterally: 50 mg I.V. or I.M. q 6 to 8 hours. When administering I.V. push, dilute to a volume of 20 ml and inject over a 5-minute period. No dilution necessary when administering I.M. May also be administered by intermittent I.V. infusion: Dilute 50 mg ranitidine in 100 ml of D₅W and infuse over 15 to 20 minutes.
• Maintenance therapy of duodenal ulcer. *Adults:* 150 mg P.O. h.s.
• Gastroesophageal reflux disease. *Adults:* 150 mg P.O. b.i.d.

reserpine (Reserfia, Serpalan, Serpasil)

• Mild-to-moderate essential hypertension. *Adults:* 0.1 to 0.25 mg P.O. daily. *Children:* 5 to 20 mcg/kg P.O. daily.

salicylic acid (Calicylic, Keralyt, Salaptic Liquifilm, Salenil, Trans-Ver-Sal)

Superficial fungal infections, acne, psoriasis, seborrheic dermatitis, other scaling dermatoses, hyperkeratosis, calluses, warts. *Adults and children:* apply to affected area and cover with occlusive bandage at night.

scopolamine (Transderm-Scōp, Transderm-V)

• Prevention of nausea and vomiting associated with motion sickness. *Adults:* One Transderm-Scōp system (a circular flat unit), programmed to deliver 0.5 mg scopolamine over 3 days (72 hours), applied to the skin behind the ear several hours before the antiemetic is required.
  Not recommended for children.

sertraline hydrochloride (Zoloft)

• Obsessive-compulsive disorder. *Adults:* 50 mg P.O. daily. Adjust as needed and tolerated at intervals of at least 1 week.

silver nitrate 1%

• Prevention of gonorrheal ophthalmia neonatorum. *Neonates:* Clean lids thoroughly; instill 1 drop of 1% solution into each eye.

simethicone (Gas-X, Mylicon, Ovol, Phazyme, Silain)

• Flatulence, functional gastric bloating. *Adults and children over age 12:* 40 to 125 mg after each meal and h.s.

simvastatin (Zocor)

• Reduction of low-density lipoprotein and total cholesterol levels in patients with primary hypercholes-

DRUG DOSAGES & INDICATIONS

terolemia (types IIa and IIb). *Adults:* Initially, 5 to 10 mg h.s. Adjust dosage q 4 weeks based on patient tolerance and response. Maximum daily dosage is 40 mg.

sodium bicarbonate

• Metabolic acidosis. *Adults and children:* dosage depends on blood CO_2 content, pH, and patient's clinical condition. Usually, 2 to 5 mEq/kg I.V. is infused over 4 to 8 hours.
• Systemic or urinary alkalinization. *Adults:* 325 mg to 2 g P.O. q.i.d. *Children:* 84 to 840 mg/kg daily.

sodium biphosphate (Fleet Enema)
sodium phosphate

• Constipation. *Adults:* 20 to 30 ml solution mixed with 120 ml of cold water P.O.; or 60 to 135 ml as an enema. *Children:* 5 to 15 ml solution mixed with 120 ml of cold water P.O.; or 67.5 ml as enema.

sodium lactate

• Alkalinize urine. *Adults:* 30 ml of $^1/_6$ molar solution/kg of body weight in divided doses over 24 hours.
• Metabolic acidosis. *Adults:* usually given as ⅙ molar injection (167 mEq lactate/liter). Dosage depends on degree of bicarbonate deficit.

sodium polystyrene sulfonate (Kayexalate, SPS)

• Hyperkalemia. *Adults:* 15 g P.O. daily to q.i.d. in water or sorbitol (3 to 4 ml/g of resin). *Children:* 1 g of resin P.O. for each mEq of potassium to be removed.
• Rectal administration. *Adults:* 30 to 50 g/100 ml of sorbitol q 6 hours as warm emulsion deep into sigmoid colon (8″ or 20 cm).
• Persistent vomiting or paralytic ileus. High-retention enema of sodium polystyrene sulfonate (30 g)

suspended in 200 ml of 10% methylcellulose, 10% dextrose, or 25% sorbitol solution.

sodium thiosalicylate (Rexolate, Tusal)

• Mild pain. *Adults:* 50 to 100 mg daily or every other day, I.M. or slow I.V.
• Arthritis. *Adults:* 100 mg daily I.M. or slow I.V.

somatrem (Protropin)

• Long-term treatment of children who have growth failure because of lack of adequate endogenous growth hormone secretion. *Children (pre-puberty):* 0.1 mg/kg I.M. or S.C. given three times weekly.

streptomycin sulfate

• Primary and adjunctive treatment in tuberculosis. *Adults with normal renal function:* 1 g or 15 mg/kg I.M. daily for 2 to 3 months, then 1 g two or three times a week. Inject deeply into upper outer quadrant of buttocks. *Children with normal renal function:* 20 to 40 mg/kg I.M. daily in divided doses injected deeply into large muscle mass. Give concurrently with other antitubercular agents, but *not* with capreomycin, and continue until sputum specimen becomes negative.
• Enterococcal endocarditis. *Adults:* 1 g I.M. q 12 hours for 2 weeks, then 500 mg I.M. q 12 hours for 4 weeks with penicillin.
• Tularemia. *Adults:* 1 to 2 g I.M. daily in divided doses injected deep into upper outer quadrant of buttocks. Continue until patient is afebrile for 5 to 7 days.
• Dosage adjustments are necessary in renal failure.

sucralfate (Carafate, Sulcrate)

• Short-term (up to 8 weeks) treatment of duodenal ulcer. *Adults:* 1 g P.O. q.i.d. 1 hour before meals and h.s.

sulfacetamide sodium 10% (Bleph-10 Liquifilm Ophthalmic, Cetamide Ophthalmic, Sodium Sulamyd 10% Ophthalmic, Sulf-10 Ophthalmic)
sulfacetamide sodium 15% (Isopto Cetamide Ophthalmic)
sulfacetamide sodium 30% (Sodium Sulamyd 30% Ophthalmic)

• Inclusion conjunctivitis, corneal ulcers, trachoma, prophylaxis to ocular infection. *Adults and children:* Instill 1 to 2 drops of 10% solution into lower conjunctival sac q 2 to 3 hours during day, less often at night; or instill 1 to 2 drops of 15% solution into lower conjunctival sac q 1 to 2 hours initially, increasing interval as condition responds; or instill 1 drop of 30% solution into lower conjunctival sac q 2 hours. Instill ½" to 1" of 10% ointment into conjunctival sac q.i.d. and h.s. May use ointment at night along with drops during the day.

sulfadiazine (Microsulfon)

• UTIs. *Adults:* Initially, 2 to 4 g P.O., then 2 to 4 g daily in three to six doses q 24 hours. *Children over age 2 months:* Initially, 75 mg/kg or 2 g/m^2 P.O., then 150 mg/kg or 4 g/m^2 in four to six divided doses daily. Maximum daily dosage is 6 g.
• Adjunctive treatment in toxoplasmosis. *Adults:* 2 to 8 g P.O. daily. Usually given with pyrimethamine. *Children:* 100 to 200 mg/kg P.O. daily. Usually given with pyrimethamine.

sulfamethoxazole (Gantanol)

• UTIs. *Adults:* Initially, 2 g P.O.; then 1 g P.O. b.i.d., up to t.i.d. for severe infections. *Children and infants over age 2 months:* Initially, 50 to 60 mg/kg P.O., then 25 to 30 mg/kg b.i.d. Maximum dosage should not exceed 75 mg/kg daily.

sulfasalazine (Azulfidine)

• Mild-to-moderate ulcerative colitis, adjunctive therapy in severe ulcerative colitis. *Adults:* Initially, 3 to 4 g P.O. daily in evenly divided doses. Maintenance dosage is 1.5 to 2 g P.O. daily in divided doses q 6 hours. May need to start with 1 to 2 g initially, with a gradual increase in dose to minimize adverse reactions. *Children over age 2:* Initially, 40 to 60 mg/kg P.O. daily, divided into three to six doses; then 30 mg/kg daily in four doses. May need to start at lower dose if gastrointestinal intolerance occurs.

sulfisoxazole (Gantrisin)

• UTIs. *Adults:* Initially, 2 to 4 g P.O.; then 4 to 8 g P.O. daily in divided doses q 4 to 6 hours. *Children and infants over age 2 months:* Initially, 75 mg/kg P.O.; then 150 mg/kg (or 4 g/m^2) P.O. daily in divided doses q 4 to 6 hours. Maximum dosage should not exceed 6 g in 24 hours.
• Conjunctivitis, corneal ulcer, superficial ocular infections; adjunct in systemic treatment of trachoma. *Adults:* 2 to 3 drops in eye three or more times daily or small ribbon of ointment in lower conjunctival sac one to three times daily and h.s.

sulindac (Clinoril)

• Osteoarthritis, RA, ankylosing spondylitis. *Adults:* 150 mg P.O. b.i.d. initially; may increase to 200 mg P.O. b.i.d.
• Acute bursitis or tendinitis, acute gouty arthritis. *Adults:* 200 mg P.O. b.i.d. for 7 to 14 days. Dosage may be reduced as symptoms subside.

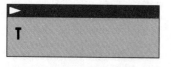

terazosin hydrochloride (Hytrin)
• Hypertension. *Adults:* Initial dose is 1 mg P.O. h.s., gradually increased according to patient response. Usual dosage range is 1 to 5 mg daily. Maximum recommended dosage is 20 mg/day.
• Symptomatic benign prostatic hyperplasia. *Adults:* Initially, 1 mg P.O. h.s. Dosage increased in a stepwise fashion to 2 mg, 5 mg, or 10 mg once daily to achieve optimal response.

terfenadine (Seldane)
• Rhinitis, allergy symptoms. *Adults and children over age 12:* 60 mg P.O. b.i.d.

tetracycline hydrochloride (Achromycin V)
• Infections caused by sensitive organisms. *Adults:* 250 to 500 mg P.O. q 6 hours. *Children over age 8:* 25 to 50 mg/kg P.O. daily, divided q 6 hours.
• Uncomplicated urethral, endocervical, or rectal infection. *Adults:* 500 mg P.O. q.i.d. for at least 7 days.
• Brucellosis. *Adults:* 500 mg P.O. q 6 hours for 3 weeks, with streptomycin 1 g I.M. q 12 hours week 1 and daily week 2.
• Gonorrhea in patients sensitive to penicillin. *Adults:* Initially, 1.5 g P.O., then 500 mg q 6 hours for 7 days.
• Syphilis in nonpregnant patients sensitive to penicillin. *Adults:* 500 mg P.O., q.i.d. for 14 days.
• Acne. *Adults and adolescents:* Initially, 250 mg P.O. q 6 hours, then 125 to 500 mg P.O. daily or every other day; apply topical ointment generously to affected areas b.i.d. until skin is thoroughly wet.
• Superficial ocular infections and inclusion conjunctivitis. *Adults and children:* Instill 1 to 2 drops of ophthalmic solution in eye b.i.d., q.i.d., or more often, depending on severity of infection.
• Trachoma. *Adults and children:* Instill 2 drops of ophthalmic solution in each eye b.i.d., t.i.d., or q.i.d.; continue for 1 to 2 months or longer. Or use 1% ointment t.i.d. or q.i.d. for 30 days.
• Prophylaxis of ophthalmia neonatorum. *Neonates:* 1 to 2 drops of ophthalmic solution in each eye shortly after delivery.
• Infection prophylaxis in minor skin abrasions and treatment of superficial infections caused by susceptible organisms. *Adults and children:* Apply topical ointment to infected area b.i.d. or t.i.d.

tetrahydrozoline hydrochloride (Tyzine, Tyzine Pediatric, Visine)
• Nasal congestion. *Adults and children over age 6:* apply 2 to 4 drops of 0.1% solution or spray to nasal mucosa q 4 to 6 hours, p.r.n. *Children ages 2 to 6:* apply 2 to 3 drops of 0.05% solution to nasal mucosa q 4 to 6 hours, p.r.n.
• Conjunctival congestion, irritation, and allergy. *Adults and children over age 2:* 1 to 2 drops of 0.05% solution up to 4 times daily or as directed.

theophylline immediate-release tablets and capsules (Bronkodyl, Elixophyllin, Slo-Phyllin)
theophylline immediate-release liquids (Aerolate, Elixophyllin)
theophylline timed-release capsules (Aerolate, Slo-Bid Gyrocaps)
theophylline timed-release tablets (Quibron-T/SR, Uniphyl)
• Prophylaxis and symptomatic relief of bronchial asthma, bronchospasm of chronic bronchitis, and emphysema. *Adults:* 6 mg/kg P.O. followed by 2 to 3 mg/kg q 4 hours for two doses. Maintenance dosage

is 1 to 3 mg/kg q 8 to 12 hours. *Children ages 9 to 16:* 6 mg/kg P.O. followed by 3 mg/kg q 4 hours for three doses. Maintenance dosage is 3 mg/kg q 6 hours. *Children ages 6 months to 9 years:* 6 mg/kg P.O. followed by 4 mg/kg q 4 hours for three doses. Maintenance dosage is 4 mg/kg q 6 hours.

Most oral timed-release forms are given q 8 to 12 hours. Several products, however, may be given q 24 hours.

thiothixene (Navane) thiothixene hydrochloride (Navane Concentrate)

• Acute agitation. *Adults:* 4 mg I.M. b.i.d. to q.i.d. Maximum dosage is 30 mg daily I.M. Change to P.O. route as soon as possible.
• Mild-to-moderate psychosis. *Adults:* Initially, 2 mg P.O. t.i.d. May increase gradually to 15 mg daily.
• Severe psychosis. *Adults:* Initially, 5 mg P.O. b.i.d. May increase gradually to 15 to 30 mg daily. Maximum recommended daily dosage is 60 mg. Alternatively, 4 mg I.M. b.i.d. or q.i.d. Maximum dosage is 30 mg I.M. daily. An oral form should supplant the injectable form as soon as possible. Not recommended for children under age 12.

thyroid USP

• Mild hypothyroidism. *Adults:* Initially, 60 mg P.O. daily, increased by 60 mg q 30 days until desired response occurs. Usual maintenance dosage is 60 to 180 mg daily as a single dose.
• Severe hypothyroidism. *Adults:* Initially, 15 mg P.O. daily, increased by 30 mg daily after 2 weeks, and 2 weeks later increased to 60 mg daily. After 2 months, dosage increased to 120 mg daily as needed for the following 2 months. Then dosage is increased to 180 mg daily as needed.
• Congenital or severe hypothyroid-

ism in children. *Children:* same as adults with severe hypothyroidism.

ticarcillin disodium/clavulanate potassium (Timentin)

• Infections of the lower respiratory tract, urinary tract, bones and joints, skin and skin structure, and septicemia when caused by susceptible organisms. *Adults:* 3.1 g (contains 3 g ticarcillin and 0.1 g clavulanate potassium) diluted in 50 to 100 ml of D_5W, 0.9% sodium chloride, or lactated Ringer's solution and administered by I.V. infusion over 30 minutes q 4 to 6 hours.
• Renal failure. Loading dose is 3.1 g (3 g ticarcillin with 100 mg clavulanate). Dosage adjustments are necessary.

timolol maleate (Blocadren)

• Hypertension. *Adults:* Initially, 10 mg P.O. b.i.d. Usual daily maintenance dosage is 20 to 40 mg. Maximum daily dosage is 60 mg. Drug is used either alone or in combination with diuretics.
• MI (long-term prophylaxis in patients who have survived acute phase). *Adults:* 10 mg P.O. b.i.d.

timolol maleate (Timoptic Solution)

• Chronic open-angle glaucoma, secondary glaucoma, aphakic glaucoma, ocular hypertension. *Adults:* Initially, instill 1 drop of 0.25% solution in each eye b.i.d.; reduce to 1 drop daily for maintenance. If patient doesn't respond, instill 1 drop of 0.5% solution in each eye b.i.d. If intraocular pressure is controlled, dosage may be reduced to 1 drop in each eye daily.

tobramycin sulfate (Nebcin)

• Infection caused by susceptible organisms; serious infections caused by sensitive *Escherichia coli, Proteus, Klebsiella, Enterobacter, Serratia, Staphylococcus aureus, Pseudo-*

monas, Citrobacter, and *Providencia.*
Adults with normal renal function: 3
mg/kg I.M. or I.V. daily, divided q 8
hours. Up to 5 mg/kg I.M. or I.V.
daily, divided q 6 to 8 hours for
life-threatening infections. *Chil-*
dren: 6 to 7.5 mg/kg I.M. or I.V.
daily in 3 or 4 equally divided
doses. *Neonates under age 1 week:*
Up to 4 mg/kg I.M. or I.V. daily, divided q 12 hours. For I.V. use, dilute
in 50 to 100 ml of 0.9% sodium
chloride solution or D_5W for adults
and in less volume for children. Infuse over 20 to 60 minutes. *Patients*
with impaired renal function: Initial
dosage is same as for those with
normal renal function. Subsequent
doses and frequency determined by
renal function study results and
blood levels; keep peak serum concentrations between 4 and 10 mcg/
ml, and trough serum concentrations between 1 and 2 mcg/ml.
• Treatment of external ocular infection caused by susceptible gram-
negative bacteria. *Adults and chil-*
dren: In mild-to-moderate infections, instill 1 or 2 drops into affected eye q 4 hours. In severe infections, instill 2 drops into the affected eye hourly.

tocainide hydrochloride (Tonocard)

• Suppression of symptomatic ventricular arrhythmias, including frequent PVCs and ventricular tachycardia. *Adults:* Initially, 400 mg P.O.
q 8 hours. Usual dosage is between
1,200 and 1,800 mg daily in three
divided doses.

tolazamide (Tolamide, Tolinase)

• Adjunct to diet to lower the blood
glucose level in patients with non-
insulin-dependent diabetes mellitus
(Type II). *Adults:* initially, 100 mg
P.O. daily with breakfast if fasting
blood sugar is under 200 mg/dl; or
250 mg if fasting blood sugar is
over 200 mg/dl. May adjust dosage

at weekly intervals by 100 to
250 mg. Maximum dosage is 500
mg b.i.d. before meals.
• To change from insulin to oral
therapy. *Adults:* if insulin dosage is
under 20 units daily, insulin may be
stopped and oral therapy started at
100 mg P.O. daily with breakfast. If
insulin dosage is 20 to 40 units
daily, insulin may be stopped and
oral therapy started at 250 mg P.O.
daily with breakfast.

tolbutamide (Mobenol, Oramide, Orinase)

• Non-insulin-dependent (Type II)
diabetes mellitus uncontrolled by diet
alone. *Adults:* Initially, 1 to 2 g P.O.
daily or in divided doses. May adjust
dosage to maximum of 3 g daily.
• To change from insulin to oral
therapy. *Adults:* if insulin dosage is
under 20 units daily, insulin may be
stopped and oral therapy started at
1 to 2 g daily. If insulin dosage is
20 to 40 units daily, insulin is reduced 30% to 50% and oral therapy started as above.

tranylcypromine sulfate (Parnate)

• Depression. *Adults:* 10 mg P.O.
b.i.d. Increase to maximum of
30 mg daily, if necessary, after
2 weeks. Not recommended for
children under age 16.

tretinoin (vitamin A acid, retinoic acid) (Retin-A)

• Acne vulgaris (especially grades I,
II, and III), fine wrinkles from pho-
todamaged skin. *Adults and children:*
clean affected area and lightly apply
solution once daily h.s.

triamcinolone acetonide (Nasacort)

• Relief of symptoms of seasonal or
perennial allergic rhinitis. *Adults*
and children age 12 and over: Initially, 2 sprays (110 mcg) in each
nostril once daily. Increased as
needed up to 440 mcg daily either

as once-daily dosage or in divided doses up to four times daily. After desired effect is obtained, dosage decreased, if possible, to as little as one spray (55 mcg) in each nostril daily.

triamcinolone acetonide (Aristocort, Kenalog)

• Inflammation of corticosteroid-responsive dermatoses. *Adults and children:* clean affected area and apply cream, ointment, lotion, foam, or aerosol sparingly b.i.d. to q.i.d. For aerosol application, shake can well. Direct spray onto affected area from a distance of approximately 6″ (15 cm) and apply for only 3 seconds.

• Inflammation associated with oral lesions. *Adults and children:* Apply paste h.s. and, if needed, two to three times daily, preferably after meals. Apply a small amount without rubbing and press to lesion in mouth until a thin film develops.

trimipramine maleate (Surmontil)

• Treatment of depression. *Adults:* Initially, 75 mg daily in divided doses, increased to 200 mg daily. Dosages over 300 mg daily not recommended.

tripelennamine citrate (PBZ)

• Rhinitis, allergy symptoms. *Adults:* 25 to 50 mg P.O. q 4 to 6 hours; or 100 mg (timed-release) b.i.d. or t.i.d. Maximum dosage is 600 mg/day. *Children:* 5 mg/kg P.O. daily in four to six divided doses. Maximum dosage is 300 mg/day.

Children under age 12 should use only as directed by a doctor.

triprolidine hydrochloride (Actidil)

• Allergy symptoms. *Adults and children over age 12:* 2.5 mg P.O. t.i.d. or q.i.d. Maximum dosage is 10 mg/day. *Children ages 6 to 12:* 1.25 mg P.O. t.i.d. or q.i.d. Maximum dosage is 5

mg/day. *Children ages 4 to 6:* 0.938 mg P.O. t.i.d. or q.i.d. Maximum dosage is 3.75 mg/day. *Children ages 2 to 4:* 0.625 mg P.O. t.i.d. or q.i.d. Maximum dosage is 2.5 mg/day. *Children ages 4 months to 2 years:* 0.3 mg P.O. t.i.d. or q.i.d. Maximum dosage is 1.25 mg/day.

Children under age 12 should use only as directed by a doctor.

tropicamide (Mydriacyl)

• Cycloplegic refraction. *Adults and children:* Instill 1 to 2 drops of 1% solution in each eye; repeat in 5 minutes. Additional drops may be instilled in 20 to 30 minutes.

• Fundus examination. *Adults and children:* Instill 1 to 2 drops of 0.5% solution in each eye 15 to 20 minutes before examination.

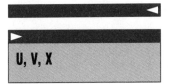

U, V, X

ursodiol (Actigall)

• Dissolution of gallstones less than 20 mm in diameter in patients who are poor surgical candidates or who refuse surgery. *Adults:* 8 to 10 mg/kg P.O. daily in two or three divided doses. Most patients receive 300 mg P.O. b.i.d. Therapy is usually long-term, with ultrasound images of the gallbladder at 6-month intervals. If partial stone dissolution is not seen within 12 months, eventual success is unlikely. Safe ursodiol use for longer than 2 years has not been established.

valproate sodium (Depakene Syrup, Myproic Acid Syrup) valproic acid (Dalpro, Depakene, Myproic Acid) divalproex sodium (Depakote)

• Simple and complex absence seizures, mixed seizure types (including absence seizures), investigationally in tonic-clonic seizures. *Adults and children:* initially, 15 mg/kg P.O. daily, divided b.i.d. or t.i.d.; then may increase by 5 to 10 mg/kg daily at weekly intervals up to a maximum of 60 mg/kg daily, divided b.i.d. or t.i.d.

vasopressin (Aqueous Pitressin) vasopressin tannate (Pitressin Tannate)

• Pituitary diabetes insipidus. *Adults:* 5 to 10 units I.M. or S.C. b.i.d. to q.i.d., p.r.n.; or intranasally (spray or cotton balls) in individualized doses, based on response. For long-term therapy, inject 5 to 10 units Pitressin Tannate in oil suspension I.M. or S.C. q 2 to 4 days. *Children:* 2.5 to 10 units I.M. or S.C. b.i.d. to q.i.d., p.r.n.; or intranasally (spray or cotton balls) in individualized doses. For long-term therapy, inject 1.25 to 2.5 units Pitressin Tannate in oil suspension I.M. or S.C. q 2 to 3 days.

verapamil hydrochloride Calan, Calan SR, Isoptin, Isoptin SR, Verelan)

• Vasospastic (Prinzmetal's or variant) angina and classic chronic, stable angina pectoris. *Adults:* Starting dosage is 80 mg P.O. t.i.d. or q.i.d. Dosage may be increased at weekly intervals. Some patients may require up to 480 mg daily.
• Atrial arrhythmias. *Adults:* 0.075 to 0.15 mg/kg (5 to 10 mg) I.V. push over 2 minutes with ECG and blood pressure monitoring. Repeat dose in 30 minutes if no response. Follow bolus injection with maintenance infusion of 0.005 mg/kg/minute. *Children ages 1 to 15:* 0.1 to 0.3 mg/kg as I.V. bolus over 2 minutes. *Children under age 1:* 0.1 to 0.2 mg/kg as I.V. bolus over 2 minutes under continuous ECG

monitoring. Dose can be repeated in 30 minutes if no response.
• Hypertension. *Adults:* Usual starting dose is 80 mg P.O. t.i.d. or 1 240-mg sustained-release tablet or capsule daily in the morning. Dosage may be increased at weekly intervals. For patients taking sustained-release tablets, dosage may be increased in 120-mg increments, with second dose added in the evening. Elderly patients or patients of smaller stature may initiate therapy at 120 mg P.O. b.i.d.

Maximum dosage is 480 mg daily. Sustained-release capsules should be given only once daily. Antihypertensive effects are usually seen within the first week of therapy. Most patients respond to 240 mg daily.

vidarabine (Vira-A Ophthalmic)

• Acute keratoconjunctivitis, superficial keratitis, and recurrent epithelial keratitis resulting from herpes simplex types I and II. *Adults and children:* Instill ½" ointment into lower conjunctival sac five times daily at 3-hour intervals.

xylometazoline hydrochloride (Otrivin)

• Nasal congestion. *Adults and children age 12 and over:* apply 2 to 3 drops or 1 to 2 sprays of 0.1% solution to nasal mucosa q 8 to 10 hours. *Children under age 12:* apply 2 to 3 drops or 1 spray of 0.05% solution to nasal mucosa q 8 to 10 hours.

CHAPTER 12

Drug hazards:
Recognizing and responding to them

DRUG HAZARDS

DRUG HAZARDS

Adverse or toxic drug reactions

Identifying and treating toxic drug reactions

TOXIC REACTIONS AND CLINICAL EFFECTS	INTERVENTIONS	SELECTED CAUSATIVE DRUGS
Anemia, aplastic • Bleeding from mucous membranes, ecchymoses, petechiae • Fatigue, pallor, progressive weakness, shortness of breath, tachycardia progressing to congestive heart failure (CHF) • Fever, oral and rectal ulcers, sore throat without characteristic inflammation	• Stop drug, if possible, as ordered. • Give vigorous supportive care, including transfusions, neutropenic isolation, antibiotics, and oxygen. • Colony-stimulating factors may be given. • In severe cases, bone marrow transplant may be needed.	• altretamine • aspirin (long-term) • carbamazepine • chloramphenicol • co-trimoxazole • ganciclovir • gold salts • hydrochlorothiazide • mephenytoin • penicillamine • phenothiazines • phenylbutazone • triamterene • zidovudine
Anemia, hemolytic • Chills, fever, back and abdominal pain (hemolytic crisis) • Jaundice, malaise, splenomegaly • Signs of shock	• Stop drug, as ordered. • Give supportive care, including transfusions and oxygen. • Obtain a blood sample for Coombs' tests, as ordered.	• carbidopa-levodopa • levodopa • mefenamic acid • penicillins • phenazopyridine • primaquine • sulfonamides
Bone marrow toxicity (agranulocytosis) • Enlarged lymph nodes, spleen, tonsils • Septicemia; shock • Progressive fatigue and weakness, then sudden overwhelming infection with chills, fever, headache, and tachycardia • Pneumonia • Ulcers in the colon, mouth, and pharynx	• Stop drug, as ordered. • Begin antibiotic therapy while awaiting blood culture and sensitivity results. • Give supportive therapy, including neutropenic isolation, warm saline gargles, and oral hygiene.	• ACE inhibitors • aminoglutethimide • carbamazepine • co-trimoxazole • flucytosine • gold salts • penicillamine • phenothiazines • phenylbutazone • phenytoin • procainamide • propylthiouracil • sulfonylureas

(continued)

DRUG HAZARDS

Identifying and treating toxic drug reactions *(continued)*

TOXIC REACTIONS AND CLINICAL EFFECTS	INTERVENTIONS	SELECTED CAUSATIVE DRUGS
Bone marrow toxicity (thrombocytopenia) • Fatigue, weakness, lethargy, malaise • Hemorrhage, loss of consciousness, shortness of breath, tachycardia • Sudden onset of ecchymoses or petechiae; large blood-filled bullae in the mouth	• Stop drug or reduce dosage, as ordered. • Administer corticosteroids and platelet transfusions.	• anistreplase • ciprofloxacin • cisplatin • colfosceril • etretinate • floxuridine • flucytosine • ganciclovir • gold salts • heparin • interferons alfa-2a and alpha-2b • lymphocyte immune globulin • methotrexate • penicillamine • procarbazine • tetracyclines • valproic acid
Cardiomyopathy • Acute hypertensive reaction • Atrial and ventricular arrhythmias • Chest pain • CHF • Chronic cardiomyopathy • Pericarditis-myocarditis syndrome	• Discontinue drug, as ordered, if possible. • Closely monitor patients receiving concurrent radiation therapy. • Institute cardiac monitoring at earliest sign of problems. • If patient is receiving doxorubicin, limit cumulative dose to less than 500 mg/m^2.	• cytosine arabinoside • daunorubicin • doxorubicin • idarubicin • mitoxantrone

Identifying and treating toxic drug reactions *(continued)*

TOXIC REACTIONS AND CLINICAL EFFECTS	INTERVENTIONS	SELECTED CAUSATIVE DRUGS
Dermatologic toxicity • May vary from phototoxicity to acneiform eruptions, alopecia, exfoliative dermatitis, lupus erythematosus-like reactions, toxic epidermal necrolysis	• Stop drug, as ordered. • Administer topical antihistamines and analgesics, as ordered.	• androgens • barbiturates • corticosteroids • gold salts • hydralazine • interferons • iodides • pentamidine • phenolphthalein • phenothiazines • phenylbutazone • procainamide • psoralens • sulfonamides • sulfonylureas • tetracyclines • thiazides
Hepatotoxicity • Abdominal pain, hepatomegaly • Abnormal levels of alanine aminotransferase (ALT), formerly SGPT; aspartate aminotransferase (AST), formerly SGOT; serum bilirubin; and lactate dehydrogenase • Bleeding, low-grade fever, mental changes, weight loss • Dry skin, pruritus, rash • Jaundice	• Reduce dosage or stop drug, as ordered. • Monitor vital signs, blood levels, weight, intake and output, fluids and electrolytes. • Promote rest. • Assist with hemodialysis, if needed. • Give symptomatic care: vitamins A, B complex, D, and K; potassium for alkalosis; salt-poor albumin for fluid and electrolyte balance; neomycin for GI flora; stomach aspiration for blood; reduced dietary protein; and lactulose for blood ammonia.	• amiodarone • asparaginase • carbamazepine • chlorpromazine • chlorpropamide • ciprofloxacin (parenteral) • cytosine arabinoside • dantrolene • erythromycin estolate • ifosfamide • ketoconazole • leuprolide • methotrexate • methyldopa • mitoxantrone • niacin • plicamycin • sulindac

(continued)

DRUG HAZARDS

Identifying and treating toxic drug reactions *(continued)*

TOXIC REACTIONS AND CLINICAL EFFECTS	INTERVENTIONS	SELECTED CAUSATIVE DRUGS
Nephrotoxicity • Altered creatinine clearance (decreased or increased) • Blurred vision, dehydration (depending on part of kidney affected), edema, mild headache, pallor • Casts, albumin, or red or white blood cells in urine • Dizziness, fatigue, irritability, slowed mental processes • Electrolyte imbalance • Elevated blood urea nitrogen level • Oliguria	• Reduce dosage or stop drug, as ordered. • Assist with hemodialysis, if needed. • Monitor vital signs, weight changes, and urine volume. • Give symptomatic care: fluid restriction and loop diuretics to reduce fluid retention, I.V. solutions to correct electrolyte imbalance.	• aminoglycosides • cephalosporins • cisplatin • contrast media • corticosteroids • cyclosporine • gallium • gold salts (parenteral) • nitrosoureas • nonsteroidal anti-inflammatory drugs • penicillin • pentamidine isethionate • plicamycin • vasopressors or vasoconstrictors
Neurotoxicity • Akathisia • Bilateral or unilateral palsies • Muscle twitching, tremor • Paresthesia • Seizures • Strokelike syndrome • Unsteady gait • Weakness	• Notify doctor as soon as changes appear. • Reduce dosage or stop drug, as ordered. • Monitor carefully for any changes in the patient's condition. • Give symptomatic care: Remain with the patient, reassure him, and protect him during seizures. Provide a quiet environment, draw shades, and speak in soft tones. Maintain the airway, and ventilate the patient as needed.	• aminoglycosides • cisplatin • cytosine arabinoside • isoniazid • nitroprusside • polymyxin B injection • vinca alkaloids

DRUG HAZARDS

Identifying and treating toxic drug reactions *(continued)*

TOXIC REACTIONS AND CLINICAL EFFECTS	INTERVENTIONS	SELECTED CAUSATIVE DRUGS
Ocular toxicity • Acute glaucoma • Blurred, colored, or flickering vision • Cataracts • Corneal deposits • Diplopia • Miosis • Mydriasis • Optic neuritis • Scotomata • Vision loss	• Notify doctor as soon as changes appear. • Stop drug, as ordered. (Some oculotoxic drugs used to treat serious conditions may be given again at a reduced dosage after the eyes are rested and have returned to near normal.) • Monitor carefully for changes in symptoms. • Treat effects symptomatically.	• amiodarone • antibiotics, such as chloramphenicol • anticholinergic agents • chloroquine • clomiphene • corticosteroids • cyclophosphamide • cytarabine • digitalis glycosides • ethambutol • lithium carbonate • methotrexate • phenothiazines • quinidine • quinine • rifampin • tamoxifen • vinca alkaloids
Ototoxicity • Ataxia • Hearing loss • Tinnitus • Vertigo	• Notify doctor as soon as changes appear. • Stop drug or reduce dosage, as ordered. • Monitor carefully for symptomatic changes.	• aminoglycosides • antibiotics, such as colistimethate sodium, gentamicin, kanamycin, and streptomycin • chloroquine • cisplatin • loop diuretics • minocycline • quinidine • quinine • salicylates • vancomycin

(continued)

DRUG HAZARDS

Identifying and treating toxic drug reactions *(continued)*

TOXIC REACTIONS AND CLINICAL EFFECTS	INTERVENTIONS	SELECTED CAUSATIVE DRUGS
Pseudomembranous colitis • Abdominal pain • Colonic perforation • Fever • Hypotension • Severe dehydration • Shock • Sudden, copious diarrhea (watery or bloody)	• Notify doctor as soon as changes appear. • Immediately discontinue drug, as ordered. • Give another antibiotic, such as vancomycin, metronidazole, or bacitracin. • Maintain fluid and electrolyte balance. Check serum electrolyte levels daily. If pseudomembranous colitis is mild, give an ion exchange resin as ordered. • Record intake and output. • Monitor vital signs, skin color and turgor, urine output, and level of consciousness. • Immediately report signs of shock. • Observe for signs of hypokalemia, especially malaise and weak, rapid, irregular pulse.	• antibiotics

Preventing drug overdose in renal failure

Impaired renal function can modify a drug's bioavailability, distribution, pharmacologic action, or elimination. To prevent accidental overdose in a patient with renal failure, adjust dosages according to the severity of renal impairment, as shown in the chart below. (*Note:* "GFR" refers to glomerular filtration rate.)

DRUG	MILD RENAL IMPAIRMENT (GFR > 50 ml/min)		MODERATE RENAL IMPAIRMENT (GFR 10 to 50 ml/min)		SEVERE RENAL IMPAIRMENT (GFR < 10 ml/min)	
	% of normal dose	Interval	% of normal dose	Interval	% of normal dose	Interval
Acetaminophen	100%	q 4 hr	100%	q 6 hr	100%	q 8 hr
Acetazolamide	100%	q 6 hr	100%	q 12 hr	Avoid	Avoid
Acetohexamide	100%	q 12 hr	Avoid	Avoid	Avoid	Avoid
Acyclovir	100%	q 8 hr	100%	q 24 hr	100%	q 48 hr
Allopurinol	100%	q 8 hr	75%	q 8 hr	50%	q 8 hr
Amantadine	100%	q 12 to 24 hr	100%	q 48 to 72 hr	100%	q 7 days
Amikacin	60% to 90%	q 12 hr	30% to 70%	q 12 to 24 hr	20% to 30%	q 24 hr
Amoxicillin	100%	q 6 hr	100%	q 6 to 12 hr	100%	q 12 to 16 hr
Amphotericin B	100%	q 24 hr	100%	q 24 hr	100%	q 24 to 36 hr
Ampicillin	100%	q 6 hr	100%	q 6 to 12 hr	100%	q 12 to 16 hr
Aspirin	100%	q 4 hr	100%	q 4 to 6 hr	Avoid	Avoid
Atenolol	100%	q 24 hr	100%	q 48 hr	100%	q 96 hr
Azathioprine	100%	q 24 hr	100%	q 24 hr	100%	q 36 hr
Betaxolol	100%	q 24 hr	100%	q 24 hr	50%	q 24 hr
Bleomycin	100%	Varies	100%	Varies	50%	Varies
Bretylium	100%	Continuous infusion	25% to 50%	Continuous infusion	Avoid	Avoid
Captopril	100%	t.i.d.	100%	t.i.d.	50%	t.i.d.

(continued)

Preventing drug overdose in renal failure *(continued)*

DRUG	MILD RENAL IMPAIRMENT (GFR > 50 ml/min)		MODERATE RENAL IMPAIRMENT (GFR 10 to 50 ml/min)		SEVERE RENAL IMPAIRMENT (GFR < 10 ml/min)	
	% of normal dose	Interval	% of normal dose	Interval	% of normal dose	Interval
Carbamazepine	100%	q 6 to 8 hr	100%	q 6 to 8 hr	75%	q 6 to 8 hr
Carbenicillin	100%	q 8 to 12 hr	100%	q 12 to 24 hr	100%	q 24 to 48 hr
Cefaclor	100%	q 6 hr	50% to 100%	q 6 hr	33%	q 6 hr
Cefadroxil	100%	q 8 hr	100%	q 12 to 24 hr	100%	q 24 to 48 hr
Cefamandole	100%	q 6 hr	100%	q 6 to 8 hr	100%	q 8 hr
Cefonicid	50%	q 24 hr	25%	q 24 hr	25%	q 3 to 5 days
Cefotaxime	100%	q 6 to 8 hr	100%	q 8 to 12 hr	100%	q 24 hr
Cefoxitin	100%	q 8 hr	100%	q 8 to 12 hr	100%	q 24 to 48 hr
Cephalexin	100%	q 6 hr	100%	q 6 to 8 hr	100%	q 12 hr
Cephalothin	100%	q 6 hr	75%	q 6 hr	50%	q 6 hr
Cephapirin	100%	q 6 hr	100%	q 6 to 8 hr	100%	q 12 hr
Cephradine	100%	q 6 hr	50% to 100%	q 6 hr	50%	q 6 to 12 hr
Chloral hydrate	100%	At bedtime	Avoid	Avoid	Avoid	Avoid
Chlorpropamide	100%	q 24 hr	Avoid	Avoid	Avoid	Avoid
Chlorthalidone	100%	q 24 hr	100%	q 24 hr	100%	q 48 hr
Cimetidine	100%	q 6 hr	100%	q 8 hr	100%	q 12 hr
Ciprofloxacin	100%	q 12 hr	100%	q 12 to 24 hr	100%	q 24 hr

Preventing drug overdose in renal failure *(continued)*

DRUG	MILD RENAL IMPAIRMENT (GFR > 50 ml/min)		MODERATE RENAL IMPAIRMENT (GFR 10 to 50 ml/min)		SEVERE RENAL IMPAIRMENT (GFR < 10 ml/min)	
	% of normal dose	Interval	% of normal dose	Interval	% of normal dose	Interval
Cisplatin	100%	Varies	75%	Varies	50%	Varies
Clofibrate	100%	q 6 to 12 hr	100%	q 12 to 18 hr	100%	q 24 to 48 hr
Clonidine	100%	b.i.d.	100%	b.i.d.	50% to 75%	b.i.d.
Colchicine	100%	Varies	100%	Varies	50%	Varies
Cyclophospha-mide	100%	q 12 hr	100%	q 12 hr	100%	q 18 to 24 hr
Diflunisal	100%	q 12 hr	100%	q 12 hr	50%	q 12 hr
Digitoxin	100%	q 24 hr	100%	q 24 hr	50% to 75%	q 24 hr
Digoxin	100%	q 24 hr	100%	q 36 hr	100%	q 48 hr
Diphenhydra-mine	100%	q 6 hr	100%	q 6 to 9 hr	100%	q 9 to 12 hr
Disopyramide	100%	q 6 hr	100%	q 12 to 24 hr	100%	q 24 to 40 hr
Doxycycline	100%	q 12 hr	100%	q 12 to 18 hr	100%	q 18 to 24 hr
Ethacrynic acid	100%	q 6 hr	100%	q 6 hr	Avoid	Avoid
Ethambutol	100%	q 24 hr	100%	q 24 to 36 hr	100%	q 48 hr
Ethosuximide	100%	q 12 hr	100%	q 12 hr	75%	q 12 hr
Flucytosine	100%	q 6 hr	100%	q 12 to 24 hr	100%	q 24 to 48 hr
Ganciclovir	100%	q 12 hr	100%	q 24 hr	100%	q 24 hr
Gemfibrozil	100%	b.i.d.	50%	b.i.d.	25%	b.i.d.
Gentamicin	60% to 90%	q 8 to 12 hr	30% to 70%	q 12 hr	20% to 30%	q 24 hr
Guanethidine	100%	q 24 hr	100%	q 24 hr	100%	q 24 to 36 hr

(continued)

DRUG HAZARDS

Preventing drug overdose in renal failure *(continued)*

DRUG	MILD RENAL IMPAIRMENT (GFR >50 ml/min) % of normal dose	Interval	MODERATE RENAL IMPAIRMENT (GFR 10 to 50 ml/min) % of normal dose	Interval	SEVERE RENAL IMPAIRMENT (GFR <10 ml/min) % of normal dose	Interval
Hydralazine	100%	q 8 hr	100%	q 8 hr	100%	q 8 to 16 hr or q 12 to 24 hr* *depending on whether patient is a fast or slow acetylator
Hydroxyurea	100%	Varies	100%	Varies	50%	Varies
Isoniazid	100%	q 24 hr	100%	q 24 hr	66% to 75%	q 24 hr
Kanamycin	60% to 90%	q 8 to 12 hr	30% to 70%	q 12 hr	20% to 30%	q 24 hr
Ketorolac	100%	p.r.n.	100%	p.r.n.	50%	p.r.n.
Lincomycin	100%	q 6 hr	100%	q 12 hr	100%	q 24 hr
Lisinopril	100%	q 24 hr	50%	q 24 hr	25%	q 24 hr
Lithium carbonate	100%	t.i.d. to q.i.d.	50% to 75%	t.i.d. to q.i.d	25% to 50%	t.i.d. to q.i.d.
Loracarbef	100%	q 12 to 24 hr	50%	q 12 to 24 hr	100%	q 3 to 5 days
Lorazepam	100%	t.i.d. to q.i.d.	100%	t.i.d. to q.i.d.	50%	t.i.d. to q.i.d.
Meperidine	100%	Varies	75%	Varies	50%	Varies
Meprobamate	100%	q 6 hr	100%	q 9 to 12 hr	100%	q 12 to 18 hr
Methadone	100%	q 6 to 8 hr	100%	q 6 to 8 hr	50% to 75%	q 6 to 8 hr
Methotrexate	100%	Varies	50%	Varies	Avoid	Avoid
Methyldopa	100%	q 6 hr	100%	q 8 to 18 hr	100%	q 12 to 24 hr
Metoclopramide	100%	Varies	75%	Varies	50%	Varies

Preventing drug overdose in renal failure *(continued)*

DRUG	MILD RENAL IMPAIRMENT (GFR > 50 ml/min)		MODERATE RENAL IMPAIRMENT (GFR 10 to 50 ml/min)		SEVERE RENAL IMPAIRMENT (GFR < 10 ml/min)	
	% of normal dose	Interval	% of normal dose	Interval	% of normal dose	Interval
Metronidazole	100%	q 8 hr	100%	q 8 to 12 hr	100%	q 12 to 24 hr
Mexiletine	100%	q 12 hr	100%	q 12 hr	50% to 75%	q 12 hr
Mezlocillin	100%	q 4 to 6 hr	100%	q 6 to 8 hr	100%	q 8 hr
Mithramycin	100%	Varies	75%	Varies	50%	Varies
Mitomycin	100%	Varies	100%	Varies	75%	Varies
Moricizine	100%	q 8 hr	100%	q 8 hr	50% to 75%	q 8 hr
Nadolol	100%	q 24 hr	50%	q 24 hr	25%	q 24 hr
Nalidixic acid	100%	q.i.d.	Avoid	Avoid	Avoid	Avoid
Neostigmine	100%	q 6 hr	100%	q 6 hr	100%	q 12 to 18 hr
Netilmicin	60% to 90%	q 8 to 12 hr	30% to 70%	q 12 hr	20% to 30%	q 24 hr
Nicotinic acid	100%	t.i.d.	50%	t.i.d.	25%	t.i.d.
Nitrofurantoin	100%	q.i.d.	Avoid	Avoid	Avoid	Avoid
Oxazepam	100%	q.i.d.	100%	q.i.d.	75%	q.i.d.
Penicillin G	100%	q 6 to 8 hr	100%	q 8 to 12 hr	Avoid over 10 million units/day	q 12 to 16 hr
Pentamidine isethionate (parenteral)	100%	q 24 hr	100%	q 24 to 36 hr	100%	q 48 hr
Phenobarbital	100%	t.i.d.	100%	t.i.d.	100%	q 12 to 16 hr
Phenylbutazone	100%	t.i.d. to q.i.d.	100%	t.i.d. to q.i.d.	Avoid	Avoid
Piperacillin	100%	q 4 to 6 hr	100%	q 6 to 8 hr	100%	q 8 hr

(continued)

DRUG HAZARDS

Preventing drug overdose in renal failure *(continued)*

DRUG	MILD RENAL IMPAIRMENT (GFR >50 ml/min)		MODERATE RENAL IMPAIRMENT (GFR 10 to 50 ml/min)		SEVERE RENAL IMPAIRMENT (GFR <10 ml/min)	
	% of normal dose	Interval	% of normal dose	Interval	% of normal dose	Interval
Primidone	100%	q 8 hr	100%	q 8 to 12 hr	100%	q 12 to 24 hr
Probenecid	100%	q.i.d.	Avoid	Avoid	Avoid	Avoid
Procainamide	100%	q 4 hr	100%	q 6 to 12 hr	100%	q 8 to 24 hr
Propoxyphene	100%	q 4 hr	100%	q 4 hr	25%	q 4 hr
Reserpine	100%	q 24 hr	100%	q 24 hr	Avoid	Avoid
Spironolactone	100%	q 6 to 12 hr	100%	q 12 to 24 hr	Avoid	Avoid
Streptomycin	100%	q 24 hr	100%	q 24 to 72 hr	100%	q 72 to 96 hr
Streptozocin	100%	Varies	75%	Varies	50%	Varies
Sulfamethoxazole	100%	q 12 hr	100%	q 18 hr	100%	q 24 hr
Sulfisoxazole	100%	q 6 hr	100%	q 8 to 12 hr	100%	q 12 to 24 hr
Sulindac	100%	b.i.d.	100%	b.i.d.	50%	b.i.d.
Terbutaline	100%	t.i.d.	50%	t.i.d.	Avoid	Avoid
Thiazides	100%	Daily to b.i.d.	100%	Daily to b.i.d.	Avoid	Avoid
Ticarcillin	100%	q 8 to 12 hr	100%	q 12 to 24 hr	100%	q 24 to 48 hr
Tobramycin	60% to 90%	q 8 to 12 hr	30% to 70%	q 12 hr	20% to 30%	q 24 hr
Triamterene	100%	q 12 hr	100%	q 12 hr	Avoid	Avoid
Trimethoprim	100%	q 12 hr	100%	q 18 hr	100%	q 24 hr
Vancomycin	100%	q 1 to 3 days	100%	q 3 to 10 days	100%	q 10 days
Vidarabine	100%	Continuous infusion	100%	Continuous infusion	75%	Continuous infusion

> **LIFE-THREATENING EFFECTS**

Reversing anaphylaxis

Anaphylaxis – the sudden, extreme reaction to a foreign antigen – requires immediate treatment. Generally, the faster the onset of symptoms, the more severe the reaction. This chart lists drugs useful in reversing anaphylactic reactions.

DRUG AND DOSAGE	ACTION	NURSING CONSIDERATIONS
Aminophylline (Aminophyllin) *Severe anaphylaxis I.V.:* 5 to 6 mg/kg as loading dose, followed by 0.4 to 0.9 mg/kg/min by infusion.	• Causes bronchodilation • Stimulates respiratory drive • Dilates constricted pulmonary arteries • Causes diuresis • Strengthens cardiac contractions • Increases vital capacity • Causes coronary vasodilation	• Monitor blood pressure, pulse, and respirations. • Monitor intake and output, hydration status, and aminophylline and electrolyte levels. • Monitor patient for arrhythmias. • Use I.V. controller to reduce risk of overdose. • Maintain serum levels at 10 to 20 mcg/ml.
Cimetidine (Tagamet) *Severe anaphylaxis* (experimental use in refractory cases) *I.V.:* 600 mg diluted in dextrose 5% in water (D$_s$W) and administered over 20 min.	• Competes with histamine for H$_2$-receptor sites • Prevents laryngeal edema	• Be aware that drug is incompatible with aminophylline. • Reduce dosage for patients with impaired renal or hepatic function.
Diphenhydramine (Benadryl) *Mild anaphylaxis P.O.:* 25 to 100 mg t.i.d. *I.V.:* 25 to 50 mg q.i.d.	• Competes with histamine for H$_1$-receptor sites • Prevents laryngeal edema • Controls localized itching	• Administer I.V. doses slowly to avoid hypotension. • Monitor patient for hypotension and drowsiness. • Give fluids as needed. Drug causes dry mouth.

(continued)

DRUG HAZARDS

Reversing anaphylaxis *(continued)*

DRUG AND DOSAGE	ACTION	NURSING CONSIDERATIONS
Epinephrine (Adrenalin) *Severe anaphylaxis (drug of choice)* *Initial infusion:* 0.2 to 0.5 mg (0.2 to 0.5 ml of 1:1,000 strength diluted in 10 ml of 0.9% sodium chloride solution) given I.V. slowly over 5 to 10 min, followed by continuous infusion. *Continuous infusion:* 1 to 4 mcg/min (mix 1 ml of 1:1,000 epinephrine in 250 ml of D_5W to get concentration of 4 mcg/ml).	*Alpha-adrenergic effects:* • Increases blood pressure • Reverses peripheral vasodilation and systemic hypotension • Considered the drug of choice for treating anaphylaxis • Decreases angioedema and urticaria • Improves coronary blood flow by raising diastolic pressure • Causes peripheral vasoconstriction *Beta-adrenergic effects:* • Causes bronchodilation • Causes positive inotropic and chronotropic cardiac activity • Decreases synthesis and release of chemical mediators	• Select large vein for infusion. • Use infusion controller to regulate drip. • Check blood pressure and heart rate frequently. • Monitor patient for arrhythmias. • Check solution strength, dosage, and label before administration. • Watch for signs of extravasation at infusion site. • Monitor intake and output. • Assess color and temperature of extremities.
Hydrocortisone (Solu-Cortef) *Severe anaphylaxis* *I.V.:* 100 to 200 mg q 4 to 6 hr.	• Prevents neutrophil and platelet aggregation • Inhibits synthesis of mediators • Decreases capillary permeability	• Monitor fluid and electrolyte balance, intake and output, and blood pressure closely. • Maintain patient on ulcer and antacid regimen prophylactically.

> ## Recognizing common adverse reactions in elderly patients

Elderly patients are especially susceptible to adverse reactions, such as urticaria, impotence, incontinence, GI upset, and rashes. Less common adverse reactions, such as anxiety, confusion, and forgetfulness, may be mistaken for typical elderly behaviors. The reactions described below are serious—you need to know how to recognize and deal with them.

Altered mental status

Agitation or confusion may follow use of anticholinergics, diuretics, antihypertensives, and antidepressants. Paradoxically, depression may result from antidepressant drugs.

Anorexia

This is a warning sign of toxicity—especially from digitalis glycosides such as digoxin. That's why the doctor usually prescribes a very low initial dose.

Blood disorders

If the patient takes an anticoagulant, watch for signs of easy bruising or bleeding (such as excessive bleeding after toothbrushing). Such signs may signal thrombocytopenia or blood dyscrasias. Other drugs that may cause these reactions include antineoplastics such as methotrexate, antibiotics such as nitrofurantoin, and anticonvulsants such as valproic acid and phenytoin. Tell your patient to report easy bruising to his doctor immediately.

Dehydration

If the patient is taking diuretics, be alert for dehydration and electrolyte imbalance. Monitor blood levels of the drug, and give potassium supplements as ordered. Many drugs, such as anticholinergics, cause a dry mouth. Suggest sucking on sugarless candy for relief.

Orthostatic hypotension

Marked by light-headedness or faintness and unsteady footing, orthostatic hypotension can occur with the use of sedatives, antidepressants, antihypertensives, and antipsychotics. To prevent falls, warn the patient not to sit up or get out of bed too quickly, and to call for help in walking if he feels dizzy or faint.

Tardive dyskinesia

Characterized by abnormal tongue movements, lip pursing, grimacing, blinking, and gyrating motions of the face and extremities, this disorder may be triggered by psychotropic drugs such as haloperidol or chlorpromazine.

► LIFE-THREATENING EFFECTS

> ## Identifying the most dangerous drugs

Almost any drug can cause an adverse reaction in some patients. But the following drugs cause roughly 90% of all reported reactions.

Anticoagulants
• heparin
• warfarin

Antimicrobials
• cephalosporins
• penicillins
• sulfonamides

Bronchodilators
• sympathomimetics
• theophylline

DRUG HAZARDS

Cardiac drugs
- antihypertensives
- digoxin
- diuretics
- quinidine

Central nervous system drugs
- analgesics
- anticonvulsants
- neuroleptics
- sedative-hypnotics

Diagnostic agents
- X-ray contrast media

Hormones
- corticosteroids
- estrogens
- insulin

Reporting reactions to the FDA

Drug manufacturers monitor adverse drug reactions and report them to the Food and Drug Administration (FDA). That's the law.

The FDA also wants to hear from nurses whose patients have experienced serious reactions associated with drugs—especially drugs that have been on the market for 3 years or less. After all, you and your colleagues are the ones most likely to see the reactions, so you can give the best clinical descriptions. But unlike the manufacturers, you aren't required by law to make a report.

What constitutes a serious reaction? According to the FDA, it's one that:
- is life-threatening.
- causes death.
- leads to or prolongs hospitalization.
- results in permanent or severe disability.

The FDA also wants to know about drugs that don't produce a therapeutic response. It doesn't need to hear about inappropriate drug use, prescriber errors, or administration errors. (But the United States Pharmacopeia does want to know about medication errors—especially those caused by sound-alike or look-alike drug names. See your hospital pharmacist for more information.)

You can submit a report to the FDA even when you aren't sure whether your patient's reaction was serious or when you suspect, but you don't know for certain, that a

To file a report, use the MED-WATCH form, which should be available in your pharmacy. When you fill it out, be as complete as possible. You don't have to include the patient's name or initials, but you should be able to identify the patient if the FDA requests follow-up information.

Some 60,000 reports on adverse reactions are collected annually; more than 400,000 are currently in the FDA's data base. This translates into improved patient safety because the more reports submitted, the more information the FDA will have. The agency can then alert health care professionals to these problems.

What the JCAHO requires

To meet standards set by the Joint Commission on Accreditation of Healthcare Organizations (JCAHO), a hospital must have an adverse drug reaction reporting program in place. The hospital's pharmacy and therapeutics committee is required to review "all significant untoward drug reactions" to ensure quality patient care.

What is a "significant" reaction? According to the JCAHO, it's one in which:
• the drug suspected of causing the reaction must be discontinued.
• the patient requires treatment with another drug, such as an antihistamine, a steroid, or epinephrine.
• the patient's hospital stay is prolonged—for example, because surgery had to be delayed or more diagnostic tests had to be done.

Why is such a reporting program important? For one thing, the quality of care improves when you know which patients are at higher risk for an adverse drug reaction and which drugs are most likely to cause these reactions. You'll be more alert for the early signs and symptoms of problems, and you'll be prepared to intervene before things get out of hand.

Second, the hospital will get more mileage out of its health care dollars because the lengthy stays and extra treatments associated with adverse drug reactions will be decreased.

Third, reducing drug-induced injuries will decrease the number of malpractice lawsuits brought against the hospital and staff. That saves money, time, and aggravation.

Managing I.V. extravasation

Extravasation is the leakage of infused solution from a vein into surrounding tissue. The result of a needle puncturing the vessel wall or leakage around a venipuncture site, extravasation causes local pain and itching, edema, blanching, and decreased skin temperature in the affected extremity. Extravasation of I.V. solution may be referred to as infiltration because the fluid infiltrates the tissues.

Extravasation of a small amount of isotonic fluid or nonirritating drug usually causes only minor discomfort. Treatment involves routine comfort measures, such as the application of warm compresses. However, extravasation of some drugs can severely damage tissue through irritative, sclerotic, vesicant, corrosive, or vasoconstrictive action. In these cases, emergency measures must be taken to minimize tissue damage and necrosis, prevent the need for skin grafts or, rarely, avoid amputation.

Equipment and preparation
• Three 25G ⅝″ needles • antidote for extravasated drug in appropriate syringe • 5-ml syringe • three tuberculin syringes • alcohol sponge or gauze pad soaked in antiseptic cleaning agent • 4″ × 4″ gauze pad • cold and warm compresses.
• Optional: anti-inflammatory drug, 8.4% sodium bicarbonate, 0.9% sodium chloride solution.

Attach one 25G ⅝″ needle to the syringe containing the antidote. Connect the two remaining needles to two tuberculin syringes. Then fill the remaining tuberculin syringe with the anti-inflammatory drug, if needed.

DRUG HAZARDS

Implementation

Hospital policy dictates extravasation treatment steps, which may include some or all of these steps.
• Stop the infusion, and remove the I.V. needle unless you need the route to infiltrate the antidote. Carefully estimate the amount of extravasated solution, and notify the doctor.
• Disconnect the tubing from the I.V. needle. Attach the 5-ml syringe to the needle and try to withdraw 3 to 5 ml of blood to remove any medication or blood in the tubing or needle and to provide a path to the infiltrated tissues.
• Clean the area around the I.V. site with an alcohol sponge or 4" × 4" gauze pad soaked in an antiseptic agent. Then insert the needle of the empty tuberculin syringe into the subcutaneous tissue around the site, and gently aspirate as much solution as possible from the tissue.
• Instill the prescribed antidote into the subcutaneous tissue around the site. Then, if ordered, slowly instill an anti-inflammatory drug subcutaneously to help reduce inflammation and edema.
• If ordered, instill the prescribed antidote through the I.V. needle.
• Apply cold compresses to the affected area for 24 hours, or apply an ice pack for 20 minutes every 4 hours, to cause vasoconstriction that may localize the drug and slow cell metabolism. After 24 hours, apply warm compresses, and elevate the affected extremity to reduce discomfort and promote fluid reabsorption. If the extravasated drug is a vasoconstrictor, such as norepinephrine or metaraminol bitartrate, apply warm compresses only.
• Continuously monitor the I.V. site for signs of abscess or necrosis.

Special considerations

• If you're administering a potentially tissue-damaging drug by I.V. bolus or push, first start an I.V. infusion, preferably with 0.9% sodium chloride solution. Infuse a small amount of this solution, and check for signs of infiltration before injecting the drug.
• Know the antidote (if any) for an I.V. drug that can cause tissue necrosis, in case extravasation occurs. Make sure you're familiar with your hospital's policy regarding the administration of such drugs and their antidotes.
• Tell the patient to report any discomfort at the I.V. site. During infusion, frequently check the site for signs of infiltration.

Antidotes for extravasation

ANTIDOTE	DOSE	EXTRAVASATED DRUG
Ascorbic acid injection	50 mg	• dactinomycin
Edetate calcium disodium (calcium EDTA)	150 mg	• cadmium • copper • manganese • zinc
Hyaluronidase 15 units/ml Mix a 150-unit vial with 1 ml 0.9% sodium chloride solution for injection. Withdraw 0.1 ml, and dilute with 0.9 ml of the sodium chloride solution to get 15 units/ml.	0.2 ml injected subcutaneously five times around site of extravasation	• aminophylline • calcium solutions • contrast media • dextrose solutions (concentrations of 10% or more) • nafcillin • potassium solutions • total parenteral nutrition solutions • vinblastine • vincristine • vindesine
Hydrocortisone sodium succinate 100 mg/ml Usually followed by topical application of hydrocortisone cream 1%	50 to 200 mg or 25 to 50 mg/ml of extravasate injected locally around site of extravasation	• doxorubicin • vincristine
Phentolamine Dilute 5 to 10 mg with 10 ml of sterile 0.9% sodium chloride solution for injection.	5 to 10 ml injected locally around site of extravasation	• dobutamine • dopamine • epinephrine • metaraminol bitartrate • norepinephrine
Sodium bicarbonate 8.4%	5 ml injected locally around site of extravasation	• carmustine • daunorubicin • doxorubicin • vinblastine • vincristine
Sodium thiosulfate 10% Dilute 4 ml with 6 ml of sterile water for injection.	10 ml injected locally around site of extravasation	• dactinomycin • mechlorethamine • mitomycin

DRUG HAZARDS

Drug overdoses

General guidelines

If your patient has signs of acute drug toxicity, institute advanced life support measures as indicated. Administer the prescribed antidote, if available, and institute measures to block absorption and speed elimination of the drug, as ordered. Consult with a regional poison control center for additional information about treatment of specific toxins. The steps below outline how to manage an acute overdose of ingested systemic drugs.

Starting advanced life support
• Establish and maintain an airway. This is usually done by inserting an oropharyngeal or endotracheal airway.
• If the patient is not breathing, start ventilation with a bag-valve mask until a mechanical ventilator is available. Administer oxygen as indicated by pulse oximetry or arterial blood gas levels.
• Maintain circulation. Start an I.V. infusion and obtain laboratory specimens to assess for toxic drug levels, electrolytes, and glucose levels as indicated. *For hypotension:* Administer fluids and vasopressors such as dopamine (Intropin). *For hypertension:* Prepare to administer antihypertensive agents (usually beta blockers if catecholamines were ingested). Prepare to treat arrhythmias as indicated for the specific toxin.
• Protect the patient from injury and monitor for seizures. Observe the patient, and provide supportive care. Prepare to administer lorazepam, diazepam, or phenytoin, as ordered.

Administering the antidote
The antidote is administered as soon as possible. As ordered, administer the prescribed antidote according to the class of drugs the patient has taken. The specific antidotes are described in the following pages.

Blocking drug absorption
• Gastric emptying is effective 1 to 2 hours after drug ingestion. Two methods are used: syrup of ipecac for a conscious patient who is not expected to deteriorate, and gastric lavage for a comatose patient or one who does not respond to syrup of ipecac.
• Adsorption with activated charcoal is used in place of emesis or lavage if the drug is well adsorbed by activated charcoal or after emesis or lavage to adsorb co-ingestants if the primary toxin is not well adsorbed by activated charcoal.
• A cathartic may be given to speed transit of the poison through the GI tract. Whole bowel irrigation with a balanced polyethylene glycol electrolyte solution may be ordered if a sustained-release product was ingested.

Speeding drug elimination
• Gastric dialysis uses timed doses of activated charcoal for 1 to 2 days. The charcoal binds to the drug, thereby facilitating its removal in feces.
• Diuresis is effective for some drug overdoses. Forced diuresis uses furosemide and osmotic diuretics; alkaline diuresis uses I.V. sodium bicarbonate; and acid diuresis uses oral or I.V. ascorbic acid or ammonium chloride.
• Peritoneal dialysis and hemodialysis are occasionally used in severe overdose.

► LIFE-THREATENING EFFECTS

Administering antidotes in poisoning or overdose

ANTIDOTE AND INDICATIONS	DOSAGE	NURSING CONSIDERATIONS
Acetylcysteine (Airbron, Mucomyst, Mucosol, Parvolex) • Treatment of acetaminophen toxicity	• *Adults and children:* 140 mg/kg P.O. initially, followed by 70 mg/kg q 4 hr for 17 doses (total of 1,330 mg/kg).	• Use cautiously in elderly or debilitated patients and in patients with asthma or severe respiratory insufficiency. • Don't use with activated charcoal. • Don't combine with amphotericin B, ampicillin, chymotrypsin, erythromycin lactobionate, hydrogen peroxide, iodized oil, oxytetracycline, tetracycline, or trypsin. Administer separately.
Activated charcoal (Actidose-Aqua, Charcoaide, Charcocaps, Liqui-Char, Superchar) • Treatment of poisoning or overdose with most orally administered drugs, except caustic agents and hydrocarbons	• *Adults:* initially, 1 g/kg (30 to 100 g) P.O., or 5 to 10 times the amount of poison ingested as a suspension in 180 to 240 ml of water. • *Children ages 1 to 12:* 20 to 50 g P.O. as single dose. • *Children under age 1:* 1 g/kg P.O. as single dose.	• Don't give to semiconscious or unconscious patients. • If possible, administer within 30 minutes of poisoning. Administer larger dose if patient has food in his stomach. • Don't give with syrup of ipecac because charcoal inactivates ipecac. If a patient needs syrup of ipecac, give charcoal after he has finished vomiting. • Don't give in ice cream, milk, or sherbet because they reduce adsorption capacities of charcoal. • Powder form is most effective. Mix with tap water to form thick syrup. You may add small amount of fruit juice or flavoring to make syrup more palatable. • You may need to repeat dose if patient vomits shortly after administration.

(continued)

DRUG HAZARDS

Administering antidotes in poisoning or overdose *(continued)*

ANTIDOTE AND INDICATIONS	DOSAGE	NURSING CONSIDERATIONS
Aminocaproic acid (Amicar) • Antidote for alteplase, anistreplase, streptokinase, or urokinase toxicity	• *Adults:* initially, 5 g P.O. or as slow I.V. infusion, followed by 1 to 1.25 g/hr until bleeding is controlled. Don't exceed 30 g daily.	• Use cautiously with oral contraceptives and estrogens because they may increase risk of hypercoagulability. • For infusion, dilute solution with sterile water for injection, 0.9% sodium chloride injection, dextrose 5% in water (D_5W), or Ringer's solution. • Monitor coagulation studies, heart rhythm, and blood pressure.
Amyl nitrite • Antidote for cyanide poisoning	• *Adults:* 0.2 or 0.3 ml by inhalation for 30 to 60 sec q 5 min until patient regains consciousness.	• Amyl nitrite is effective within 30 seconds, but its effects last only 3 to 5 minutes. • To administer, wrap ampule in cloth and crush. Hold near the patient's nose and mouth so that he can inhale vapor. • Monitor the patient for orthostatic hypotension. • The patient may experience headache after administration.
Atropine sulfate • Antidote for anticholinesterase toxicity	• *Adults:* initially, 1 to 2 mg by direct I.V. injection, then 2 mg q 5 to 60 min until symptoms subside. In severe cases, initial dose may be as much as 6 mg q 4 to 60 min, as needed. Administer over 1 to 2 min.	• Atropine sulfate is contraindicated for patients with glaucoma, myasthenia gravis, obstructive uropathy, or unstable cardiovascular status. • Monitor intake and output to assess for urine retention.

Administering antidotes in poisoning or overdose *(continued)*

ANTIDOTE AND INDICATIONS	DOSAGE	NURSING CONSIDERATIONS
Botulism antitoxin, trivalent equine • Treatment of botulism	• *Adults and children:* 2 vials I.V. Dilute antitoxin 1:10 in D_5W, dextrose 10% in water, or 0.9% sodium chloride solution before administration. Give first 10 ml of diluted solution over 5 min; after 15 min, you may increase rate.	• Obtain an accurate patient history of allergies, especially to horses, and of reactions to immunizations. • Test the patient for sensitivity (against a control of 0.9% sodium chloride solution in opposing extremity) before administration. Read results after 5 to 30 minutes. A wheal indicates a positive reaction, requiring patient desensitization. • Keep epinephrine 1:1,000 available in case of allergic reaction.
Deferoxamine mesylate (Desferal) • Adjunctive treatment of acute iron intoxication	• *Adults and children:* initially, 1 g I.M. or I.V., followed by 500 mg I.M. or I.V. q 4 hr for two doses; then 500 mg I.M. or I.V. q 4 to 12 hr. Don't infuse more than 15 mg/kg/hr. Don't administer more than 6 g in 24 hr.	• Don't administer the drug to patients with severe renal disease or anuria. Use cautiously in patients with impaired renal function. • Keep epinephrine 1:1,000 available in case of allergic reaction. • Use I.M. route if possible. Use I.V. route only when the patient is in shock. • To reconstitute for I.M. administration, add 2 ml of sterile water for injection to each ampule. Make sure the drug dissolves completely. To reconstitute for I.V. administration, dissolve as for I.M. use but in 0.9% sodium chloride solution, D_5W, or lactated Ringer's solution. • Monitor intake and output carefully. Warn patient that his urine may turn red. • Reconstituted solution can be stored for up to 1 week at room temperature. Protect from light. *(continued)*

Administering antidotes in poisoning or overdose *(continued)*

ANTIDOTE AND INDICATIONS	DOSAGE	NURSING CONSIDERATIONS
Digoxin immune Fab (ovine) (Digibind) • Treatment of potentially life-threatening digoxin or digitoxin intoxication	• *Adults and children:* give I.V. over 30 min or as a bolus if cardiac arrest is imminent. Dosage varies according to amount of drug ingested; average dose is 10 vials (400 mg), but if toxicity resulted from acute digoxin ingestion and neither serum digoxin level nor estimated ingestion amount is known, increase dose to 20 vials (800 mg).	• Use cautiously in patients allergic to ovine proteins because the drug is derived from digoxin-specific antibody fragments obtained from immunized sheep. Perform skin test before administering. • Use only in patients in shock or cardiac arrest with ventricular arrhythmias, such as ventricular tachycardia or fibrillation; with progressive bradycardia, such as severe sinus bradycardia; or with second- or third-degree atrioventricular block unresponsive to atropine. • Infuse through a 0.22-micron membrane filter, if possible. • Refrigerate powder for reconstitution. If possible, use reconstituted drug immediately, although you may refrigerate it for up to 4 hours. • Drug interferes with digitalis immunoassay measurements, resulting in misleading standard serum digoxin levels until the drug is cleared from the body (about 2 days). • Total serum digoxin levels may rise after administration of this drug, reflecting Fab-bound (inactive) digoxin. • Monitor potassium levels closely.

Administering antidotes in poisoning or overdose *(continued)*

ANTIDOTE AND INDICATIONS	DOSAGE	NURSING CONSIDERATIONS
Edetate calcium disodium (Calcium Disodium Versenate, Calcium EDTA) • Treatment of lead poisoning in patients with blood levels >50 mcg/dl	*For blood levels of 51 to 100 mcg/dl* • *Adults and children:* 1 g/m² I.M. or I.V. daily for 3 to 5 days. For I.V. infusion, dilute in D₅W or 0.9% sodium chloride solution and give over 1 to 2 hr. *For blood levels >100 mcg/dl* • *Adults and children:* 1.5 g/m² I.M. or I.V. daily for 3 to 5 days, usually with dimercaprol. For I.V. infusion, dilute in D₅W or 0.9% sodium chloride solution and administer over 1 to 2 hr. If necessary, repeat course 2 to 3 weeks later.	• Don't give to patients with severe renal disease or anuria. • Avoid using I.V. route in patients with lead encephalopathy because intracranial pressure may increase; use I.M. route. • Avoid rapid infusion; I.M. route is preferred, especially for children. • If giving a high dose, give with dimercaprol to avoid toxicity. • Force fluids to facilitate lead excretion except in patients with lead encephalopathy. • Before giving, obtain baseline intake and output, urinalysis, blood urea nitrogen, and serum alkaline phosphatase, calcium, creatinine, and phosphorus levels. Then monitor these values on first, third, and fifth days of treatment. Monitor electrocardiogram (ECG) periodically. • If procaine hydrochloride has been added to I.M. solution to minimize pain, watch for local reaction.
Methylene blue • Treatment of cyanide poisoning	• *Adults and children:* 1 to 2 mg/ kg of 1% solution by direct I.V. injection over several minutes. May repeat dose in 1 hr.	• Don't give to patients with severe renal impairment or hypersensitivity to drug. • Use with caution in glucose-6-phosphate dehydrogenase deficiency; may cause hemolysis. • Avoid extravasation; S.C. injection may cause necrotic abscesses. • Warn the patient that methylene blue will discolor his urine and stools and stain his skin. Hypochlorite solution rubbed on his skin will remove stains.

(continued)

DRUG HAZARDS

Administering antidotes in poisoning or overdose *(continued)*

ANTIDOTE AND INDICATIONS	DOSAGE	NURSING CONSIDERATIONS
Naloxone hydrochloride (Narcan) • Treatment of respiratory depression caused by opioid drugs • Treatment of postoperative narcotic depression • Treatment of asphyxia neonatorum	*For respiratory depression caused by opioid drugs* • *Adults:* 0.4 to 2 mg I.V., S.C., or I.M. May repeat q 2 to 3 min p.r.n. *For postoperative narcotic depression* • *Adults:* 0.1 to 0.2 mg I.V. q 2 to 3 min p.r.n. • *Children:* 0.01 mg/kg I.V., I.M., or S.C. Repeat as necessary q 2 to 3 min. If patient doesn't improve with initial dose of 0.01 mg/kg, he may need up to 10 times this dose (0.1 mg/kg). *For asphyxia neonatorum* • *Neonates:* 0.01 mg/kg I.V. into umbilical vein. Repeat q 2 to 3 min for three doses, if necessary.	• Use cautiously in patients with cardiac irritability or narcotic addiction. • Monitor respiratory depth and rate. Be prepared to provide oxygen, ventilation, and other resuscitative measures. • If neonatal concentration (0.02 mg/ml) isn't available, dilute adult concentration (0.4 mg) by mixing 0.5 ml with 9.5 ml of sterile water or 0.9% sodium chloride injection. • Respiratory rate increases within 2 min. Effects last 1 to 4 hours. • Duration of narcotic may exceed that of naloxone, causing the patient to relapse into respiratory depression. • You may administer drug by continuous I.V. infusion to control adverse effects of epidurally administered morphine. • You may see "overshoot" effect—the patient's respiratory rate after receiving drug exceeds his rate before respiratory depression occurred. • Naloxone is the safest drug to use when the cause of respiratory depression is uncertain. • This drug doesn't reverse respiratory depression caused by diazepam. • Although generally believed ineffective in treating respiratory depression caused by nonopioid drugs, naloxone may reverse coma induced by alcohol intoxication, according to recent reports.

Administering antidotes in poisoning or overdose *(continued)*

ANTIDOTE AND INDICATIONS	DOSAGE	NURSING CONSIDERATIONS
Pralidoxime chloride (Protopam Chloride) • Antidote for organophosphate poisoning and cholinergic drug overdose	• *Adults:* I.V. infusion of 1 to 2 g in 100 ml of 0.9% sodium chloride solution over 15 to 30 min. If the patient has pulmonary edema, administer by slow I.V. push over 5 min. Repeat in 1 hr if weakness persists. If the patient needs additional doses, administer them cautiously. If I.V. administration isn't possible, give I.M. or S.C., or 1 to 3 g P.O. q 5 hr. • *Children:* 20 to 40 mg/kg I.V.	• Don't give to patients poisoned with carbaryl (Sevin), a carbamate insecticide, because it increases Sevin's toxicity. • Use with caution in patients with renal insufficiency, myasthenia gravis, asthma, or peptic ulcer. • Use in hospitalized patients only; have respiratory and other supportive equipment available. • Administer antidote as soon as possible after poisoning. Treatment is most effective if started within 24 hours of exposure. • Before administering, suction secretions and make sure airway is patent. • Dilute drug with sterile water without preservatives. Give atropine along with pralidoxime. • If the patient's skin was exposed, remove his clothing and wash his skin and hair with sodium bicarbonate, soap, water, and alcohol as soon as possible. He may need a second washing. When washing the patient, wear protective gloves and clothes to avoid exposure. • Observe the patient for 48 to 72 hours if he ingested poison. Delayed absorption may occur. • Watch for signs of rapid weakening in the patient with myasthenia gravis being treated for overdose of cholinergic drugs. He may pass quickly from cholinergic crisis to myasthenic crisis and require more cholinergic drugs to treat the myasthenia. Keep edrophonium available.

(continued)

DRUG HAZARDS

Administering antidotes in poisoning or overdose *(continued)*

ANTIDOTE AND INDICATIONS	DOSAGE	NURSING CONSIDERATIONS
Protamine sulfate • Treatment of heparin overdose	• *Adults:* usually 1 mg for each 78 to 95 units of heparin, based on coagulation studies. Dilute to 1% (10 mg/ml) and give by slow I.V. injection over 1 to 3 min. Don't exceed 50 mg in 10 min.	• Use cautiously after cardiac surgery. • Administer slowly to reduce adverse reactions. Have equipment available to treat shock. • Monitor the patient continuously, and check vital signs frequently. • Watch for spontaneous bleeding (heparin "rebound"), especially in patients undergoing dialysis and in those who have had cardiac surgery. • Protamine sulfate may act as an anticoagulant in extremely high doses.
Syrup of ipecac (ipecac syrup) • Induction of vomiting in poisoning	• *Adults:* 15 ml P.O., followed by 200 to 300 ml of water. • *Children over age 1:* 15 ml P.O., followed by about 200 ml of water or milk. • *Children under age 1:* 5 to 10 ml P.O., followed by 100 to 200 ml of water or milk. Repeat dose once after 20 min, if necessary.	• Ipecac syrup is contraindicated for semicomatose, unconscious, and severely inebriated patients and for those with seizures, shock, or absent gag reflex. • Don't give after ingestion of petroleum distillates or volatile oils because of the risk of aspiration pneumonitis. Don't give after ingestion of caustic substances such as lye because further injury can result. • Before giving, make sure you have ipecac syrup, not ipecac fluid extract (14 times more concentrated, and deadly). • If two doses don't induce vomiting, notify doctor, who will probably order gastric lavage. • If the patient also needs activated charcoal, give charcoal after he has vomited or charcoal will neutralize emetic effect. • Suggest to parents of children over age 1 that they keep 1 oz (30 ml) of syrup available.

► LIFE-THREATENING EFFECTS

Acetaminophen overdose

In an acute overdose, plasma levels of 300 mcg/ml 4 hours after ingestion or 50 mcg/ml 12 hours after ingestion are associated with hepatotoxicity. Clinical findings in an overdose include cyanosis, anemia, jaundice, skin eruptions, fever, emesis, central nervous system stimulation, delirium, and methemoglobinemia progressing to CNS depression, coma, vascular collapse, seizures, and death. Acetaminophen poisoning develops in stages:
• *Stage 1* (12 to 24 hours after ingestion): nausea, vomiting, diaphoresis, anorexia
• *Stage 2* (24 to 48 hours after ingestion): clinically improved but elevated liver function tests
• *Stage 3* (72 to 96 hours after ingestion): peak hepatotoxicity
• *Stage 4* (7 to 8 days after ingestion): recovery.

To treat acetaminophen toxicity, immediately induce emesis with ipecac syrup if patient is conscious, or with gastric lavage. Administer activated charcoal via a nasogastric tube. Oral acetylcysteine, a specific antidote for acetaminophen poisoning, is most effective if started within 12 hours after ingestion but can help if started as late as 24 hours after ingestion. Administer an acetylcysteine loading dose of 140 mg/kg P.O., followed by maintenance doses of 70 mg/kg P.O. every 4 hours for an additional 17 doses. Doses vomited within 1 hour of administration must be repeated. Remove charcoal by lavage before administering acetylcysteine because it may interfere with this antidote's absorption.

Acetylcysteine minimizes hepatic injury by supplying sulfhydryl groups that bind with acetaminophen metabolites. Hemodialysis may be helpful in removing acetaminophen from the body. Monitor laboratory parameters and vital signs closely. Cimetidine has been used investigationally to block acetaminophen's metabolism to toxic intermediates. Provide symptomatic and supportive measures (respiratory support and correction of fluid and electrolyte imbalances). Determine plasma acetaminophen levels at least 4 hours after overdose. If they indicate hepatotoxicity, perform liver function tests every 24 hours for at least 96 hours.

◄

► LIFE-THREATENING EFFECTS

Analeptic drug overdose (amphetamines, cocaine)

Individual responses to overdose vary widely. Toxic doses also vary, depending upon the drug and the route of ingestion.

Signs and symptoms of overdose include restlessness, tremor, hyperreflexia, tachypnea, confusion, aggressiveness, hallucinations, and panic; fatigue and depression usually follow excitement stage. Other effects may include arrhythmias, shock, altered blood pressure, nausea, vomiting, diarrhea, and abdominal cramps; death is usually preceded by seizures and coma.

Treat overdose symptomatically and supportively: If oral ingestion is recent (within 4 hours), use gastric lavage or ipecac syrup to empty the stomach and reduce further absorption. Follow with activated charcoal. Monitor vital signs and fluid and electrolyte balance. If drug was smoked or injected, interventions are focused on enhanced drug elimination and providing supportive care. Administer sedatives as needed. Urine acidification may

DRUG HAZARDS

enhance excretion. A saline cathartic (magnesium citrate) may hasten GI evacuation of unabsorbed sustained-release drug.

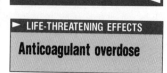

► LIFE-THREATENING EFFECTS
Anticholinergic overdose

Clinical effects of an overdose include such peripheral effects as dilated, nonreactive pupils; blurred vision; flushed, hot, dry skin; dry mucous membranes; dysphagia; decreased or absent bowel sounds; urine retention; hyperthermia; tachycardia; hypertension; and increased respiratory rate.

Treatment is primarily symptomatic and supportive, as needed. If patient is alert, induce emesis (or use gastric lavage), and follow with a saline cathartic and activated charcoal to prevent further drug absorption. In severe cases, physostigmine may be administered to block central antimuscarinic effects. Give fluids as needed to treat shock. If urine retention occurs, catheterization may be necessary.

► LIFE-THREATENING EFFECTS
Anticoagulant overdose

Clinical effects of an oral anticoagulant overdose vary with severity. They may include internal or external bleeding or skin necrosis, but the most common sign is hematuria. Excessively prolonged prothrombin time or minor bleeding mandates withdrawal of therapy; withholding one or two doses may be adequate in some cases. Treatment to control bleeding may include oral or I.V. phytonadione (vitamin K_1) and, in severe hemor-

rhage, fresh frozen plasma or whole blood. Menadione (vitamin K_3) isn't as effective. Use of phytonadione may interfere with subsequent oral anticoagulant therapy.

► LIFE-THREATENING EFFECTS
Antihistamine overdose

Drowsiness is the usual clinical sign of overdose. Seizures, coma, and respiratory depression may occur with severe overdose. Certain histamine$_1$ antagonists, such as diphenhydramine, also block cholinergic receptors and produce modest anticholinergic symptoms, such as dry mouth, flushed skin, fixed and dilated pupils, and GI symptoms, especially in children. Phenothiazine-type antihistamines, such as promethazine, also block dopamine receptors. Movement disorders mimicking Parkinson's disease may be seen.

Treat overdose with gastric lavage followed by activated charcoal. Ipecac syrup is generally not recommended because acute dystonic reactions may increase risk of aspiration. In addition, phenothiazine-type antihistamines may have antiemetic effects. Treat hypotension with fluids or vasopressors, and treat seizures with phenytoin or diazepam. Watch for arrhythmias, and treat accordingly.

► LIFE-THREATENING EFFECTS
Barbiturate overdose

An overdose causes unsteady gait, slurred speech, sustained nystagmus, somnolence, confusion, respiratory depression, pulmonary edema, areflexia, and coma. Typical shock syndrome with tachycardia and hypotension, jaundice, hypothermia followed by fever, and oliguria may occur.

Maintain and support ventilation and pulmonary function as necessary; support cardiac function and circulation with vasopressors and I.V. fluids as needed. If patient is conscious and gag reflex is intact, induce emesis (if ingestion was recent) by administering ipecac syrup. If emesis is contraindicated, perform gastric lavage while a cuffed endotracheal tube is in place to prevent aspiration. Follow with administration of activated charcoal and saline cathartic. Measure intake and output, vital signs, and laboratory parameters; maintain body temperature. Patient should be rolled from side to side every 30 minutes to avoid pulmonary congestion.

Alkalinization of urine may be helpful in removing drug from the body; hemodialysis may be useful in severe overdose.

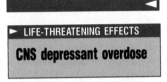

► LIFE-THREATENING EFFECTS
Benzodiazepine overdose

An overdose of benzodiazepines produces somnolence, confusion, coma, hypoactive reflexes, dyspnea, labored breathing, hypotension, bradycardia, slurred speech, and unsteady gait or impaired coordination.

Support blood pressure and respiration until drug effects subside; monitor vital signs. Mechanical ventilatory assistance via endotracheal tube may be required to maintain a patent airway and support adequate oxygenation. Flumazenil, a specific benzodiazepine antagonist, may be useful. Use I.V. fluids or vasopressors such as dopamine and phenyl-

ephrine to treat hypotension as needed. If the patient is conscious and his gag reflex is intact, induce emesis (if ingestion was recent) by administering ipecac syrup. If emesis is contraindicated, perform gastric lavage while a cuffed endotracheal tube is in place to prevent aspiration. After emesis or lavage, administer activated charcoal with a cathartic as a single dose. Dialysis is of limited value.

► LIFE-THREATENING EFFECTS
CNS depressant overdose

Signs of central nervous system (CNS) depressant overdose include prolonged coma, hypotension, hypothermia followed by fever, and inadequate ventilation even without significant respiratory depression. Absence of pupillary reflexes, dilated pupils, loss of deep tendon reflexes, tonic muscle spasms, and apnea may occur.

Treatment of overdose involves support of respiration and cardiovascular function; mechanical ventilation may be necessary. Maintain adequate urine output with adequate hydration while avoiding pulmonary edema. Empty gastric contents by inducing emesis. For lipid-soluble drugs such as glutethimide, charcoal and resin hemoperfusion are effective in removing the drug; hemodialysis and peritoneal dialysis are of minimal value. Because of the significant storage of glutethimide in fat tissue, blood levels commonly show large fluctuations with worsening of symptoms.

DRUG HAZARDS

► LIFE-THREATENING EFFECTS
Digitalis glycoside overdose

Clinical effects of an overdose primarily affect the GI, cardiac, and central nervous systems.

Severe overdose may cause hyperkalemia, which may develop rapidly and result in life-threatening cardiac effects. Cardiac signs of digoxin toxicity may occur with or without other toxicity signs and commonly precede other toxic effects. Because cardiotoxic effects also can occur in heart disease, determining whether these effects result from an underlying heart disease or digoxin toxicity may be difficult. Digoxin has caused almost every kind of arrhythmia; various combinations of arrhythmias may occur in the same patient. Patients with chronic digoxin toxicity commonly have ventricular arrhythmias, atrioventricular (AV) conduction disturbances, or both. Patients with digoxin-induced ventricular tachycardia have a high mortality because ventricular fibrillation or asystole may result.

If toxicity is suspected, the drug should be discontinued and serum drug level measurements obtained. Usually, the drug takes at least 6 hours to be distributed between plasma and tissue and reach equilibrium; plasma levels drawn earlier may show higher digoxin levels than those present after the drug is distributed into the tissues.

Other treatment measures include immediate emesis induction, gastric lavage, and administration of activated charcoal to reduce absorption of the remaining drug. Multiple doses of activated charcoal (such as 50 g q 6 hours) may help reduce further absorption, especially of any drug undergoing enterohepatic

recirculation. Some clinicians advocate cholestyramine administration if digoxin was recently ingested; however, it may not be useful if the ingestion is life-threatening. Any interacting drugs probably should be discontinued. Ventricular arrhythmias may be treated with I.V. potassium (replacement doses; but not in patients with significant AV block), I.V. phenytoin, I.V. lidocaine, or I.V. propranolol. Refractory ventricular tachyarrhythmias may be controlled with overdrive pacing. Procainamide may be used for ventricular arrhythmias that do not respond to the above treatments. In severe AV block, asystole, and hemodynamically significant sinus bradycardia, atropine restores a normal rate.

Administration of digoxin-specific antibody fragments (digoxin immune Fab [Digibind]) is a promising new treatment for life-threatening digoxin toxicity. Each 40 mg of digoxin immune Fab binds about 0.6 mg of digoxin in the bloodstream. The complex is then excreted in the urine, rapidly decreasing serum levels and therefore cardiac drug concentrations.

► LIFE-THREATENING EFFECTS
Iron supplement overdose

Iron supplements represent a major source of poisoning, especially in small children. In fact, as little as 1 g of ferrous sulfate can kill an infant.

Symptoms of poisoning result from iron's acute corrosive effects on the GI mucosa, as well as the adverse metabolic effects caused by iron overload. Four stages of acute iron poisoning have been identified, and signs and symptoms may occur within the first 10 to 60 minutes of ingestion or may be delayed several hours.

The first findings reflect acute GI irritation and include epigastric pain, nausea, and vomiting. Diarrhea may present as green, followed by tarry, stools, then as melena. Hematemesis may be accompanied by drowsiness, lassitude, shock, and coma. Local erosion of the stomach and small intestine may further enhance the absorption of iron. If death does not occur in the first phase, a second phase of apparent recovery may last 24 hours. A third phase, which can occur 4 to 48 hours after ingestion, is marked by central nervous system abnormalities, metabolic acidosis, hepatic dysfunction, renal failure, and bleeding diathesis. This may progress to circulatory failure, coma, and death. If the patient survives, the fourth phase consists of late complications of acute iron intoxication and may occur 2 to 6 weeks after overdose. Severe gastric scarring, pyloric stenosis, or intestinal obstruction may be present.

Patients who develop vomiting, diarrhea, leukocytosis, or hyperglycemia and have an abdominal radiograph positive for iron within 6 hours of ingestion are likely to be at risk for serious toxicity. Empty the stomach by inducing emesis with ipecac syrup, and perform gastric lavage. If patients have had multiple episodes of vomiting or the vomitus contains blood, avoid ipecac and perform lavage. Some clinicians add sodium bicarbonate to the lavage solution to convert ferrous iron to ferrous carbonate, which is poorly absorbed. Disodium phosphate has also been used; however, some children may develop life-threatening hyperphosphatemia or hypercalcemia. Other possible treatments include lavage with 0.9% sodium chloride solution, administration of a saline cathartic, surgical removal of tablets, and chelation therapy with deferoxamine mesylate. Hemodialysis is of little value. Supportive treatment includes monitoring acid-base balance, maintaining a patent airway, and controlling shock and dehydration with appropriate I.V. therapy.

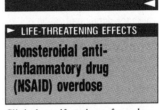

► LIFE-THREATENING EFFECTS
Nonsteroidal anti-inflammatory drug (NSAID) overdose

Clinical manifestations of overdose include dizziness, drowsiness, paresthesia, vomiting, nausea, abdominal pain, headache, sweating, nystagmus, apnea, and cyanosis.

To treat overdose of ibuprofen, empty stomach immediately by inducing emesis with ipecac syrup or by gastric lavage. Administer activated charcoal via a nasogastric tube. Provide symptomatic and supportive measures (respiratory support and correction of fluid and electrolyte imbalances). Monitor laboratory parameters and vital signs closely. Alkaline diuresis may enhance renal excretion. Dialysis is of minimal value because ibuprofen is strongly protein-bound.

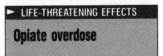

► LIFE-THREATENING EFFECTS
Opiate overdose

Rapid I.V. administration may result in overdose because of the delay in maximum central nervous system (CNS) effect (30 minutes). The most common signs of morphine overdose are respiratory depression with or without CNS depression and miosis (pinpoint pupils). Other acute toxic effects include hypoten-

DRUG HAZARDS

sion, bradycardia, hypothermia, shock, apnea, cardiopulmonary arrest, circulatory collapse, pulmonary edema, and seizures.

To treat acute overdose, first establish adequate respiratory exchange via a patent airway and ventilation, as needed; administer a narcotic antagonist (naloxone) to reverse respiratory depression. (Because the duration of action of morphine is longer than that of naloxone, repeated doses of naloxone are necessary.) Naloxone should not be given unless clinically significant respiratory or cardiovascular depression is present. Monitor vital signs closely.

If the patient presents within 2 hours of an oral overdose, empty the stomach immediately by inducing emesis (with ipecac syrup) or using gastric lavage. Use caution to avoid any risk of aspiration. Administer activated charcoal via a nasogastric tube for further removal of the drug in an oral overdose.

Provide symptomatic and supportive treatment (continued respiratory support and correction of fluid or electrolyte imbalance). Monitor laboratory parameters, vital signs, and neurologic status closely.

▶ LIFE-THREATENING EFFECTS
Phenothiazine overdose

Central nervous system depression is characterized by deep, unarousable sleep and possible coma, hypotension or hypertension, extrapyramidal symptoms, abnormal involuntary muscle movements, agitation, seizures, arrhythmias, electrocardiogram changes, hypothermia or hyperthermia, and autonomic nervous system dysfunction.

Treatment is symptomatic and supportive, including maintaining vital signs, a patent airway, stable body temperature, and fluid and electrolyte balance.

Do not induce vomiting; because phenothiazines inhibit the cough reflex, aspiration may occur. Use gastric lavage, then activated charcoal and saline cathartics. Dialysis does not help. Regulate body temperature as needed. Treat hypotension with I.V. fluids: *Don't give epinephrine.* Treat seizures with parenteral diazepam or barbiturates; arrhythmias with parenteral phenytoin; and extrapyramidal reactions with benztropine or parenteral diphenhydramine.

▶ LIFE-THREATENING EFFECTS
Salicylate overdose

Clinical effects of an overdose include metabolic acidosis with respiratory alkalosis, hyperpnea, and tachypnea, due to increased carbon dioxide production and direct stimulation of the respiratory center.

To treat aspirin overdose, empty the patient's stomach immediately by inducing emesis with ipecac syrup if patient is conscious, or by gastric lavage. Administer activated charcoal via a nasogastric tube. Provide symptomatic and supportive measures (respiratory support and correction of fluid and electrolyte imbalances). Closely monitor laboratory values and vital signs. Enhance renal excretion by administering sodium bicarbonate to alkalinize urine. Use cooling blanket or sponging if patient's rectal temperature is above 104° F (40° C). Hemodialysis is effective in removing aspirin but is used only in severely poisoned individuals or those at risk for pulmonary edema.

► LIFE-THREATENING EFFECTS

Tricyclic antidepressant overdose

This overdose is commonly life-threatening, particularly when combined with alcohol. The first 12 hours after ingestion are a stimulatory phase characterized by excessive anticholinergic activity (agitation, irritation, confusion, hallucinations, hyperthermia, parkinsonian symptoms, seizures, urine retention, dry mucous membranes, pupillary dilation, constipation, and ileus). This phase precedes central nervous system (CNS) depressant effects, including hypothermia, decreased or absent reflexes, sedation, hypotension, cyanosis, and cardiac irregularities, including tachycardia, conduction disturbances, and quinidine-like effects on the electrocardiogram.

Severity of overdose is best indicated by a widening of the QRS complex, which usually represents severe toxicity; obtaining serum measurements is usually not helpful. Metabolic acidosis may follow hypotension, hypoventilation, and seizures.

Treatment is symptomatic and supportive, including maintaining a patent airway, stable body temperature, and fluid and electrolyte balance. Induce emesis if patient is conscious; follow with gastric lavage and activated charcoal to prevent further absorption. Dialysis is of little use. Treat seizures with parenteral diazepam or phenytoin; arrhythmias with parenteral phenytoin or lidocaine; and acidosis with sodium bicarbonate. Do not give barbiturates; they may enhance CNS and respiratory depressant effects.

►

Dangers of uncontrolled I.V. flow

Let's suppose that you're caring for a patient who's receiving a drug through an electronic infusion device. His gown needs changing, but it doesn't have sleeve snaps. So you have to deactivate the device, clamp and remove the tubing, remove the fluid bag from the I.V. pole, and pull the I.V. bag and tubing through the sleeve—a tiresome job.

Actually, the task is more than tiresome: It's dangerous. In one documented case, a nurse deactivated the infusion device, and her patient died. Either she didn't secure the roller clamp correctly or it malfunctioned, causing rapid, uncontrolled drug flow into the patient.

No standards

No standards exist for I.V. devices and sets, so many systems don't have free-flow protection. Because safer systems are more expensive, hospitals may use them only in labor and delivery units or critical areas, or to give drugs with narrow therapeutic windows. This increases your risk for error because you may get used to using the safer equipment and mistake one system for another.

To protect your patients and yourself, be extremely careful when using infusion sets—especially if you're unfamiliar with a hospital's equipment because you're floating to a temporary assignment. This will have to do until free-flow protected equipment becomes the standard.

DRUG HAZARDS

Interactions

Compatibility of drugs combined in a syringe

KEY
Y = compatible for at least 30 minutes
P = provisionally compatible; administer within 15 minutes
P(5) = provisionally compatible; administer within 5 minutes
N = not compatible
* = conflicting data

(A blank space indicates no available data.)

	atropine sulfate	benzquinamide HCl	butorphanol tartrate	chlorpromazine HCl	cimetidine HCl	codeine phosphate	dimenhydrinate	diphenhydramine HCl	droperidol	fentanyl citrate	glycopyrrolate	heparin Na	hydromorphone HCl	hydroxyzine HCl	meperidine HCl	metoclopramide HCl
atropine sulfate	■	Y	Y	Y	Y		P	P	P	P	Y	P(5)	Y	Y	Y	P
benzquinamide HCl	Y	■									Y			Y	Y	
butorphanol tartrate	Y		■	Y	Y		N	Y	Y	Y				Y	P	
chlorpromazine HCl	Y		Y	■	N		N	P	P	P	Y	N	Y	P	P	P
cimetidine HCl	Y		Y	N	■			Y	Y	Y	Y	Y	Y	Y	Y	
codeine phosphate						■					Y			Y		
dimenhydrinate	P		N	N			■	P	P	P	N	P(5)	N	P	P	
diphenhydramine HCl	P		Y	P	Y		P	■	P	P	Y		Y	P	P	Y
droperidol	P		Y	P	Y		P	P	■	P	Y	N		P	P	P
fentanyl citrate	P		Y	P	Y		P	P	P	■		P(5)	Y	Y	P	P
glycopyrrolate	Y	Y		Y	Y	Y	N	Y	Y	Y	■		Y	Y	Y	
heparin Na	P(5)			N	Y		P(5)		N	P(5)		■			N	P(5)
hydromorphone HCl	Y			Y	Y			Y		Y	Y		■	Y		
hydroxyzine HCl	Y	Y	Y	P	Y	Y	N	P	P	Y	Y		Y	■	P	P
meperidine HCl	Y	Y	P	P	Y		P	P	P	P	Y	N		P	■	P
metoclopramide HCl	P			P			P	Y	P	P		P(5)		P	P	■
midazolam HCl	Y	Y	Y	Y	Y		N	Y	Y	Y	Y		Y	Y	Y	Y
morphine sulfate	P	Y	Y	P	Y		P	P	P	P	Y	N*		Y	N	P
nalbuphine HCl	Y			Y				Y			Y			Y		
pentazocine lactate	P	Y	Y	P	Y		P	P	P	P	N	N	Y	Y	P	P
pentobarbital Na	P	N	N	N	N		N	N	N	N	N		Y	N	N	
perphenazine	Y		Y	Y	Y		Y	Y	Y	Y					P	P
phenobarbital Na		N										P(5)				
prochlorperazine edisylate	P		Y	Y	Y		N	P	P	P	Y		N*	P	P	P
promazine HCl	P			P	Y		N	P	P	P	Y			P	P	P
promethazine HCl	P		Y	P	Y		N	P	P	P	Y	N	Y	P	Y	P
ranitidine HCl	Y			Y			Y	Y		Y	Y		Y	N	Y	Y
scopolamine HBr	P	Y	Y	P	Y		P	P	P	P	Y		Y	Y	P	P
secobarbital Na		N			N					N						
sodium bicarbonate										N						N
thiethylperazine maleate			Y											Y		
thiopental Na		N		N			N	N		N				N		

midazolam HCl	morphine sulfate	nalbuphine HCl	pentazocine lactate	pentobarbital Na	perphenazine	phenobarbital Na	prochlorperazine edisylate	promazine HCl	promethazine HCl	ranitidine HCl	scopolamine HBr	secobarbital Na	sodium bicarbonate	thiethylperazine maleate	thiopental Na	
Y	P	Y	P	P	Y		P	P	P	Y	P					atropine sulfate
Y	Y		Y	N		N					Y	N			N	benzquinamide HCl
Y	Y		Y	N	Y		Y		Y		Y			Y		butorphanol tartrate
Y	P		P	N	Y		Y	P	P	Y	P				N	chlorpromazine HCl
Y	Y	Y	Y	N	Y		Y	Y	Y		Y	N				cimetidine HCl
																codeine phosphate
N	P		P	N	Y		N	N	N	Y	P				N	dimenhydrinate
Y	P		P	N	Y		P	P	P	Y	P				N	diphenhydramine HCl
Y	P	Y	P	N	Y		P	P	P		P					droperidol
Y	P		P	N	Y		P	P	P	Y	P					fentanyl citrate
Y	Y		N	N			Y	Y	Y	Y	Y	N	N		N	glycopyrrolate
	N*		N			P(5)			N							heparin Na
Y			Y	Y			N*		Y	Y	Y			Y		hydromorphone HCl
Y	Y	Y	Y	N			P	P	P	N	Y					hydroxyzine HCl
Y	N		P	N	P		P	P	Y	Y	P				N	meperidine HCl
Y	P		P		P		P	P	P	Y	P		N			metoclopramide HCl
■	Y	Y		N	N		N	Y	Y	N	Y			Y		midazolam HCl
Y	■		P	N*	Y		P*	P	P*	Y	P				N	morphine sulfate
Y		■		N			Y		Y	Y	Y			Y		nalbuphine HCl
	P		■	N	Y		P	Y	Y	Y	P					pentazocine lactate
N	N*	N	N		■		N	N	N		Y		Y		Y	pentobarbital Na
N	Y		Y	N	■		Y			Y						perphenazine
						■				N						phenobarbital Na
N	P*	Y	P	N	Y		■	P	P	Y	P				N	prochlorperazine edisylate
Y	P		Y	N			P	■	P	P						promazine HCl
Y	P*	Y	Y	N			P	P	■	Y	P				N	promethazine HCl
N	Y	Y	Y		Y	N	Y	P	Y	■	Y			Y		ranitidine HCl
Y	P	Y	P	Y			P		P	Y	■				Y	scopolamine HBr
												■				secobarbital Na
			Y										■		N	sodium bicarbonate
Y		Y								Y				■		thiethylperazine maleate
	N			Y			N		N		Y		N		■	thiopental Na

Compatibility of I.V. drugs

Use this chart only as a guide to drug compatibilities. Compatibility varies with the type, temperature, and volume of diluting solutions. Never com-

KEY	
24	Compatible (numbers indicate compatible only for hours indicated)
■	Incompatible
?	Questionable compatibility
(blank)	Data unavailable
◺	Identical drug

Compatibility matrix of I.V. drugs. Column headings (left to right): acyclovir, albumin, amikacin, amino acid injection, aminophylline, ampicillin, bretylium, calcium gluconate, cefamandole, cefazolin, cefoxitin, ceftazidime, chloramphenicol, cimetidine, ciprofloxacin, clindamycin, corticotropin, dexamethasone, dextrose 5% in water (D₅W), D₅W in lactated Ringer's, D₅W in 0.9% NaCl solution, diazepam, diphenhydramine, dobutamine, dopamine, epinephrine, erythromycin lactobionate, esmolol, gentamicin, heparin sodium.

Row headings (top to bottom): acyclovir, albumin, amikacin, amino acid injection, aminophylline, ampicillin, bretylium, calcium gluconate, cefamandole, cefazolin, cefoxitin, ceftazidime, chloramphenicol, cimetidine, ciprofloxacin, clindamycin, corticotropin, dexamethasone, dextrose 5% in water (D₅W), D₅W in lactated Ringer's, D₅W in 0.9% NaCl solution, diazepam, diphenhydramine, dobutamine, dopamine, epinephrine, erythromycin lactobionate, esmolol, gentamicin, heparin sodium, hydrocortisone Na succinate, insulin (regular), isoproterenol, lactated Ringer's, lidocaine, methylprednisolone, mezlocillin, multiple vitamin infusion, nafcillin, netilmicin, norepinephrine, 0.9% NaCl solution, ondansetron, oxacillin, oxytocin, penicillin G potassium, phenytoin, phytonadione, piperacillin, potassium chloride, procainamide, ranitidine, sodium bicarbonate, thiamine, ticarcillin, tobramycin, vancomycin, verapamil, vitamin B complex with C.

bine two drugs if you're uncertain of their compatibility. Check appropriate references, or ask a pharmacist to be sure.

Column key (left to right):

1. hydrocortisone Na succinate
2. insulin (regular)
3. isoproterenol
4. lactated Ringer's
5. lidocaine
6. methylprednisolone
7. mezlocillin
8. multiple vitamin infusion
9. nafcillin
10. netilmicin
11. norepinephrine
12. 0.9% NaCl solution
13. ondansetron
14. oxacillin
15. oxytocin
16. penicillin G potassium
17. phenytoin
18. phytonadione
19. piperacillin
20. potassium chloride
21. procainamide
22. ranitidine
23. sodium bicarbonate
24. thiamine
25. ticarcillin
26. tobramycin
27. vancomycin
28. verapamil
29. vitamin B complex with C

Drug	1	2	3	4	5	6	7	8	9	10	11	12	13	14	15	16	17	18	19	20	21	22	23	24	25	26	27	28	29
acyclovir																													
albumin																													
amikacin	24			24							24	24		8		8	24		4			24	24				24	24	
amino acid injection	24	24		24	24		24	24	24		24	24		24		24	24					12			24	4			
aminophylline	24			24	24							24										24	24						
ampicillin												8									?	?						?	
bretylium		48			48	24					48						48	24		48							48	
calcium gluconate		24	24								24													1				48	
cefamandole											12																	24	
cefazolin				24							24										?							24	
cefoxitin	24		24		24						24											24			24		24	24	
ceftazidime			24								24											6						24	
chloramphenicol		24	24		24	20					24																	24	
cimetidine	24	24		24	24						24											24			24		24	24	48
ciprofloxacin		24		24							24														24			24	
clindamycin	24		24		24			24			24					48	24		24				48		24	24			
corticotropin																													
dexamethasone																												24	
dextrose 5% in water (D₅W)	24			24	6	24	24	24	24	24	48	6	6	24		24	24		48	24	24	24	24	24	24		24		
D₅W in lactated Ringer's		24			24			24			24			24		24			24			24			24			24	
D₅W in 0.9% NaCl solution	24	24		24		24	24			48	6		24		24	24			24	24		48		24		24			
diazepam																												24	
diphenhydramine					72						24	24		24								24	24	48		24				
dobutamine	24	24	24		48	24	18				48		24				24		48				24				24		
dopamine	18		48	24	18						48		24				24		48				24				24		
epinephrine	24				24						24																24		
erythromycin lactobionate	18				22						24												24				24		
esmolol	24				24						24																24		
gentamicin	24			24	24						24								24			24	24				24	24	
heparin sodium		24		24	24														24		24	24				24			
hydrocortisone Na succinate		24									24					24			24			24				24			
insulin (regular)			24								24																48		
isoproterenol			24		24						24																24		
lactated Ringer's	24		24	24		72	24				24			6		24			24	24	24						48		
lidocaine	24	24		24							24								24	24	24						48		
methylprednisolone						6					24					24											24			?
mezlocillin					72						48																24			?
multiple vitamin infusion					24					24	24												24				24			?
nafcillin	24										24											24				24			
netilmicin					24						24															24			
norepinephrine	24		24		24	6	48	24	24	24	24		24	6		24			24	24	24	48	24	24	48	24	24		
0.9% NaCl solution					24						24																24			
ondansetron		6									6												24				?			
oxacillin											24												24				24			
oxytocin		24		24							24											24				24			
penicillin G potassium											24											24				48			
phenytoin											24											24				24			
phytonadione	24										24							24								24			
piperacillin									24		24					24			48	24						24			
potassium chloride			24		24						24																48			
procainamide			24						48	48	24							48				24	24	24				24	
ranitidine	24			24		24	24			24	24	24		24					24								24		
sodium bicarbonate			24								24							24									24		
thiamine			24								24											24				24			
ticarcillin			24								48											24				24			
tobramycin			24								24											24				24			
vancomycin	24	48	24	24	48	24	?	24	?		24	24	24	48		24	24	48		24	24	48		24	24	24	24		24

► LIFE-THREATENING EFFECTS

Dangerous drug interactions

Drugs can interact to produce undesirable, even hazardous, effects. Such interactions can decrease therapeutic efficacy or cause toxicity. If possible, avoid administering the combinations shown here.

DRUG	INTERACTING DRUG	POSSIBLE EFFECT
Aminoglycosides amikacin gentamicin kanamycin neomycin netilmicin streptomycin tobramycin	parenteral cephalosporins • ceftazidime • ceftizoxime • cephalothin	Possible enhanced nephrotoxicity
	loop diuretics • bumetadine • ethacrynic acid • furosemide	Possible enhanced ototoxicity
Amphetamines amphetamine benzphetamine dextroamphetamine methamphetamine	urine alkalinizers • potassium citrate • sodium acetate • sodium bicarbonate • sodium citrate • sodium lactate • tromethamine	Decreased urinary excretion of amphetamine
Angiotensin-converting enzyme (ACE) inhibitors captopril enalapril lisinopril	indomethacin	Decreased or abolished effectiveness of antihypertensive action of ACE inhibitors
Barbiturate anesthetics methohexital thiamylal thiopental	opiate analgesics	Enhanced central nervous system and respiratory depression
Barbiturates amobarbital aprobarbital butabarbital mephobarbital pentobarbital phenobarbital primidone secobarbital	valproic acid	Increased serum barbiturate levels

Dangerous drug interactions *(continued)*

DRUG	INTERACTING DRUG	POSSIBLE EFFECT
Beta-adrenergic blockers acebutolol atenolol betaxolol carteolol esmolol levobunolol metoprolol nadolol penbutolol pindolol propranolol timolol	verapamil	Enhanced pharmacologic effects of both beta-adrenergic blockers and verapamil
Captopril	food	Possible diminished GI absorption
Carbamazepine	erythromycin	Increased risk of carbamazepine toxicity
Carmustine	cimetidine	Enhanced risk of bone marrow toxicity
Ciprofloxacin	antacids containing magnesium or aluminum hydroxide	Decreased plasma levels and effectiveness of ciprofloxacin
Clonidine	beta-adrenergic blockers	Enhanced rebound hypertension following rapid clonidine withdrawal
Cyclosporine	hydantoins	Reduced plasma levels of cyclosporine
Digitalis glycosides	loop and thiazide diuretics	Increased risk of cardiac arrhythmias due to hypokalemia
	thiazide-like diuretics	Increased therapeutic or toxic effects *(continued)*

DRUG HAZARDS

Dangerous drug interactions *(continued)*

DRUG	INTERACTING DRUG	POSSIBLE EFFECT
Digitoxin	quinidine	Decreased digitoxin clearance
Digoxin	verapamil	Elevated serum digoxin levels
	quinidine	Enhanced clearance of digoxin
Dopamine	phenytoin	Hypertension and bradycardia
Epinephrine	beta-adrenergic blockers	Increased systolic and diastolic pressures; marked decrease in heart rate
Erythromycin	astemizole terfenadine	Increased risk of arrhythmia
Ethanol	• disulfiram • furazolidone • metronidazole	Acute alcohol intolerance reaction
Furazolidone	amine-containing foods anorexiants	Inhibits monoamine oxidase, possibly leading to hypertensive crisis
Heparin	salicylates	Enhanced risk of bleeding
Levodopa	furazolidone	Enhanced toxic effects of levodopa
Lithium	thiazide diuretics	Decreased lithium excretion
Meperidine	monoamine oxidase (MAO) inhibitors	Cardiovascular instability and increased toxicity
Methotrexate	probenecid	Decreased methotrexate elimination
	salicylates	Increased risk of methotrexate toxicity

Dangerous drug interactions *(continued)*

DRUG	INTERACTING DRUG	POSSIBLE EFFECT
MAO inhibitors	amine-containing foods anorexiants meperidine	Risk of hypertensive crisis
Nondepolarizing muscle relaxants	aminoglycosides inhalational anesthetics	Enhanced neuromuscular blockade
Nonsedating antihistamines astemizole terfenadine	erythromycin ketoconazole	Decrease metabolism of antihistamine; risk of cardiac arrhythmia
Warfarin	amiodarone	Increased risk of bleeding
	androgens • testosterone	Possible enhanced bleeding caused by increased hypoprothrombinemia
	barbiturates carbamazepine	Reduced effectiveness of warfarin
	certain cephalosporins chloral hydrate cholestyramine cimetidine clofibrate co-trimoxazole dextrothyroxine disulfiram erythromycin glucagon metronidazole phenylbutazone quinidine quinine salicylates sulfinpyrazone thyroid drugs tricyclic antidepressants	Increased risk of bleeding

(continued)

Dangerous drug interactions *(continued)*

DRUG	INTERACTING DRUG	POSSIBLE EFFECT
Warfarin *(continued)*	ethchlorvynol glutethimide griseofulvin	Decreased pharmacologic effect
	rifampin trazodone	Decreased risk of bleeding
	methimazole propylthiouracil	Increased or decreased risk of bleeding
Potassium supplements	potassium-sparing diuretics	Increased risk of hyperkalemia
Quinidine	amiodarone	Increased risk of quinidine toxicity
Sympathomimetics	MAO inhibitors	Increased risk of hypertensive crisis
Tetracyclines	antacids containing magnesium, aluminum, or bismuth salts iron supplements	Decreased plasma levels and effectiveness of tetracyclines

Drug-smoking interactions

Smoking—or living and working in a smoke-filled environment—can affect a patient's drug therapy, especially if he's taking one of the drugs listed here. If your patient is using any of these drugs, monitor plasma drug levels closely, and watch for possible adverse reactions.

Ascorbic acid (vitamin C)
Possible effects:
• Low serum vitamin C levels
• Decreased oral absorption of vitamin C

Nursing considerations:
• Tell the patient to increase his vitamin C intake.

Chlordiazepoxide hydrochloride, chlorpromazine hydrochloride, diazepam
Possible effects:
• Increased drug metabolism, which results in reduced plasma levels
• Decreased sedative effects
   Nursing considerations:
• Watch for a decrease in the drug's effectiveness.
• Adjust the patient's drug dosage, if ordered.

Propoxyphene hydrochloride
Possible effects:
• Increased drug metabolism and diminished analgesic effects

Nursing considerations:
• Watch for a decrease in the drug's effectiveness.

Propranolol hydrochloride
Possible effects:
• Increased metabolism, which decreases drug's effectiveness
• Propranolol's effectiveness hampered by the effects of smoking, which increases heart rate, stimulates catecholamine release from the adrenal medulla, raises arterial blood pressure, and increases myocardial oxygen consumption
Nursing considerations:
• Monitor the patient's blood pressure and heart rate.
• To reduce drug and smoking interaction, the doctor may order a selective beta blocker, such as atenolol.

Oral contraceptives containing estrogen and progestogen
Possible effects:
• Increased adverse reactions, such as headache, dizziness, depression, libido changes, migraine, hypertension, edema, worsening of astigmatism or myopia, nausea, vomiting, and gallbladder disease
Nursing considerations:
• Inform the patient of increased risk of myocardial infarction and cerebrovascular accident.
• Suggest that the patient stop smoking or use a different birth control method.

Theophylline
Possible effects:
• Increased theophylline metabolism (due to induction of liver microsomal enzymes)
• Lower plasma theophylline levels
Nursing considerations:
• Monitor plasma theophylline levels, and watch for decreased therapeutic effect.
• Increase drug dosage, if ordered.

▶

Drug-food interactions

Acebutolol (Sectral): Food in general. *Slightly decreases drug absorption and peak concentrations.*

Amiloride hydrochloride (Midamor): Potassium-rich diet. *May rapidly increase serum potassium levels.*

Antihypertensive drugs: Licorice. *Decreases antihypertensive effect.*

Astemizole (Hismanal): Food in general. *Reduces drug absorption by 60%.*

Bacampicillin hydrochloride (Spectrobid Powder for Oral Suspension): Food in general. *Decreases drug absorption.*

Buspirone hydrochloride (BuSpar): Food in general. *May decrease presystemic drug clearance.*

Caffeine (Caffedrine, No Doz, Quick Pep, Tirend, Vivarin): Caffeine-containing beverages and food. *May cause sleeplessness, irritability, nervousness, and rapid heartbeat.*

Calcium glubionate (Neo-Calglucon Syrup): Bran, cereals (whole grain), dairy products, rhubarb, spinach. *Large quantities interfere with calcium absorption.*

Captopril (Capoten): Food in general. *Reduces drug absorption by 30% to 40%.*

Cefuroxime axetil (Ceftin Tablets): Food in general. *Increases drug absorption.*

DRUG HAZARDS

Choline and magnesium salicylate (Trilisate): Food that lowers urinary pH. *Decreases urinary salicylate excretion and increases plasma levels.*

Food that raises urinary pH. *Enhances renal salicylate clearance and diminishes plasma salicylate concentration.*

Demeclocycline hydrochloride (Declomycin): Dairy products, food in general. *Interfere with absorption of oral forms of demeclocycline.*

Dextroamphetamine sulfate (Dexedrine Elixir): Fruit juice. *Lowers blood drug levels and efficacy.*

Dicumarol: Diet high in vitamin K. *Decreases prothrombin time.*

Digoxin (Lanoxin Tablets, Lanoxicaps): Food high in bran fiber. *May reduce bioavailability of oral digoxin.*
Food in general. *Slows drug absorption rate.*

Dyclonine hydrochloride (Dyclone 0.5% and 1% Topical Solutions, USP): Food in general. *Topical anesthesia may impair swallowing and thus enhance danger of aspiration; food should not be ingested for 60 minutes.*

Erythromycin base (Eryc, PCE Dispertab Tablets): Food in general. *Optimum blood levels are obtained on a fasting stomach; administration is preferable 30 minutes before or 2 hours after meals.*

Estramustine phosphate sodium (Emcyt): Dairy products, calcium-rich foods. *Impair drug absorption.*

Etodolac (Lodine): Food in general. *Reduces peak concentration by approximately 50% and increases time to peak concentration by 1.4 to 3.8 hours.*

Etretinate (Tegison Capsules): Dairy products, high-lipid diet. *Increase drug absorption.*

Famotidine (Pepcid Oral Suspension): Food in general. *Slightly increases bioavailability.*

Felodipine (Plendil): Grapefruit juice, doubly concentrated. *Increases bioavailability more than twofold.*

Fenoprofen calcium (Nalfon Pulvules and Tablets): Dairy products, food in general. *Delay and diminish peak blood levels.*

Ferrous sulfate (Feosol, Slow-Fe): Dairy products, eggs. *Inhibit iron absorption.*

Fluoroquinolone antibiotics, such as ciprofloxacin (Cipro), norfloxacin (Noroxin), ofloxacin (Floxin): Food in general. *May decrease absorption of oral fluoroquinolones.*

Flurbiprofen (Ansaid): Food in general. *Alters rate of absorption but not extent of drug availability.*

Fosinopril sodium (Monopril): Food in general. *May slow rate but not extent of drug absorption.*

Glipizide (Glucotrol): Food in general. *Delays absorption by about 40 minutes.*

Hydralazine hydrochloride (Apresoline Tablets): Food in general. *Increases plasma levels.*

Hydrochlorothiazide (Esidrix, HydroDIURIL): Food in general. *Enhances GI drug absorption.*

Ibuprofen (Advil, Children's Advil Suspension, Motrin, Nuprin, PediaProfen Suspension, Rufen): Food in general. *Reduces rate but not extent of drug absorption.*

Isotretinoin (Accutane): Dairy products, food in general. *Increase absorption of oral isotretinoin.*

Isradipine (DynaCirc): Food in general. *Significantly increases time to peak by about 1 hour with no effect on bioavailability.*

Ketoprofen (Orudis Capsules): Food in general. *Slows absorption rate, delays and reduces peak concentrations.*

Levodopa-carbidopa (Sinemet Tablets): High-protein diet. *May impair levodopa absorption.*

Food in general. *Increases the extent of availability and peak concentrations of sustained-release levodopa-carbidopa.*

Levothyroxine sodium (Synthroid Injection): Soybean formula (infant's). *May cause excessive fecal loss.*

Lidocaine hydrochloride (Xylocaine): Food in general. *Topical anesthesia may impair swallowing and thus enhance danger of aspiration; avoid food ingestion for 60 minutes.*

Liotrix (Euthroid, Thyrolar): Soybean formula (infant's). *May cause excessive fecal loss.*

Meclofenamate (Meclomen): Food in general. *Decreases rate and extent of drug absorption.*

Methenamine mandelate (Mandelamine Granules): Food that raises urinary pH. *Reduces essential antibacterial activity.*

Methotrexate sodium (Rheumatrex): Food in general. *Delays absorption and reduces peak concentration of oral methotrexate sodium.*

Minocycline hydrochloride (Minocin): Dairy products. *Slightly decrease peak plasma concentration levels and delay them by 1 hour.*

Misoprostol (Cytotec): Food in general. *Diminishes maximum plasma concentrations.*

Monoamine oxidase (MAO) inhibitors, such as isocarboxazid (Marplan Tablets), phenelzine (Nardil), or tranylcypromine (Parnate Tablets); drugs that also inhibit MAO, such as amphetamines, furazolidone (Furoxone), isoniazid (Laniazid), or procarbazine (Matulane Capsules): Anchovies, avocados, bananas, beans (broad, fava), beer (including alcohol-free and reduced-alcohol), caviar, cheese (especially aged, strong, unpasteurized), chocolate, cream (sour), figs (canned), herring (pickled), liqueurs, liver, meat extracts, meat prepared with tenderizers, raisins, sauerkraut, sherry, soy sauce, red wine, yeast extract, yogurt. *Can cause hypertensive crisis.*

Moricizine hydrochloride (Ethmozine): Food in general. *Administration 30 minutes after a meal delays rate but not extent of drug absorption.*

Nifedipine (Procardia XL Tablets): Food in general. *Slightly alters early rate of drug absorption.*

Nitrofurantoin (Macrodantin Capsules): Food in general. *Increases drug bioavailability.*

Pancrelipase (Creon Capsules): Food with a pH greater than 5.5. *Dissolves protective enteric coating.*

Pentoxifylline (Trental): Food in general. *Delays drug absorption, but doesn't affect total absorption.*

DRUG HAZARDS

Phenytoin: Charcoal-broiled meats. *May decrease blood drug levels.*

Polyethylene glycol electrolyte solution (GoLYTELY, NuLYTELY): Food in general. *For best results, no solid food should be consumed during 3- to 4-hour period before drinking solution.*

Propafenone hydrochloride (Rythmol): Food in general. *Increased peak blood levels and bioavailability in a single-dose study.*

Propranolol hydrochloride (Inderal): Food in general. *Increases bioavailability of oral propranolol.*

Ramipril (Altace): Food in general. *Reduces rate but not extent of drug absorption.*

Salsalate (Disalcid, Mono-Gesic, Salflex): Food that lowers urinary pH. *Decreases urinary excretion and increases plasma levels.*

Food that raises urinary pH. *Increases renal clearance and urinary excretion of salicylic acid.*

Selegiline hydrochloride (Eldepryl): Food with high concentration of tyramine. *May precipitate hypertensive crisis if daily dosage exceeds recommended maximum.*

Sodium fluoride (Luride): Dairy products. *Form calcium fluoride, which is poorly absorbed.*

Sulindac (Clinoril Tablets): Food in general. *Slightly delays peak plasma concentrations of biologically active sulfide metabolite.*

Tetracycline hydrochloride (Achromycin V): Dairy products, food in general. *Interfere with absorption of oral tetracycline.*

Theophylline (Constant-T, Quibron T, Quibron SR, Respbid, Slo-Bid, Theo-Dur, Theo-24, Theolair-SR, TheoX, Uniphyl): Caffeine-containing beverages, chocolate, cola. *Large quantities increase adverse effects of theophylline.*

High-lipid diet. *Reduces plasma concentration levels and delays time of peak plasma levels.*

Charcoal-broiled foods, especially meats; cruciferous (cabbage family) vegetables; high-protein and low-carbohydrate diets. *Large quantities may increase hepatic metabolism of theophylline.*

Tolmetin sodium (Tolectin): Dairy products. *Decrease total tolmetin bioavailability by 16%.*

Food in general. *Decreases total tolmetin bioavailability by 16% and reduces peak plasma concentrations by 50%.*

Trazodone hydrochloride (Desyrel): Food in general. *May affect bioavailability, including amount of drug absorbed and peak plasma levels.*

Verapamil hydrochloride (Calan SR, Isoptin SR): Food in general. *Decreases bioavailability but narrows peak-to-trough ratio.*

Warfarin sodium (Coumadin, Panwarfin): Diet high in vitamin K. *Decreases prothrombin time.*

Charcoal-broiled meats. *May decrease blood drug levels.*

► LIFE-THREATENING EFFECTS

Drug-alcohol interactions

DRUG	EFFECTS
• Analgesics • Antianxiety drugs • Antidepressants • Antihistamines • Antipsychotics • Hypnotics	Deepened central nervous system (CNS) depression
• Monoamine oxidase inhibitors	Deepened CNS depression; possible hypertensive crisis with certain types of beer and wine containing tyramine (Chianti, Alicante)
• Oral antidiabetics	Disulfiram-like effects (facial flushing, headache), especially with chlorpropamide; inadequate food intake may trigger increased antidiabetic activity
• Cephalosporins • Metronidazole	Disulfiram-like effects

►

Compatibility of drugs with tube feedings

Some feeding formulas, such as Ensure, may chemically break down when combined with a drug such as Dimetapp Elixir. Increased formula viscosity – and a clogged tube – can occur from giving Klorvess, Neo-Calglucon Syrup, Dimetane Elixir, Phenergan Syrup, or Sudafed Syrup with a feeding formula.

Drug preparations such as ferrous sulfate or potassium chloride liquids are incompatible with some formulas, causing clumping and other problems when mixed in a tube. Still other combinations may alter the bioavailability of some drugs, such as phenytoin.

To avoid incompatibility problems, follow these guidelines.
• Never add a drug to a feeding formula container.
• Always check the compatibility of an ordered drug and the feeding formula before administering.
• Infuse 30 ml of water before and after giving a single drug dose through the tube.
• Flush the feeding tube with 5 ml of water between drug doses if you're giving more than one drug.
• Dilute highly concentrated liquids with 60 ml of water before giving.
• Instill drugs in liquid form when possible. If you must crush a tablet, crush it into fine dust and dissolve it in warm water. (Never crush and liquefy enteric-coated tablets or timed-release capsules.)
• Time drug and formula administration intervals appropriately. Or you may need to withhold tube feeding and supply medication by mouth to an empty stomach or with food.

DRUG HAZARDS

▶

Drug interference with test results

Drugs can interfere with the results of blood or urine tests in two ways. A drug in a blood or urine specimen may interact with the chemicals used in the laboratory test, causing a false result. Or a drug may cause a physiologic change in the patient, resulting in an actual increased or decreased blood or urine level of the substance being tested. This chart identifies drugs that can cause these two types of interference in some common blood and urine tests.

TEST AND DRUGS CAUSING CHEMICAL INTERFERENCE	DRUGS CAUSING PHYSIOLOGIC INTERFERENCE	
Alkaline phosphatase • albumin • fluorides	*Increased test values* • anticonvulsants • hepatotoxic drugs	*Decreased test values* • clofibrate
Ammonia, blood	*Increased test values* • acetazolamide • ammonium chloride • asparaginase • barbiturates • diuretics, loop and thiazide • ethanol	*Decreased test values* • kanamycin, oral • lactulose • neomycin, oral • potassium salts
Amylase, serum • chloride salts • fluorides	*Increased test values* • asparaginase • cholinergic agents • contraceptives, oral • contrast media with iodine • drugs inducing acute pancreatitis: azathioprine, corticosteroids, loop and thiazide diuretics • methyldopa • narcotics	
Aspartate aminotransferase • erythromycin • methyldopa	*Increased test values* • cholinergic agents • hepatotoxic drugs • opium alkaloids	
Bilirubin, serum • ascorbic acid • dextran • epinephrine • pindolol	*Increased test values* • hemolytic agents • hepatotoxic drugs • methyldopa • rifampin	*Decreased test values* • barbiturates

Drug interference with test results *(continued)*

TEST AND DRUGS CAUSING CHEMICAL INTERFERENCE	DRUGS CAUSING PHYSIOLOGIC INTERFERENCE	
Blood urea nitrogen • chloral hydrate • chloramphenicol • streptomycin	*Increased test values* • anabolic steroids • nephrotoxic drugs	*Decreased test values* • tetracyclines
Calcium, serum • aspirin • heparin • hydralazine • sulfisoxazole	*Increased test values* • asparaginase • calcium salts • diuretics, loop and thiazide • lithium • thyroid hormones • vitamin D	*Decreased test values* • acetazolamide • anticonvulsants • calcitonin • cisplatin • contraceptives, oral • corticosteroids • laxatives • magnesium salts • plicamycin
Chloride, serum	*Increased test values* • acetazolamide • androgens • estrogens • nonsteroidal anti-inflammatory drugs	*Decreased test values* • corticosteroids • diuretics, loop and thiazide
Cholesterol, serum • androgens • aspirin • corticosteroids • nitrates • phenothiazines • vitamin D	*Increased test values* • beta-adrenergic blocking agents • contraceptives, oral • corticosteroids • diuretics, thiazide • phenothiazines • sulfonamides	*Decreased test values* • androgens • captopril • chlorpropamide • cholestyramine • clofibrate • colestipol • haloperidol • neomycin, oral
Creatine kinase (CK)	*Increased test values* • aminocaproic acid • amphotericin B • chlorthalidone • clofibrate • ethanol (chronic use)	
Creatinine, serum • cefoxitin • cephalothin • flucytosine	*Increased test values* • cimetidine • nephrotoxic drugs	

(continued)

DRUG HAZARDS

Drug interference with test results *(continued)*

TEST AND DRUGS CAUSING CHEMICAL INTERFERENCE	DRUGS CAUSING PHYSIOLOGIC INTERFERENCE	
Glucose, serum • acetaminophen • ascorbic acid (urine) • cephalosporins (urine)	*Increased test values* • antidepressants, tricyclic • beta-blockers • corticosteroids • dextrothyroxine • diazoxide • diuretics, loop and thiazide • epinephrine • estrogens • isoniazid • lithium • phenothiazines • phenytoin • salicylates	*Decreased test values* • acetaminophen • anabolic steroids • clofibrate • disopyramide • ethanol • gemfibrozil • monoamine oxidase (MAO) inhibitors • pentamidine
Magnesium, serum	*Increased test values* • lithium • magnesium salts	*Decreased test values* • aminoglycosides • amphotericin B • calcium salts • cisplatin • digitalis glycosides • diuretics, loop and thiazide • ethanol
Phosphates, serum	*Increased test values* • vitamin D (excessive amounts)	*Decreased test values* • antacids, phosphate-binding • mannitol
Potassium, serum	*Increased test values* • aminocaproic acid • angiotensin-converting enzyme (ACE) inhibitors • antineoplastics • diuretics, potassium-sparing • isoniazid • lithium • mannitol • succinylcholine	*Decreased test values* • ammonium chloride • amphotericin B • corticosteroids • diuretics, potassium-wasting • glucose • insulin • laxatives • penicillins, extended-spectrum • salicylates

Drug interference with test results *(continued)*

TEST AND DRUGS CAUSING CHEMICAL INTERFERENCE	DRUGS CAUSING PHYSIOLOGIC INTERFERENCE	
Protein, serum	*Increased test values* • anabolic steroids • corticosteroids • phenazopyridine	*Decreased test values* • contraceptives, oral • estrogens • hepatotoxic drugs
Protein, urine • aminoglycosides • cephalosporins • contrast media • magnesium sulfate • miconazole • nafcillin • phenazopyridine • sulfonamides • tolbutamide • tolmetin	*Increased test values* • cephalosporins • contrast media with iodine • corticosteroids • nafcillin • nephrotoxic drugs • sulfonamides	
Prothrombin time	*Increased test values* • anticoagulants • asparaginase • aspirin • azathioprine • certain cephalosporins • chloramphenicol • cholestyramine • colestipol • cyclophosphamide • hepatotoxic drugs • propylthiouracil • quinidine • quinine • sulfonamides	*Decreased test values* • anabolic steroids • contraceptives, oral • estrogens • vitamin K
Sodium, serum	*Increased test values* • clonidine • diazoxide • guanabenz • guanadrel • guanethidine • methyldopa • nonsteroidal anti-inflammatory drugs • steroids	*Decreased test values* • ammonium chloride • carbamazepine • desmopressin • diuretics • lypressin • vasopressin *(continued)*

DRUG HAZARDS

Drug interference with test results (continued)

TEST AND DRUGS CAUSING CHEMICAL INTERFERENCE	DRUGS CAUSING PHYSIOLOGIC INTERFERENCE	
Uric acid, serum	*Increased test values*	*Decreased test values*
• ascorbic acid	• acetazolamide	• acetohexamide
• caffeine	• cisplatin	• allopurinol
• levodopa	• diazoxide	• clofibrate
• theophylline	• diuretics	• contrast media with iodine
	• epinephrine	• diflunisal
	• ethambutol	• glucose infusions
	• ethanol	• guaifenesin
	• levodopa	• phenothiazines
	• niacin	• phenylbutazone
		• salicylates (small doses)
		• uricosuric agents

Drug additives

Drugs with ethanol additives

Many liquid drug preparations for oral use contain ethanol, which produces a slight sedative effect but isn't harmful to most patients and can in fact be beneficial. But ingesting ethanol can be undesirable and even dangerous in some circumstances. The list below identifies generic drugs that commonly contain ethanol. Note that some manufacturers of these drugs also produce ethanol-free (alcohol-free) formulations. Check with your pharmacist for more information.

• acetaminophen, acetaminophen with codeine elixir
• belladonna tincture
• bitolterol mesylate
• brompheniramine maleate elixir
• butabarbital sodium
• chlorpheniramine maleate elixir
• chlorpromazine hydrochloride
• clemastine fumarate
• co-trimoxazole
• cyproheptadine hydrochloride
• dexchlorpheniramine maleate
• dextroamphetamine sulfate
• diazepam
• diazoxide
• digoxin
• dihydroergotamine mesylate injection
• diphenhydramine hydrochloride
• epinephrine
• ergoloid mesylates
• esmolol hydrochloride
• ferrous sulfate elixirs
• fluphenazine hydrochloride
• hydromorphone hydrochloride cough syrup
• hyoscyamine sulfate
• indomethacin suspension
• isoetharine mesylate
• isoproterenol hydrochloride

- mesoridazine besylate
- methadone hydrochloride oral solution
- methdilazine hydrochloride
- methyldopa suspension
- minocycline hydrochloride
- molindone hydrochloride
- nitroglycerin infusion
- nystatin
- opium alkaloid hydrochlorides
- oxycodone hydrochloride
- paramethadione
- pentobarbital sodium elixir, pentobarbital sodium injection
- perphenazine
- phenobarbital injection
- phenytoin sodium injection
- promethazine hydrochloride
- pyridostigmine bromide
- thioridazine hydrochloride
- thiothixene hydrochloride
- trimeprazine tartrate
- trimethoprim
- tripelennamine hydrochloride
- triprolidine hydrochloride

Drugs with sulfite additives

Used as a drug preservative, sulfites can cause allergic reactions in certain patients. The list below identifies generic drugs that commonly contain sulfites. A pharmacist can provide definitive information on brand-name drugs.

- amikacin sulfate
- aminophylline
- amrinone lactate
- atropine sulfate with meperidine hydrochloride
- betamethasone sodium phosphate
- bupivacaine hydrochloride with epinephrine 1:200,000
- carisoprodol with aspirin and codeine phosphate
- chlorpromazine, chlorpromazine hydrochloride
- dexamethasone acetate, dexamethasone sodium phosphate
- diphenhydramine hydrochloride
- dobutamine hydrochloride
- dopamine hydrochloride
- epinephrine, epinephrine bitartrate, epinephrine bitartrate with pilocarpine hydrochloride, epinephrine hydrochloride
- etidocaine hydrochloride with epinephrine bitartrate 1:200,000
- heparin calcium, heparin sodium
- hydralazine hydrochloride
- hydrocortisone sodium phosphate
- hyoscyamine sulfate
- imipramine hydrochloride
- influenza virus vaccine
- isoetharine hydrochloride, isoetharine mesylate
- isoproterenol hydrochloride isoproterenol sulfate
- lidocaine hydrochloride with epinephrine hydrochloride
- mafenide acetate
- metaraminol bitartrate
- methotrimeprazine hydrochloride
- methyldopa; methyldopate hydrochloride
- metoclopramide hydrochloride
- orphenadrine citrate, orphenadrine hydrochloride
- oxycodone hydrochloride with acetaminophen
- pentazocine hydrochloride, pentazocine hydrochloride with acetaminophen
- perphenazine
- phenylephrine hydrochloride
- procainamide hydrochloride
- procaine hydrochloride
- prochlorperazine, prochlorperazine edisylate, prochlorperazine maleate
- promazine hydrochloride
- propoxycaine hydrochloride with procaine hydrochloride 2% and levonordefrin 1:20,000
- ritodrine hydrochloride
- scopolamine hydrobromide with phenylephrine hydrochloride 10%
- tetracycline hydrochloride 0.22% topical

DRUG HAZARDS

- theophylline
- thiethylperazine maleate
- trifluoperazine hydrochloride
- tubocurarine chloride

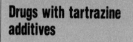

Drugs with tartrazine additives

Also known as FD&C Yellow No. 5, tartrazine is a dye used as an additive in certain drugs. It can provoke a severe allergic reaction in some people, especially those who are also allergic to aspirin. The list below identifies some drugs containing tartrazine, although not all dosage forms may contain the dye. Check with your pharmacist for more information:

- benzphetamine HCl (Didrex tablets)
- butabarbital sodium (Butisol elixir and tablets)
- carisoprodol (Rela)
- chlorphenesin carbonate (Maolate)
- chlorprothixene (Taractan)
- clindamycin HCl (Cleocin capsules)
- desipramine HCl (Norpramin)
- dextroamphetamine sulfate (Dexedrine elixir, spansule, and tablets)
- dextrothyroxine HCl (Choloxin)
- fluphenazine HCl (Prolixin)
- haloperidol (Haldol tablets)
- hydralazine HCl (Apresoline tablets)
- hydromorphone HCl (Dilaudid cough syrup)
- imipramine (Janimine, Tofranil-PM)
- mepenzolate bromide (Cantil tablets)
- methamphetamine HCl (Desoxyn Gradumet)
- methenamine hippurate (Hiprex tablets)
- methysergide maleate (Sansert tablets)
- niacin (Nicolar)
- paramethadione (Paradione)
- penicillin G potassium (Pentids syrup, Pentids 400 syrup, Pentids 800)
- penicillin V potassium (Veetids 125 oral solution)
- pentobarbital sodium (Nembutal Sodium)
- procainamide HCl (Pronestyl)
- promazine HCl (Sparine)
- rauwolfia serpentina (Raudixin)
- uracil mustard.

How aging increases the risk of drug hazards

The physiologic changes of aging make geriatric patients more susceptible to drug-induced illnesses, adverse effects, toxicity, and interactions than younger adults. Other conditions common to many geriatric patients also increase the risk of these problems.

To help prevent these problems or detect them early, check the patient's history for the following risk factors when developing your teaching plan:

- altered mental status
- patient is a woman
- small build
- financial problems
- frail health
- poor nutritional status
- patient lives alone
- history of previous adverse effects
- history of allergies
- multiple chronic illnesses
- renal failure
- treatment by several doctors
- polypharmacy or complex medication regimens.

Substance abuse

▶ LIFE-THREATENING EFFECTS

Recognizing and treating acute toxicity

SUBSTANCE	SIGNS AND SYMPTOMS	INTERVENTIONS
Alcohol (ethanol) • Beer and wine • Distilled spirits • Other preparations, such as cough syrup, aftershave, or mouthwash	• Ataxia • Seizures • Coma • Hypothermia • Alcohol breath odor • Respiratory depression • Bradycardia • Hypotension • Nausea and vomiting	• Expect to induce vomiting or perform gastric lavage if ingestion occurred in the previous 4 hours. Give activated charcoal and a saline cathartic, as ordered. • Start I.V. fluid replacement and administer dextrose 5% in water, thiamine, B-complex vitamins, and vitamin C, as ordered, to prevent dehydration and hypoglycemia and to correct nutritional deficiencies. • Pad bed rails and apply cloth restraints to protect the patient from injury. • Give an anticonvulsant such as diazepam, as ordered, to control seizures. • Watch the patient for signs and symptoms of withdrawal, such as hallucinations and alcohol withdrawal delirium. If these occur, give chlordiazepoxide, chloral hydrate, or paraldehyde, as ordered. (Be sure to administer paraldehyde with a glass syringe or glass cup to avoid a chemical reaction with plastic.) • Auscultate the patient's lungs frequently to detect crackles or rhonchi, possibly indicating aspiration pneumonia. If you note these breath sounds, expect to give antibiotics. • Monitor the patient's neurologic status and vital signs every 15 minutes until he's stable. Assist with dialysis if his vital functions are severely depressed. *(continued)*

DRUG HAZARDS

Recognizing and treating acute toxicity *(continued)*

SUBSTANCE	SIGNS AND SYMPTOMS	INTERVENTIONS
Amphetamines • Amphetamine sulfate (Benzedrine) – bennies, greenies, cartwheels • Dextroamphetamine sulfate (Dexedrine) – dexies, hearts, oranges • Methamphetamine (Methadrin) – speed, meth, crystal	• Dilated reactive pupils • Altered mental status (from confusion to paranoia) • Hallucinations • Tremors and seizure activity • Hyperactive deep tendon reflexes • Exhaustion • Coma • Dry mouth • Shallow respirations • Tachycardia • Hypertension • Hyperthermia • Diaphoresis	• If the drug was taken orally, induce vomiting or perform gastric lavage; give activated charcoal and a sodium or magnesium sulfate cathartic, as ordered. • Lower the patient's urine pH to 5 by adding ammonium chloride or ascorbic acid to his I.V. solution, as ordered. • Force diuresis by giving the patient mannitol, as ordered. • Expect to give a short-acting barbiturate, such as pentobarbital, to control stimulant-induced seizures. • Restrain the patient, especially if he's paranoid or hallucinating, so he won't injure himself and others. • Give haloperidol I.M., as ordered, to treat agitation or assaultive behavior. • Give an alpha-adrenergic blocker such as phentolamine for hypertension, as ordered. • Watch for cardiac arrhythmias. Notify the doctor if these develop, and expect to give propranolol or lidocaine to treat tachyarrhythmias or ventricular arrhythmias, respectively. • Treat hyperthermia with tepid sponge baths or a hypothermia blanket, as ordered. • Provide a quiet environment to avoid overstimulation. • Be alert for signs and symptoms of withdrawal, such as abdominal tenderness, muscle aches, and long periods of sleep. • Observe suicide precautions, especially if the patient shows signs of withdrawal.

Recognizing and treating acute toxicity *(continued)*

SUBSTANCE	SIGNS AND SYMPTOMS	INTERVENTIONS
Antipsychotics • Chlorpromazine (Thorazine) • Phenothiazines • Thioridazine (Mellaril)	• Constricted pupils • Photosensitivity • Extrapyramidal effects (dyskinesia, opisthotonos, muscle rigidity, ocular deviation) • Dry mouth • Decreased level of consciousness (LOC) • Decreased deep tendon reflexes • Seizures • Hypothermia or hyperthermia • Dysphagia • Respiratory depression • Hypotension • Tachycardia	• Expect to perform gastric lavage if the patient ingested the drug within the past 6 hours. (Don't induce vomiting, because phenothiazines have an antiemetic effect.) Give activated charcoal and a cathartic, as ordered. • Give diphenhydramine or benztropine, as ordered, to treat extrapyramidal effects. • Give physostigmine salicylate, as ordered, to reverse anticholinergic effects in severe cases. • Replace fluids I.V., as ordered, to correct hypotension; monitor the patient's vital signs often. • Monitor his respiratory rate, and give supplemental oxygen to treat respiratory depression. • Give an anticonvulsant, such as diazepam, or a short-acting barbiturate, such as pentobarbital sodium, as ordered, to control seizures. • Keep the patient's room dark to avoid exacerbating his photosensitivity.
Anxiolytic sedative-hypnotics • Benzodiazepines (Valium, Librium)	• Confusion • Drowsiness • Stupor • Decreased reflexes • Seizures • Coma • Shallow respirations • Hypotension	• Induce vomiting or perform gastric lavage; give activated charcoal and a cathartic, as ordered. • Give supplemental oxygen to correct hypoxia-induced seizures. • Replace fluids I.V., as ordered, to correct hypotension; monitor the patient's vital signs often. • If the patient has severe toxicity, give physostigmine salicylate, as ordered, to reverse respiratory and central nervous system (CNS) depression.

(continued)

DRUG HAZARDS

Recognizing and treating acute toxicity *(continued)*

SUBSTANCE	SIGNS AND SYMPTOMS	INTERVENTIONS
Barbiturate sedative-hypnotics • Amobarbital sodium (Amytal Sodium)—blue angels, blue devils, blue birds • Phenobarbital (Luminal)—phennies, purple hearts, goofballs • Secobarbital sodium (Seconal)—reds, red devils, seccy	• Poor pupil reaction to light • Nystagmus • Depressed LOC (from confusion to coma) • Flaccid muscles and absent reflexes • Hyperthermia or hypothermia • Cyanosis • Respiratory depression • Hypotension • Blisters or bullous lesions	• Induce vomiting or perform gastric lavage if the patient ingested the drug within 4 hours; give activated charcoal and a saline cathartic, as ordered. • Maintain his blood pressure with I.V. fluid challenges and vasopressors, as ordered. • If the patient has taken a phenobarbital overdose, give sodium bicarbonate I.V., as ordered, to alkalinize his urine and to speed the drug's elimination. • Apply a hyperthermia or hypothermia blanket, as ordered, to help return the patient's temperature to normal. • Prepare your patient for hemodialysis or hemoperfusion if toxicity is severe. • Perform frequent neurologic assessments, and check your patient's pulse rate, temperature, skin color, and reflexes often. • Notify the doctor if you see signs of respiratory distress or pulmonary edema. • Watch for signs and symptoms of withdrawal, such as hyperreflexia, tonic-clonic seizures, and hallucinations. Provide symptomatic relief of withdrawal symptoms, as ordered. • Protect the patient from injuring himself.
Cocaine • Cocaine hydrochloride • Crack • freebase	• Dilated pupils • Confusion • Alternating euphoria and apprehension • Hyperexcitability	• Calm the patient down by talking to him in a quiet room. • If cocaine was ingested, induce vomiting or perform gastric lavage; give activated charcoal followed by a saline cathartic, as ordered.

Recognizing and treating acute toxicity *(continued)*

SUBSTANCE	SIGNS AND SYMPTOMS	INTERVENTIONS
Cocaine *(continued)*	• Visual, auditory, and olfactory hallucinations • Spasms and seizures • Coma • Tachypnea • Hyperpnea • Pallor or cyanosis • Respiratory arrest • Tachycardia • Hypertension or hypotension • Fever • Nausea and vomiting • Abdominal pain • Perforated nasal septum or mouth sores	• Give the patient a tepid sponge bath, and administer an antipyretic, as ordered, to reduce fever. • Monitor his blood pressure and heart rate. Expect to give propranolol for symptomatic tachycardia. • Administer an anticonvulsant such as diazepam, as ordered, to control seizures. • Scrape the inside of his nose to remove residual amounts of the drug. • Monitor his cardiac rate and rhythm— ventricular fibrillation and cardiac standstill can occur as a direct cardiotoxic result of cocaine ingestion. Defibrillate the patient, and initiate cardiopulmonary resuscitation, if indicated.
Glutethimide (Doriden) Cibas, CD, blues	• Small, reactive pupils • Nystagmus • Drowsiness • Irritability • Impaired thought processes (memory, judgment, attention span) • Slurred speech • Twitching, spasms, and seizures • Hypothermia • CNS depression (from unresponsiveness to deep coma)	• If the drug was taken orally, induce vomiting or perform gastric lavage; give activated charcoal and a cathartic, as ordered. • Maintain the patient's blood pressure with I.V. fluid challenges and vasopressors, as ordered. • Assist with hemodialysis or hemoperfusion if the patient has hepatic or renal failure or is in a prolonged coma. • Administer an anticonvulsant such as diazepam for seizures, as ordered. • Perform hourly neurologic assessments: Coma may recur because of the drug's slow release from fat deposits. *(continued)*

Recognizing and treating acute toxicity *(continued)*

SUBSTANCE	SIGNS AND SYMPTOMS	INTERVENTIONS
Glutethimide *(continued)*	• Apnea • Respiratory depression • Hypotension • Paralytic ileus • Poor bladder control	• Be alert for signs of increased intracranial pressure, such as decreasing LOC and widening pulse pressure. Give mannitol I.V., as ordered. • Watch for signs and symptoms of withdrawal, such as hyperreflexia, tonic-clonic seizures, and hallucinations, and provide symptomatic relief of withdrawal symptoms. • Protect the patient from injuring himself.
Hallucinogens • Lysergic acid diethylamide (LSD) – hawk, acid, sunshine • Mescaline (peyote) – mese, cactus, big chief	• Dilated pupils • Intensified perceptions • Agitation and anxiety • Synesthesia • Impaired judgment • Hyperactive movement • Flashback experiences • Hallucinations • Depersonalization • Moderately increased blood pressure • Increased heart rate • Fever	• Reorient the patient repeatedly to time, place, and person. • Restrain the patient to protect him from injuring himself and others. • Calm the patient down by talking to him in a quiet room. • If the drug was taken orally, induce vomiting or perform gastric lavage; give activated charcoal and a cathartic, as ordered. • Give diazepam I.V., as ordered, to control seizures.
Narcotics • Codeine • Heroin – junk, smack, H, snow	• Constricted pupils • Depressed LOC (but the patient is usu-	• Give naloxone as ordered until the drug's CNS depressant effects are reversed. • Replace fluids I.V., as ordered, to increase circulatory volume.

Recognizing and treating acute toxicity *(continued)*

SUBSTANCE	SIGNS AND SYMPTOMS	INTERVENTIONS
Narcotics *(continued)* • Hydromorphone hydrochloride (Dilaudid) – D, lords • Morphine – mort, monkey, M, Miss Emma	ally responsive to persistent verbal or tactile stimuli) • Seizures • Hypothermia • Slow, deep respirations • Hypotension • Bradycardia • Skin changes (pruritus, urticaria, and flushed skin)	• Correct hypothermia by applying extra blankets; if the patient's body temperature doesn't increase, use a hyperthermia blanket, as ordered. • Reorient the patient often. • Auscultate the lungs often for crackles, possibly indicating pulmonary edema. (Onset may be delayed.) • Administer oxygen via nasal cannula, mask, or mechanical ventilation to correct hypoxemia from hypoventilation. • Monitor cardiac rate and rhythm, being alert for atrial fibrillation. (This should resolve when hypoxemia is corrected.) • Be alert for signs of withdrawal, such as piloerection (goose flesh), diaphoresis, and hyperactive bowel sounds. • Institute safety measures to prevent patient injury.
Phencyclidine (PCP) Angel dust, peace pill, hog	• Blank stare • Nystagmus • Amnesia • Decreased awareness of surroundings • Recurrent coma • Violent behavior • Hyperactivity • Seizures • Gait ataxia • Muscle rigidity	• If the drug was taken orally, induce vomiting or perform gastric lavage; instill and remove activated charcoal repeatedly, as ordered. • Acidify the patient's urine with ascorbic acid, as ordered, to increase drug excretion. • Expect to continue to acidify urine for 2 weeks because signs and symptoms may recur when fat cells release PCP stores. • Give diazepam and haloperidol, as ordered, to control agitation or psychotic behavior. • Institute safety measures to protect patient from injury. *(continued)*

DRUG HAZARDS

Recognizing and treating acute toxicity *(continued)*

SUBSTANCE	SIGNS AND SYMPTOMS	INTERVENTIONS
Phencyclidine (PCP) *(continued)*	• Drooling • Hyperthermia • Hypertensive crisis • Cardiac arrest	• Administer diazepam, as ordered, to control seizures. • Institute seizure precautions. • Provide a quiet environment and dimmed light. • As ordered, give propranolol for hypertension and tachycardia, and give nitroprusside for severe hypertension. • Closely monitor urine output and serial renal function tests—rhabdomyolysis, myoglobinuria, and renal failure may occur in severe intoxication. • If renal failure develops, prepare the patient for hemodialysis.

DRUG HAZARDS

CHAPTER 13

Complications:
Spotting and correcting life-threatening conditions

Common complications

► Air embolism

Air embolism refers to the migration of a bolus of gas from the systemic circulation into the microvasculature. Obstruction occurs when the gas reaches the capillary system. Besides impairing blood flow, an air embolus causes a physiologic response as fibrin, platelets, and red blood cells congregate at the occlusion site. This further restricts blood flow and contributes to an inflammatory vasospasm of the affected vessel.

Arterial air emboli may lodge in the small vessels supplying major organs or peripheral circulation. Venous air emboli frequently occlude pulmonary blood flow. Venous air emboli also may obstruct arterial circulation in the presence of an intracardiac defect or a microvascular shunt between arterioles and venules of the lungs.

Causes

A bolus of air may enter the bloodstream during positive pressure ventilation in the presence of a lung tear, or when air enters an artery or vein through an I.V. cannula during insertion, maintenance, or removal of the line. Air emboli also have been associated with oral-vaginal sex, laser surgery, pneumoperitoneum, and as a complication of needle biopsies. Air emboli also result from rapid decompression following underwater diving.

Venous air emboli may occur as a complication of surgery or blunt or penetrating trauma to the head, neck, chest, heart, or abdomen.

Signs and symptoms

The first symptom of a venous air embolism may be cardiopulmonary collapse, especially in the presence of a rapid infusion of a large volume of air.

If the embolus moves into the arterial circulation, central nervous system and cardiac symptoms may develop. The patient may complain of dyspnea, vertigo, anxiety, or impending doom. A "gasp" reflex (cough, short exhalation and prolonged inhalation) has been documented.

Other signs include tachycardia, tachypnea, and elevated central venous and pulmonary artery pressures. Electrocardiograms show S-T segment changes reflecting ischemia. A transient churning heart murmur has been noted. Hypotension and decreased peripheral vascular resistance indicate progressive shock. Crepitus occasionally is palpable, and wheezes and crackles may be auscultated when pulmonary edema is present.

Treatment

Treatment aims to mitigate life-threatening symptoms and promote reabsorption of trapped air. In the event of cardiac arrest, cardiopulmonary resuscitation (CPR) is initiated immediately. External cardiac massage improves circulation and may help break up right ventricular bubbles, increasing blood flow to the pulmonary vasculature.

An air embolus may be removed through a central venous catheter or by needle aspiration. Bubble size may be reduced by administering 100% oxygen (which reduces the amount of nitrogen in the bubble), or by administering hyperbaric oxygen; the latter approach also may improve sequelae by oxygenating ischemic tissue.

Nursing interventions

• Prevention of air embolism is the key to nursing care. Ensure that all air is purged from catheters and I.V. lines before connecting them.
• Keep closed systems as airtight as possible; tape all tubing connections or use luer-lock devices for all connections.
• Place the patient in the Trendelenburg position when inserting all central venous line catheters. Have the patient perform Valsalva's maneuver during catheter insertion and tubing changes.
• Position the patient on his left side in the Trendelenburg position so air can enter the right atrium and be dispersed by the pulmonary artery.
• Initiate CPR immediately if cardiac collapse occurs.

Atelectasis

In atelectasis, alveolar clusters (lobules) or lung segments fail to expand completely during respiration, causing part or all of the affected lung to collapse. Because the collapsed lung tissue is effectively isolated from gas exchange, unoxygenated blood passes unchanged through these tissues and produces hypoxia.

Causes

Atelectasis can result from bronchial occlusion by mucus plugs—a special problem in patients with chronic obstructive pulmonary disease, bronchiectasis, or cystic fibrosis. Atelectasis also may result from occlusion caused by foreign bodies, bronchogenic cancer, and inflammatory lung disease.

Other causes include idiopathic respiratory distress syndrome of the newborn, oxygen toxicity, and pulmonary edema.

External compression, which inhibits full lung expansion, or any condition that makes deep breathing painful also may cause atelectasis. Compression or pain may result from upper abdominal surgical incisions, rib fractures, pleuritic chest pain, tight chest dressings, and obesity (which elevates the diaphragm and reduces tidal volume).

Lung collapse or reduced expansion may accompany prolonged immobility or mechanical ventilation; central nervous system depression eliminates periodic sighing and predisposes the patient to progressive atelectasis.

Signs and symptoms

Clinical effects vary with the causes of lung collapse, the degree of hypoxia, and the underlying disease. If atelectasis affects a small lung area, symptoms may be minimal and transient. However, with massive collapse, the patient may report severe symptoms—for example, dyspnea, anxiety, and pleuritic chest pain.

Inspection may disclose decreased chest wall movement, cyanosis, diaphoresis, and substernal or intercostal retractions. Palpation may detect decreased fremitus and mediastinal shift to the affected side. Percussion may disclose dullness or flatness over lung fields. Auscultation may disclose crackles during the last part of inspiration and decreased (or absent) breath sounds with major lung involvement. Auscultation also may disclose tachycardia.

Chest X-rays are the primary diagnostic tool. Other diagnostic tests may include bronchoscopy to rule out an obstructing neoplasm or a foreign body; arterial blood gas analysis to detect respiratory acidosis and hypoxemia resulting from atelectasis; and pulse oximetry, which may show deteriorating arterial oxygen saturation levels.

Treatment

Incentive spirometry, chest percussion, postural drainage, mucolytics, and frequent coughing and deep-breathing exercises may improve oxygenation. If these measures fail, bronchoscopy may help remove secretions. Humidity and bronchodilating medications can improve mucociliary clearance and dilate airways.

To minimize the risk for atelectasis after thoracic and abdominal surgery, the patient requires analgesics to facilitate deep breathing. If the patient has atelectasis secondary to an obstructing neoplasm, he may need surgery or radiation therapy.

Nursing interventions

• Offer reassurance and emotional support because the patient may be frightened by his limited ability to breathe.
• Encourage the patient recovering from surgery to perform coughing and deep-breathing exercises and incentive spirometry every 1 to 2 hours while splinting the incision. Encourage these procedures in any other patients who are at high risk for atelectasis.
• Assess breath sounds and respiratory status frequently. Report any changes immediately; monitor pulse oximetry readings and arterial blood gas values for evidence of hypoxia.
• *Gently* reposition the patient often, and help him walk as soon as possible. Administer adequate analgesics to control pain.
• If the patient is receiving mechanical ventilation, maintain tidal volume at 10 to 15 cc/kg of body weight to ensure adequate lung expansion. Use the ventilator's sigh mechanism, if appropriate, to intermittently increase tidal volume at the rate of 10 to 15 sighs per hour.
• Humidify inspired air, and encourage adequate fluid intake to mobilize secretions. Use postural drainage and chest percussion to remove secretions. Provide suctioning as needed.
• Administer sedatives cautiously because they depress respirations and the cough reflex; they also suppress sighs.

Bone marrow suppression

Bone marrow suppression is characterized by reduced numbers of hematopoietic (blood-forming) stem cells in the bone marrow. Impaired hematopoiesis leads to reduced numbers of peripheral blood leukocytes and neutrophils (neutropenia), thrombocytes (thrombocytopenia), and erythrocytes (anemia).

Causes

Many chemotherapeutic agents injure the rapidly proliferating stem cells. Other drugs, such as sulfa compounds, anticonvulsants, and immunosuppressants, also may suppress bone marrow.

Radiation to large marrow-bearing areas, such as the pelvis, ribs, spine, and sternum, may produce significant and permanent bone marrow damage.

Bone marrow suppression and depressed peripheral blood cell counts occur in patients with tumor replacement of the bone marrow (leukemia, myeloma, or metastatic deposits from solid tumors). Additional causes of bone marrow suppression include autoimmune disor-

▶

Nursing interventions in bone marrow suppression

The chart below summarizes essential nursing interventions for patients experiencing anemia, neutropenia, or thrombocytopenia.

CONDITION	INTERVENTIONS
Anemia (hemoglobin < 14 gm/dl in males; < 12 gm/dl in females) Severe anemia (hemoglobin < 8 gm/dl)	• Monitor complete blood count (CBC). • Monitor for signs of inadequate oxygenation (pallor, tachypnea, decreased capillary refill). • Instruct on nutritional supplementation (such as iron or folic acid). • Assess for source of blood loss, if applicable. • Teach energy conservation measures. • Teach patient to avoid driving or hazardous activities if dizziness is present. • Teach patient to change positions slowly to avoid syncopal episodes. • Administer transfusions of packed red blood cells, as ordered. Monitor for transfusion reactions. • Administer recombinant erythropoetin, as ordered.
Neutropenia (neutrophil count < 1,500/mm³) (Severe neutropenia < 500/mm³)	• Monitor temperature and vital signs. Report fever ≥ 101.3° F (38.5° C). • Monitor CBC, blood chemistries. • Assess for localized signs of infection. • Assess for symptoms of sepsis. • Obtain cultures of blood, urine, throat, sputum, and stool, as ordered (blood cultures with temperature spike ≥ 101.3° F [38.5° C]). • Avoid invasive procedures or rectal manipulation. • Avoid contact with persons with viral or bacterial infections. • Administer broad-spectrum antibiotics, as indicated. • Teach patient or caregiver rationale for use of hematopoietic growth factors and self-administration if indicated. • Teach proper storage and precautions for hematopoietic growth factors.

(continued)

▶

Nursing interventions in bone marrow suppression *(continued)*

CONDITION	INTERVENTIONS
Thrombocytopenia (Platelet count < 100,000/mm³) (Severe thrombocyto- penia platelet count < 20,000/mm³)	• Teach patient to avoid injury and sharp objects. • Teach patient to avoid straining or Valsalva's maneuver. • Avoid invasive procedures (no I.M. injections, enemas or suppositories). • Apply direct pressure for 5 minutes to needle puncture sites. • Assess for signs of bleeding, increased petechiae, or increased bruising. • Monitor for internal bleeding (blood in stool, hematuria); signs of intracranial bleeding, such as headache, restlessness, decreased level of consciousness, pupillary changes, and seizures. • Administer platelet transfusions, as ordered. • Monitor for transfusion reactions. Check posttransfusion platelet count.

◁

ders, certain congenital disorders, and exposure to pesticides, benzene-containing solvents, or other toxins.

Signs and symptoms

Manifestations of bone marrow suppression are related to its severity. The patient with *neutropenia* is at risk for infection from bacteria, viruses, or fungi. The neutropenic patient may exhibit fever, chills, malaise, or other localized signs of infection.

Thrombocytopenia is associated with bleeding (especially from the gums and nose), bruising, petechiae, ecchymoses, hematuria, and possibly hematochezia. Spontaneous bleeding is likely to occur if the platelet count drops below 20,000/mm³.

Signs and symptoms of *anemia* include fatigue, weakness, pallor, tachycardia, shortness of breath on exertion, and headache.

Treatment

Improved antimicrobial therapy has dramatically reduced morbidity and mortality of patients with neutropenia. Chemotherapy-induced neutropenia can be reduced by use of myeloid growth factors (granulocyte colony-stimulating factor [filgrastim] or granulocyte-macrophage colony-stimulating factor [sargramostin]).

Removal of the offending agents in drug-induced thrombocytopenia or proper treatment of the underlying cause (when possible) is essential. Corticosteroids or lithium carbonate or folate may be used to increase platelet production. Platelet transfusions may be used to stop episodic abnormal bleeding caused by a low platelet count. However, if platelet destruction results from an immune disorder, platelet infusions may have only a minimal effect and may be reserved for life-threatening bleeding.

Recombinant erythropoietin may help improve anemia due to chronic disease or renal dysfunction. Packed red blood cells and platelets are administered to support the patient until bone marrow function recovers.

Nursing interventions

Nursing interventions for the patient with bone marrow suppression are summarized in *Nursing interventions in bone marrow suppression*.

Brain herniation

This neurologic complication results from distortion and displacement of brain tissue through a natural opening in the intracranial cavity.

There are three types of brain herniation syndromes: cingulate, central, and transtentorial. *Cingulate herniation* occurs across the midline where the hemisphere is distorted beneath the falx cerebri. Few symptoms are associated with this type of herniation because it rarely occurs in isolation. *Central herniation* occurs when the medial aspects of the temporal lobe, the diencephalon, and the midbrain are pushed downward into the posterior fossa. In *transtentorial herniation*, the most common type of brain herniation, the medial aspect of the temporal lobe is pushed over the tentorium. Signs and symptoms reflect pressure on the midbrain and surrounding structures.

Causes

Brain herniation results from space-occupying lesions, cerebral edema due to trauma or stroke, or hydrocephalus. It also can be caused by excessive drainage of cerebrospinal fluid (CSF) from a ventricular catheter or a lumbar puncture.

Signs and symptoms

Signs and symptoms vary with the type of herniation. General early signs include decreasing level of consciousness, pupillary abnormalities, impaired motor function, and impaired brain stem reflexes. Signs of central herniation include small reactive pupils (early phase), roving eye movements with loss of upward gaze, intermittent agitation and drowsiness progressing to stupor, contralateral hemiparesis, and Cheyne-Stokes respirations. Signs of transtentorial herniation include ipsilateral pupil dilatation, paralysis of eye movements, restlessness progressing to loss of consciousness, contralateral hemiparesis, decorticate or decerebrate posturing, and bilateral Babinski's sign. Altered vital signs become evident late in the syndrome.

Treatment

If herniation results from a space-occupying lesion such as a hematoma or tumor, surgical removal of the lesion will relieve the pressure and allow adjacent structures to resume their normal shape. If herniation is related to increased intracranial pressure (ICP) resulting from cerebral edema, treatment involves reducing the edema using osmotic diuretics or steroids, CSF drainage, hyperventilation, and, in extreme cases, barbiturates. Maintenance of temperature control and normal fluid balance also are important. In some situations, such as cerebral edema resulting from traumatic injury, the patient may have an ICP monitor in place to help guide treatment.

Nursing interventions

• Perform neurologic assessments at least hourly.
• Institute precautionary measures to decrease ICP, including maintaining the head of the bed at 15 to 30 degrees to promote venous drainage. Position the patient in a neutral position, avoiding extreme hip and neck flexion.
• Institute seizure precautions and assess frequently for signs of seizures.
• Monitor vital signs frequently to ensure adequate cerebral perfusion.
• If the patient has undergone a craniotomy for a hematoma or tumor, provide postoperative craniotomy care.
• Observe carefully for other postoperative complications, such as infection, thrombophlebitis, or diabetes insipidus.

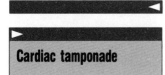

Cardiac tamponade

In cardiac tamponade, a rapid unchecked rise in intrapericardial pressure impairs diastolic filling of the heart. The increased pressure usually results from blood or fluid accumulation in the pericardial sac. If fluid accumulates rapidly, as little as 250 ml can create an emergency situation. Gradual fluid accumulation, as in pericardial effusion associated with cancer, may not produce immediate signs and symptoms because the fibrous wall of the pericardial sac can stretch to accommodate as much as 1 to 2 liters of fluid.

Causes

Cardiac tamponade may be idiopathic (Dressler's syndrome) or it may result from pleural effusion; hemorrhage from trauma; hemorrhage from nontraumatic causes (with pericarditis); acute myocardial infarction; and uremia.

Signs and symptoms

Cardiac tamponade classically produces increased venous pressure with neck vein distention, reduced arterial blood pressure, muffled heart sounds on auscultation, and pulsus paradoxus (an abnormal inspiratory drop in systemic blood pressure greater than 15 mm Hg).

Cardiac tamponade also may cause dyspnea, diaphoresis, pallor or cyanosis, anxiety, tachycardia, narrowed pulse pressure, restlessness, and hepatomegaly, but the lung fields will be clear. The patient typically sits upright and leans forward.

Chest X-rays show a slightly widened mediastinum and enlarged cardiac silhouette. Electrocardiography is done to rule out other cardiac disorders. Pulmonary artery pressure monitoring detects increases in right atrial pressure, right ventricular diastolic pressure, and central venous pressure (CVP). Echocardiography records pericardial effusion with signs of right ventricular and atrial compression.

Treatment

The goal of treatment is to relieve intrapericardial pressure and cardiac compression by removing accumulated blood or fluid. Pericardiocentesis (needle aspiration of the pericardial cavity) or surgical creation of an opening dramatically improves systemic arterial pressure and cardiac output with the aspiration of as little as 25 ml of fluid.

In the hypotensive patient, trial volume loading with 0.9% sodium chloride solution I.V. with albumin, and perhaps an inotropic drug, such as dopamine, are necessary to maintain cardiac output. Depending on the cause of tamponade, additional treatment may be needed.

Nursing interventions
• Infuse I.V. solutions and inotropic drugs (such as dopamine), as ordered, to maintain the patient's blood pressure.
• Administer oxygen therapy as needed.
• Prepare the patient for pericardiocentesis, thoracotomy, or central venous line insertion, as indicated.
• Check for signs of increasing tamponade, increasing dyspnea, and arrhythmias.
• Watch for a decrease in CVP and a concomitant rise in blood pressure following treatment, which indicate relief of cardiac compression.
• Monitor respiratory status for signs of respiratory distress, such as severe tachypnea or changes in level of consciousness.

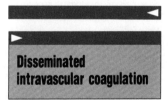

Disseminated intravascular coagulation

Also known as consumption coagulopathy or defibrination syndrome, disseminated intravascular coagulation (DIC) complicates conditions that accelerate clotting, thereby causing small vessel occlusion, organ necrosis, depletion of circulating clotting factors and platelets, and activation of the fibrinolytic system. This, in turn, can provoke severe hemorrhage.

Although usually acute, DIC may be chronic in cancer patients. The prognosis depends on early detection and treatment, the severity of the hemorrhage, and treatment of the underlying condition.

Causes
DIC results when tissue factor, a lipoprotein that helps initiate blood coagulation, is introduced into the bloodstream due to pathologic states such as infections, obstetric complications, neoplastic disease, and disorders that produce necrosis. Other causes include heatstroke, shock, poisonous snakebite, cirrhosis, fat embolism, incompatible blood transfusion, cardiac arrest, surgery necessitating cardiopulmonary bypass, giant hemangioma, severe venous thrombosis, and purpura fulminans.

Signs and symptoms
The most significant clinical feature of DIC is abnormal bleeding, *without* an accompanying history of known hemorrhagic disorder. Principal signs of such bleeding include cutaneous oozing, petechiae, ecchymoses, and hematomas caused by bleeding into the skin. Bleeding from sites of surgical or invasive procedures and from the GI tract are equally significant indications, as are acrocyanosis and signs of acute tubular necrosis.

Related symptoms and other possible effects include nausea, vomiting, dyspnea, oliguria, seizures, coma, shock, failure of major organ systems, and severe muscle, back, and abdominal pain.

The following initial laboratory findings suggest a tentative diagnosis of DIC: decreased platelet count, reduced fibrinogen levels, prolonged prothrombin time, prolonged partial thromboplastin time, and increased fibrin degradation products.

COMPLICATIONS

Treatment

Successful management of DIC requires prompt recognition and adequate treatment of the underlying disorder. If the patient isn't actively bleeding, supportive care alone may reverse DIC. However, active bleeding may require administration of blood, fresh frozen plasma, platelets, or packed red blood cells.

Nursing interventions

• Administer prescribed analgesics for pain, as needed.
• Administer oxygen therapy, as ordered.
• To prevent clots from dislodging and causing fresh bleeding, don't vigorously rub these areas when washing. If bleeding occurs, use pressure, cold compresses, and topical hemostatic agents to control it.
• After giving an I.V. injection or removing a catheter or needle, apply pressure to the injection site for at least 10 minutes. Alert other staff members to the patient's tendency to hemorrhage. Limit venipunctures whenever possible.
• Protect the patient from injury. Enforce complete bed rest during bleeding episodes. If the patient is very agitated, pad the bed rails.
• Reposition the patient every 2 hours, and provide meticulous skin care to prevent skin breakdown.
• If the patient can't tolerate activity because of blood loss, provide frequent rest periods.
• Monitor intake and output hourly. Watch for transfusion reactions and signs of fluid overload.
• Weigh dressings and linen and record drainage. Weigh the patient daily.
• Watch for bleeding from the GI and GU tracts. If you suspect intra-abdominal bleeding, measure the patient's abdominal girth at least every 4 hours, and observe closely for signs of shock.

• Monitor results of serial blood studies.
• Test all stools and urine for occult blood.
• Inform the family of the patient's progress, and provide emotional support and encouragement.

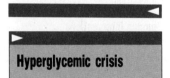

Hyperglycemic crisis

Diabetic ketoacidosis (DKA) and hyperosmolar hyperglycemic nonketotic syndrome (HHNK) are acute complications of hyperglycemic crisis that may occur in a diabetic patient. They require quick and effective treatment to avoid coma and, possibly, death. DKA occurs most often in patients with Type I diabetes; in fact, it may be the first evidence of previously unrecognized Type I diabetes. HHNK occurs most often in patients with Type II diabetes, but it also may occur in patients whose insulin tolerance is stressed and in those who've undergone certain therapeutic procedures, such as peritoneal dialysis or tube feedings.

Causes

Acute insulin deficiency (absolute in DKA; relative in HHNK) precipitates both conditions. Causes include illness, stress, infection, and failure to take insulin (*only* in a patient with DKA).

Signs and symptoms

Signs and symptoms of DKA and HHNK result primarily from soaring blood glucose levels, and include fluid loss, dehydration, shock, coma, and, possibly, death. Acetone breath; dehydration; weak, rapid pulse; and Kussmaul's respirations are seen in DKA. Polyuria, thirst, neurologic abnormalities, and stupor are evident in the patient with HHNK. Keep in mind that the patient with DKA also shows evidence of metabolic acidosis. Acidosis may start a cycle that leads to additional tissue breakdown, followed by more ketosis, more acidosis, and, eventually, shock, coma, and death.

Treatment

Both DKA and HHNK are treated with fluid and electrolyte replacement and supportive care. Sodium chloride solution (0.9% or 0.45%) is given I.V. at 1 L/hour until blood pressure is stabilized and urine output reaches 60 ml/hour. Then, regular insulin is started, initially as an I.V. bolus dose, followed by continuous infusion. The rate is adjusted until the patient's serum glucose levels decrease by 80 to 100 mg/dl/hour.

Once renal blood flow and urinary output are established, potassium is given intravenously. If acidosis is severe (pH less than 7.1), sodium bicarbonate may also be infused.

Nursing interventions

• When you recognize the signs and symptoms of DKA or HHNK, notify the doctor immediately and prepare the patient for transfer to the intensive care unit.
• Monitor the patient's vital signs, level of consciousness, electrocardiogram, and arterial blood gas, electrolyte, glucose, and osmolarity levels frequently, as ordered. Also check the patient's urine for ketones.
• Begin I.V. fluid replacement therapy as soon as possible.
• Expect to administer an injection of regular insulin immediately—either I.M. or I.V.—followed by a continuous I.V. insulin drip.

• Provide supportive care as indicated by the patient's condition.
• Prepare to administer potassium replacements, as ordered.

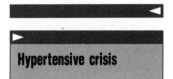

Hypertensive crisis

Hypertensive crisis refers to a severe, life-threatening form of hypertension. It is classified according to the degree of organ damage apparent at the time the patient presents for treatment.

Hypertensive emergency, the more critical crisis level, develops over hours to days and is accompanied by signs of imminent or progressing end-organ damage. Severely elevated diastolic blood pressure (DBP) must be reduced within minutes to an hour to prevent or reduce irreversible organ damage. *Hypertensive urgency*, a less critical crisis level, develops over several days to weeks and is characterized by severely elevated DBP but without evidence of end-organ damage.

Causes

Hypertensive crisis is caused by conditions or circumstances that elevate cardiac output, such as increased circulating volume due to primary aldosteronism or eclampsia; it is also caused by conditions that increase peripheral vascular resistance, such as excessive vasoconstriction due to catecholamine release accompanying pheochromocytoma, blockage of some antihypertensive drugs by monoamine oxidase (MAO) inhibitors, or release of angiotensin into the circulation (as in renal disease).

Other causes of hypertensive crisis include acute aortic dissection, coarctation of the aorta, acute left ventricular failure and pulmonary edema, renal artery stenosis, thyroid crisis, hypercalcemia, and adrenocortical disorders.

Signs and symptoms

Persons in hypertensive emergency generally present with DBP of 120 mm Hg or greater, with evidence of incipient or progressive end-organ damage. Persons with hypertensive urgency may present with elevated DBP (100 to 120 mm Hg), but with no evidence of concomitant end-organ damage.

Clinical symptoms may be absent in early stages of either hypertensive state. The patient may experience vague discomfort and fatigue or neurologic signs such as dizziness or occipital or anterior headache. In later stages of hypertensive crisis, particularly in hypertensive emergency, the patient may exhibit signs related to organs or tissues affected:

• *Eyes:* retinal changes, including arterial narrowing or papilledema, decreased acuity, and nystagmus.

• *Neurologic:* slow responses, decreased level of consciousness, cranial nerve abnormality, changes in deep tendon reflexes, nausea, vomiting, seizures, throbbing suboccipital or anterior headache, muscle weakness, and altered speech.

• *Renal:* oliguria, hematuria, azotemia, palpable enlarged kidneys, costovertebral angle tenderness.

• *Cardiopulmonary:* angina; cool, pale skin; shift in point of maximum impulse; S_3 and S_4 heart sounds; left ventricular heave; jugular vein distention; and adventitious lung sounds, such as basilar crackles.

Diagnostic tests (X-rays, electrocardiogram, computed tomography scan, urinalysis, and blood work) may determine the underlying cause.

Treatment

The priority for treating hypertensive crisis is lowering blood pressure rapidly but cautiously, to avoid sharply reducing perfusion of organs that have accommodated to higher pressures.

Some patients may require surgery to correct the underlying cause of hypertension, but most are treated conservatively with oral or parenteral antihypertensives. In hypertensive emergency, blood pressure is reduced rapidly over a few minutes to an hour. In hypertensive urgency, it's reduced gradually, over several hours to 24 hours.

Medical therapy is directed at reducing systemic vascular resistance or reducing circulating volume, as appropriate.

Nursing interventions

• The most important nursing responsibilities are accurately assessing the patient's blood pressure, detecting possible causes of the hypertension, and preventing or detecting incipient end-organ damage.

• After medication therapy is initiated, monitor blood pressure every 5 to 15 minutes, depending on the medication used.

• If mechanical or arterial line blood pressure readings are used, check their accuracy with cuff pressures at least once every 4 hours.

• Administer medications according to protocols to maintain blood pressure within a designated parameter and avoid insufficient or excessive reduction of blood pressure.

• Assess pulses, skin color, and temperature in all extremities. Note any pulse deficits; differences in rate, rhythm, and quality; bruits; or edema.

• Perform neurologic and visual checks at least once every 4 hours to determine adequate cerebral and ocular circulation. Note any changes in level of consciousness, sensory/motor changes, dizziness, visual status, and ocular fundus changes.

• Monitor closely for signs of cardiac decompensation with pulmonary edema and chest pain, which might signal the onset of angina or myocardial infarction.

• Teach the patient to avoid any stress, sudden movement, straining, and Valsalva's maneuver, to prevent sudden changes in blood pressure.

• Monitor renal status, including hourly intake and output.

• Administer pain medication and sedation, as ordered, for possible headache secondary to medication or chest pain. Institute other pain and anxiety control measures, such as quiet environment, distraction, guided imagery, and massage, to increase relaxation and comfort and relieve stress.

• Monitor the patient carefully when desired blood pressure control is attained and he is weaned from parenteral therapy to oral maintenance therapy.

• Address the patient's and family's anxiety and explain the situation and all therapy as thoroughly as possible.

• Assess the patient's knowledge of and compliance with the antihypertensive medication regimen. Plan interventions, as needed, to educate the patient and promote proper blood pressure control.

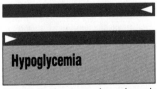

Hypoglycemia

Potentially dangerous, hypoglycemia is an abnormally low blood glucose level. It occurs when glucose burns up too rapidly, when the glucose re-

lease rate falls behind tissue demands, or when excessive insulin enters the bloodstream.

Hypoglycemia may be classified as reactive or fasting. *Reactive hypoglycemia* results from the reaction to the disposition of meals or administration of excessive insulin.

Fasting hypoglycemia causes discomfort during periods of abstinence from food, for example in the early morning hours before breakfast.

Causes

Reactive hypoglycemia may occur in several forms. In a diabetic patient, it may result from administration of too much insulin or — less commonly — too much oral hypoglycemic agent. In a mildly diabetic patient (or one in the early stages of diabetes mellitus), reactive hypoglycemia may result from delayed and excessive insulin production after carbohydrate ingestion.

Similarly, a nondiabetic patient may suffer reactive hypoglycemia from a sharp increase in insulin output after a meal. Sometimes called postprandial hypoglycemia, this form usually disappears when the patient eats something sweet.

In some patients, reactive hypoglycemia may have no known cause or may result from hyperalimentation due to gastric dumping syndrome or from impaired glucose tolerance.

Fasting hypoglycemia usually results from an excess of insulin or insulin-like substances, or from a decrease in counterregulatory hormones. It also may be exogenous, such as from alcohol or drug ingestion, or endogenous, such as from organic problems.

Other endocrine causes include destruction of the pancreatic islet cells, adrenocortical insufficiency, and pituitary insufficiency. Nonendocrine causes include severe liver disease (such as hepatitis, liver cancer, cirrhosis, and liver congestion associated with congestive heart failure).

Signs and symptoms

Reactive and fasting hypoglycemia cause fatigue, malaise, nervousness, irritability, trembling, tension, headache, hunger, cold sweats, and rapid heart rate.

Fasting hypoglycemia also may cause central nervous system (CNS) disturbances, such as blurry or double vision, confusion, motor weakness, hemiplegia, seizures, or coma. In infants and children, signs and symptoms are vague. A newborn's refusal to feed may be the primary clue to underlying hypoglycemia. Associated CNS effects include tremors, twitching, weak or high-pitched cry, sweating, limpness, seizures, and coma.

Treatment

Reactive hypoglycemia requires dietary modification to help delay glucose absorption and gastric emptying. Usually, this includes small, frequent meals; avoidance of simple carbohydrates; and ingestion of high-protein meals with added fiber. The patient also may receive anticholinergic drugs to slow gastric emptying and intestinal motility and to inhibit vagal stimulation of insulin release.

For fasting hypoglycemia, surgery and drug therapy may be required. Hormone replacement therapy may be needed for pituitary and adrenal gland insufficiency.

Nursing interventions

• Administer medications, as ordered.
• Avoid delays in meal times and provide a proper diet.
• Correct hypoglycemic episodes

quickly. Measure blood glucose to verify its presence and severity before correcting hypoglycemia.
• Monitor any I.V. infusion of hypertonic glucose solution to avoid hyperglycemia, circulatory overload, and cellular dehydration.
• Measure blood glucose levels, as ordered.
• Assess the effects of drug therapy, and watch for adverse reactions.

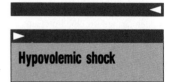

Hypovolemic shock

Potentially life-threatening, hypovolemic shock stems from reduced intravascular blood volume, which leads to decreased cardiac output and inadequate tissue perfusion. The subsequent tissue anoxia prompts a shift in cellular metabolism from aerobic to anaerobic pathways. This results in an accumulation of lactic acid, which produces metabolic acidosis.

Causes

Hypovolemic shock most commonly results from acute blood loss — about 20% of total volume. Massive blood loss may result from gastrointestinal (GI) bleeding, internal or external hemorrhage, or any condition that reduces circulating intravascular volume or other body fluids.

Other causes include intestinal obstruction, peritonitis, acute pancreatitis, ascites and dehydration from excessive perspiration, severe diarrhea or protracted vomiting, diabetes insipidus, diuresis, and inadequate fluid intake.

Signs and symptoms

The patient's history will include conditions that reduce blood volume, such as GI hemorrhage, trauma, and severe diarrhea and vomiting. A patient with cardiac disease may report anginal pain.

Inspection may reveal pale skin, decreased sensorium, and rapid, shallow respirations. Urine output usually falls below 25 ml/hour. Palpation may disclose rapid, thready peripheral pulses and cold, clammy skin. Auscultation of blood pressure usually detects a mean arterial pressure below 60 mm Hg and a narrowing pulse pressure.

Laboratory findings may include low hematocrit; decreased hemoglobin levels and red blood cell and platelet counts; elevated serum potassium, sodium, lactate dehydrogenase, creatinine, and blood urea nitrogen levels; increased urine specific gravity (greater than 1.020) and urine osmolality; decreased urine creatinine levels; and decreased pH and PaO_2 and increased $PaCO_2$.

X-rays, gastroscopy, aspiration of gastric contents through a nasogastric tube, and tests for occult blood identify internal bleeding sites. Coagulation studies may detect coagulopathy from disseminated intravascular coagulation.

Treatment

Emergency treatment relies on prompt and adequate blood and fluid replacement to restore intravascular volume and to raise blood pressure and maintain it above 60 mm Hg. Rapid infusion of 0.9% sodium chloride or lactated Ringer's solution and, possibly, albumin or other plasma expanders may expand volume adequately until whole blood can be matched.

Treatment also may include application of a pneumatic antishock garment, oxygen administration, control of bleeding, administration of dopamine or another inotropic drug and, possibly, surgery. To be effective, dopamine or other inotropic drugs must be used with vigorous fluid resuscitation.

Nursing interventions

• Check for a patent airway and adequate circulation. If the patient experiences cardiac or respiratory arrest, start cardiopulmonary resuscitation.
• Begin an I.V. infusion with 0.9% sodium chloride or lactated Ringer's solution.
• Monitor the patient's central venous pressure, right atrial pressure, pulmonary artery pressure, pulmonary artery wedge pressure (PAWP), and cardiac output at least once hourly or as ordered.
• Monitor urine output hourly; if output falls below 30 ml/hour in an adult, increase the fluid infusion rate, but watch for signs of fluid overload, such as elevated PAWP. Notify the doctor if urine output doesn't increase.
• Obtain arterial blood gas (ABG) samples as ordered. Administer oxygen by face mask or airway to ensure adequate tissue oxygenation. Adjust the oxygen flow rate as ABG measurements indicate.
• Record blood pressure, pulse and respiratory rates, and peripheral pulse rates every 15 minutes until stable. Monitor cardiac rhythm continuously.
• Also notify the doctor, and increase the infusion rate, if the patient experiences a progressive drop in blood pressure accompanied by a thready pulse.
• Obtain a complete blood count, electrolyte levels, type and crossmatching, and coagulation studies, as ordered.
• During therapy, assess skin color and temperature, and note any changes.
• Watch for signs of impending coagulopathy.

Paralytic ileus

Paralytic ileus is a physiologic form of intestinal obstruction that may develop in the small bowel after abdominal surgery. It causes decreased or absent intestinal motility that usually recovers spontaneously after 2 to 3 days.

Causes

This condition can develop as a response to trauma, toxemia, or peritonitis, or as a result of electrolyte deficiencies, especially hypokalemia, and the use of certain drugs, such as ganglionic blocking agents and anticholinergic agents. It also can result from vascular causes, such as thrombosis or embolism. Excessive air swallowing may contribute to it, but paralytic ileus brought on by this factor alone seldom lasts more than 24 hours.

Signs and symptoms

Clinical effects of paralytic ileus include severe abdominal distention, extreme distress and, possibly, vomiting. The patient may be severely constipated or may pass flatus and small, liquid stools.

Treatment

Paralytic ileus lasting longer than 48 hours requires nasogastric intubation for decompression and suctioning.

When paralytic ileus results from surgical manipulation of the bowel, treatment also may include cholinergic agents, such as neostigmine or bethanechol.

Nursing interventions

• Encourage early postoperative movement and ambulation.
• Assess for complaints of nausea and vomiting. Inspect the abdomen for signs of distention.
• Auscultate for bowel sounds; note any passage of flatus or stool.
• Monitor patients receiving cholinergic agents for possible paradoxical side effects, such as intestinal cramps and diarrhea.
• Prepare for nasogastric intubation and suctioning if indicated.
• Provide fastidious mouth and nose care if the patient has vomited or has undergone decompression by intubation.
• Assess for signs of dehydration.
• Monitor fluid and electrolyte balance closely.
• Maintain the patient on nothing by mouth, as ordered; provide I.V. fluid replacement therapy.
• Monitor intake and output. Irrigate the decompression tube with 0.9% sodium chloride solution.
• Keep the patient in Fowler's position as much as possible to promote pulmonary ventilation and ease respiratory distress.
• Check frequently for return of bowel sounds and peristalsis (passage of flatus and mucus through the rectum).

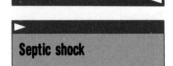

Septic shock

Usually caused by a bacterial infection, septic shock causes inadequate blood perfusion and circulatory collapse. Unless treated promptly (preferably before symptoms fully develop), it rapidly progresses to death, often within a few hours, in up to 80% of cases. Septic shock occurs most often in hospitalized patients, especially men over age 40 and women ages 25 to 45.

Causes

Many gram-positive and gram-negative bacteria, as well as actinomyces, can cause septic shock. Preexisting infections caused by viruses, rickettsiae, chlamydiae, and protozoa may be complicated by septic shock. Other predisposing factors include immunodeficiency, advanced age, trauma, burns, diabetes mellitus, cirrhosis, and disseminated intravascular coagulation.

Signs and symptoms

Indications of septic shock vary according to the stage of the shock, the organism causing it, and the age of the patient.

Early manfestations include oliguria, sudden fever (over 101° F [38.3° C]), chills, nausea, vomiting, diarrhea, and prostration.

Late manifestations include restlessness, apprehension, irritability, thirst due to reduced cerebral tissue perfusion, hypothermia, anuria, tachycardia, and tachypnea.

 In infants and elderly patients, hypotension, altered level of consciousness, and hyperventilation may be the only signs of septic shock.

Treatment

The first goal of treatment is to monitor and reverse shock through volume expansion. I.V. fluids are administered and a pulmonary artery catheter is inserted. Whole blood or plasma may be administered to raise the pulmonary artery wedge pressure (PAWP) to a satisfactory level. I.V. antibiotics are given and a urinary catheter is inserted to monitor hourly output. Mechanical ventilation may be necessary.

If shock persists after fluid infusion, vasopressors are given to maintain adequate blood perfusion. Other treatments include I.V. bicarbonate to correct acidosis and I.V. corticosteroids, to improve blood perfusion and increase cardiac output.

Nursing interventions

• Remove any I.V., intra-arterial, or urinary drainage catheters and send them to the laboratory to culture for causative organisms.
• Start an I.V. infusion of 0.9% sodium chloride or lactated Ringer's solution.
• Administer antibiotics intravenously to achieve effective blood levels rapidly; monitor serum drug levels.
• Measure hourly urine output. Watch for signs of fluid overload, such as an increase in PAWP.
• If urine output is less than 30 ml/hour, increase the fluid infusion rate. Notify the doctor if urine output doesn't improve. A diuretic may be ordered to increase renal blood flow and urine output.
• Monitor arterial blood gas (ABG) studies. Administer oxygen by face mask or airway. Adjust oxygen flow rate according to ABG measurements.
• If the patient's blood pressure drops below 80 mm Hg, increase the oxygen flow rate and notify the doctor immediately.
• Record the patient's blood pressure, pulse and respiratory rates, and peripheral pulses every 1 to 5 minutes until he is stabilized. Record hemodynamic pressure readings every 15 minutes. Monitor cardiac rhythm continuously.
• Provide emotional support to the patient and his family.
• Document the occurrence of a nosocomial infection and report it to the infection-control nurse.

Spinal cord compression

Compression of the spinal cord results in multiple disturbances that affect the individual's ability to perform activities of daily living. The onset and severity of symptoms vary with the etiology of the compression; onset may be acute (traumatic injury) or insidious (tumor growth). Outcome depends on the nature of the compression and how promptly the diagnosis is made.

Causes

Traumatic injuries are the most common cause of spinal cord compression. Hyperflexion injuries usually result from sudden deceleration, most often affecting the cervical region. Hyperextension injuries tend to cause more damage because the spine swings through a larger arc, making cord compression more likely. Rotational injuries result from extreme lateral flexion. Compression injuries result from extreme vertical pressure, usually caused by a long fall.

Spinal cord tumors are less common than other types of tumors and are most often benign. They occur most commonly in the thoracic region and usually are extradural.

Signs and symptoms

Symptoms of spinal cord compression are related to the level of the injury. Generally, sudden and complete compression causes loss of movement, spinal reflexes, and pain sensation below the level of the lesion. Bowel and bladder dysfunction also may occur, along with an inability to perspire below the level of the lesion. Incomplete, acute traumatic compression may result in any combination of these symptoms. (For more information, see *Functional loss from spinal cord injury.*)

In spinal cord tumors, the location of symptoms also is related to the level of the lesion. Pain is the most common initial symptom, along with coldness and numbness. Motor weakness usually occurs along with sensory loss. Loss of sphincter control may occur; bladder control usually is affected before bowel control.

Treatment

For traumatic injury, treatment begins with immediate stabilization followed by the basic goals of decompression, realignment, and further stabilization. The specific treatment depends on the type of injury and may be surgical, nonsurgical, or a combination. If surgery is indicated, it is usually to decrease compression and stabilize the spine.

Treatment of spinal tumors may include radiation and surgery, and depends on the tumor type, location, and rapidity of onset of the symptoms.

Nursing interventions

• With traumatic injuries, perform physical assessments with each vital sign assessment and each time the patient is moved.
• Pay special attention to respiratory status, especially with a cervical lesion; frequently measure vital capacity and tidal volume.
• Maintain a patent airway and suction as needed; perform chest physiotherapy frequently.
• Instruct the patient to cough and deep-breathe every 2 hours.
• Provide range-of-motion exercises and encourage patient participation as much as function allows.

• Reposition the patient every 2 hours and provide meticulous skin care.
• Administer analgesics and muscle relaxants, as ordered.
• Monitor intake and output to assess fluid balance. Ensure adequate oral intake.
• Provide emotional support and encouragement to the patient and his family. Assist with enhancing the patient's capabilities.
• Assist with arrangements and follow-up for rehabilitation.

Functional loss from spinal cord injury

Functional losses from spinal cord injury include variable losses of motor function, deep tendon reflexes, sensory function, respiratory function, and bowel and bladder function, depending on which vertebral level is affected.

Level C1 to C4
• Complete loss of motor function below neck
• No reflex loss
• Loss of sensory function in neck and below
• Loss of involuntary and voluntary respiratory function
• Loss of bowel and bladder control

Level C5
• Loss of all motor function below upper shoulders
• Loss of deep tendon reflexes in biceps
• Loss of sensation below clavicle and in most of chest, abdomen, and upper and lower extremities
• Phrenic nerve is intact, but not intercostal and abdominal muscles
• Loss of bowel and bladder control

Level C6
• Loss of all function below shoulders; no elbow, forearm, or hand control
• Loss of deep tendon reflexes in biceps
• Loss of sensation below clavicle and in most of chest, abdomen, and upper and lower extremities
• Phrenic nerve is intact, but not intercostal and abdominal muscles
• Loss of bowel and bladder control

Level C7
• Loss of motor control to portions of arms and hands
• Loss of deep tendon reflexes in triceps
• Loss of sensation below clavicle and in portions of arms and hands
• Phrenic nerve is intact, but not intercostal and abdominal muscles
• Loss of bowel and bladder function

Level C8
• Loss of motor control to portions of arms and hands
• Loss of deep tendon reflexes in triceps
• Loss of sensation below chest and in portions of hands
• Phrenic nerve is intact, but not intercostal and abdominal muscles
• Loss of bowel and bladder function

Level T1 to T6
• Loss of all motor function below midchest region, including trunk muscles
• No reflex loss
• Loss of sensation below midchest area
• Phrenic nerve functions independently
• Some impairment of intercostal and abdominal muscles
• Loss of bowel and bladder function

Level T6 to T12
• Loss of motor control below waist
• No reflex loss
• Loss of all sensation below waist
• No interference with respiratory function
• Impairment of abdominal muscles leading to diminished cough
• Loss of bowel and bladder control

Level L1 to L3
• Loss of most of leg and pelvis control
• Loss of knee jerk reflex (L2, L3)
• Loss of sensation to lower abdomen and legs
• No interference with respiratory function
• Loss of bowel and bladder control

Level L3 to L4
• Loss of control of portions of lower legs, ankles, and feet
• Loss of knee jerk reflex
• Loss of sensation to portions of lower legs, feet, and ankles
• No interference with respiratory function
• Loss of bowel and bladder control

Level L4 to L5
• Varying extent of motor control loss
• Loss of ankle jerk reflex (S1, S2)
• Loss of sensation in upper legs and portions of lower legs (lumbar sensory nerves) and in lower legs, feet, and perineum (sacral sensory nerves)
• No interference with respiratory function
• Possible impairment of bowel and bladder control

Superior vena cava syndrome

Superior vena cava syndrome (SVCS) arises from restriction of venous blood flow through the superior vena cava. This large, thin-walled vein is easily compressed by enlargement of adjacent lymph nodes or tumors of the mediastinum and right lung. Rapidly progressing or untreated SVCS may lead to respiratory arrest.

Causes
Malignant neoplasms account for approximately 80% of cases of SVCS. The most common malignancy associated with SVCS is small-cell carcinoma of the lung, followed by non-small-cell lung cancers, malignant lymphoma, thymoma, germ-cell tumors of the mediastinum, and metastatic breast cancer. The most common nonmalignant cause of SVCS is catheter-associated thrombosis.

Signs and symptoms
The patient with SVCS presents with dyspnea, anxiety, facial edema, cyanosis, and, possibly, edema of the arms. Physical findings include distended neck veins and dilated collateral veins on the chest, back, and, possibly, the upper abdomen as venous return circumvents the obstructed superior vena cava. Advanced SVCS is heralded by headache, changes in mental status, visual disturbances, dizziness, stridor, and respiratory distress.

Treatment
Treatment focuses on the underlying cause. In patients without a prior cancer diagnosis, needle biopsy, sputum smears, bronchoscopy, or mediastinoscopy are indicated to

COMPLICATIONS

obtain a tissue diagnosis. Computed tomography scan may reveal a mediastinal mass. Combination chemotherapy is begun promptly to control SVCS caused by small-cell lung cancer, lymphomas, and germ-cell tumors. Radiation therapy may be added for patients with bulky (> 10 cm) mediastinal lymphomas. Local radiation is the treatment of choice for SVCS associated with non-small-cell lung cancer.

Catheter-associated thrombosis may be treated with streptokinase, urokinase, or alteplase. If possible, the catheter should be removed after the patient receives anticoagulant therapy to prevent embolism.

Nursing interventions
• Elevate the head of the bed to Fowler's or high Fowler's position.
• Administer oxygen therapy, as ordered, to help reduce cardiac output and decrease venous pressure.
• Administer diuretics cautiously, as ordered, to control edema of the face and upper extremities.
• Avoid venipunctures in the upper extremities; anticipate use of a femoral catheter for giving I.V. fluids and chemotherapy.
• Monitor fluid and electrolyte balance.
• Monitor for signs and symptoms of worsening SVCS, which include progressive respiratory distress, increased edema, and mental status changes.

Syndrome of inappropriate antidiuretic hormone secretion

Syndrome of inappropriate antidiuretic hormone secretion (SIADH) is marked by excessive release of antidiuretic hormone (ADH), which disturbs fluid and electrolyte balance. Such disturbances result from an inability to excrete dilute urine, retention of free water, expansion of extracellular fluid volume, and hyponatremia. The syndrome occurs secondary to diseases that affect the osmoreceptors of the hypothalamus.

Causes
Most commonly, SIADH results from oat-cell carcinoma of the lung, which secretes excessive ADH or vasopressor-like substances. Other neoplastic diseases (such as pancreatic and prostatic cancer, Hodgkin's disease, and thymoma) also may trigger SIADH.

Additional causes include central nervous system disorders, pulmonary disorders, positive-pressure ventilation, drugs, and miscellaneous conditions, such as myxedema or psychosis.

Signs and symptoms
SIADH may produce weight gain despite appetite loss; nausea and vomiting; muscle weakness; restlessness; and, possibly, seizures and coma. Edema is rare unless water overload exceeds 4 liters, because much of the free water excess exists within cellular boundaries.

A complete medical history revealing positive water balance may suggest SIADH. Serum osmolality less than 280 mOsm/kg of water and serum sodium less than 123 mEq/L confirm it. Supportive laboratory values include high urine sodium secretion (more than 20mEq/L) without diuretics. Other diagnostic studies show normal renal function and no evidence of dehydration.

Treatment

Treatment begins with restricted water intake (500 to 1,000 ml/day). With severe water intoxication, administration of 200 to 300 ml of 3% to 5% sodium chloride solution may be needed to raise the serum sodium level. If fluid restriction is ineffective, demeclocycline or lithium may be given to help block the renal response to ADH. When possible, treatment should include correcting the root cause of SIADH. If it's related to cancer, water retention may be alleviated by surgery, irradiation, or chemotherapy.

Nursing interventions

• Restrict fluids, and provide comfort measures for thirst, including ice chips, mouth care, lozenges, and staggered water intake.
• Reduce unnecessary environmental stimuli and orient the patient, as needed.
• Provide a safe environment for the patient with an altered level of consciousness (LOC). Take seizure precautions as needed.
• Monitor the patient's serum osmolality and serum and urine sodium levels.
• Closely monitor and record intake and output, vital signs, and daily weight.
• Perform frequent neurologic checks, depending on the patient's status. Look for and report early changes in LOC.
• Observe for signs and symptoms of heart failure, which may occur as a result of fluid overload.

Thyroid storm

Also known as thyrotoxic crisis, thyroid storm is an acute manifestation of hyperthyroidism. It usually occurs in patients with preexisting (though often unrecognized) thyrotoxicosis. If thyroid storm is not promptly treated, the patient may experience hypotension, vascular collapse, coma, and death.

Causes

Onset is almost always abrupt, evoked by a stressful event, such as trauma, surgery, or infection. Less common causes include insulin-induced hypoglycemia or diabetic ketoacidosis; cerebrovascular accident; myocardial infarction; pulmonary embolism; sudden cessation of antithyroid medication; initiation of I^{131} therapy; preeclampsia; and subtotal thyroidectomy with excess intake of synthetic thyroid hormone.

Signs and symptoms

Initially, the patient may have marked tachycardia, vomiting, and stupor. Other findings include irritability and restlessness; visual disturbances, such as diplopia; tremor and weakness; angina; shortness of breath; cough; and swollen extremities. Palpation may reveal warm, moist flushed skin, and a high fever (this begins insidiously and rapidly rises to a lethal level).

Treatment

Treatment for thyroid storm includes administration of an antithyroid drug, I.V. propranolol to block sympathetic effects, a corticosteroid to inhibit conversion of thyroid hormone thyroxine (T_4) to triiodothyronine (T_3) and to replace depleted cortisol levels, and iodide to block release of thyroid hormone. Supportive measures include administration of nutrients, vitamins, fluids, and sedatives.

Nursing interventions

• Monitor vital signs, electrocardiogram, and cardiopulmonary status continuously. Assess for changes in consciousness.

• Expect to administer an antithyroid medication or a beta blocker to inhibit sympathetic effects. Monitor the patient's response to medications.

• Administer corticosteroids to inhibit conversion of T_4 and to replace depleted cortisol, as ordered; anticipate administering iodide to block release of thyroid hormones.

• Closely monitor the patient's temperature. If indicated, apply cooling measures and administer acetaminophen, as ordered. Never administer aspirin because it may further increase the patient's metabolic rate.

• Institute safety measures, including seizure precautions, to protect the patient from injury.

• Provide supportive care and administer vitamins, nutrients, fluids, and sedatives, as ordered.

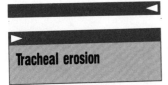

Tracheal erosion

Tracheal erosion refers to damage to the tracheal lumen through mechanical or chemical irritation. Tissue destruction most frequently progresses from interior to exterior tracheal structures, but it also may be caused or abetted by external pressure, especially to the posterior tracheal wall.

Causes

Chemical injury to tracheal tissues occurs as epithelial cells and submucosal structures are destroyed by inhalation of toxic substances (such as smoke and corrosive gases) and by direct burn injury. Edema and inflammation also occur. Mechanical injury results from lodgment of a foreign body in the airway, which may be accompanied by inflammation.

In the clinical setting, tracheal erosion most often results from traumatic intubation with cuffed or uncuffed endotracheal or tracheal tubes. High-pressure, low-volume cuffed tubes are most likely to cause damage.

Concomitant use of a nasogastric tube places additional friction on the tracheal muscle internally and externally, increasing the risk of tracheoesophageal fistula.

Signs and symptoms

Hemoptysis is the most common sign. Bleeding may be scant if only surface vessels are injured, or it may be severe if erosion penetrates the adjacent neck vessels. In patients receiving mechanical ventilation, a persistent air leak may indicate tracheal dilation and possible erosion. Tracheal erosion should be suspected when the patient aspirates food or fluid, especially during prolonged tracheal and nasogastric intubation.

Treatment

Treatment is primarily limited to allowing the affected area to heal spontaneously. For injury due to traumatic intubation, tube removal is most desirable. Otherwise, pressure on the erosion site can be reduced by cuff deflation, recannulation with a smaller airway, or replacement of a standard tracheostomy tube with a dual cuffed or longer tube. Removal of a nasogastric tube limits friction on the trachea. A gastric tube may be inserted to promote decompression or provide nutrition. Antibiotics may be given to treat infection and promote healing.

Nursing interventions
• Ensure that each patient receives an appropriately sized endotracheal or tracheal tube to avoid placing unnecessary pressure on the tracheal walls.
• Stabilize airway tubes to prevent irritation caused by movement.
• Maintain lateral wall pressures for nonatmospheric tubes at less than 18 mm Hg.
• Suction only as necessary, using a vacuum with less than 120 mm Hg of pressure; never force a suction catheter against resistance.
• Use small-bore nasogastric or gastric tubes to prevent erosion.
• If fistula is suspected, discontinue nasogastric intubation and notify the doctor.

CHAPTER 14

Documentation:
Completing forms fully and concisely

General guidelines

Nursing documentation: What to cover

With a large number of health care professionals involved in each patient's care, nursing documentation must be complete, accurate, and timely to foster continuity of care. In effect, your documentation should cover the following items:

• initial assessment using the nursing process and applicable nursing diagnoses
• nursing actions, particularly reports to the doctor
• ongoing assessment, including the frequency of assessment
• variations from the assessment and plan
• accountability information, including forms signed by the patient, the location of the patient's valuables, and any patient teaching
• notation of care by staff in other disciplines, including doctor visits, if practical
• health teaching, including content and response
• procedures and diagnostic tests performed on the patient
• the patient's response to therapy, particularly to nursing interventions and diagnostic tests
• any statements made by the patient regarding his condition or care
• patient comfort and safety measures.

Documentation timesavers

How can you document more accurately and quickly? The following suggestions will help.

Follow the nursing process

Your documentation can best substantiate quality care if it reflects this process. And the resulting record will help other caregivers provide quality care.

Use nursing diagnoses

Using standardized diagnostic labels to identify the patient's actual or potential health problems will result in less confusion and better care. Depending on your hospital's policy, you may be required to use nursing diagnoses.

Document frequently and immediately

If you chart during your shift — right after you make an observation or intervene — rather than at the end of your shift, you'll document more accurately and forget less information. You'll also provide other team members with the most current information on the patient's care and progress.

Flow sheets help you keep your documentation current, as does bedside charting. A growing number of hospitals are requiring immediate documentation.

Individualize your charting

Documenting the same information for all patients with the same diagnosis neither promotes accuracy nor demonstrates quality care. Make sure your charting demonstrates the particular care that each patient received.

Don't repeat information

Not only does this waste time, but it can be misleading. If you record data on a flow sheet, don't repeat it in the progress notes. Instead, use the progress notes to clarify information on the flow sheet. Or use them to add data, such as psychosocial information or follow-up care, that you can't chart on a flow sheet.

Sign off with initials

If the policy at your hospital allows, you can save time by signing your name, licensure, and initials on a flow sheet near the front of the chart, then using only your initials thereafter.

Don't document for other caregivers

Doctors should regularly document their own progress notes, as should other health care team members. Documenting for others may be a favor to them, but it's a liability for you.

Use the Kardex effectively

A Kardex can be made more effective by tailoring the information to the needs of a particular setting. For instance, a home care Kardex should have information on family contacts, doctors, other services, and emergency referrals.

If the Kardex is included in the clinical record at your hospital, you can save charting time because you won't need to repeat the information in another part of the record. Make sure you write in ink, revising information when the doctor writes new orders or the patient's needs change. In some hospitals, the Kardex has been eliminated, and its information has been incorporated into the nursing plan of care.

Use computerized documentation

Although not widespread yet, computer documentation will become more common as costs decrease, equipment becomes easier to use, and better software programs are developed.

Use fax machines

These machines allow you to send and receive orders, documentation forms, patient records, and test results quickly. Machines in doctors' offices can save you from taking and documenting orders over the phone.

Documenting patient assessment

▶

Standardized open-ended form

As shown below, the typical "fill-in-the blanks" assessment form comes with preprinted headings and questions. This form saves you time in two ways. Information is categorized under specific headings, so you can easily record and retrieve it. And the form can be completed using partial phrases and approved abbreviations.

Unfortunately, however, open-ended forms don't always provide the space or the instructions to encourage thorough descriptions. For instance, a nurse may write that a patient performs a certain task "within normal limits." But unless normal limits have been defined, this notation is neither clear nor legally sound.

Reason for hospitalization _"I've been having dizzy episodes and I pass out."_

Expected outcomes _By discharge, pt. and family will understand the syncopal episodes, demonstrate understanding of pacemaker therapy and adhere to self-care program._

Last hospitalization
Date _5/86_ Reason _Fx right hip_
Medical history _hypertension_

Medications and allergies

Drug	Dosage	Time of last dose	Patient's statement of drug's purpose
Cardizem CD	_180 mg_	_9:00 a.m._	_"for BP"_

Allergy	Reaction
penicillin	_hives_

Standardized close-ended form

As shown below, this form provides preprinted checklists. It saves time, avoids illegible handwriting, makes checking documented information easy, and can be incorporated into most computerized systems. And though it may use non-specific terminology, guidelines clearly define these responses.

The form also creates some problems. It may provide no place to record information that doesn't fit the preprinted choices. And it can be lengthy, especially when in-depth physical assessment data is required.

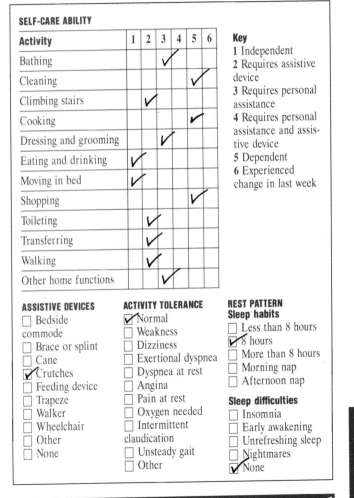

SELF-CARE ABILITY

Activity	1	2	3	4	5	6
Bathing			✓			
Cleaning				✓		
Climbing stairs		✓				
Cooking				✓		
Dressing and grooming			✓			
Eating and drinking	✓					
Moving in bed	✓					
Shopping				✓		
Toileting		✓				
Transferring		✓				
Walking		✓				
Other home functions			✓			

Key
1 Independent
2 Requires assistive device
3 Requires personal assistance
4 Requires personal assistance and assistive device
5 Dependent
6 Experienced change in last week

ASSISTIVE DEVICES
☐ Bedside commode
☐ Brace or splint
☐ Cane
☑ Crutches
☐ Feeding device
☐ Trapeze
☐ Walker
☐ Wheelchair
☐ Other
☐ None

ACTIVITY TOLERANCE
☑ Normal
☐ Weakness
☐ Dizziness
☐ Exertional dyspnea
☐ Dyspnea at rest
☐ Angina
☐ Pain at rest
☐ Oxygen needed
☐ Intermittent claudication
☐ Unsteady gait
☐ Other

REST PATTERN
Sleep habits
☐ Less than 8 hours
☑ 8 hours
☐ More than 8 hours
☐ Morning nap
☐ Afternoon nap

Sleep difficulties
☐ Insomnia
☐ Early awakening
☐ Unrefreshing sleep
☐ Nightmares
☑ None

A medical model for nursing assessment

Many hospitals still use a medical format to organize their nursing assessment forms. As shown below, the physical examination section of this form is organized according to a comprehensive review of body systems. Some hospitals have adopted formats that more readily reflect the nursing process, organizing data according to either human response patterns, functional health care patterns, or published nursing theories.

SYSTEMS REVIEW

Admission date and time: __2/11/96   2:00pm.__
Height: __5' 8"_____Weight: __150____ TPR: __99°-82-20__
BP, right arm: __110/76_____BP, left arm __110/76__

Check boxes or write descriptions as appropriate.

Mental status
- ☑ Alert
- ☑ Cooperative
- ☐ Calm
- ☐ Lethargic
- ☐ Withdrawn
- ☐ Depressed
- ☐ Agitated
- ☑ Anxious

Oriented to:
- ☑ Time
- ☑ Place
- ☑ Person

Speech
- ☑ Normal, clear
- ☐ Slurred
- ☐ Hesitant
- ☐ Hoarse
- ☐ Dysphasic

Neurologic system
- ☑ Normal
- ☑ Pupils: PERRLA
- ☐ Dizziness
- ☑ Headaches
- ☐ Numbness
- ☐ Paraplegia
- ☐ Hemiplegia, right
- ☐ Hemiplegia, left

Eyes
- ☐ Normal
Corrected:
- ☑ Glasses
- ☐ Contact lenses
- ☐ Implanted lenses
- ☐ Blind, right eye
- ☐ Blind, left eye
- ☐ Artificial prosthesis
- ☐ Discharge
- ☐ Diplopia
- ☐ Blurred vision
- ☐ Tearing
- ☐ Burning
- ☐ Itching
- ☐ Photophobia
- ☐ Pain
- ☐ Sclera color: ____
- ☐ Cataract
- ☐ Glaucoma

Ears
- ☑ Normal
- ☐ Hearing loss
- ☐ Hearing aid
- ☐ Tinnitus
- ☐ Vertigo
- ☐ Discharge
- ☐ Pain

Nose
- ☐ Normal
- ☐ Sinusitis

- ☐ Rhinitis
- ☐ Discharge
- ☐ Obstruction
- ☐ Epistaxis

Mouth and throat
- ☐ Normal
- ☐ Dentures, upper
- ☐ Dentures, lower
- ☐ Partial plate
- ☑ Dental fillings
- ☐ Sores on tongue
- ☐ Gum swelling or bleeding
- ☐ Diminished taste
- ☐ Sore throat

Respiratory system
- ☑ Normal
- ☐ Dyspnea
- ☐ Cough
- ☐ Hemoptysis
- ☐ Pain
- ☐ Orthopnea
- ☑ Breath sounds: _clear_

Cardiovascular system
- ☑ Normal
- ☐ Edema
- ☐ Cyanosis
- ☐ Cold extremities
- ☐ Palpitations

Cardiovascular system *(continued)*

Pulse:
- [x] Regular
- [ ] Irregular
- [ ] Bounding
- [ ] Weak
- [ ] Thready
- [x] Pedal pulse, right: *palpable*
- [x] Pedal pulse, left: *palpable*
- [x] Heart sounds: ___ *S₁ S₂ audible*

GI system
- [ ] Normal
- [ ] Change in appetite
- [ ] Indigestion
- [ ] Flatulence
- [ ] Nausea
- [ ] Vomiting
- [ ] Bleeding
- [ ] Abdominal pain
- [ ] Abdominal distention
- [ ] Ascites
- [ ] Hemorrhoids
- [ ] Constipation
- [ ] Diarrhea
- [x] Last bowel movement: *2/9/96*
- [ ] Number of stools per day: *1*

Bowel sounds:
- [x] Present
- [ ] Absent
- [ ] Hyperactive
- [ ] Other: ___

Nutritional status
- [ ] Special diet: *N/A*
- [x] Recent weight gain
- [ ] Recent weight loss

GU system
- [x] Normal
- [ ] Frequency
- [ ] Urgency
- [ ] Dysuria
- [ ] Nocturia

Number of times: ___
- [ ] Bleeding
- [ ] Burning

Reproductive system — female
- [x] Last menstrual period: *2/11/96*
- [ ] Cramping
- [ ] Irregular bleeding
- [ ] Discharge
- [ ] Vaginal infections
- [ ] Pain or difficulty with intercourse
- [ ] Menopause
- [ ] Other: ___

Reproductive system — male
- [ ] Prostate problems
- [ ] Lesions
- [ ] Impotence
- [ ] Other: ___

Musculoskeletal system
- [ ] Normal
- [ ] Stiffness
- [x] Pain

- [ ] Weakness
- [ ] Limited ROM
- [ ] Paralysis
- [x] Tenderness
- [ ] Swelling
- [ ] Arthritis
- [ ] Prosthesis
- [ ] Other: ___

Physical activity:
- [x] No limitations
- [ ] Walks with help
- [ ] Uses cane
- [ ] Uses crutches
- [ ] Uses walker
- [ ] Bedridden

Skin
- [ ] Turgor: ___
- [x] Temperature: *cool*
- [x] Color: *pale*
- [x] Dry
- [ ] Moist
- [ ] Diaphoretic
- [ ] Rash
- [ ] Eczema
- [ ] Acne
- [ ] Bruises
- [ ] Burns
- [ ] Lumps
- [ ] Lacerations
- [x] Abrasions
- [ ] Scars: ___
- [ ] Other: ___

Condition of:
- [x] Hair *clean and neat*
- [x] Nails *clean*

Pressure ulcers *none*
- [ ] Number ___
- [ ] Stage 1, 2, 3, 4
- [ ] Location ___
- [ ] Describe ___

Additional comments: ___

Date and time completed _2/11/96   2:00 p.m._

RN signature _Kathy Craig, R N_

> ## Assessment flow sheet

If you're developing a new assessment form or revising a current one, consider the following questions:

• What data from the health history and physical examination are currently included?
• Is this acceptable, or is more information needed to ensure quality?
• What problems exist with the current documentation system?
• What types of changes would help correct these problems?

Most assessment flow sheets cover the categories of information shown below.

Assessment flow sheet

Date __1/10/96__

DIET

Meal	Amount eaten
Breakfast	75 %
Lunch	50 %
Dinner	90 %

☐ By himself
☑ With help
☐ With NG tube

HYGIENE	7-3	3-11	11-7
By himself			
With some help	SS	PD	
With complete help			
Shower		PD	
Oral care	SS	PD	
P.M. care			
Catheter care	SS	PD	

ACTIVITY & REST

On complete bed rest			
Turn q 2 hr			CG
OOB (chair)	SS	PD	
BRP			
Walking			

ELIMINATION	7-3	3-11	11-7
Normal voiding			
Has catheter	SS	PD	CG
Incontinent			
Bowel movement	SS		
Emesis			

PULSE			
Regular			
Irregular	SS	PD	CG
Strong	SS	PD	CG
Weak			

MUSCULOSKELETAL			
Moves all limbs			
Weak	SS	PD	CG
Paralyzed			
Paresthetic			

RESPIRATORY			
Respirations			
Within normal limits	SS	PD	CG
Shallow			
Deep			
Labored			

Respiratory rate	7-3	3-11	11-7
Within normal limits	SS	PD	CG
Slow			
Rapid			
Breath sounds			
Clear	SS		
Moist		PD	CG
Wheezing			
Coughing		PD	CG
SKIN			
Temperature			
Cool			
Warm	SS	PD	CG
Hot			
Turgor			
Good			
Fair	SS	PD	CG
Poor			
Edematous			
Moisture			
Dry	SS	PD	CG
Moist			
Diaphoretic			
Color			
Within normal limits			
Pale	SS	PD	CG
Ashen			
Cyanotic			
Flushed			
Jaundiced			

MENTAL STATUS	7-3	3-11	11-7
Alert			
Oriented × 3	SS	PD	CG
Disoriented			
Lethargic	SS	PD	CG
BEHAVIOR			
Cooperative	SS	PD	CG
Uncooperative			
Anxious			
Withdrawn			
Combative			
Depressed	SS	PD	CG
SPEECH			
Clear			
Slurred	SS	PD	CG
Rambling			
Aphasic			
Inappropriate			
SLEEP			
Sleeps well			
Sleeps intermittently			CG
Awake most of time	SS	PD	
GENERAL INFORMATION			
In restraints			
Eggcrate-like mattress	SS	PD	CG
Side rails up	SS	PD	CG
In traction			
Under isolation precautions			
Above not applicable			

(continued)

DOCUMENTATION

Assessment flow sheet *(continued)*

WOUND	7-3	3-11	11-7
Type			
Size			
Appearance			
Sutures and drains			
Treatments			
Not applicable	SS	PD	CG

TUBES	7-3	3-11	11-7
Type			
Location			
Drainage			
Irrigation			
Not applicable	SS	PD	CG
I.V. THERAPY			
I.V. site	R wrist SS	L wrist PD	L wrist CG
Catheter size	#18G jelco SS	#18G jelco PD	#18G jelco CG
Tubing change	9:00 a.m. SS		
Site appearance	no redness or edema SS	no redness or edema PD	no redness or edema CG
Not applicable			

Signature and status — Initials

Signature	Initials
Steve Shaw, RN	SS
Pamela Davis, RN	PD
Cindy Gater, RN	CG

Developing a plan of care

▶
Traditional plan of care

Also called the individually developed plan of care, the traditional plan of care is written from scratch for each patient. After analyzing the assessment data, you'll either write the plan or enter it into a computer.

The basic form can vary, depending on the needs of the hospital or department. Most forms have three main columns: one for nursing diagnoses, another for patient outcomes, and a third for interventions.

What you must include on these forms also varies. Most hospitals ask you to write only short-term outcomes that the patient should reach by or before discharge. But some hospitals also want you to include long-term outcomes that reflect the maximum functional level the patient can reach.

This sample shows how a traditional plan of care organizes key information. Keep in mind that the plans of care you'll use will have wider columns to allow more room for your notes.

Date	Nursing diagnoses	Patient outcomes	Interventions	Resolution (initials and date)	Revision (initials and date)
1/3/96	Impaired gas exchange related to inadequate ventilation perfusion as evidenced by dyspnea and hypoxemia.	Decrease in dyspnea and normal ABG by 1/4/96	Auscultate chest sounds q 4 hrs and monitor for signs and symptoms. Administer bronchodilators as prescribed. Administer oxygen therapy as prescribed. Monitor arterial blood gases.		

Review dates			
Date	Signature		Initials
1/3/96	Renee Thompson, RN		RT

Standardized plan of care

Developed to save documentation time and improve the quality of care, standardized plans of care list interventions for patients with similar diagnoses. Most plans also supply root outcome statements. Current versions allow you to tailor the plan to fit your patient's specific needs.

When a patient has more than one diagnosis, the resulting combination of standardized plans can be cumbersome. But with computerized documentation, you can pull only what you need from each one and combine them to make one manageable plan. Some computer programs provide a checklist of interventions you can use to build your own plan.

The plan below concerns a patient with a nursing diagnosis of decreased cardiac output. To customize it to your patient, you'd complete the diagnosis — including signs and symptoms — and fill in the patient outcome. You'd also modify, add, or delete interventions as necessary.

Date _1/25/96_	**Nursing diagnosis** Decreased cardiac output R/T _Accelerated heart rhythm as evidenced by hypotension, diaphoresis and light-headedness._
Target date _1/27/96_	**Expected outcomes** Adequate cardiac output as evidenced by: Heart rate _< 100 beats/min_ Blood pressure _≥90/50 mm Hg and < 140/90 mmHg_ Pedal pulse _palpable and regular_ Radial pulse _palpable and regular_ Cardiac rhythm _normal sinus rhythm_ Cardiac index _NA_ Pulmonary artery wedge pressure (PAWP) _NA_ Pulmonary artery pressure (PAP) _NA_ S̄vO₂ _NA_ Urine output in ml/kg/hr _≥ 0.3 ml/kg/hr_
Date _1/27/96_	**Interventions** • Monitor the ECG for rate and rhythm; note ectopic beats. If arrhythmias occur, note the patient's response. Document and report findings and follow the appropriate arrhythmia protocol. • Monitor ~~SvO₂~~, temperature, respirations, ~~and central pressures (including PAP) continuously.~~ • ~~Monitor other hemodynamic pressures (such as PAWP) q ___ hr and p.r.n.~~ _N/A_ • Auscultate heart sounds and palpate peripheral pulses q _4_ hr and p.r.n.

Interventions *(continued)*

• Monitor I & O q ___/___ hr. Notify the doctor if urine output is less than 30 ml/hr × 2 hr.

• Administer medications and fluids as ordered, noting their effectiveness and any adverse reactions. Titrate vasoactive drugs as needed. Follow appropriate vasoactive drug protocol to wean the patient as tolerated.

• Monitor O_2 therapy or other ventilatory support measures.

• Decrease the patient's activity to reduce O_2 demands. Increase as tolerated.

• Assess and document the patient's LOC. Assess for changes q ___/___ hr and p.r.n.

• Additional interventions _____

_____

_____

_____

_____

_____

_____

Protocol format

Protocols provide specific sequential directions for treating patients with particular problems. They help ensure thorough, consistent care, teach inexperienced staff members, and can also save charting time. To use protocols effectively, follow these guidelines.

• Use the protocols that best fit your patient, and make sure you have the current versions.

• Tailor the protocol to fit your patient's needs. Cross out steps that don't apply and modify or add material as needed.

• To document properly, note in the interventions section of the plan of care that you'll follow the protocol, or list the protocols you plan to use on a flow sheet. After you intervene, write in your progress notes that you followed the protocol, or check the protocol off on your flow sheet and initial it. Include a copy of the protocol in the patient's record – especially if you've made changes to it.

As the following sample shows, protocols typically list staff requirements, patient outcomes, and supportive information, as well as appropriate nursing actions.

Protocol

Title: Altered nutrition: Less than body requirements; High risk for fluid volume deficit

Health care staff
• Assessment: RN
• Planning: RN
• Intervention: RN, LPN, nursing assistant
• Patient teaching: RN, LPN, dietitian
• Evaluation: RN
• Complications: RN, LPN, nursing assistant, dietitian
• Documentation: RN, LPN

Caregiver qualifications
The caregiver must:
• be able to identify patients at risk for nutrition and fluid volume deficits
• be able to assess patients at risk for nutrition and fluid volume deficit
• understand these problems and their treatments
• be qualified to perform necessary interventions.

Patient outcomes
The patient will:
• have decreased nausea, vomiting, or diarrhea
• take in adequate calories
• take in sufficient fluids
• demonstrate knowledge of his nutritional needs
• show signs of adequate hydration: improved skin turgor, moist mucous membranes, increased urine output
• show signs of adequate caloric intake: improved appetite, weight gain, increased energy.

Supportive data
- Risk factors:
  – hyperthermia, anorexia, nausea and vomiting, and diarrhea
  – infectious or inflammatory processes
- Signs and symptoms of nutrition and fluid volume deficit:
  – dry mucous membranes
  – poor skin turgor
  – lethargy
- Procedures for monitoring patients at risk for nutrition and fluid volume deficits include:
  – measuring intake and output and weighing patient. I.V. equipment, total parenteral nutrition equipment, and scale may be used.
  – performing a neurologic assessment to provide early clues to fluid volume deficit.

Responsibilities	Nursing actions
Assessment	• Assess general physical condition every 8 hours. • Assess neurologic status every 8 hours. Especially note subtle changes in behavior or LOC. • Assess daily caloric and fluid intake, using these guidelines: Good: Intake provides 50% or more of needed calories and fluids. Fair: Intake provides more than 20% and less than 50% of needed calories and fluids. Poor: Intake provides less than 20% of needed calories and fluids. None: Unable or refuses to eat or drink.
Planning	Collaborate with doctor to decide when to perform interventions that will help patient meet daily nutrition and fluid needs. Meet with dietitian to ensure reinforcement of nutritional counseling in preparation for discharge.
Interventions	• Monitor intake, output, and weight. • Monitor bowel function. • Monitor results of laboratory studies (serum albumin, total protein, urine protein, glucose, acetone, nitrogen). • Observe patient and help him choose amount and types of foods and liquids. • Provide smaller but more frequent meals. • Help patient to a comfortable position at mealtimes. • Help patient with meals; feed patient if necessary. • Arrange for dietitian to assess patient's caloric requirements. *(continued)*

DOCUMENTATION

Protocol format   *(continued)*

Intervention *(continued)*	• Offer fluids every 4 hours between meals; try to ensure a total daily intake of 3,000 ml unless contraindicated. • Provide parenteral fluids as ordered. • Provide nutritional supplements.
Patient teaching	• Explain the need to take in sufficient calories to maintain adequate nutrition and the need to maintain adequate fluid balance. • Instruct the patient and his family members about the patient's specific nutritional needs.
Evaluation	Evaluate nutritional and fluid status of patient every 8 hours and any time a significant change in patient status or regimen occurs.
Complications	• Observe for complications, including dehydration, anemia, malnutrition, and sepsis. • Notify the doctor, document appropriately, continue assessment and interventions, and carry out additional doctor's orders.
Documentation	Document the following: • ongoing nutritional and fluid assessment data on nurses' progress sheet • nutritional and fluid status of patient on nurses' progress sheet • intake and output every 8 hours • vital signs as ordered by doctor but at least every 8 hours • patient teaching on nutritional and fluid needs • any complications and actions taken to correct them • daily weights on graphic record • type and amount of nutritional therapy on patient care flow sheet • type and amount of fluid therapy on I.V. therapy sheet every 8 hours and at completion of infusion.

▶

Critical pathway

An abbreviated case management plan, a critical pathway covers only the key events that must occur for the patient to be discharged by the target date. Such events include consultations, diagnostic tests, physical activities the patient must perform, treatments, diet, drugs, discharge planning, and patient teaching.

At shift report each day, review the critical pathway documents with the other nurses. Before you go off duty, note any changes in the expected length of stay and point out critical events scheduled for the next shift to the nurses coming on duty. Also, discuss any variances for the pathway that may have occurred during your shift.

The sample below shows selected portions of a typical critical pathway.

Diagnosis: Partial or total parotidectomy
DRG length of stay: 2.3 days
Actual length of stay: _____
Expected outcomes
By discharge, the patient will:
• state possible complications, troubleshooting measures, and appropriate resources
• perform suture line care
• explain measures for managing his pain
• explain how to maintain his nutritional status
• demonstrate eye care measures (if applicable).

NURSE	OTHER HEALTH CARE PROVIDERS	PATIENT AND FAMILY MEMBERS
Preoperative day		
• Performs assessment • Explains case-management model and recovery pathway to patient • Completes contract with patient and his family members • Performs preoperative teaching • Notifies social worker, if appropriate, and explains assessment and possible discharge needs to her	*Primary doctor* • Performs physical examination • Orders special studies, including blood work, ECG, chest X-rays • Orders anesthesia clearance assessment *Social worker* • Consults with nurse (if appropriate)	*Patient and family members* • Sign contract • Visit immediate postoperative care unit

(continued)

Critical pathway *(continued)*

Postoperative day (POD) 1

• Provides morning care while patient is on bed rest • Sets up heparin lock on I.V. line • Teaches suture line care • Teaches eye care (if applicable) • Encourages activity • Monitors diet	*Primary doctor* • Orders laboratory tests • Orders advance in diet as tolerated • Orders heparin lock on I.V. line • Consults with ophthalmologist, radiation therapist, and dentist (as applicable) *Ophthalmologist* • Consults with doctor (if applicable) *Radiation therapist* • Consults with doctor (if applicable) *Dentist* • Consults with doctor (if applicable)	*Patient* • Performs oral hygiene and incentive spirometry • Demonstrates suture line care and eye care (if applicable) • Ambulates q 4 hr p.r.n.

POD 2

• Continues to teach suture line care and eye care • Continues to encourage activity and monitor diet.	*Dietitian* • Performs nutrition assessment *Speech pathologist* • Performs nutrition assessment (if patient has difficulty swallowing)	*Patient* • Performs morning self-care • Continues to perform oral hygiene and incentive spirometry • Demonstrates suture line care and eye care (if applicable) • Ambulates q 4 hr p.r.n.

Documenting interventions and evaluations

► Flow sheet for routine care

For years, the Joint Commission on Accreditation of Healthcare Organizations (JCAHO) has encouraged hospitals to use flow sheets for documenting routine care measures. In response, many hospitals have developed these forms for such measures as making basic assessments, giving wound care, and providing hygiene. In many hospitals, you may also use flow sheets to document vital signs checks, I.V. monitoring, equipment checks, patient education, and discharge summaries.

As this sample shows, a patient care flow sheet allows you to quickly document your routine interventions. Note that the last page of this 4-page form provides space for narrative notes.

Patient care flow sheet

DATE 1/13/96	11 p.m. to 7 a.m.	7 a.m. to 3 p.m.	3 p.m. to 11 p.m.
Respiratory			
Lung sounds	crackles left lower base SK	clear GD	clear BS
Treatments/results	chest PT q 2 hr SK	CHEST PD Q9 2HR GD	chest PT q 2 hr BS
Cough/results	small amt. of clear thin mucous SK	ō GD	ō BS
O₂ therapy nasal cannula @ 2 l/min	continuous SK	CONTINUOUS GD	continuous BS
Cardiac			
Chest pain	ō SK	ō GD	ō BS
Heart sounds	normal S₁ S₂ SK	NORMAL S₁ S₂ GD	normal S₁ S₂ BS
Telemetry	NSR SK	NSR GD	NSR BS
Pain			
Type and location	ō SK	DULL LOWER BACK PAIN GD	ō
Intervention	ō SK	DARVOCET-N 100MG P.O. GD	ō
Response	ō SK	RELIEF IN 45 MIN. GD	ō

(continued)

Flow sheet for routine care *(continued)*

DATE	11 p.m. to 7 a.m.	7 a.m. to 3 p.m.	3 p.m. to 11 p.m.
Nutrition			
Type	n/a	1500 ADA GD	1500 ada BS
Toleration %	n/a	100% GD	90% BS
Supplement	n/a	N/A	hs. snack BS
Elimination			
Stool appearance	∅ SK	∅ GD	+ soft light brown
Enema	n/a	N/A	n/a
Results	n/a	N/A	n/a
Bowel sounds	present all 4 quadrants SK	PRESENT ALL 4 QUADRANTS GD	present all 4 quadrants BS
Urine appearance	clear yellow X2 SK	CLEAR YELLOW X2 GD	clear amber x1 BS
Indwelling urinary catheter	n/a	N/A	n/a
Catheter irrigations	n/a.	N/A	n/a
I.V. Therapy			
Tubing change	n/a	8:00 a.m.	n/a
Dressing change	n/a	8:00 A.M.	n/a
Site appearance	no signs of redness or edema SK	NO SIGNS OF REDNESS OR EDEMA GD	no signs of redness or edema BS
Wound			
Type	n/a	N/A	n/a
Dressing change	n/a	N/A	n/a
Appearance	n/a	N/A	n/a
Tubes			
Type	n/a	N/A	n/a
Irrigation	↓	↓	↓
Drainage appearance	↓	↓	↓

DATE	11 p.m. to 7 a.m.	7 a.m. to 3 p.m.	3 p.m. to 11 p.m.
Hygiene			
Self/partial/complete	n/a	9:00 a.m GD PARTIAL	9:00 pm BS
Oral care	n/a	9:00 a.m. GD	9:00 pm BS
Back care	n/a	9:00 a.m. GD	9:00 pm BS
Foot care	n/a	9:00 a m GD	9:00 pm BS
Activity			
Type	BRP SK	OOB AD LIB GD	OOB ad lib BS
Toleration	Turns self SK	TOLERATES GD ACTIVITY WELL	Tolerates BS activity well
Repositioned	n/a	N/A	n/a
ROM	n/a	N/A	n/a
Sleep			
Sleeps well	1:00 a.m. 6:00 SK 5K am.	N/A	n/a
Awake at intervals	n/a	↓	↓
Awake most of the time	n/a		
Safety			
Side rails up	1:00 a.m. 6:00 a.m. SK SK	9:00 1:00 GD a.m P.m. GD	4:00 9:00 BS p.m. p.m. BS
Call light in reach	1:00 a.m. 6:00 a.m. SK SK	9:00 1:00 GD a.m. P GD p.m.	4:00 9:00 BS p.m. BS p.m.
Equipment			
Type *Gemini pump*	continuous SK	continuous GD	continuous BS
			(continued)

Flow sheet for routine care *(continued)*

DATE	11 p.m. to 7 a.m.	7 a.m. to 3 p.m.	3 p.m. to 11 p.m.
Teaching			
Diabetic Protocol	n/a	GD	BS

PROGRESS SHEET

Time	Comments
9:00 AM	Pt. admits to complaint of dull lower back pain, denies pain in legs or numbness or tingling of lower ext. Dr. Jones notified of pt.'s complaint of lower back pain. Order received for Darvocet-N 100 mg. ———————— GRACE DARNEY, RN
9:45 AM	Pt. denies complaint of pain, Darvocet effective. GRACE DARNEY, RN
2:00 PM	Reviewed signs and symptoms of hypo/hyperglycemia with pt. and family. Pt. and family receptive to information. GRACE DARNEY, RN
6:00 PM	Pt. ambulating in room. Offers no further complaint of lower back pain. Gait steady. Brooke Stevens, RN

Initials	Signature/title
SK	Sally Kendall, RN
GD	GRACE DARNEY, RN
BS	Brooke Stevens, RN

Code record

When documenting a patient emergency, follow standard guidelines, taking care to:
• be factual
• be specific about times and interventions
• include the name of the doctor you contacted, when you contacted him, and what you told him
• indicate attempts to inform the patient's family or significant other of the changes in his situation.

Use a code record to keep the progress note concise and ensure complete documentation. This specialized documentation form incorporates detailed information about a code, including observations, interventions, and medications administered. The following sample shows the typical features of a code record.

Code record

Name *Barry Craig* Body weight *183 lbs.* Date *1/23/96*

Vital signs				Bolus meds					Infused meds			Action		Blood gases			
Time a.m./p.m.	BP	Heart rate	Heart rhythm	Atropine (mg)	Calcium chloride (ampules)	Epinephrine (mg)	Lidocaine (mg)	Procainamide (mg)	Dopamine (mg/ml)	Isoproterenol (mg/ml)	Lidocaine (g/ml)	Defibrillation (joules)	CPR	Airway	PaO₂	PaCO₂	HCO₃⁻	pH

Time	BP	HR	Rhythm	Atrop	CaCl	Epi	Lido	Proc	Dopa	Isop	Lido	Defib	CPR	Airway	PaO₂	PaCO₂	HCO₃	pH
11:20	0	0											✓	mask				
11:23	0	0	VT									200						
11:25													✓					
11:26			VF									300						
11:27												360						
11:28						1	100						✓					
11:30												360						
11:31													✓					
11:31			↓									2mg 360							
11:32	100/68	96	NSR															
11:33			NSR															
11:35	110/60	92	✓												64	45	23	7.35

(continued)

Code record *(continued)*

Time   Actions

11:20 Code called, CPR initiated by C.Krane, RN and
S.Walden, RN. Ambu-bagged by S.Walden, RN.

11:25 Connected to single-channel ECG. #20 jelco
inserted via ⒧ antecubital by P.Downs, RN.

11:29 Intubation with #8 oral ETT by M.Cress,
anesthesiologist.

11:35 Converted to NSR, ABG via ⒭ femoral artery
drawn by M.White,MD. Pressure applied x 5 min.
Pt. remains unresponsive.

Time code called *11:20p.m.*

☐ Arrest witnessed
☑ Arrest unwitnessed
☑ Intubation *11:29*

☑ Arrhythmia *pulseless Vtach*
☑ Informed family
☑ Informed attending
doctor _____

Disposition

☐ SICU   ☑ CCU   ☐ Morgue
☐ MICU   ☐ OR   ☐ Other

Status after resuscitation
BP 110/60 Heart rate 92. Bagged
with 100% O₂ and transported to
ccu.

Critical care nurse
Carol Krane, RN

Code chief
M. White, MD

Patient teaching: Narrative notes

Listed below are the types of information you need to document, using a narrative format. Documentation methods may vary among facilities.

1. Date and time of each teaching session

2. Patient's name and number on every record page

3. Patient's health status and corresponding learning needs

4. Learning outcomes agreed on by health care team and patient

5. Identified learning enhancements

6. Actual teaching you carry out

7. Specific teaching techniques

8. Patient's characteristics as a learner

9. Precise description of exactly what occurred, avoiding broad

terms such as "learned well" and "seems to understand"

10. Your evaluation of patient's change or learning

11. Patient's response to teaching and learning experience, using his own words and behaviors

12. Specific teaching materials

13. Indications that patient or family member understands instructions

14. Identified learning barriers

15. Final progress notes with discharge teaching about diet, medications, activity, and follow-up care

16. Your signature

Charting progress notes

▶

Narrative format

In this paragraph approach to charting, you document ongoing assessment data, nursing interventions, and patient responses in chronological order. You'll record this information in your progress notes. Flow sheets commonly supplement these narrative notes.

This sample shows how to write a progress note using the narrative format.

Progress notes

DATE	TIME	NOTES
1/22/96	9 a.m.	Pt. complaint of Ⓛ upper quadrant abd. pain. Reports pain is an 8 on a scale of 1 to 10. Color pale, skin cool and diaphoretic, BP 84/60, T (orally) 100.2° F, P-124, R-28, abd. drsg. saturated c̄ bright red blood. Reinforced abd. drsg. c̄ 2 abd. pads. Salem connected to low continuous drainage, bright red blood noted via Salem. #18 jelco intact via Ⓡ hand, infusing c̄ no evidence of redness or infiltration. I.V. D5 ½ NSS patent. Foley draining dark amber urine; total output 10 ml in past 3 hours. Dr. O'Brien notified of pt.'s condition. Orders noted; will continue to monitor closely. I.V. solution changed to L R @ 250 ml/hr. Dr. O'Brien to see pt. — J. Paul, R N
1/22/96	9:30 a.m.	VS remain unstable, BP 80/50, P-136, R-32. Pt. anxious, trembling; color pale, skin cool and grossly diaphoretic. 100 ml of bright red bleeding noted from Salem; 4×6 cm of bright red bleeding noted on (continued on next page) – J. Paul, RN

DOCUMENTATION

▶

Problem-oriented format

The problem-oriented medical record (POMR) system of charting focuses on the patient's problems and provides a structure that's absent from narrative charting. Progress notes are organized according to the SOAP framework:

• Subjective data: information the patient tells you
• Objective data: information you gather by observation
• Assessment: your conclusions about the patient's problem, based on the subjective and objective data
• Plan: the proposed interventions to resolve the problem.

A modification, organized according to the SOAPIE framework, includes two more components:

• Intervention: the interventions you perform to resolve the problem
• Evaluation: your evaluation of the patient's response to interventions.

This sample shows how to write a progress note using the POMR system.

Progress notes

DATE	TIME	NOTES
1/22/96	2:00 p.m.	#1 Pain related to cholecystectomy surgical incision. ————
		S: "I'm having a lot of pain where they did my surgery." ————
		O: Pt. returned from postanesthesia care unit at 1:30 p.m. Pt. reports pain of 6 on a scale of 1 to 10 in abdominal RUQ. Color pale. Holding incisional area. BP 140/86. P-90. R-20. Temperature 99° orally. Abd. drsg. dry and intact. Received meperidine 50 mg I.M. at 10 a.m. ————
		A: Increased incisional pain related to wearing off of meperidine. BP and pulse increased over baseline. ————
		P: Administer meperidine 50 mg I.M. now, as ordered. Reposition pt. from back to right side to promote comfort. Reassess pain level and (continued on next page) J. Paul, RN

▶

Focus charting format

Developed by nurses who found the SOAP format awkward, Focus charting encourages you to organize your thoughts into patient-centered topics, or foci of concern, and then to document precisely and concisely. The format encourages you to use assessment data to evaluate these patient care concerns. It also helps you identify necessary revisions to the care plan as you document each entry.

This sample shows how to write progress notes using the Focus charting format.

Progress notes

Date	Time	Focus	Notes
1/22/96	2:00 p.m.	Pain related to chole- cystectomy surgical incision.	D: Patient reports pain at abdominal RUQ of 6 on a scale of 1 to 10. Color pale. Holding incisional area. BP 140/86. P. 90. R-20. Temperature 99° orally. Abd. drsg. dry and intact. Received meperidine 50mg I.M. at 10 a.m.— A: Meperidine 50mg I.M. administered, as ordered. Pt. repositioned from back to right side. Will reassess pain level and vital signs in 30 minutes and administer meperidine every 3 to 4 hours as needed (see care plan). J. Paul, RN
1/22/96	2:00 p.m.	Pt. teaching	Pt. states, "Every time I cough or move, my incision hurts." A: Splinting of surgical incision reviewed with pt. to reduce discomfort during coughing, deep breathing, and movement. R: Pt. demonstrates proper placement of hands over surgical incision site and verbalizes experiencing less incisional discomfort while coughing, deep breathing and moving. (continued on next page) J. Paul RN

▶

PIE format

Developed to simplify the documentation process, problem-intervention-evaluation (PIE) charting organizes information based on patient problems. Documentation tools for this format include a daily patient assessment flow sheet and progress notes.

By integrating the care plan into the progress notes, the PIE format eliminates the need for a separate care plan. The intention is to provide a concise, efficient record of patient care that has a nursing—not a medical—focus.

This sample shows how to write progress notes using the PIE format.

Progress notes		
Date	Time	Notes
1/22/96	2:00 p.m.	P#1: Pain related to cholecystectomy surgical incision.
		IP#1: Meperidine 50 mg I.M. administered, as ordered. Pt. repositioned from back to right side. Splinting of surgical incision reviewed with pt., and pt. demonstrated proper technique.
		EP#1: Increased postoperative incisional pain due to wearing off of meperidine. BP and pulse increased over baseline. Reassess pain level and vital signs in 30 minutes. Will give meperidine every 3 to 4 hours as needed. —————— Janice Paul, RN
1/22/96	2:00 pm.	P#2: High risk for fluid volume deficit related to nausea.
		IP#2: Prochlorperazine 10 mg I.M., administered as ordered.
		EP#2: Nausea possibly related to increased incisional pain and postanesthesia effects. Will reassess for nausea in 30 minutes. (continued on next page) J. Paul, RN

Charting-by-exception format

The charting-by-exception (CBE) format departs from traditional systems by requiring documentation of only significant or abnormal findings. It also uses military time to help prevent misinterpretations.

To use the CBE format effectively, you must know and adhere to established guidelines for nursing assessments and interventions. The CBE nursing assessment format has printed guidelines for each body system. Guidelines for interventions are derived from standardized care plans based on nursing diagnoses, protocols, doctor's orders, incidental orders, and standards of nursing practice.

Progress notes

Date	Time	Notes
1/25/96	0900	(Nursing entry)
		S "I can't remember how to use this glucose meter, I'll never be able to test my own blood sugar."
		O Pt. unable to perform blood glucose test, difficulty remembering the steps in the procedure.
		A Knowledge deficit related to use of glucose meter.
		P Review step-by-step how to use glucose meter. Assist pt. in performing self glucose monitoring. Provide pt. with information to review; teach husband how to use glucose meter; reevaluate. — M. Jones RN

Nursing-medical order flow sheet

This form documents assessments and interventions during a 24-hour period for one patient. To use the form, mark the appropriate category box with a check mark to indicate normal assessment findings, a completed intervention, or an expected patient response. Use an asterisk to indicate abnormal or significant findings or responses, and write an explanation in the comments section. Reference this note by nursing diagnosis number or doctor's order and time. If the patient's condition is unchanged, draw a horizontal arrow from the previous category box to the current one. Initial completed columns and all comments. Sign the form at the bottom of the page.

This sample shows the typical features of a nursing-medical order flow sheet.

Nursing-medical order flow sheet

Date 1/20/96

ND #/DO	Assessments and interventions	8:00am	8:10 am		
ND 1	Cardiac assessment	*	*		
ND 2	Pain/comfort intervention	8:05am ✱			
DO	12-lead ECG done	8:05am ✓			
Initials		CM	CM		

Key

DO = doctor's orders
ND = nursing diagnosis
√ = normal findings
→ = no change in condition
* = abnormal or significant finding
(See Comments section.)

ND #/DO	Time	Comments	Initials
ND 1	8:00 a.m.	Pt. admits to complaint of mid-sternal chest pain, rates pain a 4 on a scale of 1 to 10. BP 140/86, P-74, R-18.	CM
ND 2	8:05 a.m.	Medicated c̄ NTG 1/200 gr sl. for chest pain. Will reassess in 5 minutes.	CM
ND 2	8:20 a.m.	Medication effective for the relief of chest pain.	CM

Initials	Signature
CM	Carol Marker, RN

> ## Graphic record

You'll use this flow sheet to document trends in the patient's vital signs, weight, intake and output, stool, urine, appetite, and activity level. As with the nursing-medical order flow sheet, use check marks and asterisks to indicate expected and abnormal findings, respectively. Note information on abnormalities in the progress notes or on the nursing-medical order flow sheet.

In the box labeled routine standards, check off that you've carried out established nursing care interventions, such as providing hygiene. Don't rewrite these standards as orders on the nursing-medical flow sheet. Refer to the guidelines on the back of the graphic record for complete instructions.

This partial form shows how to use a typical graphic record.

Graphic record

Date	1/22/96						1/23/96								
Hour	2	6	10	14	18	22	6	10	14						
Temperature															

°F	°C
105°	40.6°
104°	40.0°
103°	39.4°
102°	38.9°
101°	38.3°
100°	37.8°
99°	37.2°
98.6°	37.0°
98°	36.7°
97°	36.1°
96°	35.6°

Pulse	76	70	78	100	84	88	76	72	
Respirations	18	18	20	22	20	18	16	18	
BP	6 146/84		18 148/86		6 140/82				
	10 152/96				10 146/84				
	14 158/90								
Appetite			✓	✓					
Routine standards	✓	✓	✓		✓	✓			
Activity 11 to 7	sleeping				sleeping				
7 to 3	OOB to chair c̄ assist x2				OOB to chair c̄ assist x1				
3 to 11									

Documenting patient discharge

▶ Discharge planning

How and where you document your discharge planning will depend on the policy at the hospital where you work. Here's one of the more common ways of documenting this information – using a designated section of an initial assessment form (usually the last page).

Discharge planning needs

Occupation _Teacher_   Language spoken _English_
Patient lives with _wife_
Self-care capabilities _independent_

Assistance available
☐ Cooking   ☐ Cleaning   ☐ Shopping
☐ Dressing changes/treatments: _N/A_

Medication administration routes
☑ P.O.   ☐ I.M.   ☐ Other: _____
☐ I.V.   ☑ S.C.

Dwelling
☐ Apartment   ☐ Inside steps   ☑ Bathrooms
☑ Private home   (number) _10_   (number) _2_
☐ Single room   ☐ Kitchen   (location) _2nd floor_
☐ Institution   (gas stove)   _1st floor (off kitchen)_
☐ Elevator   electric stove
☑ Outside steps   wood stove   ☑ Telephones
(number) _2_   other   (number) _2_
                                        (location) _bedroom_
                                        kitchen

Transportation
☑ Drives own car   ☐ Takes public   ☐ Relies on family
                   transportation   member or friend

After discharge, patient will be:
☐ Home alone   ☑ Home with family   ☐ Other: _____

Patient has had help from:
☑ Visiting nurse   ☐ Housekeeper   ☑ Other: _wife_
Anticipated needs: _Will need help with insulin_
administration and follow-up diabetic
education.

Social service requests: _visiting nurse_
Date contacted: _1/30/96_

▶

Discharge summary and patient instructions

This sample form combines your discharge summary with your postdischarge instructions for the patient. You'd give a copy of this form to the patient at discharge.

Discharge summary
Date: _1/14/96_
Time: _11 a.m._

Destination
☐ Home
☑ Nursing home
☐ Other: _____

Mobility
☐ Ambulatory
☐ Wheelchair
☑ Stretcher

PATIENT STATUS
General
TPR _98² - 84° - 18_
BP _128/76_
☐ Eating regularly
Comments: _____

Skin
☐ Good condition
☑ Wound: _____
☐ Other: _____

Bowels
☐ Regular movement
☑ Irregular movement
☐ Ostomy

Bladder
☐ Continent
☐ Urinary frequency
☐ Incontinent
☑ Catheter
Type: _Foley #16_
Date changed: _1/10/96_

Compliance
☐ Understands physical condition
☐ Willing to comply with regimen
☐ States understanding of instructions
Comments: _____
_____
_____

Medications
☐ Preadmission medications returned
_____
☐ Prescriptions given to patient
_____
☐ Medications given to patient
_____
☑ Patient or family knows of allergies
_____
Nurse's signature _Carol Brown, RN_

PATIENT INSTRUCTIONS
Diet
☐ Unrestricted
☑ Restricted _2gm low sodium — low cholesterol diet_

Activities
☑ Walking
☐ Climbing stairs
☐ Riding in car
☐ Driving car
☐ Showering
☐ Taking a tub bath
☐ Engaging in sexual intercourse
☐ Resuming regular activity
☐ Lifting
☐ Exercising
☐ Other: _____

Comments: _ambulates with walker, gradually resume activity._

(continued)

Discharge summary and patient instructions *(continued)*

Medications

Digoxin

Lasix

Darvocet – N

Dosage, route, and time

0.125 mg P.O. q.d.

40 mg P.O. bid.

100 mg P.O. prn. every
6 hours for pain

Special instructions

Saline dressings to ① leg wound
q shift.

Referral

☐ Call Dr. _____ and schedule an appointment _____
☐ Home care agency _____
☐ Other _____

If you have questions, call Dr. _Wilson_ at _251-7680_.
I've read and understood these instructions, and I've received a copy of
this form.
Date _1 / 14 / 96_

Patient or significant other _Mildred Smith (daughter)_

Nurse and doctor _Dr. H. Wilson, M.D._
Carol Brown, RN

Discharge against medical advice

When a patient wants to leave the hospital against medical advice (AMA), you can encourage him to stay by explaining the risks involved in his decision. If he still wants to leave AMA, document a detailed description of the event in the progress notes and ask him to sign a release form such as the one below.

Responsibility release form

This is to certify that I, _Karl Bird_,

a patient in _Weston Hospital_,
am being discharged against the advice of my doctor and the hospital administration. I acknowledge that I've been informed of the risks involved and hereby release my doctor and the hospital from all responsibility should I suffer any ill effects as a result of this discharge. I also understand that I may return to the hospital at any time and resume treatment.

Karl Bird
(Patient's signature)

Janet Adamson, RN
(Witness's signature)

_3/8/96_
(Date)

_432_
(Patient number)

Documenting special situations

Refusal-of-treatment release

When a patient refuses treatment, first explain the risks involved in making this choice. Then, if he still refuses to have the treatment, ask him to sign a refusal-of-treatment release form, such as the one below.

Refusal-of-treatment release form

I, _____ *John Williams* _____,
(patient's name)

refuse to allow anyone to

_____ *start an intravenous line* _____.
(insert treatment)

The risks attendant to my refusal have been fully explained to me, and I fully understand the benefits of this treatment. I also understand that my refusal of treatment seriously reduces my chances for regaining normal health and may endanger my life.

I hereby release

_____ *Weston Hospital* _____,
(name of hospital)

its nurses and employees, together with all doctors in any way connected with me as a patient, from liability for respecting and following my express wishes and direction.

Kay Jackson, RN _____   *John Williams* _____
(Witness's signature)   (Patient's or legal guardian's signature)

_____ *3/24/96* _____   _____ *32* _____
(Date)   (Patient's age)

Incident report

The incident report is used to record certain events that are inconsistent with the hospital's ordinary routine. These include patient injuries, patient complaints, medication errors, and injuries to employees and visitors.

An incident report serves two main purposes. First, it informs the hospital's administrators of the incident so changes can be considered to help prevent similar incidents. This is known as risk management. Second, the incident report alerts the administrators and the hospital's insurance company to the possibility of a liability claim and the need for further investigation. This is known as claims management.

Filing an incident report

Only a person with first-hand knowledge of an incident should file a report, and only the person making the report should sign it. Never sign a report describing circumstances or events that you didn't witness personally. Each person with first-hand knowledge should fill out and sign a separate report.

Your report should:
• identify the person involved in the incident.
• document accurately and truthfully any unusual occurrences that you witnessed.
• record details of what happened and the consequences for the person. Include sufficient information so the administrators can decide whether the matter requires further investigation.
• avoid opinions, judgments, conclusions, or assumptions about who or what caused the incident.
• avoid making suggestions on how to prevent the incident from happening again.

The incident report isn't part of the patient's clinical record, but it may be used in litigation. In general, you shouldn't note in the clinical record that an incident report has been filed. Do, however, include the clinical details of the incident in your progress notes, making sure the descriptions on the incident report and the progress notes mirror each other.

Incident report forms vary among hospitals, but most include the information shown in the sample on the following pages.

Incident report *(continued)*

INCIDENT REPORT

Name of person *Robert Wilson*

Address
643 Lincoln Street, Philadelphia, PA

| Date of report *1/9/96* | Date of incident *1/9/96* | Time of incident *10:30 a.m.* | If ED patient, give unit number: |

LOCATION OF INCIDENT
- ☑ patient room
- ☐ patient bathroom
- ☐ OR
- ☐ ED
- ☐ hospital grounds
- ☐ nurses' station
- ☐ other _____

IDENTIFICATION
- ☑ inpatient
- ☐ ED patient
- ☐ outpatient
- ☐ employee
- ☐ volunteer
- ☐ visitor
- ☐ other _____

Admitting diagnosis of patient
CHF

CONDITION BEFORE INCIDENT

Level of consciousness
(previous 4 hours)
- ☑ alert
- ☐ confused, disoriented
- ☐ uncooperative
- ☐ sedated (drug:____)
- ☐ unconscious

Ambulation
- ☐ OOB
- ☑ OOB with assistance
- ☐ bed rest with BRP
- ☐ complete bed rest
- ☐ not specified
- ☐ other (specify) ____

Side rails
- ☐ up
- ☑ partially up
- ☐ down

Restraints
Present ☐ yes ☑ no
Ordered ☐ yes ☑ no

Call system within reach
- ☑ yes
- ☐ no

Bed height
- ☐ high
- ☑ low

NATURE OF INCIDENT

Fall
- ☐ while ambulatory
- ☐ while sitting
  - ☐ chair
  - ☐ commode
- ☐ from bed
- ☐ off table, stretcher, or equipment
- ☐ found on floor
- ☐ other _____

Medication
- ☐ error in patient identification
- ☐ incorrect drug
- ☐ incorrect dosage
- ☑ incorrect route
- ☐ timing
- ☐ duplication
- ☐ omission

- ☐ incorrect I.V. solution hung
- ☐ incorrect I.V. rate
- ☐ other _____

Surgical
- [ ] consent problem
- [ ] incorrect sponge and instrument count
- [ ] foreign object left in patient
- [ ] other _____

Burn
- [ ] chemical
- [ ] cigarette
- [ ] treatment
- [ ] hot liquid
- [ ] other _____

EQUIPMENT

Type _____

Control and serial number _____

_____

- [ ] malfunction
- [ ] shock
- [ ] burn
- [ ] other _____

Date of last maintenance _____
BioMed notified [ ] yes [ ] no
Risk Management notified
[ ] yes [ ] no

Personal property
- [ ] damaged
- [ ] lost
- [ ] other _____

Describe items.

Miscellaneous
- [ ] patient refuses treatment
- [ ] needle stick
- [ ] injuries in treatment
- [ ] infection
- [ ] discharge against medical advice
- [ ] struck by door
- [ ] other _____

Describe the incident.

Digoxin 0.25 mg P.O. ordered, Digoxin 0.25 mg administered intravenously.

Witnesses: [ ] yes [✓] no
If yes, note names, addresses, and phone numbers, and indicate if they're employees, visitors, etc.

1. _____

2. _____

DISPOSITION

Seen by
- [✓] attending doctor
- [ ] ED doctor

Name:
John B. Moyer, MD

Treatment
- [✓] not indicated
- [ ] treatment given
- [ ] treatment refused
- [ ] X-ray ordered
- [ ] admitted to hospital
- [ ] follow-up care indicated

Examination findings:
NSR rate 80; BP 122/76

Doctor's signature: *John B. Moyer, MD*

Notification
(include your name, the date, and the time)
Attending doctor notified
[✓] yes [ ] no

Roxanne Smith, RN
1/9/96   10:50 am.
(continued)

Incident report *(continued)*

DISPOSITION *(continued)*

Supervisor notified
☑ yes ☐ no

Roxanne Smith, 1/9/96 10:50a.m.
RN

Noted in chart
☑ yes ☐ no

Roxanne Smith, RN 1/9/96
10:50a.m. ☑ Documented in progress notes

Sick call request completed
☐ yes ☑ no

Patient or family notified
☐ yes ☑ no

GENERAL DATA

Attending doctor _____ John B. Moyer, MD _____

Room number   Bed number   Shift ☑ 1 ☐ 2 ☐ 3
305   /

Additional details of incident

_____
_____
_____
_____

Signature *Roxanne Smith*
Title   R N
Date   1 / 9 / 96

Director's summary
(detail follow-up to above incident and action taken)

_____
_____
_____
_____
_____

Signature _____
Title _____
Date _____

Home care:
A caregiver's survival guide

Basic principles

▶

What is home health care?

Home health care is a component of comprehensive health care in which services are provided to patients of all ages and their families in their homes in order to restore, maintain, or promote health and to minimize the effects of illness and disability. Based on the patient's and family's needs, the appropriate care is planned, coordinated, and supplied by a home health care agency, a kind of "hospital without walls."

With the speedy discharge of patients from hospitals (the "quicker and sicker" syndrome), the increasing number of elderly patients, and the availability of safe, easily operated health care equipment, home health care has a bright future. Between 1989 and 1994, the number of home health care agencies (both Medicare-certified and noncertified) increased by 26% to over 15,000 entities, according to the National Association for Home Care. As hospitals continue to diversify into outpatient services and form integrated delivery systems, the number of home health care agencies is expected to increase.

The home health care industry may conceivably become the primary supplier of health care in the United States. Because skilled nursing service lies at the heart of any successful home health care program, it's important for you to understand home health care principles and practices.

Certification and accreditation

Home health care agencies, except for hospices and home health aide agencies, are regulated by the Medicare Conditions of Participation. Hospices are certified as Medicare providers under a separate federal standard.

Federal law requires that the state health department conduct an unannounced Medicare survey of each home health care agency every year. At the time of this survey, the agency is also licensed by the state. Medicare certification is critical to the success of a home health care agency. For more information, see "Case management and quality improvement" later in this chapter.

In addition to Medicare certification, agencies may opt for accreditation by the Joint Commission on Accreditation of Healthcare Organizations (JCAHO) or the National League for Nursing's Community Health Accreditation Program (CHAP). Although JCAHO and CHAP accreditation are not currently required, managed care insurance companies may eventually mandate this accreditation for their contracted agencies.

An agency applying for accreditation must demonstrate compliance with established standards. Every 3 years, the accrediting body reviews the agency's operations, policies, and procedures; interviews staff; and evaluates home visits and compliance with clinical practice standards, such as those set by the American Nurses' Association for home health nursing practice.

Determining the patient's eligibility

To be eligible for home care, the patient must be recognized by the provider as being homebound (able to leave the home infrequently, primarily for medical care) and requiring intermittent *skilled care* services (nursing, physical therapy, and speech therapy). Home health aide services, occupational therapy, and medical social services are *ancillary* services that can only be provided under the auspices of skilled care services.

Patients are referred for home health care services primarily by hospital discharge planners. They may also be referred by doctors, their families, community agencies, skilled nursing facilities, or insurance case managers. In any case, the home health care agency must obtain a doctor's order prior to initiating service, and the doctor must review a progress report and recertify the need for continued service every 2 months (not more than 62 days).

Future developments

Several major trends are emerging as the home health care industry continues to evolve.

• *Accountability pressures.* Today, home care services are reimbursed by Medicare, Medicaid, and managed care private insurers. More and more private insurers require that home health care services be preauthorized. This cost-conscious environment confronts the nurse with challenges ranging from loss of control over patient care to ethical dilemmas and quality improvement issues.

• *Consolidation.* Home health care agencies will be forced to merge with hospital networks to form integrated delivery systems. The independent agency will cease to exist as insurance companies seek contracts with those agencies that can provide diverse services to a wide geographic area.

• *Emphasis on outcomes.* Disease-specific management programs — such as those now in place for diabetes and congestive heart failure —

will require home health care agencies to develop critical pathways that incorporate patient outcome analysis. In the future, an agency's quality will be measured by outcome data.

• *Computerizing care.* Increasingly, home care nurses are coping with an expanding paperwork load by using laptop computers. These are equipped with software that speeds clinical documentation to develop the plan of care, formulate goals, monitor patient progress, update medications, and generate visit notes. The new technology also expedites the exchange of current clinical data and other information among doctors, other care providers, and reimbursers.

Ethical and legal aspects of home care

The Code for Nurses of the American Nurses' Association (ANA) includes standards of ethical conduct and practice that are relevant to home care. As in any other health care setting, you're expected to provide services while respecting the patient's human dignity and uniqueness without regard to his or her socioeconomic status, personal attributes, or nature of the health problem. Specific ethical principles include autonomy, beneficence, veracity, fidelity, justice, and respect for others. Each of these principles helps to define the quality and adequacy of health care delivered in the home setting. (See *Applying ethical principles in home health nursing,* page 632.)

Many factors can complicate ethical decisions, such as the legal right of a competent adult to refuse care, increasing patient sophistication, living wills, confidentiality issues, and limited financial resources.

You should be aware that ethical concerns are being strongly emphasized in the home care field. In its accreditation process, the JCAHO is looking for agencies to establish committees that handle ethical issues arising in the home.

Ethical guidelines are supported by a network of federal and state laws relating to home nursing care. For example, you won't lose your nursing license if you fail to abide by the ANA's Code for Nurses — a voluntary guide document. However, you will lose your license if you violate your state's nurse practice act, which sets *legal* practice standards in your state. Federal and state laws relevant to home care are briefly reviewed below.

Federal legislation

Federal legislation sets requirements for all home health care nurses. The Omnibus Budget Reconciliation Act (OBRA), as amended in 1987, substantially changed the law relating to participating Medicare agencies. The law requires that patients be screened for eligibility; that they be informed of their legal rights before signing the home care contract; and that they be fully informed in advance about the agency's plan of care and about changes in care or treatment that may affect their well-being. In addition, the law gives the patient a voice in planning his or her care and treatment and addresses confidentiality and grievance issues.

A separate OBRA provision sets strict criteria for home health care aides, who typically provide a large share of hands-on patient care. An agency may not use any individual who is not a licensed health care professional unless he or she has successfully completed a training program that meets minimum federal standards and is deemed competent to provide assigned services. For more information, see "Working with home health aides" later in this chapter.

The Older Americans Act was amended in 1987 to strengthen home care consumer protections, such as the rights of developmentally disabled persons.

The Patient Self-Determination Act of 1991 requires federally funded home health agencies to abide by the terms of a patient's living will or other special directive, such as a durable power of attorney. If a patient lacks such an instrument but wants to obtain it, the agency must instruct the patient how to do so.

State legislation

As you might expect, your state's nurse practice act governs the standards of practice and standards of care in the patient's home as in other health care settings. You should also be aware of your state's laws in such areas as tenants' rights, protection of uninsured persons, and abused or homeless persons. For example, you should know how and when to report cases of suspected abuse. Also familiarize yourself with family law issues, such as guardians' rights, implementing a durable power of attorney, and obtaining consent to perform procedures on minors or incompetent persons.

Common legal issues
Standing orders

Because the home health setting is usually isolated, your agency should have written standing orders in place to allow you to deal with emergencies or unexpected needs of patients when an attending doctor isn't available. Standing orders should be reviewed and updated regularly; they must be signed by the attending doctor before being implemented.

If you obtain a verbal order, document it, have the doctor co-sign it as soon as possible, and insert it in the patient's record. If a patient is injured while you were relying on a verbal order, and no documentation of the order can be found, you may have trouble proving that you accurately implemented the doctor's order. Also, be sure you've obtained the verbal order and had it approved *before* the approved plan of care expires. Medicare will not cover a home visit that takes place outside the approved time period.

Contracts

Home health nurses must honor contracts made with patients. Contracts include both written and oral agreements of understanding made between the agency and the prospective patient. Be aware that the services offered in the agency's brochures and other advertisements can also be construed as part of the formal contract.

A home care contract should specify the following elements: the provider's and patient's respective roles and responsibilities; the duration, type, frequency, and limitations of services; discharge planning; cost and payment schedules; and provisions for obtaining informed consent from the patient or patient's surrogate for specific interventions.

Before the contract is signed, the patient should be informed about the availability of 24-hour staffing, how to contact staff during off-hours, and reasons why this service may be needed.

If necessary, a patient may be transferred to another site by the agency after the contract has been signed. All aspects of a transfer (physical, psychological, and financial) should be discussed with the patient beforehand.

The agency must develop and implement a satisfactory discharge plan to avoid liability in the event of perceived patient "abandonment" or "dumping" at termination or discharge. Discharge planning should be started with the initial patient evaluation, and the patient should be involved in the plan throughout the care period.

When a patient is to be discharged, he or she must be given reasonable notice and adequate health care services up to the discharge date. However, the agency is not obligated to provide ongoing services without due compensation. Nor must the agency continue to care for a patient who is a threat to the physical safety of the staff.

Confidentiality

As a general rule, you must protect the confidentiality of the patient's medical record. In most states, all health care records, including clinical data obtained from examinations, treatments, observations, and conversations, are considered confidential. Specific state laws may restrict disclosure of this information.

Nevertheless, you may have to share the patient's record with other members of the home care team, as well as third-party payers. You may also be legally required to disclose confidential information in exceptional instances, such as child abuse cases, matters of public health and safety, and criminal cases. To address these issues, obtain written consent from your patient beforehand, preferably at contract signing. If no provision was made for sharing of information, have the patient sign a release form. This form should specify what information is to be released,

Applying ethical principles in home health nursing

PRINCIPLE	MEANING	EXAMPLE OF NURSING APPLICATION
Autonomy	Personal freedom	Allowing the patient to decide when to implement care or to refuse treatment.
Beneficence	Duty to promote good	Allowing the patient to die without life-sustaining treatment if that is what he or she desires.
Veracity	Being truthful	Providing the patient with enough information to allow him or her to make informed choices about care.
Fidelity	Keeping one's promise	Refraining from promising the patient that you or another health care worker will be at the bedside when death comes (it may not be possible to keep such a promise).
Justice	Treating others fairly	Ensuring that you will provide the care that the patient needs even if there are other, more seriously ill patients that you need to see.
Respect for others	Right of individuals to be treated equally	Treating all patients with the same level of empathy and competent care, even when they are noncompliant or of another culture or race.

to whom it will be given, and the time period during which the release is valid.

Because the patient may also request information from the record, the agency should have a written policy concerning release of information to the patient or patient's surrogate. Although the original record is the property of the agency, a copy may be given to the patient for his or her records.

Refusal of care

An issue of growing concern is the patient's right to refuse treatment. Even if the patient has previously consented to treatment, a mentally competent patient can later withdraw consent if the patient has been fully informed about his or her medical condition and the likely consequences of refusal. Verbal withdrawal of consent is adequate, and this should be immediately communicated to other members of the home care team. The patient's refusal or withdrawal of consent must be documented, along with any patient education measures, and placed in the patient's medical record.

Implementation

▶

Ensuring safe home care visits

When providing patient care in the home, you're faced with two challenges that don't normally arise in a hospital setting: First, making sure you're not harmed before, during, and after the home visit; and second, making sure the patient can receive care in a safe home environment. This section will help you meet these challenges.

Personal safety guidelines

Most home health agencies have specific policies and procedures to ensure staff safety. You should discuss any safety concerns with your supervisor as soon as they arise so that appropriate corrective action can be taken. The chart on the next page summarizes what you can do to protect yourself. (See *Personal safety pointers,* page 634.)

Assessing the home environment

You're legally responsible for ensuring that the home is indeed the best place for your patient to receive his or her prescribed care and treatment. Begin checking the patient's home environment for actual and potential safety problems at your first visit. Document your findings regarding room layout, accessibility, bathroom facilities, storage areas, provision for medical waste disposal, and availability of support persons. You'll be assessing and correcting safety concerns for the duration of the contract period. You'll also be teaching the patient and family about specific safety measures to implement in your ab-

sence. The information below will help you assess possible safety hazards and provide appropriate teaching.

General safety

• Make sure stairs have secure railings and nonslip tread surfaces.
• Provide good lighting in halls and stairways.
• Install a bedside telephone. Provide phone numbers of emergency contact person(s), the doctor, 911 (local fire and police), and the agency (agencies must be accessible 24 hours a day). If necessary, install a telephone alert system.
• Make sure pathways are clear and unobstructed; rugs, if used, should have nonslip backings. Avoid using rugs in high-traffic areas.
• Provide nonskid slippers or shoes for the patient to use when out of bed.

Bathroom safety

• Adjust water heater temperature to below 120° F (48.8° C); instruct the patient or family member to check water temperature before getting into the tub or shower.
• Install rubber mats or nonslip strips in the tub and shower.
• Install grab bars in the tub and shower.

Patient care safety

• Determine availability of support person(s).
• Demonstrate storage of medications in a safe place, out of the reach of children, and disposal of old or expired medications.
• Instruct the patient to use bed rails when in bed; use seat belts, if necessary, when in a chair; and keep wheelchair brakes locked and footrests out of the way when transferring to a wheelchair.
• If ordered, apply patient restraints properly.

Personal safety pointers

As a home health care nurse, you'll serve many patients who may be scattered over a wide area in a variety of settings. The suggestions below will help you avoid potential problems.

BEFORE YOU GO

• Know your agency's safety protocols.
• Verify where the patient lives; call the family or use a map.
• Leave a copy of your itinerary at the office.
• If the patient lives in an unsafe area, try planning your visit early in the day; if possible, bring a nurse "buddy" along.
• If you don't wear a uniform, dress in business clothes, wear a name tag, and carry agency identification; make it easy for the patient to identify you.
• Carry an extra set of keys with you (in case you lock yourself out of your car), bring just enough money for emergency calls and transportation, and have a list of important phone numbers (agency, police, fire).

ON THE ROAD

• Make sure your car runs well, and fill the gas tank before a visit. Consider joining an automobile club for quick access to road service.
• Always use your seat belt; practice defensive driving.
• If you're taking public transportation, make sure you know the route; if you must walk, don't accept rides from strangers.
• Be prepared for poor weather and delays on the road. Have a flashlight, blanket, and extra snacks handy.

WHEN YOU ARRIVE

• Don't park your car near the patient's home if it's in an unsafe area. Instead, park in a public area and walk to the home along well-lit streets. If you must visit in the evening, park in an open, well-lit area.
• Before you get out of your car, look around. If you feel unsafe, drive to a safe place to phone the agency about your concern.
• If you have any doubts about the safety of entering the patient's home or building, don't enter. Contact the agency immediately.
• If the patient doesn't answer the door, call the patient from a pay phone or car phone, or have the agency contact the patient.
• When entering the home, observe all the exits. If you're uneasy or if you suspect anyone in the home is using alcohol or drugs, do what is necessary for the patient and leave. If this is not possible, leave immediately.
• If a pet is obnoxious or hostile, politely ask that it be moved to another room. Always be respectful of the patient's attachment to the pet. After your visit, document the animal's presence in the home to warn other caregivers.

• Advise the patient to set electrical heating pads on low to medium and to keep them covered.
• Place bedside items within the patient's reach.
• Institute and teach infection control measures.

Fire safety
• Warn the patient against smoking in bed or while oxygen is in use, and tell patient to make sure all cigarettes and matches are out before throwing them away.
• Install smoke or heat detectors on each level of the home.
• Place portable heaters in well-ventilated areas.
• Make sure appliances' electric cords are intact, not frayed or split, and have straight plug prongs.

Medical equipment
• Instruct the patient or family in function and proper use of prescribed equipment, and how to report malfunctions.
• Explain possible hazards related to electrical, mechanical, and fire safety aspects of equipment.
• Store medical gases, supplies, and drugs in a safe, protected area.

Medical waste disposal
• Make sure appropriate containers are available for disposal of needles, syringes, and other contaminated medical supplies.
• Teach proper handling of medical wastes.

Document your actions
Document your home care safety recommendations. Be sure to enclose a statement in the patient's record listing what was taught or recommended, and record any instances of the patient's or family's refusal or failure to follow your recommendations. For example, they may balk at the extra expense of

installing smoke detectors or a tub rail. Or the patient may continue to smoke when oxygen is being used. Carefully documenting noncompliance will help protect you and your agency from possible liability.

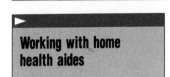

Working with home health aides

If the patient's condition and situation warrant it, you may assign a paraprofessional home health aide (HHA) to assist the patient intermittently with personal care and activities of daily living. The HHA's role is crucial because he or she may spend more time with the patient and family than any other member of the health care team. Typically, you'll determine the need for HHA services during the initial home visit.

Criteria for HHA services
For planning and reimbursement purposes, the use of HHAs is considered ancillary (not skilled care) service. The National Association for Home Care has identified three levels of home health aide services. An HHA I performs housekeeping services only; an HHA II performs nonmedical personal care as well as level I tasks; and an HHA III may perform medically supervised tasks, such as nonsterile wound care, assisting with prescribed rehabilitation therapy, and assisting with self-administered medications, in addition to level I and II tasks.

Depending on the patient's situation, you may elect to use HHA services at level I, II, or III. However, Medicare will reimburse a home care agency only for care provided by a certified level III home health aide. An HHA III may become certified after completing a training program of at least 75 hours, 16 of which must be in laboratory and clinical settings. To justify HHA III services, you must be able to demonstrate that skilled care is being provided on an intermittent basis, thereby creating a need for hands-on personal care and assistance with the patient's treatment.

In any case, the continued need for HHA services must be documented at least every 2 weeks. The doctor must confirm the type and frequency of HHA service in the plan of care and must also recertify the order for HHA service every 2 months.

Be sure to explain to the patient and family that HHA services will only be reimbursed if the above criteria are met. Often, the patient and family become dependent on the HHA and have difficulty adjusting when HHA services are discontinued.

What home health aides do

Most of an HHA's tasks are related to personal care. This includes bathing, dressing, grooming, and oral hygiene; changing bed linens of an incontinent patient; shaving; skin care; and routine foot care.

The HHA may also help with feeding and elimination; he or she may administer an enema or give routine catheter and colostomy care, unless the patient's condition requires skilled care (for example, if the patient has a heart disorder). The HHA also can assist the patient with ambulation, changing position in bed, and transfers.

Examples of reimbursable HHA services include the following:
• a simple dressing change that does not require skilled care, such as a dry, nonsterile dressing change

• helping to give medications that the patient would normally take unaided and that do not require a nurse's skills to achieve safe, accurate administration
• helping with activities related to skilled therapy services that do not require the therapist to be present, such as maintenance exercises and speech exercises
• performing routine care of prosthetic and orthotic devices.

The HHA may perform other activities during a home visit, but these aren't reimbursable unless they're performed during that same visit. Such activities, labeled by Medicare as "incidental," may include light housekeeping, light cleaning of the patient's immediate area, meal preparation and cleanup, laundry related to the patient's care, essential grocery shopping and errands, and taking out the trash.

Supervising HHAs

When HHA services are ordered, plan to meet with the aide during one of your home care visits. This allows the aide and the patient to get acquainted and lets you all discuss the plan of care together. The plan of care will specify the HHA's duties. At the end of the visit, you'll leave a copy with the patient.

Typically, you're responsible for communicating with the HHA about any changes in the patient's condition or care and communicating with the patient and family about the care provided. However, if another skilled service (such as physical or speech therapy) is involved and skilled nursing is not, you can delegate supervisory responsibility to the therapist.

You can monitor the HHA's performance during a home visit while the aide is present to directly observe, to instruct the HHA, and to make recommendations and suggestions for care. Also plan a visit when the HHA is not present, so that you can get additional feedback. Often, patients are reluctant to say anything about the HHA while he or she is present.

Managed care organizations and private insurers have reimbursement and supervisory criteria for HHA services similar to Medicare's. Consult your case manager about specific requirements.

Documenting HHA services

Most home care agencies use a standardized form for documenting HHA supervision. This data should also be entered in the patient's care record. Include information relating to assessment of the patient's health status, rapport of the patient and HHA, and determination of goal achievement. Include any recommendations and suggestions. If teaching is involved, document what was taught and the HHA's response to the teaching, including a return demonstration, if appropriate.

◀

▶

Documentation and reimbursement

In no other health care setting are you as responsible for ensuring reimbursement payments as you are in the home health care setting. Your success or failure largely depends on your documentation skills. For this reason, home health care agencies have a highly structured documentation system.

The federal Health Care Financing Administration (HCFA), which monitors Medicare and Medicaid disbursements, requires home health care agencies to standardize

their documentation. Required data for each certified patient are collected using a Home Health Certification and Plan of Treatment form (HCFA-485) and a Medical Update and Patient Information form (HCFA-486). These forms allow Medicare reviewers to evaluate each claim in accordance with the established criteria for coverage. Medicare will not provide payment unless these forms are properly completed, signed by the nurse and the attending doctor, and submitted.

Developing the plan of care

Many home health agencies use HCFA-485 as the patient's official plan of care (POC). Be aware that because the patient's care occurs in the home—usually with the family participating—you have less control than you would in an institutional setting. The patient and his family become the decision makers in many aspects and have greater control of the situation. These factors must be addressed realistically when developing the POC, and you may need to readjust your interventions, patient goals, and teaching accordingly.

To maximize reimbursement, to support the patient's need for services and supplies, and to justify any change in the POC, your documentation must be clear, thorough, and accurate. Good documentation also facilitates medical review and continuity of care and helps protect you legally.

The initial home visit

During the initial home visit, you'll evaluate the patient's eligibility for home care based on Medicare guidelines. You'll also obtain a complete health history and assess the patient's psychosocial and physiologic status in the context of his or her environment.

The history and assessment should focus primarily on acute medical instabilities (especially those that influence the patient's homebound status). Be sure to document any and all functional limitations of the patient and caregiver, including (but not limited to) mobility, dexterity, vision, hearing, and strength. Also assess and document any home safety needs.

When documenting the patient's psychosocial status, include data on living conditions, economic situation, culture, primary language of patient and caregiver, ability of patient and caregiver to learn, availability of caregiver, coping styles, support systems, and availability of transportation.

Also obtain a medication history. Because Medicare reimburses for teaching related to new medications (and, in some instances, for old and changed medications as well), the POC must indicate whether each medication (prescription and over-the-counter) is new, old, or changed.

Obtaining a doctor's order

The POC that results from the initial visit must be signed by the attending doctor to become a valid order. This signature must be obtained prior to submitting the claim for payment. The doctor's order must specify the type of skilled and unskilled services required and the frequency of those services. Amended orders must clearly indicate what is to be changed and the reason for the changes.

A verbal order for skilled services must be documented in the patient's record to cover the services rendered from the initial visit (start of certification period) to the time the POC is signed by the doctor. Amendments to the POC must also be signed and placed in the

patient's record within 10 days of receiving verbal orders.

Justifying visit frequency

The number of home visits per week is specified during the initial home visit. Daily or multiple daily visits (5 or more visits per week) are allowed only when the visits will not be required for an indefinite period of time. Visits are usually less frequent as the patient's condition improves. Typically, a range of visit frequency is specified in the POC to provide some flexibility and ensure that the most appropriate level of care is being provided.

Once a frequency has been incorporated into the POC, it can only be altered by the doctor's order. Any change in frequency (increase or decrease) must be justified by a change in the patient's medical condition. For example, a stage III wound that is no longer draining may warrant fewer visits (if the wound is the only current diagnosis). Conversely, worsening edema and shortness of breath in an acute exacerbation of chronic obstructive pulmonary disease could require additional visits.

When documenting each home visit, you'll need to clearly explain to the payer why the provided service is reasonable and necessary. Do this by charting the "negative" (the illness or disability), thereby focusing on the patient's problems and the skilled care needed to deal with them. For example, include detailed information about why the patient or caregiver can't or won't learn to perform a skilled procedure or comply with a medication regimen.

▶
Understanding skilled and ancillary home care services

This chart gives examples of skilled and ancillary services used in home health care and how they may be reimbursed.

SERVICES	INDICATIONS AND EXAMPLES	NOTES
Physical therapy (skilled service)	Indicated for functional limitations and deficits in safety, mobility, strength, and range of motion. Examples: gait training, strengthening exercises.	Some states allow trained physical therapists to perform wound debridement.
Speech therapy (skilled service)	Indicated for dysphasia and dysphagia. Examples: assessment and evaluation, diagnostic testing, teaching and training, aural rehabilitation, and maintenance therapy.	Medicare will not reimburse for repetition and reinforcement, work-related therapy, or a nondiagnostic or nontherapeutic routine.
Occupational therapy (not considered a skilled service)	Indicated for functional limitation of activities of daily living that relates to the primary or secondary diagnosis. Examples: therapeutic activities, energy conservation methods, task simplification.	Skilled nursing, physical therapy, or speech therapy must be ordered and provided for occupational therapy services to be reimbursed.
Medical social service (not considered a skilled service)	Indicated for social or emotional difficulties of patient or caregiver that affect treatment or rate of recovery. Examples: referrals, counseling, and long-term care planning.	Skilled nursing, physical therapy, or speech therapy must be ordered and provided for medical social services to be reimbursed.
Home health aide care (not considered a skilled service)	Need is determined by home care nurse, usually at initial visit. Aide may assist with personal hygiene, patient transfers, light meal preparation, light housekeeping, and, possibly, medications (check state laws).	Skilled nursing, physical therapy, or speech therapy must be ordered and provided for home health aide care services to be reimbursed.

◀

Documenting ancillary services

If ancillary services (occupational therapy, medical social services, or home health aides) are needed and ordered, a referral for the appropriate service must be completed. It should outline the type of ancillary service required and explain why it's needed. The patient's rehabilitation potential must be judged as at least "fair" to qualify for reimbursement. (See *Understanding skilled and ancillary home care services.*)

Documenting patient teaching

Medicare reimburses for teaching as a skilled service. Certain guidelines must be followed and documented:

• Identify precisely what was taught and to whom it was taught (patient or caregiver).

• Document the patient or caregiver's ability to learn, especially if he or she is slow or overwhelmed.

• Describe the teaching outcome. What was the level of understanding? Evaluate and document the patient's or caregiver's return demonstration performance.

Medicare will not reimburse for repeated instruction unless the patient or caregiver states that he or she forgot the teaching or is unsure of a specific instruction, or if the caregiver has changed. When documenting this, avoid using terms that suggest repetitive instruction (such as "reinforced," "reviewed," "reinstructed," and "reminded"). Also avoid using the word "encourage" because it is interpreted by Medicare and other payers to be unskilled care.

Obtaining recertification

Documentation requesting recertification must clearly support the need for continued care within Medicare guidelines. Every 2 months, a progress report summarizing the patient's condition and stating any proposed changes in the POC must be sent to the doctor for review. At that point, a new HCFA-485 is completed and signed by the doctor.

Discharge notification

If the patient is deemed ready for discharge from home health care services, the doctor is consulted, appropriate orders are obtained, and a discharge summary is completed. The summary should state the patient's condition at discharge, the reason for discharge, the extent to which the goals of care were met, and any instructions for patient follow-up with the doctor.

Case management and quality improvement

Case management and quality improvement are concepts central to providing professional home health care services. They are intended to provide a structure for providing care according to standards established by government regulation, voluntary accreditation agencies, professional organizations, third-party payers, and individual agencies. This section will examine the two concepts in turn.

Case management

Case management involves prioritizing care among the patients in a caseload and delivering that care according to procedural steps that ensure successful patient outcomes. These steps are based on the nursing process and include information gathering and assessment; establishing a multidisciplinary plan of care; and implementing and evaluating the plan of care.

You may feel that a managed care environment impairs your agency's flexibility in responding to changing patient needs or that much of the decision-making you were accustomed to is curtailed. In addition, you may have to deal with several case managers from different managed care organizations with different policies and procedures. Case managers, for their part, may be frustrated by the need to constantly explain and justify their role when they feel they should be treated as valued customers. Effective communication can reduce the level of mutual distrust and frustration. At its best, external case management matches the home care nurse's strengths — knowledge of the patient and the community resources available — with the case manager's strengths — knowledge of reimbursement procedures and efficient use of available resources.

Suggestions for working with managed care providers

These pointers will help you work well with managed care providers and maintain quality care for patients.
• Learn as much as possible about trends in reimbursement for home health care, the various types of managed care organizations, and the ways your agency has adapted to this new type of health care.
• Work with an understanding of the managed care organization's interest in finding the most efficient way of meeting patient needs. You need to know the most current treatment strategies and patient-teaching methods, and you need to be aware of the cost of various treatment alternatives.
• Redouble your efforts to be familiar with community resources that can help patients become more independent. Services coordinated by area agencies on aging frequently can help a patient make the transition to home care service. Churches are a largely untapped resource for help in meeting patient needs.
• Be aware of the need to document successful patient outcomes. Present the patient's needs with a clear explanation of the specific actions you've requested and the specific outcomes you believe will result. Support this with evidence that the outcome will prevent a complication or a recurring problem.

Quality improvement

Health care agencies' quality control efforts have advanced from static reviews of patient care documentation to ongoing integration of quality improvement measures into all procedures. The term quality assurance (QA) has given way to total quality management (TQM), followed by total quality improvement (TQI) and, finally, continuous quality improvement (CQI).

The CQI process can be seen as yet another variation of the nursing process. Data is gathered; problems are defined; goals are set; actions are selected; evaluations are made using structure, process, and outcome indicators; and variances are identified. This, in turn, cues a new round of the CQI process. Nurses have multiple opportunities to become involved in the CQI process. If chosen to participate on a quality improvement committee, you would work with other caregivers to set the course for the CQI program for a significant time period. Many agencies have a quality improvement coordinator or director who chairs the committee.

On another quality front, many health care providers are developing sets of standard interventions, based on medical diagnoses or surgical procedures, to ensure that patients receive care that is normative for the specific condition. These standard interventions are known as clinical paths, critical paths, care tracks, and coordinated care guides.

Clinical paths resemble standardized nursing plans of care in some respects. They are multidisciplinary tools that need to be accepted by all involved in the patient's care, particularly the doctor. Clinical paths can reduce documentation requirements and streamline the quality improvement process.

Medicare site visits

When home health agencies are reviewed to certify them for Medicare reimbursement, the aspects of care that are examined are determined by the conditions of participation in the Medicare program documented in the Home Health Agency Health Insurance Manual (HIM-11). To prepare for a Medicare site visit, you should review your practices to make sure Medicare guidelines are followed for every Medicare-reimbursed case.

• Check admission practices to ensure that the patient and family understand the conditions of Medicare eligibility, their rights with regard to Medicare service, and how to access information about these rights.

• Document that a copy of the patient's bill of rights was given to the patient, and place a copy in the patient's record.

• Document that the patient's wishes with regard to advance medical directives was discussed.

• Review the patient's record for adherence to standards of timeliness of documentation, for visit frequency, and for completion of all necessary forms, particularly doctor's orders (Health Care Financing Administration Form 485).

• Ensure that visit records reflect the skilled care given, the homebound status of the patient, and the coordination of all services provided by the agency.

• Perform supervision of home health aides according to your agency's policy. Documentation always includes the patient's or caregiver's satisfaction with the service, the rationale for continued home health aide service, and the nurse's recommendation to continue or modify the service.

CHAPTER 16

Abbreviations and acronyms:
Learning their meanings

ABBREVIATIONS AND TERMS

Medical abbreviations and acronyms

ā	before	AICD	automatic implantable cardioverter-defibrillator
āā	of each	AIDS	acquired immunodeficiency syndrome
AAA	abdominal aortic aneurysm	ALL	acute lymphocytic leukemia
Ab	antibody		
ABC	airway, breathing, circulation	ALS	amyotrophic lateral sclerosis
ABG	arterial blood gas	ALT	alanine aminotransferase (formerly called SGPT)
a.c.	before meals		
ACE	angiotensin-converting enzyme	a.m., A.M.	morning
ACh	acetylcholine	AMA	against medical advice
ACLS	advanced cardiac life support	AMI	acute myocardial infarction
a.d., AD	auris dextra (right ear)	AML	acute myelocytic leukemia
AD	Alzheimer's disease	ANA	antinuclear antibody
ADH	antidiuretic hormone	AP	anteroposterior apical pulse
ADL	activities of daily living		
AER	aldosterone excretion rate	APTT	activated partial thromboplastin time
AFIB	atrial fibrillation	aq	aqueous (watery)
AFL	atrial flutter	ara-A	adenine arabinoside (vidarabine)
AFP	alpha-fetoprotein		
Ag	antigen	ara-C	cytosine arabinoside (cytarabine)
A-G	albumin-globulin (ratio)	ARDS	acute respiratory distress syndrome adult respiratory distress syndrome
AGA	appropriate for gestational age		
AHD	arteriosclerotic heart disease autoimmune hemolytic disease	ARF	acute renal failure acute respiratory failure acute rheumatic fever
AHF	antihemophilic factor (factor VIII)	a.s., AS	auris sinistra (left ear)

AS	aortic sounds aqueous solution astigmatism	**CABG**	coronary artery bypass grafting
ASA	acetylsalicylic acid (aspirin)	**CAD**	coronary artery disease
		CAFT	Clinitron air-fluidized therapy
ASD	atrial septal defect		
ASO	antistreptolysin-O	**cAMP**	cyclic adenosine monophosphate
AST	aspartate aminotransferase (formerly called SGOT)	**CAPD**	continuous ambulatory peritoneal dialysis
		caps	capsules
ATP	adenosine triphosphate	**CBC**	complete blood count
A.U.	each ear	**cc**	cubic centimeter
AV	arteriovenous atrioventricular	**CC**	Caucasian child chief complaint common cold creatinine clearance critical care critical condition
AVM	arteriovenous malformation		
BBB	bundle branch block		
BCG	bacille Calmette-Guérin	**CCNU**	lomustine
BCNU	carmustine	**CCU**	cardiac care unit critical care unit
BE	barium enema base excess	**CDC**	Centers for Disease Control and Prevention
b.i.d.	twice daily		
BJ	Bence Jones	**CEA**	carcinoembryonic antigen
BLS	basic life support	**CF**	cardiac failure cystic fibrosis
BMR	basal metabolic rate		
BP	blood pressure	**CFS**	chronic fatigue syndrome
BPH	benign prostatic hyperplasia (or hypertrophy)		
		CGL	chronic granulocytic leukemia
BPM	beats per minute		
BSA	body surface area	**CHB**	complete heart block
BUN	blood urea nitrogen	**CHD**	childhood disease congenital heart disease congenital hip disease
C	Celsius centigrade certified cervical		
		CHF	congestive heart failure
c̄	with	**CK**	creatine kinase
Ca	calcium	**CK-BB**	creatine kinase, brain
CA	cardiac arrest	**CK-MB**	creatine kinase, heart

CK-MM	creatine kinase, skeletal muscle
cm	centimeter
CML	chronic myelogenous leukemia
CMV	continuous mandatory ventilation cytomegalovirus
CNS	central nervous system
CO	carbon monoxide cardiac output
COEPS	cortically originating extrapyramidal system
CO_2	carbon dioxide
COLD	chronic obstructive lung disease
comp	compound
COPD	chronic obstructive pulmonary disease
CP	capillary pressure cerebral palsy cor pulmonale creatine phosphate
CPAP	continuous positive airway pressure
cpm	counts per minute cycles per minute
CPR	cardiopulmonary resuscitation
CRIS	controlled-release infusion system
CSF	cerebrospinal fluid
CT	clotting time coated tablet compressed tablet computed tomography corneal transplant
CV	cardiovascular central venous
CVA	cerebrovascular accident costovertebral angle

CVP	central venous pressure
d	day
/d	per day
D	dextrose
dB	decibel
D/C	discharge discontinue
D & C	dilatation and curettage
DD	differential diagnosis discharge diagnosis dry dressing
D & E	dilatation and evacuation
DES	diethylstilbestrol
DIC	disseminated intravascular coagulation
dil	dilute
disp	dispense
DJD	degenerative joint disease
DKA	diabetic ketoacidosis
dl	deciliter
DNA	deoxyribonucleic acid
DNR	do not resuscitate
DOA	date of admission dead on arrival
DS	double strength
DSA	digital subtraction angiography
DSM-III-R	Diagnostic and Statistical Manual of Mental Disorders, 3rd ed., revised
DTP	diphtheria and tetanus toxoids and pertussis vaccine
DVT	deep vein thrombosis
D_5W	5% dextrose in water
EBV	Epstein-Barr virus
EC	enteric-coated

ECF	extended care facility extracellular fluid		**FFP**	fresh frozen plasma
ECG	electrocardiogram		**FHR**	fetal heart rate
ECHO	echocardiography		**fl, fld**	fluid
ECMO	extracorporeal mem- brane oxygenator		**FRC**	functional residual capacity
ECT	electroconvulsive therapy		**FSH**	follicle-stimulating hormone
ED	emergency department		**FSP**	fibrinogen-split products
EDTA	ethylenediaminetetra- acetic acid		**FT₃**	free triiodothyronine
EEG	electroencephalogram		**FT₄**	free thyroxine
EENT	eyes, ears, nose, throat		**FTA**	fluorescent treponemal antibody (test)
EF	ejection fraction		**FTA- ABS**	fluorescent treponemal antibody absorption (test)
ELISA	enzyme-linked immuno- sorbent assay		**FUO**	fever of undetermined origin
elix	elixir		**FVC**	forced vital capacity
EMG	electromyography		**G**	gauge
EMIT	enzyme-multiplied im- munoassay technique		**g, gm, GM**	gram
ENG	electronystagmography			
EOM	extraocular movement		**GFR**	glomerular filtration rate
ER	emergency room expiratory reserve		**GI**	gastrointestinal
ERCP	endoscopic retrograde cholangiopancreatogra- phy		**G6PD**	glucose-6-phosphate dehydrogenase
			gr	grain
ERV	expiratory reserve vol- ume		**gtt**	drop
ESR	erythrocyte sedimenta- tion rate		**GU**	genitourinary
			GVHD	graft-versus-host disease
ESWL	extracorporeal shock- wave lithotripsy		**GYN**	gynecologic
et	and		**h, hr**	hour
ext.	extract		**Ⓗ**	hypodermic injection
F	Fahrenheit		**HAV**	hepatitis A virus
FDA	Food and Drug Adminis- tration		**Hb**	hemoglobin
			HBD	α-hydroxybutyrate dehy- drogenase
FEF	forced expiratory flow		**HBIG**	hepatitis B immuno- globulin
FEV	forced expiratory volume			

HBsAg	hepatitis B surface antigen
HBV	hepatitis B virus
hCG	human chorionic gonadotropin
Hct	hematocrit
HDL	high-density lipoprotein
HDN	hemolytic disease of the newborn
hGH	human growth hormone
HHNK	hyperosmolar hyperglycemic nonketotic syndrome
HIV	human immunodeficiency virus
HLA	human leukocyte antigen
HMO	health maintenance organization
hPL	human placental lactogen
h.s.	at bedtime
HS	half strength hour of sleep house surgeon
HSV	herpes simplex virus
HVA	homovanillic acid
Hz	hertz
HZV	herpes zoster virus
IA	internal auditory intra-arterial intra-articular
IABP	intra-aortic balloon pump
IC	inspiratory capacity
ICF	intracellular fluid
ICHD	Inter-Society Commission for Heart Disease
ICP	intracranial pressure
ICU	intensive care unit

ID	identification initial dose inside diameter intradermal
I&D	incision and drainage
IDDM	insulin-dependent diabetes mellitus
Ig	immunoglobulin
IM	infectious mononucleosis
I.M.	intramuscular
IMV	intermittent mandatory ventilation
in., "	inch
IND	investigational new drug
IPPB	intermittent positive-pressure breathing
IQ	intelligence quotient
IRV	inspiratory reserve volume
IU	International Unit
IUD	intrauterine device
I.V.	intravenous
IVGTT	intravenous glucose tolerance test
IVH	intravenous hyperalimentation (now called total parenteral nutrition)
IVP	intravenous pyelogram
IVPB	intravenous piggyback
J	joule
JCAHO	Joint Commission on Accreditation of Healthcare Organizations
JVD	jugular venous distention
JVP	jugular venous pressure
kg	kilogram
17-KGS	17-ketogenic steroids
17-KS	17-ketosteroids
KUB	kidneys-ureters-bladder

KVO	keep vein open
L	liter lumbar
Ⓛ	left
LA	left atrium long-acting
LAP	left atrial pressure leucine aminopeptidase
lb., #	pound
LD	lactate dehydrogeuase
LDL	low-density lipoproteins
LE	lupus erythematosus
LES	lower esophageal sphincter
LGL	Lown-Ganong-Levine variant syndrome
LH	luteinizing hormone
LLQ	left lower quadrant
LOC	level of consciousness
LR	lactated Ringer's solution
LSB	left scapular border left sternal border
LTC	long-term care
LUQ	left upper quadrant
LV	left ventricle
LVEDP	left ventricular end-diastolic pressure
LVET	left ventricular ejection time
LVF	left ventricular failure
m	meter
M	molar (solution)
m²	square meter
mm³	cubic millimeter
MAO	maximal acid output monoamine oxidase

MAST	medical antishock trousers (pneumatic antishock garment)
mcg	microgram
MCH	mean corpuscular hemoglobin
MCHC	mean corpuscular hemoglobin concentration
MCV	mean corpuscular volume
MD	manic depressive medical doctor muscular dystrophy
mEq	milliequivalent
mg	milligram
mgtt	microdrip or minidrop
MI	mental illness mitral insufficiency myocardial infarction myocardial ischemia
ml	milliliter
μg	microgram
μL	microliter
MLC	mixed lymphocyte culture
mm	millimeter
MMEF	maximal midexpiratory flow
mmol	millimole
MRI	magnetic resonance imaging
M.R.×1	may repeat once
MS	mitral sounds mitral stenosis morphine sulfate multiple sclerosis musculoskeletal
MUGA	multiple-gated acquisition scanning

ABBREVIATIONS & ACRONYMS

MVI	multivitamin infusion	**O₂**	oxygen
MVP	mitral valve prolapse	**OB**	obstetric
MVV	maximal voluntary ventilation	**OD**	occupational disease overdose right eye
Na	sodium		
NaCl	sodium chloride	**OGTT**	oral glucose tolerance test
NCV	nerve conduction velocity	**OR**	operating room
ng	nanogram	**OS**	left eye
NG	nasogastric	**O₂ sat.**	oxygen saturation
NICU	neonatal intensive care unit	**OTC**	over-the-counter
		OU	each eye
NIDDM	non-insulin-dependent diabetes mellitus (Type II diabetes)	**oz**	ounce
		p̄	after
NKA	no known allergies	**PA**	pernicious anemia posteroanterior pulmonary artery
NMR	nuclear magnetic resonance		
Noct.	night	**PABA**	para-aminobenzoic acid
NP	nasopharynx nerve palsy new patient not palpable	**PAC**	premature atrial contraction
		PaCO₂	partial pressure of carbon dioxide in arterial blood
NPN	nonprotein nitrogen		
NPO	nothing by mouth	**PaO₂**	partial pressure of oxygen in arterial blood
NR	nerve root nonreactive no refills no report no respirations	**PAP**	Papanicolaou smear passive-aggressive personality primary atypical pneumonia pulmonary artery pressure
N/R	not remarkable		
NS, NSS	normal saline solution (0.9% sodium chloride)		
		PAT	paroxysmal atrial tachycardia
¼NS	¼ normal saline solution (0.225% sodium chloride)	**PAWP**	pulmonary artery wedge pressure
½NS	½ normal saline solution (0.45% sodium chloride)	**p.c.**	after meals
		PCA	patient-controlled analgesia
NSAID	nonsteroidal anti-inflammatory drug	**PDA**	patent ductus arteriosus

PE	pelvic examination
	physical examination
	pulmonary embolism
PEEP	positive end-expiratory pressure
PEFR	peak expiratory flow rate
PEP	pre-ejection period
per	by or through
PET	positron-emission tomography
pg	picogram
PID	pelvic inflammatory disease
PKU	phenylketonuria
p.m. **P.M.**	afternoon
PMI	point of maximum impulse
PML	progressive multifocal leukoencephalopathy
PMS	premenstrual syndrome
PND	paroxysmal nocturnal dyspnea
	postnasal drip
P.O.	by mouth
	postoperative
PP	partial pressure
	peripheral pulses
	postpartum
	postprandial
	presenting problem
p.r.n.	as needed
PROM	passive range of motion
	premature rupture of the membranes
pt.	pint
PT	prothrombin time
PTCA	percutaneous transluminal coronary angioplasty
PTH	parathyroid hormone

PTT	partial thromboplastin time
PUD	peptic ulcer disease
	pulmonary disease
PVC	premature ventricular contraction
	polyvinylchloride
q	every
QA	quality assurance
q a.m.	every morning
q.d.	every day
q.h.	every hour
q.i.d.	four times daily
q.n.	every night
QNS	quantity not sufficient
q.o.d.	every other day
QS	quantity sufficient
qt.	quart
R, PR	by rectum
Ⓡ	right
RA	renal artery
	rheumatoid arthritis
	right arm
	right atrium
RAF	rheumatoid arthritis factor
RAP	right atrial pressure
RAST	radioallergosorbent test
RBB	right bundle branch
RBC	red blood cell
RDA	recommended daily allowance
RE	rectal examination
	right ear
REM	rapid eye movement
RES	reticuloendothelial system
Rh	rhesus blood factor

RHD	relative hepatic dullness rheumatic heart disease	**SHBG**	sex hormone-binding globulin
RIA	radioimmunoassay	**SI**	Système International d'Unités
RL	right lateral right leg Ringer's lactate (lactated Ringer's solution)	**SIADH**	syndrome of inappropriate antidiuretic hormone
RLQ	right lower quadrant	**SIDS**	sudden infant death syndrome
RNA	ribonucleic acid		
ROM	range of motion right otitis media	**Sig**	write on label
RSV	respiratory syncytial virus right subclavian vein Rous sarcoma virus	**SIMV**	synchronized intermittent mandatory ventilation
		SL, sl.	sublingual
RUQ	right upper quadrant	**SLE**	systemic lupus erythematosus
RV	residual volume right ventricle	**SOB**	shortness of breath
RVEDP	right ventricular end-diastolic pressure	**sol., soln.**	solution
RVEDV	right ventricular end-diastolic volume	**sp.**	spirits
		SR	sustained release
RVP	right ventricular pressure	**SRS-A**	slow-reacting substance of anaphylaxis
Rx	prescription	**stat.**	immediately
s̄	without	**STD**	sexually transmitted disease
s̄s̄	one-half		
SA	sinoatrial	**supp.**	suppository
sat.	saturated	**susp.**	suspension
S.C., SQ	subcutaneous	**Sv̄o₂**	mixed venous oxygen saturation
SCID	severe combined immunodeficiency syndrome		
		syr.	syrup
sec	second	**T, Tbs., tbsp.**	tablespoon
SGOT	serum glutamic oxaloacetic transaminase (now called aspartate aminotransferase [AST])		
		t, tsp.	teaspoon
		tab.	tablet
SGPT	serum glutamic pyruvic transaminase (now called alanine aminotransferase [ALT])	**TBG**	thyroxine-binding globulin
		TCA	tricyclic antidepressant

TENS	transcutaneous electrical nerve stimulation	**vag., V, PV**	vaginal
TIA	transient ischemic attack	**VDRL**	Venereal Disease Research Laboratory (test)
t.i.d.	three times daily		
TIL	tumor-infiltrating lymphocytes	**VLDL**	very low-density lipoprotein
tinct., tr.	tincture	**VMA**	vanillylmandelic acid
		VO	verbal order
TLC	total lung capacity	**V/Q**	ventilation-perfusion ratio
TM	temporomandibular tympanic membrane		
TMJ	temporomandibular joint	**VSD**	ventricular septal defect
TNF	tumor necrosis factor	**VT**	tidal volume
t-PA	tissue plasminogen activator	**WBC**	white blood cell
		WPW	Wolff-Parkinson-White syndrome
TPN	total parenteral nutrition	**Z/G or ZIG**	zoster immune globulin
TRH	thyrotropin-releasing hormone		
TSH	thyroid-stimulating hormone	**×**	times, multiply
		eD	dram
UCE	urea cycle enzymopathy	**z or ℥**	ounce
USP	United States Pharmacopeia	**>**	greater than
		<	less than
UTI	urinary tract infection	**↑**	increase
UV	ultraviolet	**↓**	decrease
VAD	vascular access device ventricular assist device	**≈**	approximately equal

▶

Abbreviations to avoid

The Joint Commission on Accreditation of Healthcare Organizations requires hospitals to list approved abbreviations for staff use. Certain abbreviations, such as the ones below, should *never* be used because they're easily misunderstood, especially when handwritten.

ABBREVIATION	MISINTERPRETATION	CORRECTION
Apothecaries' symbols fluidounce fluidram minim scruple	Frequently misinterpreted	Use the metric equivalents.
auris uterque each ear	Frequently misinterpreted as "OU" (*oculus uterque*– each eye)	Write it out.
Drug names AZT	azathioprine (Immuran), aztreonam (Azactam, an antibiotic)	Use "zidovudine" (Retrovir). AZT is its old trademark.
methotrexate	mustargen (mechlorethamine hydrochloride)	Spell out drug names.
Compazine (prochlorperazine)	chlorpromazine	
hydrochloric acid	potassium chloride ("H" is misinterpreted as "K")	
digoxin	digitoxin	
multivitamins *without* fat-soluble vitamins	multivitamins *with* fat-soluble vitamins	
hydrochlorothiazide	hydrocortisone (HCT)	
vidarabine	cytarabine (ara-C)	
microgram	Frequently misinterpreted as "mg"	Use "mcg."

Abbreviations to avoid *(continued)*

ABBREVIATION	MISINTERPRETATION	CORRECTION
once daily	Frequently misinterpreted as "OD" (*oculus dexter* – right eye).	Don't abbreviate "daily." Write it out.
orange juice	Frequently misinterpreted as "OD" (*oculus dexter* – right eye) or "OS" (*oculus sinister* – left eye). Medications that were meant to be diluted in orange juice and given orally have been given in a patient's right or left eye.	Write it out.
once daily	Misinterpreted as "t.i.d."	Write it out.
orally	The "os" is frequently misinterpreted as "OS" (*oculus sinister* – left eye).	Use "P.O." or "by mouth" or "orally."
every day	The period after the "q" has sometimes been misinterpreted as "i," and the drug has been given q.i.d. rather than daily.	Write it out.
nightly or at bedtime	Misinterpreted as "q.h." (every hour)	Use "h.s." or "nightly."
every other day	Misinterpreted as "q.d." (daily) or "q.i.d."	Use "q other day" or "every other day."
subcutaneous	The "q" has been misinterpreted as every. For example, a prophylactic heparin dose meant to be given 2 hours before surgery may be given *every* 2 hours before surgery.	Use "S.C." or "SQ" or write out "subcutaneous."
unit	Misinterpreted as a "0" or a "4," causing a tenfold or greater overdose.	Write it out.

Acknowledgments

p. 24-26   *The Mini-Mental State Examination*
Adapted from *Journal of Psychiatric Research* 12(3), Folstein, M.F., et al., "Mini-mental State: A Practical Method for Grading the Cognitive State of Patients for the Clinician," pp. 189-198, copyright 1975, with kind permission from Pergamon Press Ltd., Headington Hill Hall, Oxford OX3 OBW, UK.

p. 192-194   *NANDA taxonomy I*
North American Nursing Diagnosis Association, *NANDA Nursing Diagnoses: Definitions and Classification 1995-1996.* (Philadelphia: NANDA, 1994). Used with permission.

p. 337-342   *Recommended barriers to infection*
Adapted from Pugliese, G. (ed.), *Universal Precautions: Policies, Procedures, and Resources.* Chicago: American Hospital Publishing, Inc., 1991. Used with permission.

p. 430   *Estimating body-surface area in adults*
Reprinted from Lentner, C. (ed.), *Geigy Scientific Tables,* 8th ed., vol. 1, p. 227, copyright 1981. Courtesy Ciba-Geigy, Basel, Switzerland. Used with permission.

p. 634   *Personal safety pointers*
Adapted from Humphrey, Carolyn J., *Home Care Nursing Handbook,* pages 5-7. Gaithersburg, Md.: Aspen Publishers, Inc., 1994. Used with permission.

Index

A

i refers to an illustration; t refers to a table

H

I

i refers to an illustration; t refers to a table

i refers to an illustration; t refers to a table